Phil:

It has been a pleasure to work with you.

Pete

PRESCRIBING FOR THE ELDERLY

Peter P. Lamy, PhD, FCP

Professor and Director
Institutional Pharmacy Programs

Chairman, Department of Pharmacy
Practice and Administrative Science

School of Pharmacy
University of Maryland at Baltimore

PSG Publishing Company, Inc.
Littleton, Massachusetts

Library of Congress Cataloging in Publication Data

Lamy, Peter P
  Prescribing for the elderly.

  Includes bibliographies and index.
  1. Geriatric pharmacology. 2. Drugs—Prescribing.
I. Title. [DNLM: 1. Drug therapy—In old age. WT100.3
L242p]
RC953.7.L35   615'.58   78-55289
ISBN 0-88416-208-7

Second printing 1981.

Copyright © 1980 by PSG Publishing Company, Inc.

All rights reserved. No part of this publication may be reproduced or transmitted in any form or by any means, electronic or mechanical, including photocopying, recording, or any information storage or retrieval system, without permission in writing from the publisher.

Printed in the United States of America.

International Standard Book Number: 0-88416-208-7

Library of Congress Catalog Card Number: 78-55289

DEDICATION

I dedicate this book to the women in my life who have been so supportive, encouraging, helpful, and some of whom have found their way into the pages of this book; and to my father, the late Rudolf Lamy, M.D., Fellow, American Geriatrics Society, who, as primary physician to the German Old Folks Home in Franklin Square, L.I., long ago gave me my first inkling that the elderly deserve and have a right to the full support of us all.

THE AUTHOR

Peter P. Lamy, PhD, FCP is editor of the *Geriatrics* column in "Drug Intelligence and Clinical Pharmacy" and has been active in the fields of gerontology and geriatrics for over a decade. He has written over 35 papers on aging which have appeared in international scientific and professional journals and books, including chapters in works by Dr. Busse and Dr. Reichel. Dr. Lamy is a consultant to the John L. Deaton Medical Center in Baltimore, Maryland and was formerly a consultant at the Levindale Hebrew Geriatric Center and Hospital in Baltimore. Currently, Dr. Lamy is a special advisor to the 1981 White House Conference on Aging and the Maryland Governor's Conference on Aging.

A member of the UMAB Task Force on Aging, Dr. Lamy has made numerous presentations on geriatrics and gerontology to physicians, nurses, pharmacists, and nursing home administrators, including television and radio appearances. He has testified before US House Select Committee on Aging and the Maryland Legislature. He has been a consultant to the Department of Health, Education and Welfare, the State of Maryland, and the Baltimore City PSRO, Long Term Care Committee.

Dr. Lamy is a Fellow, *American Geriatrics Society*, a member of the *Gerontological Society*, and is a Fellow, *American College of Clinical Pharmacology* and a Fellow, *American Association for the Advancement of Science*.

He who is of a calm and happy nature will hardly feel the pressure of age, but to him who is of an opposite disposition, youth and age are equally a burden.

Cephalus
in
Plato's *Republic*
ca. 387 BC

The long-term survival personality most frequently is a middle-of-the-roader, a moderate, friendly, social, active, wise or practical person who cares about life and seems to "program" herself/himself for the future and for living to enjoy it.

Robert J. Samp, M.D.
University of Wisconsin Hospitals
1976

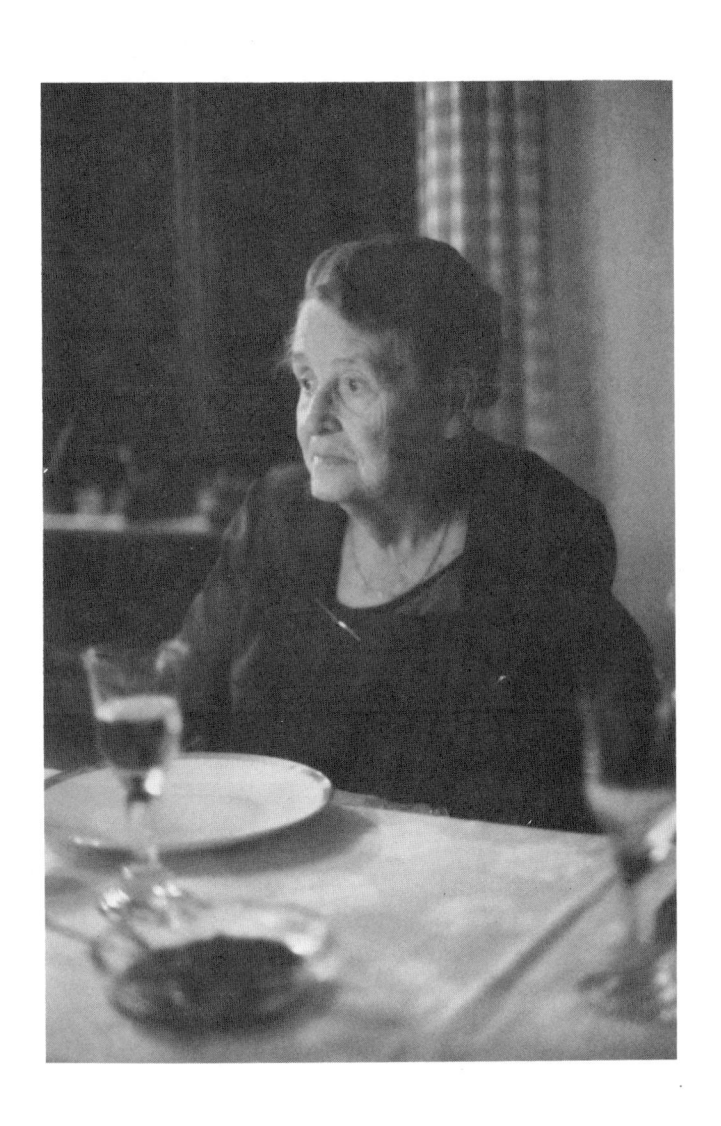

Pharmacology is an ever-changing science. As new research and clinical experience broaden our knowledge, changes in treatment and drug therapy are required. The author and the publisher of this work have made every effort to ensure that the treatment and drug dosage schedules herein are accurate and in accord with the standards accepted at the time of publication. Readers are advised, however, to check the product information sheet included in the package of each drug they plan to administer to be certain that changes have not been made in the recommended dose or in the indications and contraindications for administration. This recommendation is of particular importance in regard to new or infrequently used drugs.

CONTENTS

Foreword ix
　Murray M. Kappelman

Preface xi

Introduction xiii

1　Some Demographic and Other Data 1

2　Theories of Aging 19

3　Primary and Secondary Aging 27

4　Sociogenic Aging 73

5　Can Aging Be Decelerated? 81

6　Health Care Expenditures and Drugs 89

7　The Health Status of the Elderly 109

8　Diagnosis 143

9　Some Patient Factors Governing Responses to Drugs 151

10　Some Considerations Before Prescribing 169

11　The Little White Pill 177

12　Nutrition and Drug-Food Interactions 183

13　Altered Pharmacokinetics in the Elderly 249

14	Adverse Effects of Drugs in the Elderly	293
15	Nonprescription Drugs	313
16	Analgesic and Antiinflammatory Drugs	345
17	Anticonvulsants	363
18	Antimicrobials	365
19	Cardiovascular Drugs	385
20	Diabetes and Its Management in the Elderly	463
21	Ophthalmic Drugs	489
22	Psychopharmacologic Drugs	501
23	Management of Respiratory Problems	593
24	Skin Problems of the Elderly	601
25	Pressure Sores	607
26	Drugs and Surgery	627
27	Patient Counseling and Compliance	633
28	A New Care System is Needed	649
	Index	661

FOREWORD

The elderly can no longer be dismissed as middle-aged adults grown older. Individuals who have passed through their middle years and entered the final decades are a distinctive and specific group requiring a thorough and complete understanding of their age-related problems. For far too long, the elderly have been stereotyped as frail, institutionalized, non-comprehending persons suffering through the twilight of their lives. Because of their multiple medical, social, economic, and nursing related problems, health professionals have quietly avoided their responsibilities toward our older generation. Avoidance behavior by professionals has alienated and intimidated the older person so that the search for appropriate health care is often disregarded by the elderly as hopeless and embarrassing. As health professionals, we stand condemned by our negligence, our lack of thorough understanding and knowledge, our tendency to categorize older individuals as a group rather than as persons, and our readiness to remove the elderly from our domain by resorting to institutionalization long before this last step is necessary.

The time has come to take stock of our position in the health care system. Each of us, physician, pharmacist, nurse, dentist, social worker, is a vital advocate for a large segment of our population—the elderly. We have cared for these persons for years. Is it appropriate suddenly to stop caring and treating and knowing about them because they have passed a landmark measured in years? Without our assiduous attention, the elderly face their remaining years adrift in a health and social system unable to fight their way to proper care and attention. As professionals overlooking the elderly, we are condemning them to early institutionalization and senescence. How often do the frail elderly only become that way because we have not exerted the time, effort, and knowledge to keep them strong?

Too frequently, the elderly are dismissed as being or behaving like "children." The only similarity between the child and the older adult is the common need for a professional team approach to advocate the proper health and social care of each group. The elderly have multiple problems. These problems are so tightly interwoven that they form a tapestry of woes, often unable to be dissected one from the other. The social and medical problems overlap significantly. Drug problems involve the pharmacist, the physician, the nurse, and the dentist. The social worker must enter the health care team to assure the availability and accessibility of the necessary medications. The elderly person who depends upon only one professional for all of the care in his or her life is short-changing him or herself. The professional who assumes that he or she can fulfill all of the needs of the older person has inappropriate delusions of adequacy. There is no one professional who is omnipotent nor omnipresent to the degree that he or she can minister to the varied and complex needs of the older person. Caring for the elderly must be an interdisciplinary team effort.

But first, we must learn. Professional schools are on the threshold of the realization that teaching the care of the older person is an absolute necessity. Generations of professionals practice their specialty without proper background information on the aging process and the aged. These professionals must seek the additional training necessary to render appropriate care to the rapidly increasing older generation. The ideal is for the various health and social care professionals to learn together. If the physician, pharmacist, social worker, nurse, and dentist experience learning about the aging process and the aged in an interdisciplinary environment, then each will be better prepared to join the others in rendering total, thorough, multi-professional care.

This book is a major step in that direction. It deals not only in depth with pharamacologic aspects of drugs on each of the various organ systems of the aging individual; it explores the physiology, demography, psychology, and social problems of the elderly that impact upon drugs and their importance and misuse in our older population. In no way is this a discipline-specific work. It should prove of immeasurable value to all professions which must and should confront the daily problem of successfully and properly treating the elderly.

There is dignity and success in growing old which must be nurtured and encouraged by every professional who deals with an older individual. Only with proper knowledge and sensitivity of the aging process and the aged can we feel comfortable and fully equipped to approach the older person intelligently and humanely. We only avoid and dismiss those medical, dental, and social problems about which we feel incompetent and unsure. This book will go a long way to alleviate that sense of insecurity among all professionals. As a physician, I am delighted to have read this work, and enlarged and intensified my knowledge and concern about the older generation. Not only have I learned a great deal about drugs and the elderly, but I have deepened my understanding about aging and the aged in many additional ways.

Murray M. Kappelman, M.D.

PREFACE

Little did I know of the complexities of preparing a book, much less a book of the special needs of the elderly, with an emphasis on the health care needs of the geriatric patient.

I want to express my appreciation to the many individuals who, through their help and participation, furthered the writing and completion of this book. I am especially grateful for the continuing support of my immediate family, particularly my son Carl who helped with typing and organizing. I am most appreciative of the support of Dr. William J. Kinnard, Jr., Dean of the School of Pharmacy, University of Maryland at Baltimore, and the many other faculty and staff as well as past and present graduate students from the University of Maryland. My thanks go to Mr. Henry Derewicz, Mr. Don Fedder, Dr. Gary Hollenbeck, and Dr. Ralph Shangraw. I was greatly helped by the efforts of Mrs. Faustina Drummond, Mr. Michael Gentry, Mrs. Monica Johnson, Mr. Philip Szczepanski, and Mrs. Linda Thomas.

Special thanks to Miss Alice Haywood of the National Center for Health Statistics, and Mrs. Phyllis Fansler of Baltimore, Md. Finally, for his help, my thanks to Mr. John Jordan, Chief, Pharmacy Service, VA Medical Center, Baltimore, Md.

INTRODUCTION

Geriatric medicine is complex and difficult. In the elderly, sociogenic factors may combine with effects of primary and secondary aging to produce a complex clinical picture. The clinical presentation of the patient may be confused. Many classical signs and symptoms may be absent or exacerbated.

Therapeutic management of the elderly patient involves more than a response to medical needs. It demands an understanding of personal attributes, which may be deeply rooted in the patient's religious, cultural, or ethnic background and beliefs. This understanding is vital to the successful medical management of older patients, but may be difficult to achieve because many misconceptions about the elderly have been fostered and are perpetuated.

Thus, prescribing for the elderly is, at best, difficult. Problems encountered may range from inappropriate prescribing by the primary provider to inappropriate drug use by the patient. This may be due to the fact that "appropriate" prescribing in many instances is still ill-defined or not defined at all.

The British National Formulary addresses these problems in an introductory statement. No similar statement is found in any US compendium:

Prescribing for the Elderly*

It is a convention that the standard advice on the choice and dosage of drugs applies to adults and that modifications have to be made for children. But it is sometimes forgotten that the elderly are also in a special case, with the result that they may get drugs that do them no good, or which are dangerous or may be harmful.

The Patient's Mentality Most elderly patients have poor memories and get confused. They may live alone, or with a partner who is no better. They find it difficult to follow even simple instructions and the complicated schedules sometimes offered, with many drugs to be taken at different times, are quite beyond them. They are also creatures of habit and once they have been on tablets for a long time it may be difficult or unkind to stop them. Although it may be reasonable for a doctor to try various drugs, he should satisfy himself that benefit has resulted, otherwise the patient remains indefinitely on them merely because they were started.

The Patient's Reactions The capacities of old people fail progressively and this applies also to their ability to deal with drugs. This may show itself in two ways. First, there may be an enhanced or prolonged effect as is common with digoxin or hypoglycaemic agents. It will also occur with any drug that has to be excreted or metabolised by failing kidneys or liver. It follows that in general drugs should be

---

*Reprinted with permission from: *The British National Formulary, 1976–1978*, British Medical Association and Pharmaceutical Society of Great Britain, London, 1976.

started in low doses, and the dose be kept low if they are to be continued for long. Second, the threshold for unwanted effects may be reduced. Hypnotics and sedatives are particularly difficult and the phenothiazine tranquilizers are especially hazardous as they impair the already unreliable powers of regulating temperature and blood pressure.

The Time Span   A great deal of treatment that is given to the young and middle aged is intended to prevent troubles in the distant future and some nuisance in the present may be accepted to obtain this end. The rigid control of hypertension and diabetes are examples. It is of course obvious that old people have no distant future, yet they are often continued on treatment which, however correct it might have been, can no longer benefit them.

Multiplicity of Symptoms   From the nature of things old people may have several diseases and many symptoms so that the doctor may be tempted to give a drug for each. It is better to decide which can really be improved and concentrate on those. It would not be unusual to find an elderly patient suffering at one and the same time from hypertension, cardiac failure, pruritus, angina, bronchitis, cystitis, glycosuria, insomnia, arthritis, and depression. These cannot all be treated at once and it is best not to be over-ambitious or one may easily add to the patient's burdens.

Conclusions   Drug schedules should be simple and never beyond the patient's understanding. Doses should be low. No treatment should be continued that does not clearly give relief.

Aging has physical and socioenvironmental concomitants that often give rise to medical problems. More so than in any other age group, socioeconomic factors and psychosocial factors can influence the outcome of a particular disease state.

The geriatric patient is frequently in need of continuous care. It is not always possible to reverse a disease process, but it can be made more tolerable (Goldman 1978).

This care must be offered with thought and consideration. The primary provider must ascertain the stresses to which a patient is exposed, as well as the patient's ability to deal with these (Mechanic 1976). Events causing maladaptive responses may contribute to traditional disease entities, and environmental, rather than medical manipulation may be necessary to eliminate stressful situations and, thus, prevent or at least mollify potential disease states (Cassel 1970; Mechanic 1974). In general, the elderly will be cooperative, particularly when faced with the prospect of institutionalization. They will make every effort to maintain themselves in their own homes and in their accustomed lifestyle. Universally, the elderly select institutional care only as a last resort (Schultz 1976), and so should the health provider.

Health care for the elderly encompasses four stages: acute care, continuing care, rehabilitation, and home care. Institutionalization, often viewed as synonymous with continuing or long-term care, is one alternative. Others, such as rehabilitation and home care are often pursued less vigorously.

Drugs are a mainstay in long-term care, and there is renewed interest in the effects of chronic drug treatment contrasted with the effects of acute drug administration. Yet there is still an astounding dearth of data on the pharmacology of drugs used chronically in the elderly (Gitman and Williams 1970).

The multitude of drugs often prescribed for the elderly has been called a "geriatric confectionary." Although drugs are remarkably nontoxic in relation to their extensive use (Jick 1974), nevertheless, the elderly person is more vulnerable to drug effects, both therapeutic and adverse. A host of factors combine to produce an increasingly unpredictable drug effect (Figure I-1) with advancing age.

Even an extensive knowledge of physiologic changes with aging is not always sufficient to assess the possible risk involved in geriatric

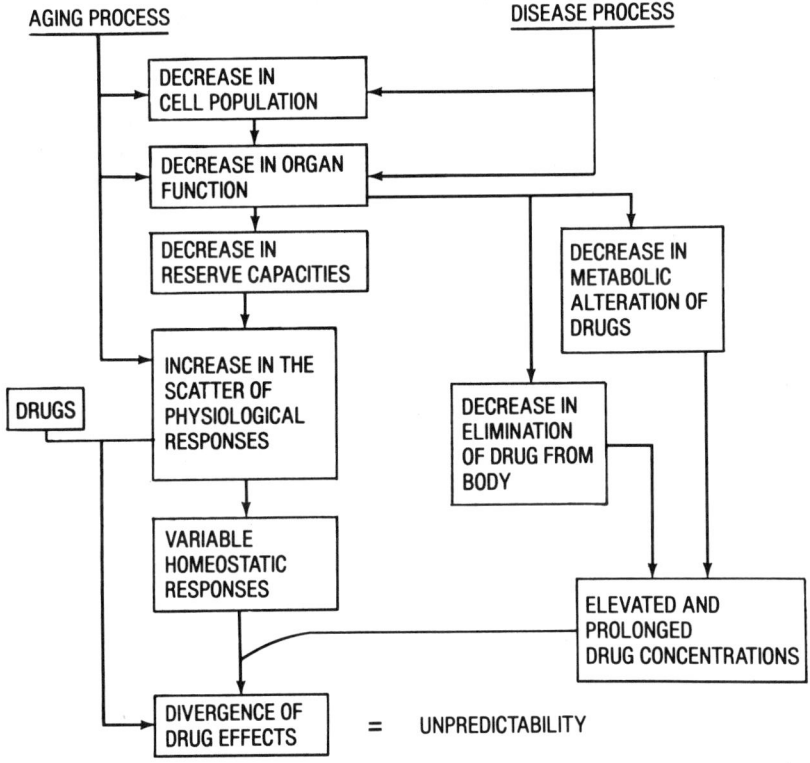

Figure I-1 Flow diagram leading to unpredictability of drug effects in the aged.*

*Reprinted with permission from: G.A. Riley, The influence of aging on drug therapy, US Pharmacist 2(10):28, 1977.

drug therapy. Failure to accommodate the "distant" effect that a medication may have in a compromised host can seriously complicate management. For example, hypotension is rapidly induced in the presence of arteriosclerotic disease in patients treated with antihypertensives. Thus, the response of an elderly patient to a drug primarily depends on the functional status of the target organ. If this functional status changes with age or is changed by disease, the reaction to the drug also changes (Heim 1976).

The use of drugs in geriatric patients has the potential to reduce the quality of life for the patient. Nearly all classes of drugs pose potential and special problems in geriatric medicine. Certain drugs deserve special attention because of their increased use by these patients or because they pose a particular challenge for the clinician. It is, therefore, distressing that some drugs used for elderly patients are sometimes continued indefinitely, even though there may be no further indication for their use. This group includes the steroids, used to treat rheumatoid arthritis or chronic bronchitis (Eastwood 1974), digoxin (Dall 1970), and the oral hypoglycemic agents (Tompkins and Bloom 1972).

The purpose of this work is to bring to the clinician not the usual indications for which drugs can be used, but to attempt to highlight the various factors which can influence drug response of elderly patients and the patient variables which make this drug response increasingly unpredictable with advancing age.

Before prescribing any drug for an elderly patient, the clinician should be able to answer three questions (Powell 1977):

1. Should this disease be treated?
2. Should this patient be treated?
3. Should this drug be used?

REFERENCES

Cassel, J. Edited by S. Levine, and N. Scotch. In *Social Stress*. Chicago: Aldine Publishing Co., 1970.

Dall, J.L.C. Maintenance digoxin in elderly patients. *Br Med J*. 1:706, 1970.

Eastwood, H.D.H. Steroid therapy in the elderly. *Gerontol Clin*. 16:163, 1974.

Gitman, E.L., and Williams, E.W. *Research, Training and Practice in Clinical Medicine of Aging*. Basel: S. Karger Verlag, 1970.

Goldman, R. Care of the aging veteran and the national implications. *Geriatrics* 33(2):25, 1978.

Heim, F. Die Altersabhaengigkeit von Pharmakawirkungen. *Aktuel Gerontol*. 6:329, 1976.

Jick, H. Drugs–remarkably nontoxic. *N Engl J Med*. 291:824, 1974.

Mechanic, D. Edited by G. Coelho, D. Hamburg, and J.E. Adams. In *Coping and Adaptation*. New York: Basic Books, 1974.

Mechanic, D. Stress, illness, and illness behavior. *J Hum Stress.* 2(2):2, 1976.

Powell, C. Edited by W. Ferguson Anderson, and J.R. Carlton-Ashton. In *Brain Failure in Old Age. Age Ageing.* 6(suppl):83, 1977.

Schultz, R. Effects of control and predictability on the physical and psychological well-being of the institutionalized aged. *J Pers Soc Psychol.* 33:563, 1976.

Tompkins, A.M., and Bloom, A. Assessment of the need for continued oral therapy in diabetics. *Br Med J.* 1:649, 1972.

1 Some Demographic and Other Data

The world population is increasing dramatically. It quadrupled in the years 1 AD to 1850 AD (Table 1-1), and quadrupled again in the next 125 years. In the United States, similar statistics hold true.

In addition, the statistics concerning the United States elderly population are being carefully evaluated. Obviously, the baby boom of the recent past is being replaced by the senior citizen explosion (Charatan 1975); the four-generation family is rapidly becoming common, and the country is experiencing the "rise of the elders" (Wheeler 1978). The power of the elderly is increasing, and while nobody lives a great deal longer than elders in the past, everybody has the potential of living longer than ever before.

Similar changes have been observed throughout the world. Nations have been classified according to the percentage of their elderly citizens (Laslett 1977) (Table 1-2). According to population statistics, many Western nations would therefore be classified as ancient (Table 1-3).

This increase in the elderly population has brought about major misgivings in certain circles. In a Christmas message in 1977, Poland's Roman Catholic bishops predicted a "population catastrophe" in

Table 1-1
World Population

Year	Population in billions
Birth of Christ	0.25
1850	1
1930	2
1960	3
1975	4

Table 1-2
Classification of Nations According to Percentage of Elderly

	Percent Population over 65 years
Mature	4
Aged	7
Ancient	13

Source: P. Laslett. *New Society.* October 27, 1977, p. 171.

Table 1-3
Some Population Statistics

	Percent Population over 65 years
East Germany	15.6
Austria	
France	
Sweden	
West Germany	13.4
Wales	13.3
England	13.3
Scotland	12.3
N. Ireland	10.8
United States	10.0

Source: P. Laslett. *New Society.* October 27, 1977, p. 171.

Poland unless the birth rate increased, as the younger generation is no longer fully replacing the older one. There are fears of demographic stagnation and adverse economic effects. An aging society, it has been said, slides toward inevitable decline. There is no question that transition to an older society causes social and economic dislocations, but the ultimate effect need not be damaging.

What changes may occur? Some are obvious. For example, a stable, older society will need fewer baby foods, fewer toys, fewer teachers, and fewer maternity clinics. On the other hand, the demand for retirement homes will increase; there will be strong demands for a different health care system, for more recreational facilities, and for additional social services.

It has been predicted that both per-capita income and consumption will rise in a stable, older population. There has also been concern that an older society may be less creative, less innovative, and more conservative. Much concern has been expressed that the number of dependents per active worker in the United States would increase sharply, leading to a breakdown of the current Social Security system. Actually, a stable, older society would have the same proportion of people in the working ages, 18 to 65 years, compared to the dependent young and old as it does today, ie, three workers to every two dependents. However, the preponderant number of dependents would be the elderly.

No doubt, the needs and demands of these dependents would differ greatly, particularly in the health care field. While communicable diseases and diseases of childhood would still demand attention, in the stable, older society chronic diseases of middle age and later life would be most prevalent.

Obviously, these changes would demand a reappraisal of the current devaluation of the elderly and their potential contribution to society at large. The values and beliefs of the elderly, currently often in conflict with those of the younger population, would be a potent political force (Bozzetti and MacMurray 1977).

THE ELDERLY—AN OVERVIEW

In 1790, one-half the population of the United States was 16 years of age or younger. The median age in 1970 was below 28 years; it will pass 30 years in 1981, reach 35 years by the year 2000, and approach 40 years by the year 2030.

Statistics about the elderly are confusing and sometimes even contradictory. Nevertheless, it is clear that only about 4% to 5% of the elderly are in nursing homes. Over 50% of older people live with their spouses. Nearly 15% are single individuals living with relatives, and 20% to 30% have no families and live alone.

Living alone is one of the strongest indicators of risk of institutionalization, for it is the elderly living alone who require most social support. It is also true that need and desire for services are not synonymous. Many of the aged may neither want services nor seek them. Measures of perceived needs, based on objective conditions, are not necessarily related to measures of expressed needs. For example, in one study, residents of center city hotels were, as a group, not very healthy. However, their dominant cultural norms included self-reliance, fear of dependence, and a strong desire for privacy and freedom. Therefore, they did not use available social and health services external to their environment (Eckert 1977).

Of the elderly living in the community, 2% are probably bedfast, 6% are housebound, and another 6% can leave their houses only with difficulty. In one study of 1000 elderly, 236 had at least one unmet need, while 80 of 1000 had multiple unmet needs (Massachusetts Department of Public Health, 1976), and it has been suggested that the typical "well" at-home elderly individual may, in fact, have more than six undetected chronic conditions. In general, though, the characterization of older Americans as impoverished, debilitated, and depressed fails to describe 85% of the elderly Americans. The elderly are most afraid of crime, poor health, lack of money, and loneliness. They are afraid of outliving their capacity to cope with daily living and health problems.

At all ages, men have a shorter life expectancy than women. Three of every five aged Americans are females. At most ages, blacks have a shorter life expectancy than whites. However, by the time a black male reaches 75 years of age, his life expectancy is greater than that of a white male of the same age. Elderly blacks tend to have lower incomes, be underenrolled in federal programs such as Social Security Supplemental Income (SSSI), and black elderly males more often live alone than do white or Spanish-American males.

Economic statistics must be viewed with caution. While the percentage of older Americans living below the poverty line has decreased from 25% in 1969 to 16% in 1974, there is a question as to the reasonableness of the poverty line. Families with heads aged 65 years and older have incomes slightly over half the incomes of families with younger heads. In 1975, of the nation's 8.2 million families headed by persons 65 years and older, approximately 7% (460,000) had yearly incomes of less than $3000. One-third (2.7 million) of the families with older heads of family had yearly incomes of less than $6000.

Aged single persons run a greater risk of living in poverty than elderly persons living with families. In 1975, of the almost 6.9 million older persons living alone or with nonrelatives, approximately 8% had yearly incomes of less than $1500. In fact, less than 20% of these persons had incomes of $6000 or more.

In the nation, the most prevalent sources of income for the elderly are retirement benefits (Social Security and public and private pensions). Retirement payments provide at least one-half the income for the majority of elderly couples with a head of household over 65 years of age. Retirement benefits provide nearly two-thirds of the total income of elderly persons living alone. Wages served as sole income for only 7% of aged couples, and for even fewer elderly individuals, and as less than one-half of the income of one-quarter of the nation's elderly couples. Public assistance is the fourth ranking source of income for the elderly.

Most senior citizens do not move to Florida and to retirement cities. In general, higher proportions of the elderly than of the general population live in rural areas; the elderly are also concentrated in the inner cities. In both the country and the inner city, the elderly have remained while younger people have moved to the suburbs. Thus, the elderly are not a very mobile group. Over 90% of the elderly in the United States made no residential move at all in 1970 to 1971 and of those who did, most remained in the same county. Only slightly more than 1% moved to another state. These statistics certainly document a strong domicile stability of the elderly, which may well be economically mandated.

On the average, the elderly have completed fewer years of formal education than younger adults. For example, in 1970 about 4% of those 65 years of age and over had no formal schooling at all, and another 53% had completed less than the eighth grade. In contrast, of those between 25 and 64 years of age, only 1% had had no schooling and only 21% had less than an eighth grade education. The lower educational status of the elderly is changing rapidly, as younger persons with more education move into the older age cohorts. By 1990, about half the population over 65 years of age is expected to have at least a high school education. This will be more noticeable in older women than in men, following a national trend for women of all ages to have higher levels of educational attainments than men.

THE ELDERLY—A HOMOGENEOUS GROUP?

The elderly are most often viewed as a homogeneous group. For example, the elderly, as a group, will avoid seeing a physician rather than risk being stereotyped as complainers. As a group, the elderly often deny their own aging and see themselves as middle-aged or even young, possibly as occupancy of an aged status in American society is degrading (Bultena and Powers 1978). But, contrary to popular belief, the elderly are not a homogeneous group at all (Sukosky 1977). As many different types and categories have been identified among the elderly as among younger people (Maddox 1973; Neugarten 1973; Kimmel 1974) and recognition of this fact is basic to the understanding of the elderly and their needs.

POPULATION CHARACTERISTICS OF THE UNITED STATES

Longevity of humans has steadily increased over the centuries. In ancient Rome, the longevity curve peaked at approximately 20 years of age. The current US life expectancy is shown in Figure 1-1.

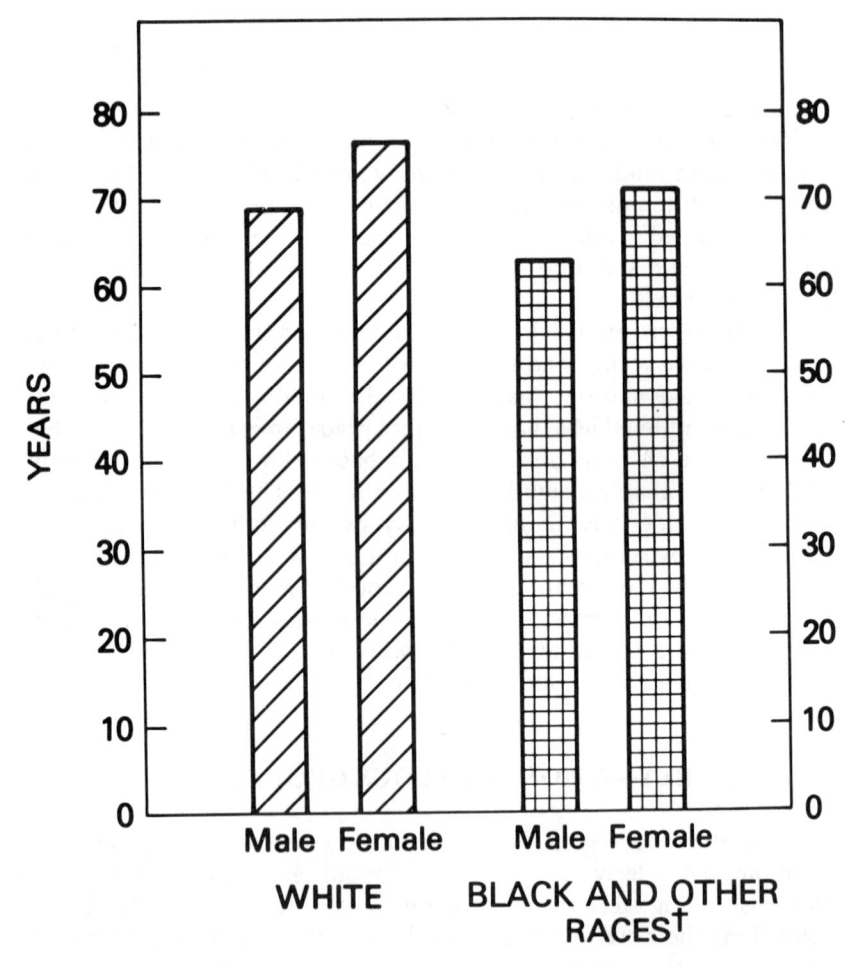

Figure 1-1 Life expectancy at birth in 1974. Note: † Black only for 1929–1931 and 1900–1902.

Longevity, of course, is related to both the birthrate and the mortality rate. Birthrates differ sharply throughout the world. In Europe, where birth control is very effective, the rate is 0.8%. In the United States, the rate is estimated to be 1.1%. In Latin America, it is 2.9%, similar to the rates in Africa and Asia. Thus, it has been predicted that by the year 2000, 80% of the world's population will live in three regions of the world: South America, Asia, and Africa.

In the United States, the birthrate continues to decline. At the same time, the death rate in 1976 was the lowest ever recorded, having declined by 2.9% from 1975. The age-adjusted rate for men was 1.8 times that for women. If the 1975 mortality rates continue, 75% of babies born in 1975 will reach 65 years, 50% will reach age 75, and 25% will reach age 85. These figures vary with race and sex, with white women having the best chance of survival (Figures 1-2 and 1-3).

In general, the black population is younger than the white one, because its life expectancy is seven years shorter. Among the causes for this discrepancy is the fact that diseases which can be controlled are still predominant among the blacks (Volinn 1974). Therefore, it has been suggested that for blacks, age 45 years should be the appropriate legal base for admission to publicly funded social and health services

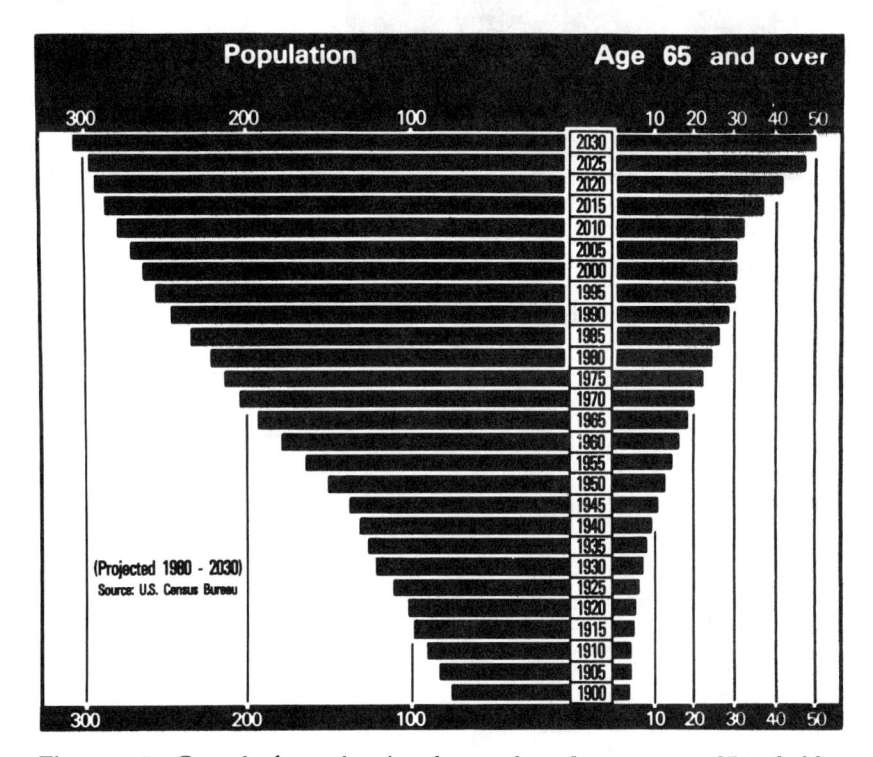

Figure 1-2 Growth chart, showing the number of persons age 65 and older compared with the total population, from 1900 through 2030.

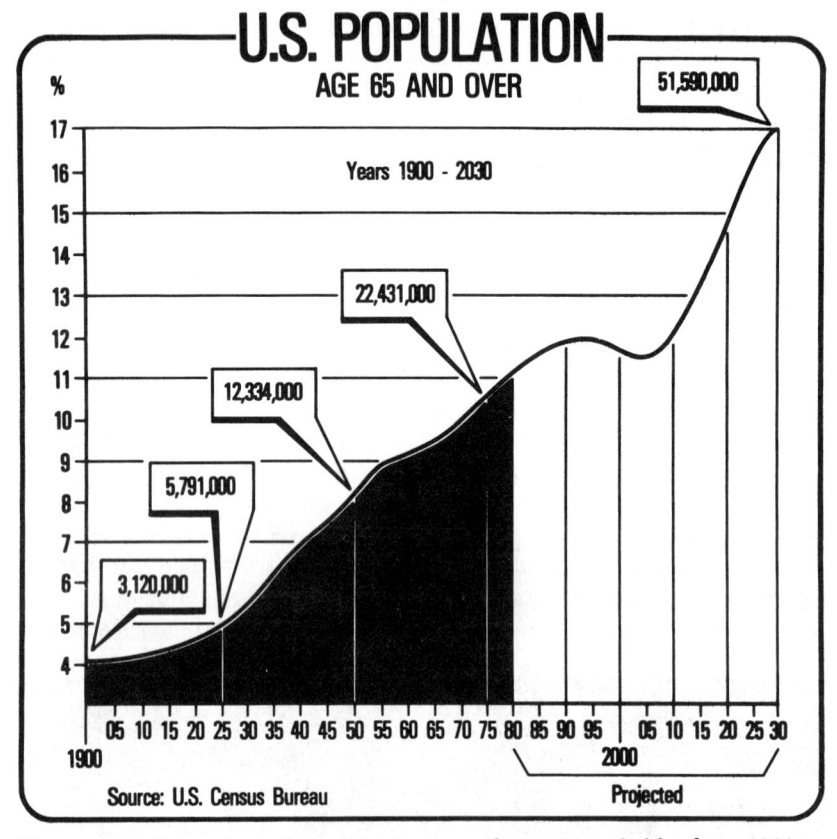

Figure 1-3 Percentage of the American population 65 and older from 1900 to 1975, with predictions for 1980 and 2030.

(Jackson 1971). Similarly, the American Indian, representing less than 1% of the total US population, belongs to a relatively young population group. The American Indians have a high birthrate and a high death rate. Their life expectancy is estimated to be 44 years, one-third shorter than the national average. It has been suggested that this ethnic group be considered "old" at a much earlier chronologic age than nonminority groups. The conventional approach to aging has been to alter survival so that more people live to 70 to 80 years of age. In 1900, life expectancy at birth was 49 years, and increased to 68 years in 1950, but there are significant variations among different groups. For example, the difference in life expectancy between men and women continues to increase. If current death rates continue unchanged, the life expectancy of white females born in 1975 will be 77.2 years, almost eight years longer than that of white males. A similar difference will be seen between black women and black men.

Life expectancy is increased by controlling or eliminating disease. Indeed, it is postulated that a great reduction in the death rate of children is still possible, as about one-third of those under four years of age are still not protected against measles, rubella, diphtheria-tetanus-pertussis, and polio. On the other hand, since 1950 only about 2.4 years have been added to the average life expectancy and most of the major and important advances in medicine have taken place after 1950. The projected effects of elimination of various causes of death on life expectancy are shown in Table 1-4. Life expectancy may peak at 100 years by the end of this century. This prediction may correlate with the results of a study sponsored by the US Public Health Service which showed that men can increase longevity by 11 years and women can add seven years to their life by observing certain rules, which include the right amount of sleep, good nutritional intake, exercise, weight control, and abstinence from drinking and smoking. The effects of this increase in longevity are shown by the fact that 20% of all deaths occurred in the age group of 65 years and older some 200 years ago, while currently 80% of all deaths occur in this age group. Thus, the mean lifespan has been substantially increased by prevention and cure of diseases that formerly led to deaths at relatively early ages. Control of the major causes of infant mortality produced the largest gain in life expectancy. Although the disease-oriented approach to medicine has increased life expectancy, that same approach will most likely not impact on human lifespan. Indeed, lifespan has remained essentially unchanged. What has changed is that more people live longer and reach the mean maximum lifespan.

Table 1-4
Gain in Expectation of Life at Birth and at the Age of 65 Due to Elimination of Various Causes of Death*

Cause of death	Gain (yr.) in expectation of life if cause was eliminated	
	At birth	*At age 65*
Major cardiovascular-renal diseases	10.9	10.0
Heart diseases	5.9	4.9
Vascular diseases affecting central nervous system	1.3	1.2
Malignant neoplasms	2.3	1.2
Accidents, excluding those caused by motor vehicles	0.6	0.1
Motor vehicle accidents	0.5	0.2
Influenza and pneumonia	0.5	0.2
Infectious diseases (excluding tuberculosis)	0.2	0.1
Diabetes mellitus	0.2	0.2
Tuberculosis	0.1	0.0

*Source: National Center for Health Statistics. *Some Demographic Aspects of Aging in the United States.* February, 1973.

Population Projections for the Elderly

While projections on life expectancy and the growth of the elderly population (Bureau of the Census 1976) have been made (Figure 1-4), it has also been suggested that these projections may change with altered survival probabilities, for instance, the elimination of cancer and cardiovascular disease (Myers 1976) and further decreases in the mortality rate of the young (Spiegelman and Erhardt 1974). Survival probabilities have increased with the eradication of such diseases as smallpox, yellow fever, cholera, dysentery, typhoid, diphtheria, measles, and mumps. In the middle-aged population, the death rates from heart conditions, stroke, arteriosclerosis, and kidney disease have shown significant declines in the past 25 years. Since 1950, the mortality rate from stroke has fallen by 39%, and from rheumatic fever and rheumatic heart disease by 66%, according to the National Heart, Lung and Blood Institute. Furthermore, since 1970 the

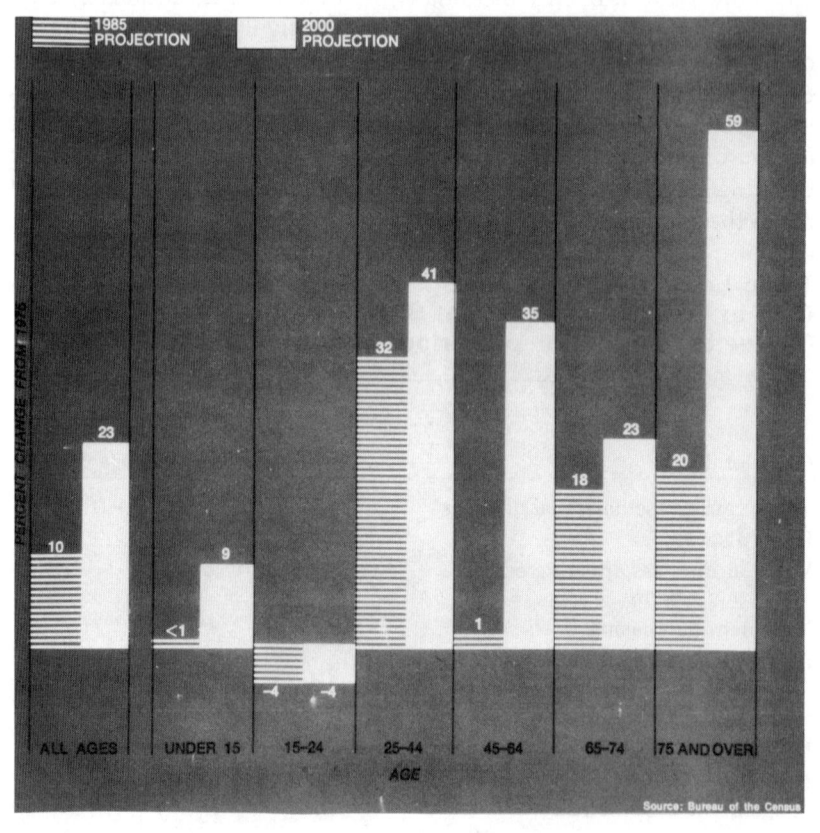

Figure 1-4 Percent changes in population for different ages, for 1985 and 2000.

mortality rate from hypertension and hypertensive heart disease has declined by 28%. Yet, as shown previously, even the elimination of cancer would increase life expectancy only slightly, particularly after age 65. At this age, every added year exposes a person to sharply increased risks of death from heart conditions or strokes. By age 55, the risk of death in American males increases appreciably because of risk of heart attack (Fuchs 1974), and 34% of all deaths in those over 65 years of age are attributed to heart disease (Pomerance 1974).

Thus, the main determinant of the proportion of the aged in the US population remains the birthrate (Hermalin 1966), and present predictions for the growth of the elderly population are based on the currently low birthrate, with provisions made for an even greater decrease in the current birthrate (Fowles 1978).

By the year 2000 there will be 260 million people in the United States if current mortality rates prevail and women continue to have, on the average, 2.1 children. There will then be almost 50 million additional people in the United States, or 23% more than in 1975.

The elderly are the fastest growing minority in the United States and will continue to grow at a faster rate than any other age group. Every day, the number of elderly increases by about 1000. Currently, one person in 10 is classified as "elderly." By 1985, 50% of the population will be older than 50 years of age. Population projections are presented in Tables 1-5 and 1-6. The age group of 75 years and over increases by nearly 40% each year, that of over 65 years by more than 20%, while the population under 65 years of age grows by only 12%. Thus, the greatest percentage increase will be in the older ages (Table 1-7). About 20% of the population over 65 years of age is now over 80 years of age (4.5 million) and by the year 2000, there will be six million people 80 years or older, the most vulnerable age, medically and socially (Figure 1-5). Between 1975 and 2000, the number of people aged 75 years and over will increase by 60% (Brotman 1977). The second largest increase will occur in the working age population. The

Table 1-5
Population Projection: United States

	Population in millions			
	1975	2000	2025	2050
All ages	213	264	302	320
0–19	75	80	84	88
20–64	116	154	173	183
65–74	22	30	45	49
75+	8.4	13	16	20

Source: US Census Population Reports, Series P-25 No. 470.

Table 1-6
Estimated Population Increase from 1975 to 2050

Age (yrs)	Percent increase
All ages	50.2
0–19	17.3
20–64	57.8
65–74	122.8
75+	138.1

Source: US Census Population Reports, Series P-25 No. 470.

Table 1-7
Elderly Population in the United States

Year	Total no. (in millions)	% of total 75 yrs and over
1900	3.1	29
1940	9.0	
1965	18.5	
1970		38
1975	22.4	
2000*	31.8	45
2030*	55.0	

*Projected.
Source: US Census Population Reports, Series P-25, No. 470.

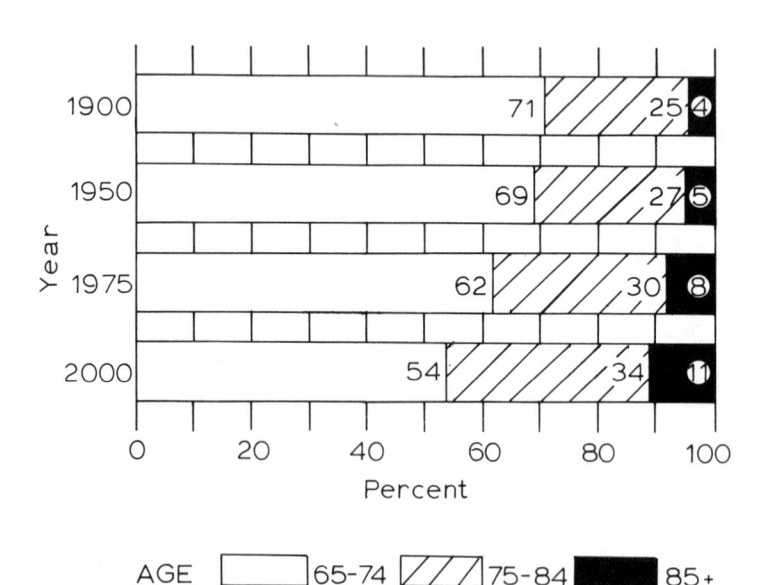

Figure 1-5 Changing demographic characteristics of the elderly.

group between 45 and 64 years of age will increase by 41%. The current low birth rate in the United States is reflected in the projected decrease in the number of young adults between the ages of 15 and 24 years, from 40 million to 38.8 million.

Unless there is a new baby boom, current demographic trends will lead to a stabilized age structure, in which all generations and age groups are of about the same size. The demographic profile by the year 2000 will have changed from the traditional triangle to almost a rectangle (Maxwell 1975) (Figure 1-6).

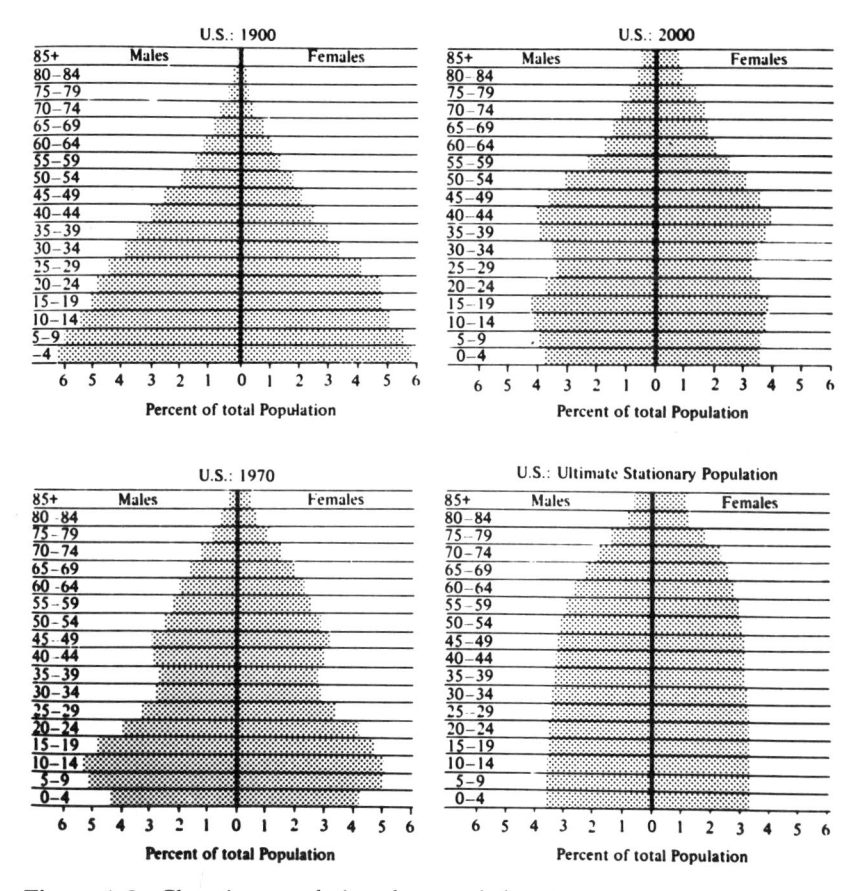

Figure 1-6 Changing population characteristics. From R. Maxwell. The case for intervention. Edited by D.A. Ehrlich. In *The Health Care Cost Explosion: Which Way Now?* Bern: Hans Huber Publishers, 1975. Reprinted with permission.

WHO ARE THE ELDERLY?

Chronologic age is a convenient personal and societal marker. However, age can be described in chronologic, sociologic, psychologic, and biologic terms (Riley et al 1972). It is not clear which age represents the particular one at which a person would be classified as "elderly." It is still common to classify as "elderly" someone past the age of 65 (DHEW Task Force on Prescription Drugs 1968).

Many people credit Chancellor Bismarck with establishing a system of old age pensions and a retirement age of 65. Sometimes this is related to Bismarck's known custom to retire Prussian generals at age 65, and it is felt that this custom was simply extended to the population at large. At other times, a more cold-hearted approach is seen. Life expectancy at that time was below 65 years and it has been suggested that Bismarck set retirement at an age that would not overburden the national treasury. However, it is clear that Bismarck set retirement age at 70 years, and eligibility for old-age pension started at age 70. An Imperial law (June 12, 1916) reduced this to age 65. Obviously, then, Bismarck was not responsible for the age 65 provision in the US Social Security Act.

The criterion for chronologic age is arbitrary, and in terms of health care, is not very helpful. Other classifications have been suggested, but age 65 is a significant year. Statistics purport to show that about 15% of people between 45 and 65 years of age must limit their major activities because of health, while almost 40% of people over 65 years of age must restrict theirs (Neugarten and Havighurst 1976). This type classification, based on the health status of an individual, has been extended (Koutsopoulous and Smith 1976). Those who suffer no major handicap, either physical, emotional, social, or economic would be classified as chronologically aged, while those with visual or hearing problems, mental or physical problems and economic problems would be categorized as impaired aged. Obviously, from an administrative point of view and from the point of view of an individual who may feel the "impaired" classification as a stigma, this classification is not the answer.

There are many suggestions. For example, the Food and Drug Administration, in its review of nonprescription antacids, determined the maximum safe dose of sodium-containing antacids for persons 60 years and older (Federal Register 1973). The British often refer to those 75 years of age and older as frail-old, but it has also been said that those under 75 years of age are young and that old age hardly starts until age 80 (Brocklehurst 1968). The New York State Assembly, in debating a bill to protect elderly citizens from crime, defined the elderly as persons aged 62 years or older, while the New York State Senate chose 60 years as the determining age. Young middle age has been suggested for those between 25 and 39 years, older middle age for those between 40 and 59 years, the designation of "elderly" for people between 60 and 74 years, and old age happens after age 75 (Breslow and Somers 1977). Still another classification views human maturity between the ages of 20 and 40 years, middle age lasting from 41 to 60 years, and senescence starting with 80 years (Finch 1976). Middlescence, it has been proposed, ranges from 30 to 70 years (Stevenson 1977), age 30 has been called early middle age (Garcia et al 1977) and, starting with age 50, people are thought to enter "senior adulthood" (Peterson and Thomas 1975). In the USSR, middle age is considered to last from age 45 to 59; those between 60 and 74 years are classified as elderly, those between 75 and 89 years are aged or old, and those 90 years and older as longevous (Chebotarev 1969). Recently, it has been speculated that, ultimately, middle age may extend from 40 to 70 years, the young-old from 70 to 90 years, and the old-old from 90 to 110 years.

Apparently, many of these classifications are based on personal convictions, the perceived need of those now classified as "elderly," changing societal concepts, and an attempt to change societal concepts of aging and the aged.

Age classification is necessary for purposes of statistics and delivery of support services. One useful attempt is the division of the elderly into the young-old and the old-old (Neugarten 1974, 1975; Youmans 1978). The young-old are all persons between the ages of 55 and 74 years, while the old-old are those older than 75 years of age. Strong differences between these two groups are apparent. The young-old, compared to the old-old, are a vigorous group, completely deviating from the stereotypic view of the elderly. They include a larger proportion of married persons, report a higher annual income, and have fewer health problems. Interestingly, the lower age group of 55 years was included as more and more women drop out of the labor market at that age and seek retirement, a somewhat doubtful reason for designating a person as old, even if it is only young-old. This classification system will be used in the remainder of this book.

Few, if any of these classifications, would be helpful in patient management. They do not provide a sound basis, given the possibility that physiologic changes may produce an "elderly" person long before age 65. Premature aging syndromes have been documented. It is well known that changes dealing with the dioptric media can be observed as early as age 40 and that the risk of dying for the American male between the ages of 55 and 65 is much higher than during the entire span of 15 to 55 years. Thus, dependency on chronologic age in assessing a patient is not only undesirable but impossible. Assessment of the health status of the elderly person must be based on the understanding that problems of living, general health factors, and a decrease in the efficiency of several organ systems combine to determine the elderly's status. More so than in any other age group, socioeconomic and physiologic factors can cause or influence the outcome of a particular disease and possibly the patient's status as elderly or nonelderly.

REFERENCES

Bozzetti, L.P., and MacMurray, J.P. Contemporary concepts of aging: an overview. *Psychiatr Ann.* 7:117, 1977.

Breslow, L., and Somers, A.R. The lifetime health-monitoring program. *N Engl J Med.* 296:601, 1977.

Brocklehurst, J.C. The general health of the elderly. Edited by A.N. Exton-Smith, and D.L. Scott. In *Vitamins in the Elderly.* Bristol, England: John Wright and Sons, Ltd., 1968.

Brotman, H.B. Population projections. I. Tomorrow's older population (to 2000). *Gerontologist* 17:203, 1977.

Bultena, G.L., and Powers, E.A. Denial of aging: age identification and reference group orientations. *J Gerontol.* 33:748, 1978.

Bureau of the Census. *Demographic Aspects of Aging and the Older Population in the United States, Current Population Reports.* Special Studies, Series P-23, No. 59. Washington, D.C.: U.S. Government Printing Office, 1976.

Charatan, F.B. Depression in old age. *NY State J Med.* 75:2505, 1975.

Chebotarev, D.F. Longevity and the role of its investigation in the evaluation of aging processes. Proceedings of the Eighth International Congress of Gerontology, Vol I. Washington, D.C., 1969.

Department of Health, Education and Welfare Task Force on Prescription Drugs. *The Drug Users.* Washington, D.C.: U.S. Government Printing Office, 1968.

Eckert, J.K. Health status, adjustments, and social supports of older people living in center city hotels. Presented at the 30th Annual Meeting of the American Gerontological Society. San Francisco, 1977.

Federal Register 38(65):8719, 1973.

Finch, C.E. The regulation of physiological changes during mammalian aging. *Q Rev Biol.* 51:49, 1976.

Fowles, D.G. *Some Prospects for Future Elderly Population.* DHEW Publ. No. (OHDS) 78-20288. Washington, D.C.: U.S. Government Printing Office, 1978.

Fuchs, V.R. *Who Shall Live.* New York: Basic Books, 1974.

Garcia, P.A., Battese, G.E., and Brewer, W.D. Longitudinal study of age and cohort influences on dietary patterns. *J Gerontol.* 30:349, 1977.

Hermalin, A.J. The effect of changes in mortality rates on population and age distribution in the US. *Milbank Mem Fund Q.* 44:451, 1966.

Jackson, J.J. National caucus on the black aged: a progress report. *Aging Hum Dev.* 2:226, 1971.

Kimmel, D.C. *Adulthood and Aging.* New York: John Wiley and Sons, Inc., 1974.

Koutsopoulous, K.C., and Smith, C.G. Mobility constraints of the carless. *Traffic Q.* 30(1):67, 1976.

Laslett, P. In an aging world. *New Society.* Vol. 42, No. 786, Oct. 27, 1977, pp 171-173.

Maddox, G.L. Themes and issues in sociological theories of human aging. Edited by V.M. Brantl, and M.R. Brown. In *Readings in Gerontology.* St. Louis: C.V. Mosby Co., 1973.

Massachusetts Department of Public Health. Determining the needs of the elderly and the chronically disabled. *N Engl J Med.* 294:110, 1976.

Maxwell, R. The case for intervention. Edited by D.A. Ehrlich. In *The Health Care Cost Explosion: Which Way Now?* Bern: Hans Huber Publishers, 1975.

Myers, G.C. Demographic data on the elderly. *Science* 193:358, 1976.

Neugarten, B.L. Developmental perspectives. Edited by V.M. Brantl, and M.R. Brown. In *Readings in Gerontology.* St. Louis: C.V. Mosby Co., 1973.

Neugarten, B.L. Age groups in American society and the rise of the young-old. *Ann Am Acad Pol Soc Sci.* 415:187, 1974.

Neugarten, B.L. The future of the young-old. *Gerontologist* 15:4, 1975.

Neugarten, B.L., and Havighurst, R.J. Aging and the future. Edited by B.L. Neugarten, and R.J. Havighurst. In *Social Policy, Social Ethics, and the Aging Society.* Washington, D.C.: U.S. Government Printing Office, 1976.

Peterson, D.M., and Thomas, C.W. Acute drug reactions among the elderly. *J Gerontol.* 5:552, 1975.

Pomerance, A. Pathology of heart disease in the elderly. *Br J Hosp Med.* 11(2):245, 1974.

Riley, M.W., Johnson, M., and Foner, A. (eds.). *Aging and Society.* New York: Russell Sage Foundation, 1972.

Spiegelman, M., and Erhardt, C.L. Mortality and longevity in the United States. Edited by C.L. Erhardt, and J.E. Berlin. In *Mortality and Morbidity in the United States.* Cambridge: Harvard University Press, 1974.

Stevenson, J.S. *Issues and Crises During Middlescence.* New York: Appleton-Century-Crofts, 1977.

Sukosky, D.G. Sociological factors of friendship: relevance for the aged. *J Gerontol Nurs.* 3(6):25, 1977.

Volinn, I.J. Gerontological research and public health. *Public Health Rev.* 3(1):73, 1974.

Wheeler, H. Goodbye to mandatory retirement. *Modern Maturity* 21(3):9, 1978.

Youmans, E.G. Attitudes: young-old and old-old. *Gerontologist* 17:175, 1978.

2 Theories of Aging

An understanding of the aging process may lead to a modification of this process, the development of anti-aging drugs, an extension of the life span, a better quality of life for the aged, and finally, a different societal concept of aging.

Many different theories conceptualize the aging process (Bakerman 1969). In general, aging is thought to follow an entropic or decremental model (Strumpf 1978), which documents the decline of biologic, cognitive, and psychomotor function (Butler 1974). This concept views aging as an inevitable process which leads to irreversible decline and, concurrently, to the widely-accepted stereotype of aging. Even psychosocial theories of aging, such as the theory of disengagement, have overtones of a decremental model; age results in a decreased interaction between the aged and others in the social system (Cumming and Henry 1961). Therefore, efforts have been made to describe aging as a negentropic or open and progressive model. Aging then would be viewed as a maturation process. Based on this model, aging is not simply an accumulation of decrements and losses but is a continued accumulation of gains.

A clearer understanding of the aging process is needed in order to gain a better knowledge of the so-called diseases of old age. Pathologic conditions that normally accompany old age are not easily distinguishable from the normal process of senescence as the diseases of old age are superimposed on the normal physiologic decrements. Age-associated physiologic decrements, in addition, increase the elderly's vulnerability to disease and make the occurrence of disease more likely (Hayflick 1976). In turn, certain diseases like diabetes, living conditions, and characteristics like being overweight can adversely influence the aging process (Curtis 1966). The interdependence of aging and disease is clear. The aging process diminishes functional capacity and increases the incidence of pathologic conditions exponentially. In senescence, risk of these pathologic changes increases rapidly.

AGING—HOW IS IT DEFINED?

In societal terms, aging is that stage in life when a person loses interest in new things and thoughts and stops relating to the present and prefers to think about the good old days. In biologic terms, aging is a complex phenomenon correlated with the passage of time (Tuchweber and Salas 1975). Structural and functional changes occur (Mooney 1978), which might be likened to a wearing-out process accelerated by abuse and decelerated by care (Ochsner 1976). Physiologically, aging may be viewed as an ontogenetic cycle, starting with conception and leading to decline; pathologically, it is the result of an accumulation of stresses and strains, injuries and infections, immunologic reactions, nutritional deficiencies, metabolic disturbances, neglect and abuse (Smith and Sethi 1975).

Aging is a normal, genetically determined part of the life cycle. It is said to have two distinct components: the nuisance factor (muscular weakness) and the mortality factor, which results from degenerative diseases. Although heredity seems influential in normal longevity to age 70, at older ages there is far less evidence of a genetic pattern, and a strong influence of individual life styles, habits, and personal actions in favor of survival.

The process of aging has also been summarized as a gradual loss of functional cells and a gradual biochemical impairment of the remaining cells. Diminished sensorimotor speed, which involves all processes integrated by the central nervous system, is partially responsible for aging. Some describe aging as a decline in the energy needed by the cell to perform its function, or as a process of deterioration, degeneration, and atrophy at the molecular, cellular, and organic levels. During this process, no proteins, matrices, or organs with new structures or functions arise. As a consequence, physiologic regulation declines in efficiency, leading to an organism less resistant to stress.

Aging has no defined limits. It is an insidious, progressive process with no single cause. Many aging phenomena are universal, but a common denominator has not yet been found. People grow old at different rates and at different ages. These rates and ages change from generation to generation and vary between populations, as well as with living and working conditions. The differences depend, to some degree, on genetic (intrinsic) and environmental (extrinsic) factors. The extent to which human physiology responds to these factors is not clearly understood.

STUDY OF AGING

Animal models often provide the basis for the development of theories of aging. There has been pronounced interest in some of the premature aging syndromes shown in Table 2-1.

In people, progeria (Hutchinson-Gilford disease) has been studied as a model of the aging process. Only about 80 cases have been recorded. Progeria represents a severe growth deceleration in young patients.

Table 2-1
Premature Aging Syndromes

Syndrome	Age of onset	Prognosis
Acrogeria	In early life	Somatic and sexual development is normal. Atrophic skin with mottled pigmentation, mostly on limbs. Normal life expectancy.
Pangeria (Werner's syndrome)	Second decade	Sexual maturation at puberty incomplete. Atherosclerosis in early adult life. Diabetes mellitus around 30. Mean life span 47 years.
Progeria (Hutchinson-Gilford disease)	During first year	Severely retarded growth. No sexual maturation. Atrophic skin, loss of hair. Atherosclerosis. Life expectancy 16 years.
Metageria	Evident at birth	Atrophic skin with mottled hyperpigmentation. Generalized loss of subcutaneous fat on limbs. Normal sexual maturation. Early atherosclerosis and diabetes mellitus. Life expectancy 25 years(?)

Children affected by this syndrome, at the end of their first decade, exhibit signs which are normally found in adults at the end of their seventh decade. The disease affects weight more than height. The skin, the musculoskeletal system, the cardiovascular system, and the metabolism are all affected. Extensive atherosclerosis is usually present, bones are fragile, and the cranium is very thin. The skin is old and wrinkled and there is joint flexion deformity. Patients exhibit relative insulin resistance, comparable to glucose tolerance in the elderly. Collagen is highly cross-linked and cardiac findings are characteristic of findings in the elderly. Symptoms of angina and heart failure are observed, and the patient usually dies of coronary disease.

Pangeria (Werner's syndrome) is very much like progeria, but manifestations occur later. There is early graying and loss of hair, cataracts, diabetes, atherosclerosis, osteoporosis, and a high incidence of neoplasm. Therefore, Werner's syndrome has been considered as a case of accelerated aging, but while there are remarkable consistencies with the aging process, there are also some differences (Fulder 1977).

THEORIES OF AGING

Many different theories of aging have been proposed and described (Comfort 1974; Emanuel 1976; Curtis 1971). One of the earlier theories suggested was the rate-of-living theory, which was very similar to the wear-and-tear theory of aging. In short, it proposed that each individual had a certain reserve of vitality, which could be used up quickly, leading to a short life, or slowly, thereby prolonging life.

In an effort to elucidate the relationship between aging and disease, all theories of aging are divided into two classes. Reduction theories propose that changes occur at the molecular and cellular levels; theories dealing with the total organism usually focus on the homeostatic mechanisms (Blumenthal 1978). Aging theories have also been divided into two major categories depending on which aging process they attempt to explain (Finch 1976):

1. Intrinsic changes: those independent of other cells or extracellular factors.
2. Extrinsic changes: those that occur in hormones outside cells.

A number of theories address the fact that aging is genetically induced, either preprogrammed or in a random fashion.

The somatic mutation theory (Szilard 1959), addressing the intrinsic aging mechanism, proposed that spontaneous mutations occur in somatic cells, which would lead to changed cell functions. Some cells might exhibit uncontrolled growth characteristics (cancer), some altered cholesterol metabolism (arteriosclerosis), and others altered immune mechanisms (autoimmune diseases). Ultimately, the mutated cells would accumulate to cause chromosomal inactivation and cell death. This theory cannot account for the entire aging process and it is no longer accepted. However, it has led to the development of the error theories, which describe mishaps in the fidelity of information flow.

The error catastrophe theory (Orgel 1970) proposes that the aging process is characterized not only by an increasing error rate in the translation of the genetic code for protein synthesis, but also by a progressive increase in the half-life of enzyme proteins. Both transcriptional and translational errors occur. There is then progressive disruption of cellular function because of defective enzymes that are normally responsible for the fidelity of the genetic information flow. Correlation between this theory and intrinsic aging mechanisms has been disputed.

Another error theory, which views aging as a degenerative process, proposes a sophisticated mechanism of codon modulation and speculates that aging is the result of the loss of the original transfer RNA species (Strehler et al 1971). Similarly, it has been posited that error accumulation and life span depend on redundant DNA sequences. As regulatory genes mutate, new genes replace the faulty ones. Assuming finite gene redundancy, the error accumulation is regulated at the transcriptional level (Medvedev 1972). It has been further hypothesized that a specific control mechanism, at the level of transcription, is responsible for the initiation and sequence of primary aging events (Von Hahn 1970).

The theory of the finite limit of cell division (Hayflick and Moorhead 1962; Hayflick 1965, 1968, 1970, 1974) seemingly supports the error theory. According to Hayflick's theory, a clock, most likely situated in the cell nucleus, dictates a cell's capacity to replicate. The doubling potential is inversely related to age, and correlates with the mean life span in various species. Accordingly, cell death and probably aging appear to be genetically programmed. At one time, it was assumed that aging occurred only in tissues composed of fixed postmitotic cells. There is now evidence, though that dividing cell systems are also involved in the etiology of aging symptoms. Many cells retain their capacity to replicate throughout life, among them those of the liver and intestinal mucosa. For cells capable of proliferation, it has been suggested that tissue aging might be explained by a transition of cycling to noncyling cells (Gelfant and Smith 1972).

Other aging theories address intrinsic age changes. Among them is the cross-linking theory (Verzar 1968). With time, body collagen, which makes up a large fraction of body protein, becomes more and more rigid and that process interferes with normal organ function.

This theory can be used to explain some of the "nuisance" aspects of aging, but cannot explain the etiology of degenerative diseases.

The autoimmune theory (Burnet 1970) stresses that senescence is largely mediated by autoimmune processes. Changes in the immune recognition system lead to immune reactions which, in turn, lead to various autoimmune diseases. This theory is linked to immunopathology. Normal immune function declines sharply with age (Walford 1974), while autoimmunity (the development of antibodies to inappropriate antigens) increases with age. In addition to the body becoming less resistant to diseases, the humoral machinery may turn against the mother system. This theory constitutes part of the overall aging theory, as autoimmune diseases are important degenerative diseases. However, the immune system is a rate-limiting, but not the controlling factor, in aging (Kay 1976).

The free-radical theory of aging (Harman 1961, 1969) stipulates that ionizing radiation leads to the formation of free radicals, released by polyunsaturated fats. The deleterious effects of the free radicals, liberated during energy reactions, immobilize macromolecules. Changes in free radical content in the tissue lead to various pathologic states, such as malignant growth. The thought that free radicals possess damaging activity has led to the search for the so-called "geroprotectors," such as antioxidants (vitamins C and E, 2-mercaptoethylamine) and radioprotectors (butylated hydroxytoluene). Some of these, found currently as food additives, could slow the aging process.

The accumulation of lipofuscin is a well-documented correlate of the aging process. No functional deficit has as yet been correlated to pigment accumulation, and there is no evidence that aging pigments cause defects in cell function. There is, further, no evidence that lipofuscin limits the life span of individual cells. Meclofenoxate reverses the accumulation of lipofuscin, but increases the mortality rate in mice.

Atrophy of the uterine, vaginal, and other estrogen-dependent cells illustrates the effects of the extrinsic aging mechanisms. The cybernetic pacemaker theory proposes that the central nervous system (CNS) is the pacemaker for age-related physiologic changes (Finch 1973) and that these changes may also depend on endocrine changes controlled by the hypothalamus. Thus, endocrine and neural factors, which regulate aging changes in target cells, are responsible for the extrinsic aging mechanisms. With advancing age, steroid production of the adrenal cortex and the gonads decreases, and there is a slowed turnover of thyroidal iodine. In contrast, basal levels of insulin and growth hormone do not change with age, but the secretory dynamics do change. The pancreatic set point for insulin secretion by blood glucose is progressively elevated with age in normal persons, for example.

Central nervous system monoamines are strongly implicated as the substrate for the endocrine modulation of the aging process (Finch 1976). Brain dopamine levels are reduced with age (Finch 1973), and age-related changes in brain catecholamines can trigger a series of events leading to altered cell function in those cells for which the catecholamines serve as pacemakers. There is a reduced uptake of dopamine by striatal and hypothalamic synaptosomes. The affinity of dopamine uptake is reduced, without any change in the maximum velocity.

Thus, hormonal levels fluctuate with age and specific binding of various hormones by target cells may also change during senescence (Roth and Adelman 1975). These hormonal changes cause the target cells to age faster (Everitt 1973). While there probably is no specific aging hormone, hormones in general may modulate the aging process. The theory explaining the extrinsic aging mechanisms recognizes altered regulation of neural factors, hormonal output, and target cell response. Again, these changes cannot explain all age-related changes. Thus, the composite theory of aging proposes that the symptoms of aging result from a series of changes. The first of these might be a mutation of a somatic cell, followed by stimulation for cell division, and followed in turn by many other steps which have not yet been elucidated clearly.

REFERENCES

Bakerman, S. *Aging Life Processes.* Springfield, Ill.: Charles C Thomas Co., 1969.

Blumenthal, H.T. Aging: biologic or pathologic. *Hosp Practice.* 13(4):127, 1978.

Burnet, F.M. Immunological approach to aging. *Lancet* 2:358, 1970.

Butler, R. Successful aging and the role of the life review. *J Am Geriatr Soc.* 22:533, 1974.

Comfort, A. The position of aging studies. *Mech Ageing Dev.* 3:1, 1974.

Cumming, E., and Henry, W.E. *Growing Old.* New York: Basic Books, 1961.

Curtis, H.J. *Biological Mechanisms of Aging.* Springfield, Ill.: Charles C Thomas Co., 1966.

Curtis, H.J. Genetic factors in aging. *Adv Genet.* 16:305, 1971.

Emanuel, N.M. Free radicals and the action of inhibitors of radical processes under pathological states and aging in living organisms and in man. *Q Rev Biophys.* 9:283, 1976.

Everitt, A.V. The hypothalamic-pituitary control of aging and age-related pathology. *Exp Gerontol.* 8:265, 1973.

Finch, C.E. Catecholamine metabolism in the brains of ageing male mice. *Brain Res.* 52:261, 1973.

Finch, C.E. The regulation of physiological changes during mammalian aging. *Q Rev Biol.* 51:40, 1976.

Fulder, S. A pathological race through life. *New Scientist* April 21, 1977, p. 122.

Gelfant, S., and Smith, J.G. Aging: noncycling cells-an explanation. *Science* 178:357, 1972.

Harman, D. Prolongation of the normal life span and inhibition of spontaneous cancer by antioxidants. *J Gerontol.* 16:247, 1961.

Harman, D. Prolongation of life: role of free radical reactions in aging. *J Am Geriatr Soc.* 17:721, 1969.

Hayflick, L. The limited in vitro lifetime of human diploid strains. *Exp Cell Res.* 37:614, 1965.

Hayflick, L. Human cells and aging. *Sci Am.* 218:32, 1968.

Hayflick, L. Aging under glass. *Exp Gerontol.* 5:291, 1970.

Hayflick, L. The longevity of cultured human cells. *J Am Geriatr Soc.* 22:1, 1974.

Hayflick, L. The cell biology of human aging. *N Engl J Med.* 295:1302, 1976.

Hayflick, L., and Moorhead, P.S. The serial cultivation of human diploid cell strains. *Exp Cell Res.* 25:585, 1962.

Kay, M.M.B. Autoimmune disease: the consequence of deficient T-cell functions. *J Am Geriatr Soc.* 24:253, 1976.

Medvedev, A. Repetition of molecular genetic information as a possible factor in evolutionary changes in life span. *Exp Gerontol.* 7:227, 1972.

Mooney, C.M. Psychologic problems of the aged. *J Am Geriatr Soc.* 26:268, 1978.

Ochsner, A. Aging. *J Am Geriatr Soc.* 24:385, 1976.

Orgel, L.E. The maintenance of the accuracy of protein synthesis and its relevance to aging: a correction. *Proc Natl Acad Sci USA.* 67:1476, 1970.

Roth, G.S., and Adelman, R.C. Age-related changes in hormone binding by target cells and tissues: possible role in altered adaptive responsiveness. *Exp Gerontol.* 10:1, 1975.

Smith, B.H., and Sethi, P.K. Aging and the nervous system. *Geriatrics* 30:109, 1975.

Strehler, B., Hirsch, G., Gusseck, D. et al. Codon restriction theory of aging and development. *J Theor Biol.* 33:429, 1971.

Strumpf, N. Aging–a progressive phenomenon. *J Gerontol Nurs.* 4(2):17, 1978.

Szilard, L. On the nature of the aging process. *Proc Natl Acad Sci USA.* 45:30, 1959.

Tuchweber, B., and Salas, M. Experimental pathology of aging. *Methods Achiev Exp Pathol.* 7:167, 1975.

Verzar, F. Intrinsic and extrinsic factors of molecular aging. *Exp Gerontol.* 3:69, 1968.

Von Hahn, H.P. Regulation of protein synthesis in the aging cell. *Exp Gerontol.* 5:323, 1970.

Walford, R.L. Immunologic theory of aging: current status. *Fed Proc.* 33:2020, 1974.

3 Primary and Secondary Aging

PHYSICAL CHANGES

Certain external changes take place with aging which may not have any important physiologic consequences, but which may at times have devastating psychologic effects. Undoubtedly, it is these changes which have given rise to the stereotypic presentation of the elderly.

Most older persons appear to be shorter and, in fact, a loss of one or two inches in height can occur. A changing posture, which is associated with a dehydration and flattening of the vertebral discs, contributes to that appearance. Loss of height may also be caused by a bending of the spine (kyphosis), as well as osteoporosis and emphysema (Rossman 1971). A concurrent flexing of the legs gives the arms a longer appearance.

Skin aging may appear as early as the fourth decade. Probably 90% of all people in the fifth decade of their lives have liver spots, also called senile lentigo, lentigines, or melanotic freckles. They appear most often on the cheeks, face, neck, and the backs of the hands

(Domonkos 1968; Crosby 1975). A hydroquinone preparation, applied topically, may temporarily bleach these spots. Ruby spots (cherry angioma or senile angioma) may appear, which can be removed if the patient insists. The senile skin assumes a yellowish or grayish hue.

Graying of the hair or loss of hair, particularly in elderly males, is generally accepted as one sign of aging. Similarly, there is a slowing of the nail growth rate and, to the consternation of many elderly, the nails begin to "wrinkle." A nail conditioning and polishing kit can be used to ameliorate this particular problem.*

Weight quite often remains constant up to the age of 65 to 70 years, followed frequently by a loss of overall weight. However, there is a pronounced qualitative change. The percentage of total body lipids doubles in old age, from 14% at age 25 to 30% by age 70. At the same time, there is likely to be a loss in cell population of soft tissue and muscle, for example, of between 25% to 30% between the ages of 20 and 70. Body water declines from 61% to 53% during the same time (Garth and Young 1956). These and other physiologic changes are depicted in Figure 3-1 (Lamy and Vestal 1976).

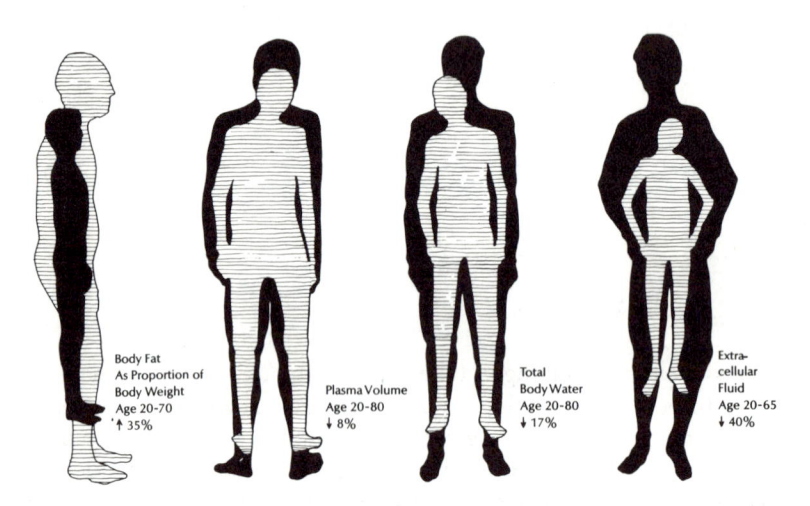

Figure 3-1 Physiologic changes in aging. From P.P. Lamy and R.E. Vestal. Drug prescribing for the elderly. *Hosp Practice.* 11(1):111, 1976. Reprinted with permission.

BIOLOGIC AGING

Although no single factor seems to be responsible for the process of aging, one fact is clear: aging does not affect the whole organism

---

*Jovan, Inc., Chicago, IL 60611

uniformly. The rate of decline of different functions varies, and it further varies from individual to individual (Lamy and Kitler 1971; Lamy 1973, 1978). In general, physiologic functions in the human decline slowly and linearly from 30 years of age. The rate constants for these losses seem to occur at about 0.8% to 0.9% per year of functional capacity present at age 30 (Hayflick 1976).

Biologic characteristics usually show earlier age decrements than do psychosocial functions. Changes depend to some degree on genetic (intrinsic) and environmental (extrinsic) factors. The human physiology responds to these factors to an extent as yet not clearly understood. Changes in physiologic functions are depicted in Tables 3-1 and 3-2. The process of biologic or primary aging probably occurs on several levels, ie, molecular, cellular, and tissue. Aging can also be characterized by anatomic, physiologic, and behavioral changes. When one considers changes taking place on the molecular and cellular levels, a great difference is found among various organs in the rates of turnover of cells and molecules. There is an age-related decrease in total cell mass and in intracellular water.

Table 3-1
Residual Physiologic Functions or Tissues of Average Male, Age 75, Compared to Average Male, Age 30

Functions or tissue	Comparative residual (percent)
Brain weight	56
Brain blood flow	80
Rapidity of blood to return to normal pH	17
Cardiac output, resting	70
Total kidney glomeruli	56
Glomerular filtration rate	69
Renal plasma flow	50
Fibers, nerve trunk	63
Nerve conduction velocity	90
Taste buds, total	36
Oxygen uptake during exercise	40
Pulmonary ventilation, exercise volume	53
Breathing capacity, maximum voluntary	43
Pulmonary vital capacity	56
Hand grip	55
Work rate, maximum	70
Work rate, short bursts	40
Basal metabolic rate	84
Water content, body	82
Weight, male	88

Source: A.B. Chinn. Working with older people, Vol. 4, PHS Publ. No. 1459, *Clinical Aspects of Aging*. Washington, D.C.: US Government Printing Office, 1971.

Table 3-2
Age-Dependent Physiologic and Pathologic Changes

System	Alterations
Cardiovascular	Coronary sclerosis and hypertension may lead to disease state. Arteriosclerotic heart disease and disturbance of heart rhythm. Decline in heart output.
Digestive	Digestive difficulties and intestinal upsets are major problems. Reduced stomach motility and reduced peristaltic activity. Increasing evidence of gastritis.
Genitourinary	Inflammatory or vascular renal pathology. Reduced blood flow through kidney. Reduced filtration rate. Water and electrolyte imbalance.
Nervous	High degree of psychiatric morbidity. Possible brain tissue breakdown and loss in total brain substance. Possible change in EEG pattern. Changes in sleep pattern. Reduction in short-term memory.
Respiratory	Decrease in lung and vital capacity. Possible calcification of costal, intercostal and intervertebral cartilages. Emphysema.
Sensory	Senses of touch and pain are reduced, as is ability to perceive odor and taste. Less sensitivity to pressure. Reflexes and reaction times are reduced.
Skeletal	Decalcification of bone and bone loss. Stiffening of joints. Ligament calcification.
Tissue	Atrophy. Regressive changes such as sclerosis and fibrosis.

Source: P.P. Lamy. Aging: how human physiology responds. In *Theory and Therapeutics of Aging*. Edited by E.W. Busse. New York: MedCom, Inc., 1973.

The collagen of the connective tissue loses osmotic swelling ability with age, its elasticity is changed and, due to intermolecular cross-linkage, its rigidity increases. Collagen makes up one-third of body proteins, provides the framework within which muscles contract, and acts as the general supporting protein of skin, the musculoskeletal system, and the vascular system.

Anatomically, the nucleus of the aging cell shrinks and there is an accumulation of vacuoles. Cross-linking of collagen impedes metabolic transfer. Biochemically, the cell shows increased lactate, histone, and lipofuscin levels, but several enzyme systems decrease. Physiologically, some organs (prostate) increase in size with age while others (brain) decrease. Sensory deprivation on a behavioral level may lead to secondary desocialization (Wallace 1977).

Perhaps the most serious physiologic change with age is the body's decreased ability to adapt to stress. All homeostatic mechanisms probably decline in functional capacity, starting shortly after onset of maturity. Under stress, older people are less able to regulate blood glucose levels, blood pH, pulse rate, blood pressure, and oxygen consumption. Thus, while many systems continue to function well in old age, because of their large reserve capacities, their ability to react to stress is impaired (Kohn 1963).

These age-related physiologic effects also create changes in responsiveness to drugs. The unpredictability of drug response increases sharply with increasing age.

PATHOLOGIC AGING

Pathologic or secondary aging encompasses disabilities from recurring injuries, trauma, stress, and loss. Diseases of adaptation caused by pollution, noise, and stress may affect elderly urban dwellers. Age-related diseases do not, of course, affect all individuals in a similar manner. The human body possesses a large reserve capacity and age decrements in biologic functions do not necessarily lead to disease.

The diseases prevalent among the elderly are caused by environmental factors that require prolonged exposure before a disease state is evident. It might also be that a long latent period is necessary before a disease becomes clinically evident. The cumulative effects of disease and environmental insults cause biologic deterioration superimposed on intrinsic or primary aging (Blumenthal 1978).

Many have claimed that there is a critical distinction between normal, age-related changes (eugenic changes) and those secondary to age-related pathologic conditions (pathogenic changes). However, pathologic conditions that accompany old age are not clearly distinguishable from the normal process of senescence. Manifestations of aging often are composite of environmental insults, disease, and intrinsic biologic aging. Since the combination of these effects may create an unpredictable drug response in the elderly, there is no valid reason to separate the effects of biologic and pathologic aging. In terms of drug therapy, drugs are foreign substances that create stress. Thus, the effects of primary and secondary aging must be taken into consideration in developing a specific therapeutic regimen for an elderly patient.

SPECIFIC CHANGES

General Tissue Changes

The most important tissue changes involve atrophy or decrease in organ weight. Regressive changes include sclerosis of vessels and fibrosis. The number and sometimes the volume of epithelial cells decrease in various organs, such as the thyroid, adrenal cortex, and the uterine endometrium. Most tissues probably respond to aging with hypertrophy and relatively little cell division (Post and Hoffman 1968). Cells which continue to divide throughout an individual's life span, such as gastrointestinal and hematopoietic cells, have been categorized as continuous mitotics. The intermittent mitotics, such as hepatic, renal tubular, and bone cells, exhibit less rapid mitotic capability with advancing age. Finally, cells that lose all mitotic capacity are called non-mitotics. They are responsible, for example, for poor and slow healing of cardiac and skeletal muscles after injury or surgery. While aged tissues heal as well as those of the young, wounds may heal more slowly because of inadequate nutrition and decreased resistance to infection.

Metabolic Changes

Metabolic functions decrease continuously from birth, and there is a gradual reduction in the metabolic rate. Physiologic activity begins to diminish during the third decade (Riccitelli 1972). Decrease in metabolic rate is about 1% per decade (Keys et al 1973).

Actually, basal oxygen consumption per unit of metabolizing tissue is not significantly altered with age (Starr 1955), but accumulation of metabolically inert fat tissue increases metabolic rate decline. Loss of ascorbic acid, calcium, potassium, sodium, and protein can lead to metabolic imbalances (Dontas 1969).

The activities of several enzymes decrease with age because of a decrease in the synthesis rate or a structural change. As cells age, they lose their ability to degrade specific enzymes. Enzymes lose from 30% to 70% of their activity during the life of an individual; however, these alterations do not change many major physical properties of enzymes, such as molecular weight. Changes have been documented for enzymes like aldolase, catalase, isocitrate lipase, and superoxide dismutase. Anaerobic glycolysis capacity is substantially reduced with age, but cathepsin levels increase. The neurohumoral chemistry is greatly affected, especially catecholamine metabolism; this creates risks when many drugs are used. There are also extensive changes in muscular enzyme systems. In the heart, there is an increase in monoamine oxidase and malic dehydrogenase, but there are decreases in dopamine beta-oxidase, dopa decarboxylase, cytochrome oxidase, and other enzymes (Finch and Hayflick 1977).

Effects of Trace Substances

Various trace substances have been implicated as contributing factors to human diseases. Cobalt, copper, zinc, manganese, selenium, tin, and cadmium can have an adverse or toxic effect on various body systems or organs. Cadmium may be responsible for emphysema or damage to the olfactory nerve, although its tissue concentration seems to diminish in the fifth and sixth decades. Cobalt and nickel in aerosol form may play a role in pulmonary disease. Brain copper concentrations increase, as do serum copper concentrations, between the ages of 20 and 70 (Louria et al 1972).

Cardiovascular System

The aging process and hemodynamic changes are responsible for anatomic and histologic changes in this system. Aging of the cardiovascular system is seldom evident before the fourth decade. Changes are most marked between the ages of 40 and 60 years, but there is little change after that (Brandfonbrenner et al 1955; Bender 1965). Cardiac tissue seems less affected by the aging process than are the blood vessels (Garbus and Lamy 1976). The aging aorta and the great muscular arteries lose their elasticity and become somewhat dilated and lengthened. Many of the changes observed are caused by elastin changes. Elastin is present in abundance in vessel walls. With advancing age, it is degraded by increasing levels of enzymes known as elastases (Ladislas 1977). The degradation of the elastic fibers is reflected on the morphologic level by lipid infiltration and the formation of calcium-containing deposits, leading to calcification of the coronary artery and the aorta. The small muscular arteries will exhibit a narrowed lumen, reducing blood supply to the various organs that they serve. However, as most organs need less oxygen with advancing age, this is not necessarily of serious clinical consequence.

Unquestionably, these changes are responsible in part for such disease states as atherosclerosis and pulmonary edema (Sandberg 1976). Changes involving blood vessels are well documented, as is the fact that there is no significant change in blood and plasma volume per unit of body weight with age (Shock 1961).

Certain anatomic and histologic changes occur in the aging heart, some of which are presented in Figure 3-2 (Lamy et al 1977a). The anatomic changes are most likely caused by alterations in collagen and connective tissues. Many changes are more prominent in the left side of the heart, probably because that side is subjected to higher pressure. With advancing age, the heart's epithelial cells increase in volume (Stoermer 1967). The heart size in old persons without hypertension or clinical heart disease remains the same as in middle age or becomes smaller as a result of decreased demand and reduced activity. Mean cardiac weight increases linearly, by about 1 gm per year in men and 1.5 gm per year in women, between the ages of 30 and 80 years. This increase is apparently accompanied by a similar increase in mean arterial blood pressure, which rises by almost 13% in men and almost 25% in women (Linzback 1975).

The gross appearance of the heart also changes. The aging heart muscle is a deeper brown and there is more subpericardial fat. The heart valves are thicker because of sclerosis and fibrosis. In general, there is increased heart valve rigidity. The mitral valve appears to be the most severely affected. It may show wear-and-tear changes, mainly in leaflet and chordal thickening. The left ventricular cavity gets smaller, presumably as cardiac output decreases with age (Roberts and Perloff 1972). In general, there is a greater amount of collagen in the valves and the endocardium.

One of the most striking physiologic changes is the decline in the heart's ability to respond to stress. During stress, the heart rate and blood flow increase, but these increases are less than those in younger

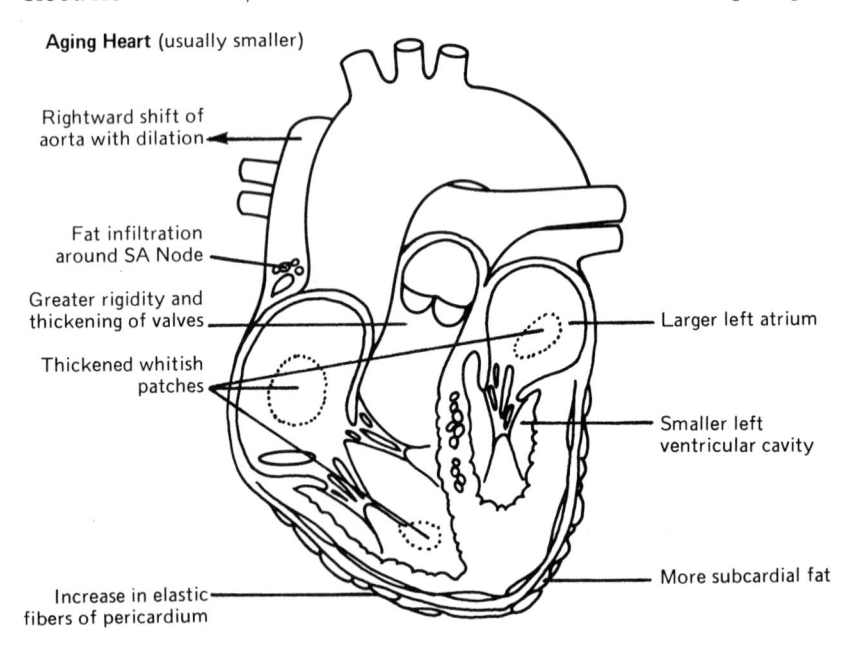

Figure 3-2 The aging heart. From P.P. Lamy et al. *The Aging Cardiovascular System.* Princeton, N.J.: E.R. Squibb & Sons, 1977. Reprinted with permission.

persons. It has been postulated that this reduced increase is caused by a reduction in the levels of catecholamines in older people or that response to catecholamines is diminished. The catecholamines increase the amount of calcium supplied to the contractile proteins of heart muscle cells and thereby cause the muscle to contract. Aging seems to affect ability of the catecholamines to alter the release of calcium rather than in the response to calcium. The heart muscle also changes its mechanical and biochemical characteristics. There is a delay in the recovery of contractility and increased irritability. The decrease in cardiac contractility with age is paralleled by a decrease in functional reserve in other major organs.

Even without disease diathesis, the aging heart at rest has a reduced output with no appreciable loss in total cardiac muscle tissue. Resting cardiac output decreases 30% to 40% between the ages of 25 and 65 (Nejat and Greif 1976), but there is not necessarily a good correlation between this decrease and the decreased capacity of the heart, as the demands on the heart also decrease because of reduced function of other organs.

The maximum blood flow through the coronary artery is reduced by 35% at age 60; there is also a reduced stroke volume, a slower heart rate, an increase in ejection time, and a relative lengthening of systole.

A contributory factor in the impairment of cardiac performance is reduced phosphorylation, a process responsible for converting chemical into mechanical energy.

These factors combine to make the older person more susceptible to arrhythmias and extrasystoles. Slowing of the electrical activity of the cardiac pacemakers with age contributes to this susceptibility. Tachycardias and arrhythmias are stressful and may be particularly detrimental in older people. There is also attenuation of ventilatory and heart rate responses to hypoxia and hypercapnia as a result of the normal aging process (Kronenberg and Drage 1973).

Yet the demands on the heart increase with age. For example, a greater peripheral resistance must be overcome and arterial pressure is higher. Thus, even the normal aging heart is burdened with the effects of numerous age changes which under stress can adversely affect an older person's health (Gruebl et al 1973). In short, the elderly heart functions well under ordinary circumstances but has lost much of its functional reserve. The elderly are prone to hypotension because of poor cardiac output, low plasma volume, and other factors. The lower the lying pressure, which is often the case in drug-induced hypotension, the smaller the fall in blood pressure before symptoms appear. The incidence of hypotension rises with age and is fairly common in the very old. Patients so afflicted will "lose the use of their legs," ie, they will be unable to walk, they will be liable to falls, and they may be bedbound with weakness and faints. Diuretics, neuroleptics, adrenergic blockers, L-dopa, and methyldopa are most often involved (Grunstein 1974).

Even in the absence of disease, the cerebral, coronary, and skeletal muscles receive proportionally more of the diminished cardiac output than do the liver and kidneys. The reduced cardiac output, coupled with a redistribution of the diminished output, may lead to unanticipated therapeutic results. The normal distribution of drugs may also change because of variations in peripheral resistance, which increases at a rate corresponding to the rate of change in cardiac output. Furthermore, as the homeostatic mechanisms in the elderly work less efficiently and respond less quickly, the elderly are particularly sensitive to excessive doses of various drugs.

The aging heart is less responsive to cardiac stimulants. The effect of atropine is also greatly reduced (Grollman and Grollman 1960). Changes in the electrical activity of the aging heart may modify its response to antiarrhythmic drugs.

The events of primary aging may be potentiated by certain disease states often associated with aging. Atherosclerosis, hypertension, kidney disease, liver disease, and obesity all cause cardiac dysfunction, so that almost one-third of people over 70 years of age have some disturbance of heart rhythm (Stoermer 1967). Cardiovascular diseases are more common in men than in women, possibly because estrogen mitigates or delays hypertension, coronary artery disease, paroxysmal tachycardia, myocardial ischemia, and certain pathologic changes in the electrocardiogram (Stumpf et al 1977). The striking and widespread pathologic conditions and processes found often in the aging heart may be caused by a great variety of factors, such as alcoholism, recurrent viral infections or infarctions, and subsequent scarring.

Central Nervous System

Integration among muscles, glands, neurons, and blood is a function of the central nervous system (CNS). With advancing age, this integration becomes less effective and efficient. Changes can be observed in motor function, adaptive responses to the environment (stress), and in sensory functions. Neuronal loss in the CNS probably begins in the fourth decade and progresses at different rates in different individuals. Yet the concept of inevitable deterioration of the nervous system is unacceptable since nerve cells have the greatest life span of any cells.

Certain decrements in CNS function do occur. For example, nerve conduction velocity declines by about 10% (Barrett 1972), although the decline may amount to as much as 30% in sensory nerves. This decrease in conduction velocity is caused by a decrease in the performance of individual nerve cells and is at least partially responsible for a slowing of reflexes (Spirduso 1975). Aging also affects the spinal cord. Spinal cord axons decline in number by as much as 37% over the years (Barrett 1972). There is a loss of nerve fibers in spinal nerve roots and peripheral nerves (Smith and Sethi 1975). The functional reserve of the CNS is reduced with aging, so that stress may activate subclinical disturbances. Even a subtle degeneration of the CNS may be responsible for terminal bronchopneumonia (Parker 1972) or increased vulnerability to drugs.

The brain is the organ of adaptation. As part of the CNS it is responsible for the regulation of many bodily functions. The brain plays a major role in the regulation of respiration, heart rate, blood pressure, and the release of hormones, as well as in the complex control of temperature and electrolyte balance (Miller and Dworkin 1977). The brain (as well as the kidney and the heart) receives less blood with advancing age, which reduces its capacity to respond to stress. Thus, psychologic stresses to an elderly patient may increase the probability of a wide range of medically adverse consequences, such as psychosomatic conditions, coronary heart disease, stroke, and diabetes.

Gross morphologic changes occur in the brain with age. There is a general widening and deepening of sulci and narrowing of gyri (Figures 3-3 and 3-4), especially evident over the frontal and upper parietal lobes (Lamy et al 1977b). Other gross changes involve a reduction in weight and volume. The female brain, which attains maximum

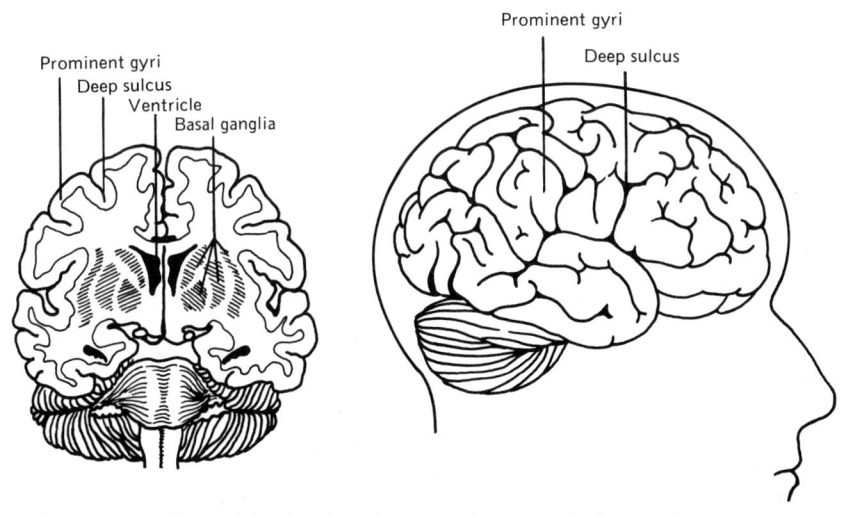

Figure 3-3 Normal brain showing prominent gyri, deep sulcus. From P.P. Lamy et al. *The Aging Brain*. Princeton, N.J.: E.R. Squibb & Sons, 1977. Reprinted with permission.

Aging Brain (smaller size)

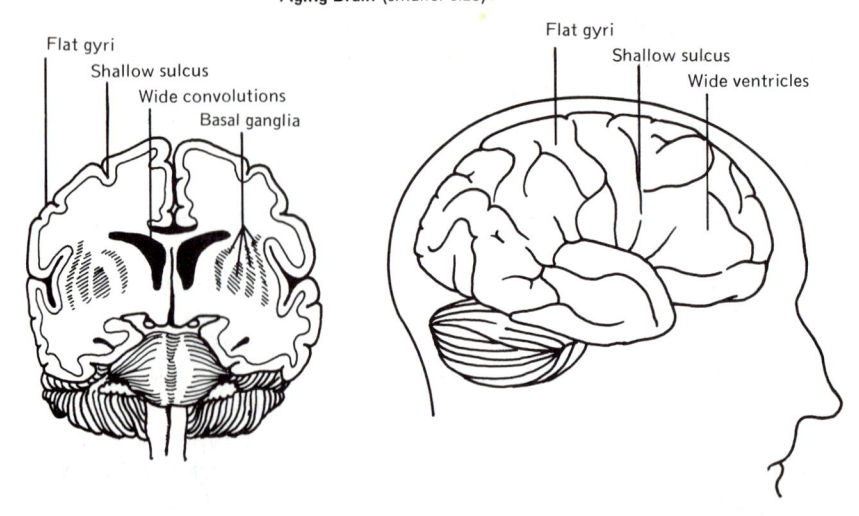

Figure 3-4 Aging brain showing flat gyri and shallow sulcus, as well as wide convolutions and wide ventricles. From P.P. Lamy et al. *The Aging Brain*. Princeton, N.J.: E.R. Squibb & Sons, 1977. Reprinted with permission.

weight earlier than does the male brain, begins to decline earlier. There is linear decrease in brain volume after age 30, evidenced by a doubling of the volume of intracranial space between 20 and 80 years of age (Barron et al 1976; Brizzee 1975). A 30% decrease in brain tissue has been suggested (Cragg 1975). A major part of this decrease, however, may come from the glial cells (connective tissue) that support the nerve cells.

The relationship between neuronal loss and decreased brain size is still being disputed. It has been said that after 50 years, the number of brain cells decreases at the rate of about 1% per year, so that the very old may retain only 40% of their brain cell volume. It is also thought that many nuclei retain their neuron population unchanged into the most advanced age, and that the number of cells in the cerebral cortex remains constant until age 65. The neurons then decrease at a rate of 1% per year. By age 70, cell loss may be 20%, with no obvious clinical sign. As much as 25% to 30% may have been lost by age 80, and in dementia that loss may amount to 40% (Nandy 1978). Different brain regions are affected to different degrees. The hippocampus appears to be particularly sensitive to age-related stress, and in the cerebral cortex the cell loss is most prominent in the prefrontal and superior temporal areas. While there is agreement that the rate of loss differs in different parts of the brain, there is still no agreement as to the amount of overall loss.

Brain cell loss does not lead to clinical manifestations. Only when a patient is exposed to stress, changing electrolyte balance, poor nutrition, or toxins (drugs) will clinical manifestations occur. The water content of the brain falls from 92% at birth to 10.5% at age 30, then declines to 7.5% in old age (Ordy 1975). Brain polyunsaturated fatty acids decrease with age, but the clinical significance of this is still unclear (Eddy and Harman 1977). Brain protein content is reduced appreciably between maturity and old age. Age-related changes in the cerebral capillaries are compensated for by a reduced cerebral blood flow. There is a 10% reduction in blood flow, but the remaining flow is sufficient for the reduced metabolic demands of the brain. The most striking microscopic change is the increase in lipofuscin pigment. Senile plaques and neurofibrillary tangles develop (Figures 3-5 and 3-6)

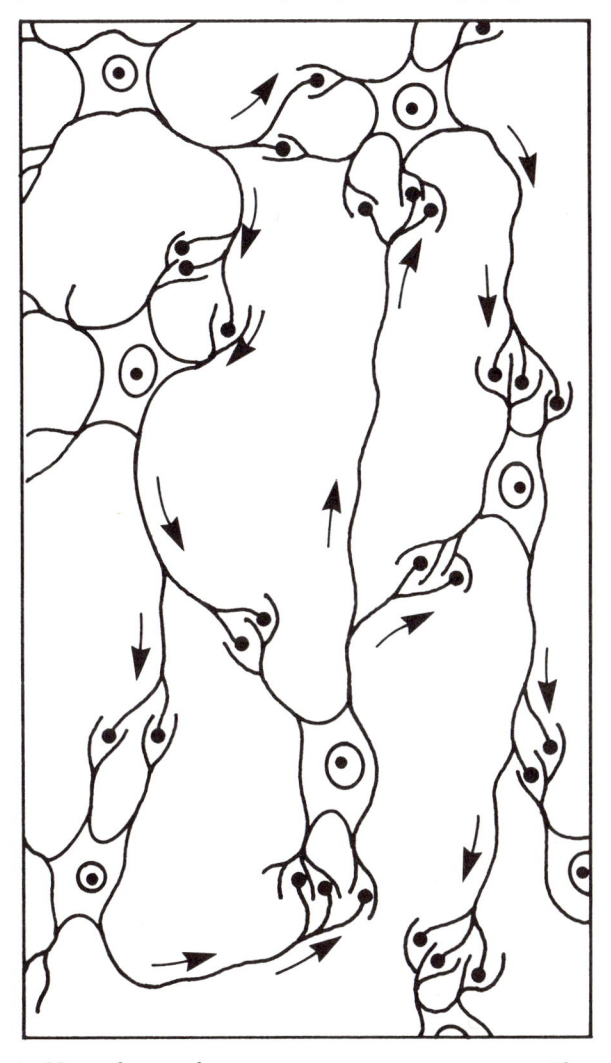

Figure 3-5 Normal neural synapse. From P.P. Lamy et al. *The Aging Brain*. Princeton, N.J.: E.R. Squibb & Sons, 1977. Reprinted with permission.

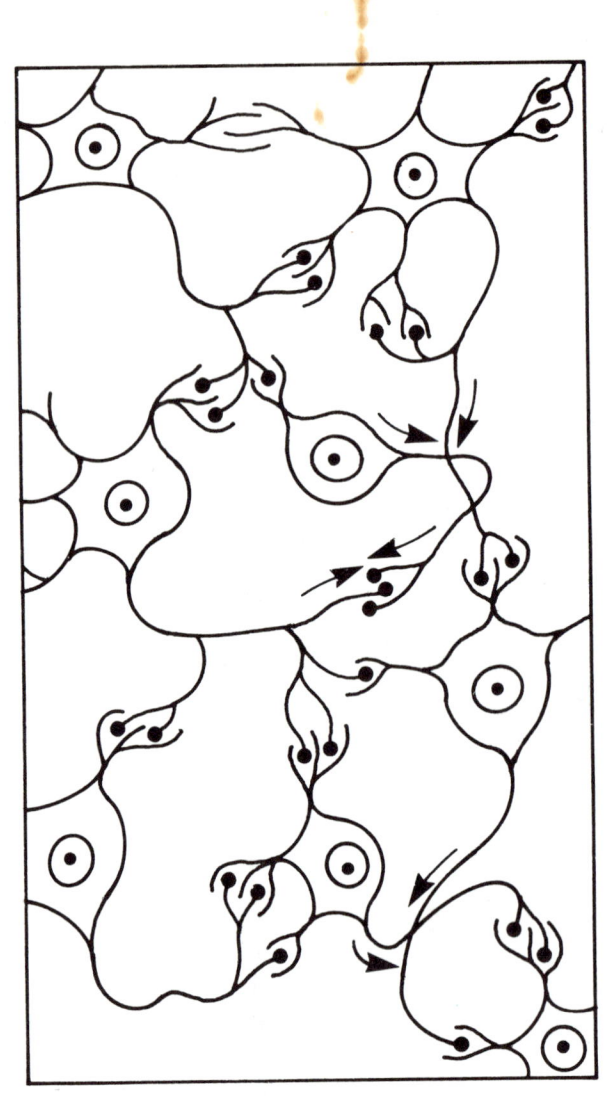

Figure 3-6 Neurofibrillar tangle, characteristic of aging brain. From P.P. Lamy et al. *The Aging Brain*. Princeton, N.J.: E.R. Squibb & Sons, 1977. Reprinted with permission.

and granulovacuolar degeneration is seen. All are highly correlated with dementia of the Alzheimer type, now regarded as senile dementia (Ball 1977). The EEG of an older person in good health is similar to that of a younger person, but the alpha frequency in the EEG slows perceptively (from more than 9 cycles/sec to less than 8 cycles/sec) in the very old, manifesting itself as a decline in intellectual function.

Slow wave foci are common and are usually maximum in the left anterior temporal area. Such foci are seen in 3.4% of the population between the ages of 20 and 29 years and increase with each passing decade, being seen in 30% of the population between the ages of 60 and 69. Fast activity also appears in women during the middle years and persists into late life (Busse 1972).

The brain tolerance for shifts in acid-base or electrolyte balance even in normal, young, healthy persons is narrow. This tolerance diminishes with age, so that slight shifts may result in a temporarily deranged sensorium. The overall basal metabolic rate decreases significantly from age 30 to age 90 (Shock and Yiengst 1955). Cerebral blood flow decreases gradually, from 61 ml/100 mg/min at 21 years to 58 ml/100 mg/min at 71 years. Uptake of oxygen decreases with age, and oxidative phosphorylation of glucose in brain mitochondria exhibits a similar decline (Ordy and Kaak 1975).

Brain biogenic amines fluctuate with age (Samorajski 1975). Brain levels of norepinephrine generally decrease during senescence, particularly in the hypothalamus. Serotonin levels increase slightly in the striatum, but decrease in the hypothalamus. Decrease in dopamine levels may bear directly upon the etiology of neurologic diseases such as parkinsonism.

Sleep-awake patterns change with age. Rapid eye movement (REM) sleep is reduced, increased wakefulness occurs and there is a reduction in the amount of stage four sleep (Feinberg 1974).

While this description of decrement and loss may lead to the inevitable conclusion of severe brain malfunction in older age, in the absence of disease, impoverished environment, or poor nutrition, the central nervous system has good potential to oppose sharp deterioration (Diamond 1978).

Brain activity depends on feedback from other systems and organs. This mechanism slows with age, delaying an individual's voluntary response to feedback information. This decrement is more pronounced as the intricacy of a task increases. The aging of the circulatory system and cerebrovascular disease can affect the brain. Even minimal arteriosclerosis may cause a significant reduction in cerebral blood flow and oxygen consumption. This could lead to deficits in physiologic, cognitive, and perceptual functions (Sokoloff 1975).

Intellectual Function

It is commonly believed that intellectual function peaks early in life and then declines progressively. According to the age-decrement model, elderly persons gradually experience cumulative intellectual deterioration (Barton et al 1975). However, recent research doubts the accuracy of this view (Labouvie-Vief and Gonda 1976). Increasing evidence shows that intellectual ability does not decrease through even the eighth decade (Kahn et al 1975) and with training, significant increments in intellectual performance can be attained (Labouvie-Vief and Gonda 1976). Although elderly persons complain about memory loss, there is evidence that the complaints do not correlate with performance (Kahn et al 1975).

It is true that general neuronal loss with aging leads to diminished receipt of information from the environment. Stimulation is necessary to maintain contact with reality, and sensory deprivation can cause perceptual disturbances. Aged persons often suffer from some sensory deprivation and paranoid states can result from, for example, loss of hearing. Thus, it is important that elderly persons receive adequate levels of thermal, olfactory, aural, and visual stimuli (Maddox 1963; Weinberg 1970). However, the elderly are likely to be exposed to sterile environments that minimize the amount of stimuli they receive.

A longitudinal study, which followed healthy men from age 71 to age 82 found no decline in intelligence quotient at age 82 compared to age 71 (Granick and Patterson 1971). The so-called impaired memory of some elderly persons may simply occur because they never fully register new information. It does take them longer to do so, and information may be presented too quickly. Although memory disorders are commonly associated with the senium, they may be much less common then assumed (Jarvick et al 1972).

There are a number of reasons for the assumption that memory does indeed decline with age. Hypothalamic changes lead to diminished stress response, so that the elderly cannot adjust quickly to changing demands. Old people fatigue quickly, which may affect performance (Atkinson et al 1977). While it is clear that the majority of the elderly have no serious memory deficit (Palmore 1977), apparent changes in intelligence may be a result of the evaluation instrument used (Bayley and Oden 1955). Performance on standardized learning tests decreases with age (Jarvick et al 1972).

It seems clear that elderly persons confronted with simple tasks show little or no change in performance speed or accuracy (Greenberg 1973). Vocabulary and verbal memory in the elderly is exceedingly stable. No memory deficit should be expected in elderly people. These elderly will retain unaltered their breadth of knowledge, practical judgment, and linguistic dexterity (Frolkis 1975). Continuous intellectual activity and sufficient stimuli, both mental and physical, assures maintenance of intellectual function in the absence of disease (Blum and Jarvick 1975; DeCarlo 1974). However, with advancing age, there may be some loss in powers of concentration and ability to reason. Abstract reasoning or conceptualizing become more difficult, as is adaptation to new situations. The elderly appear to have more trouble registering or storing new information than retrieving information from memory. The ability to code and store information for long periods of time also seems impaired (Ford and Roth 1977). There is almost always a decline in performance on speed tasks and on those tasks that exceed the immediate memory span (Smith 1977). Somatic disease seems to be the prime cause of intellectual decline in old age.

To compensate for these declining functions, the older person must simply be given a longer period of time and modified demands. The elderly, isolated person is particularly at risk for a decrease in ability to integrate information not conveyed slowly and comprehensively. This, in turn, can lead to slowed perception and decision-making. Thus, poorer memory does not necessarily result from aging, and much of what is termed "memory loss" may be a result of faulty comprehension caused by information too quickly conveyed or possibly caused by impaired sight and hearing. Furthermore, the elderly may have entirely different value systems than do younger persons and their motivation to keep up and to understand may not be sufficient to meet the demands of complex situations.

Digestive System

Extensive degenerative changes take place throughout the entire gastrointestinal system, from mouth to rectum (Lamy et al 1977c) (Figure 3-7). It should be noted first that, in general, the gut's anatomic

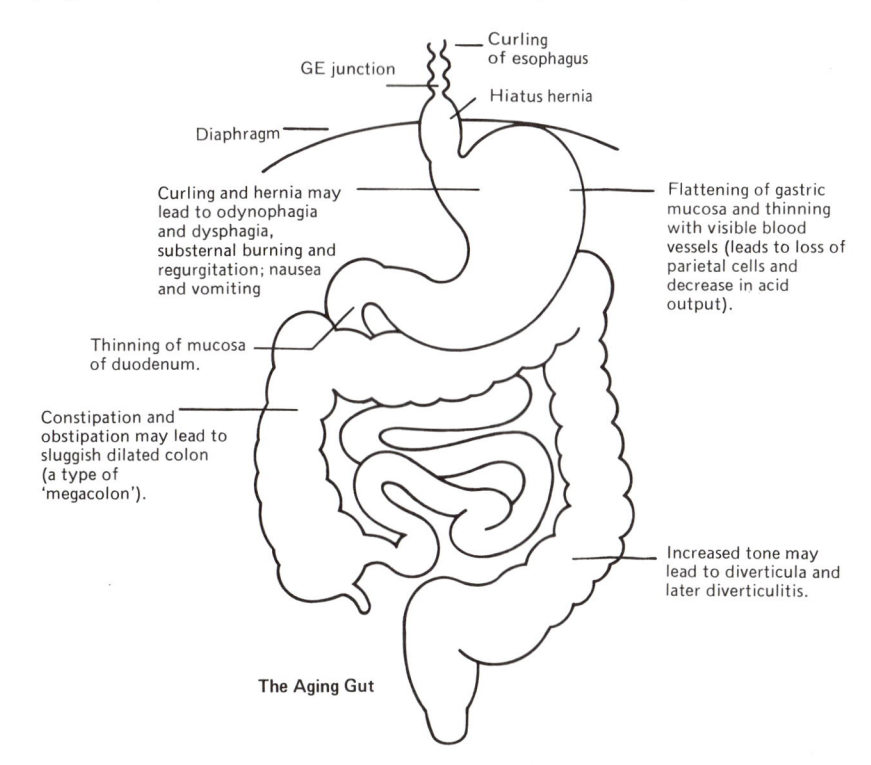

Figure 3-7 The aging gut. From P.P. Lamy et al. *The Aging Gut.* Princeton, N.J.: E.R. Squibb & Sons, 1977. Reprinted with permission.

and physiologic integrity is usually maintained at an adequate level (Berman and Kirsner 1972) and that most of the benign gastrointestinal disorders of older people may be disturbing but do not present a serious threat to their general health (Berman and Kirsner 1974). Degenerative changes in the gastrointestinal system free of disease should not complicate drug prescribing, although some precautions must be observed. In general, the healthy but aging gut can accommodate and compensate very well.

The gastrointestinal tract begins with the oral cavity, where major changes occur with aging. The National Health Survey, conducted in 1971, indicated that approximately 51% of all persons 65 years of age or older have lost all teeth in both upper and lower arches. Approximately 65% have lost all teeth in at least one arch and almost 10% completely lacked dentures or had incomplete sets of dentures (Figure 3-8). The Long-Term Care Facility Improvement Study revealed that 92% of the elderly admitted to long-term care facilities have lost some

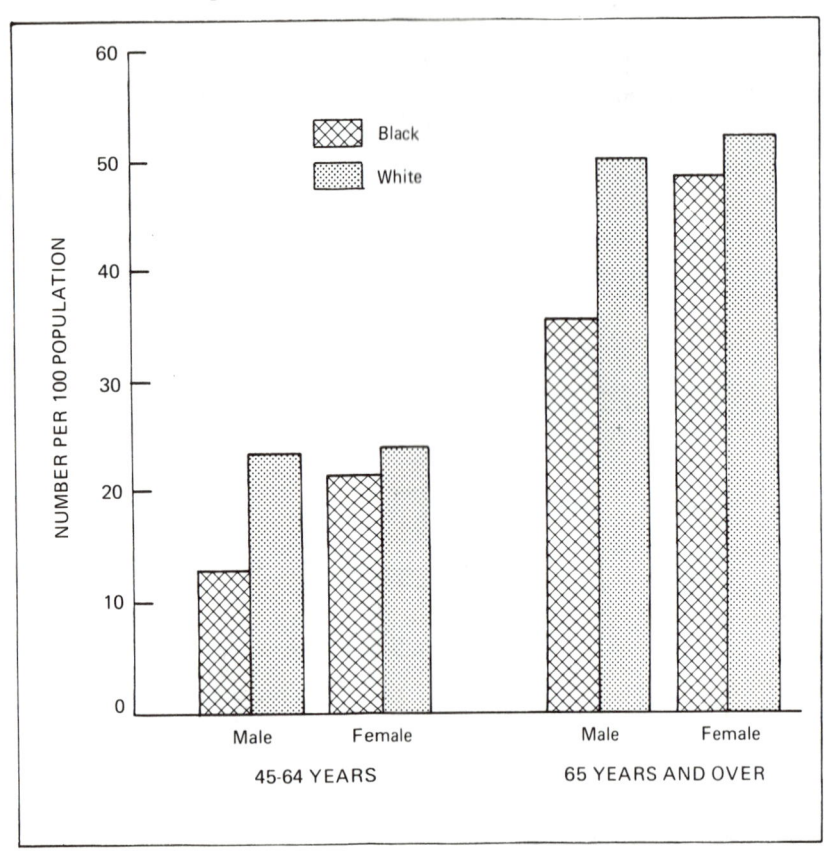

Figure 3-8 Number of edentulous persons per 100 population for persons aged 45 years and over, by age, race, and sex: United States, 1971. Source: National Center for Health Statistics.

or all teeth and 38% lack compensating restoration. The interrelation of diet, mastication, digestive tract function, and general health has long been recognized. It is necessary to provide a masticatory efficiency adequate for comminution of food and initiation of the digestive process. If an elderly patient is fitted with dentures and correct instructions are not given or instructions are not comprehended, excessive air may be swallowed, which can lead to excessive gas.

Saliva flow decreases with age, because of salivary gland degeneration and the very old may lack salivary flow completely (Stare 1977). This makes food less palatable because it is more difficult to swallow without the lubricating effect of the saliva. The number and sensitivity of taste buds are decreased, as are the olfactory cells, all of which decrease flavor sensation and make food less appealing. The elderly may, therefore, switch to more easily chewable foods and to more gratifying foods, which often means sweeter or more salty foods. Medications, especially antidepressants, reduce salivary flow. Depression (one of the most frequent psychiatric disorders of the elderly) is a strong salivary inhibitor.

There are changes in the oral mucosa with age. There may be loss of elasticity, a tendency to hyperkeratosis, and a delayed healing response (Shklar 1966). These changes may be responsible for treatment failure when sublingual or buccal tablets are prescribed.

Disturbed esophageal motility occurs in the elderly, even in the absence of disease. There may be decreased peristaltic response, increased nonperistaltic response, delayed transit time, and minor failure of the lower sphincter to relax upon swallowing (Shuster 1976). The most common esophageal problem among older people is hiatal hernia with reflux esophagitis (Berman and Kirsner 1974), which is probably present in 75% of all people between the ages of 50 and 80 years, although it is rarely symptomatic. However, if esophageal symptons become exaggerated, they can produce substernal pain and dysphagia and possibly severe emotional problems. Antacids, prescribed to treat acid-induced esophagitis, should be administered one or two hours after meals, when the stomach is empty. Antacid administration should not be tied to meals, as the elderly person will need the antacid throughout the day. Caution must be exercised when people are fed in the supine position, as aspiration pneumonia caused by abnormalities of esophageal emptying can occur (Geokas and Haverback 1969). Esophageal obstruction, such as stricture or left atrial enlargement, may be a predisposing factor to esophageal ulcers, which have been reported with the use of potassium chloride tablets, doxycycline capsules, and tetracycline capsules (Pemberton 1970; Bokey and Hugh 1975; Crowson et al 1976). Delay in passage of solid oral dosage forms can occur particularly in patients with hiatus hernia and reflux. Tablets can be retained as long as five to ten minutes and occasionally for much longer (Evans and Roberts 1976). To avoid ulceration, tablets should be taken either before or with meals or with large volumes of fluid.

Beyond the esophagus, atrophy of the alimentary canal and slowed digestive processes are common in the elderly. With aging, the numbers of absorbing cells decrease, leading to a reduction in the absorbing surface and absorption (Avioli et al 1965), which has been documented for calcium. Circulatory disturbances may affect transportation of nutrients adversely, and decreased renal excretion may affect elimination of metabolic debris. There is a great deal of atrophic change in the stomach and gastric mucosa thinning. Secretory changes also take place in the stomach. Acid and pepsin secretion decrease, which can cause lowered iron and vitamin B-12 absorption. Histamine-fast achlorhydria has been demonstrated in about 32% of patients 60 to 69 years of age, more than ten times the rate found in those 20 to 29 years of age (Polland 1933). There is an increased incidence of gastritis, paralleled by a decrease of hydrochloric acid and intrinsic factor secretion. Achlorhydria and atrophic gastritis may be associated with adenomatous polyps.

The incidence of peptic ulceration in the elderly is higher than commonly believed (Colin-Jones 1975), while the number of patients with duodenal ulcers decreases with age. In general, the risk of ulcer disease does not increase with age.

No age-related changes appear to occur in the gallbladder, and the pancreas has sufficient reserve capacity to compensate for possible decreases in digestive enzyme output. However, the mucosal lining of the duodenum becomes thin with advanced age. The intestine apparently does not change in weight or in length, although there is probably some atrophy. There may be a special problem of sprue in the small bowel of an elderly patient, which can prevent the usual exchange of nutrients and chemicals across cell walls.

The elderly often encounter colonic problems. Relaxation of the musculature may lead to constipation, which is frequent among the elderly. The general loss of elastic tissue leads to the formation of diverticula of the large bowel, affecting males between the ages of 50 and 75, and females between the ages of 50 and 89 (Chaitin 1966). Diverticula steadily increase after the age of 40. The incidence of diverticular disease has greatly increased because of the lack of cereal fiber in the diet (Painter 1975). High-fiber diets tend to increase the diameter of the colon and thus reduce pressure (Shuster 1976). Up to 40% of patients over the age of 70 can be affected. Symptomatic diverticular disease is accompanied by constipation in more than one-third of all patients. Constipation can alternate with diarrhea and periods of normal bowel behavior (Steinheber 1976; Sklar 1972).

Ischemic damage to the colon occurs characteristically in elderly patients with chronic cardiovascular disease (Turnbull and Isaacson 1977). Finally, the elderly often exhibit decreased anal sphincter tone and incontinence. On the other hand, minor pain from anal fissures may lead to voluntary withholding of the urge to defecate. Constipation in the elderly may also be caused by an enlarged prostate or it may accompany diabetes mellitus or hypothyroidism.

Liver The liver is the largest single organ in the body. Of all organs, the liver is least affected by primary aging and it will continue to function in the elderly not afflicted by disease. In general, only a small part of the organ is sufficient to perform the tasks of the entire liver. Liver weight correlates with body weight (both decrease starting in the fifth or sixth decade). As the hepatic cells decrease in number, the mitochondria increase in size. Concurrently, binucleate hepatic cells increase in number (Lamy 1973). While a majority of the elderly may have some liver function abnormality, many liver cells can be lost before liver function begins to deteriorate seriously.

Primary aging may bring about a decreased hepatic blood flow (hepatic blood flow is equal to about 25% of cardiac output or 30% of total circulating blood) and a decreased induction of enzymes. Enzyme induction, necessary for drug metabolism, has been defined as a net increase of enzymes relative to total cell protein. Decreased microsomal activity may lead to increased half-life of some drugs, and it has been suggested that medications are not as efficiently metabolized in the aged liver (Rodstein 1970). A satisfactory index to predict a person's capacity to metabolize drugs is not yet available. Elderly persons usually have a reduced level of plasma albumin, which is a reflection of the lowered activity level of the aging liver that may have implications for drugs that are protein-bound. Secondary aging of the liver caused either by inflammation of the liver (hepatitis) or scarring of the liver (cirrhosis) may have greater effects on liver function. Anoxia caused by congestive heart failure may adversely affect liver function. Thus, in cases of liver disease, drugs metabolized primarily by the liver must be prescribed with caution. The frequency of progressive liver disease increases with age (Table 3-3). Caution must be exercised. For example, among positive tuberculin reactors aged 35 years and more, the risk of hepatitis precludes the routine use of preventive tuberculosis therapy with isoniazid, unless several risk factors are present (American Thoracic Society 1974).

Table 3-3
Incidence of Liver Damage

Age (yrs)	Incidence (%)
20–34	0.3
35–49	1.2
50 and older	2.3

Source: American Thoracic Society. Preventive therapy of tuberculosis infection. *Am Rev Respir Dis.* 110:371, 1974.

Disease states of the digestive system As Table 3-4 shows, the number of patients afflicted with chronic digestive conditions increases with age. It is often difficult to differentiate between insignificant functional gastrointestinal complaints and more serious underlying disease. In one study of 276 elderly patients admitted to a hospital, almost 27% had major gastrointestinal problems, and 42% of the remaining patients demonstrated important functional or organic gastrointestinal disorders (Geboes and Bossaert 1977a).

Table 3-4
Number of Chronic Digestive Conditions per 1000 Population

Condition	All ages	45–64 years	65 years and over
Ulcer (stomach and duodenum)	17.2	33.4	29.0
Hernia (abdominal)	16.3	28.3	58.8
Upper gastrointestinal disorder	13.1	23.5	37.7
Gallbladder condition	10.3	21.4	32.8
Chronic enteritis and ulcerative colitis	9.3	17.9	32.8
Gastritis and duodenitis	8.6	16.2	24.0
Frequent constipation	23.8	35.0	96.3
Intestinal condition	4.2	8.1	12.5

Source: *Prevalence of Selected Chronic Digestive Conditions, U.S., July-Dec. 1968.* DHEW Publ. No. (HRA) 74-1510. Rockville, Md.: National Center for Health Statistics, 1973.

Nausea and vomiting are often encountered in the elderly. Many causes, including drugs, may be responsible for this. While nausea and vomiting are often relegated to the status of an intrinsic gastrointestinal disease, they may be symptomatic of a stroke or other serious clinical disease, particularly if they are of sudden onset. Therefore, a careful diagnostic procedure is necessary to elicit its origin (Lamy et al 1977c) (Figure 3-9).

Endocrine Function

Hormones play an important regulatory role in maintaining homeostasis. Changes in function and efficiency of homeostatic mechanisms may lead to increased debility. Inability to react quickly and efficiently to stress is related to changes in the body's homeostatic mechanisms that are affected by decreases in endocrine secretion.

Glucose tolerance decreases with age, as may insulin synthesis and release of insulin. Thyroid function decreases, but hypothyroidism is

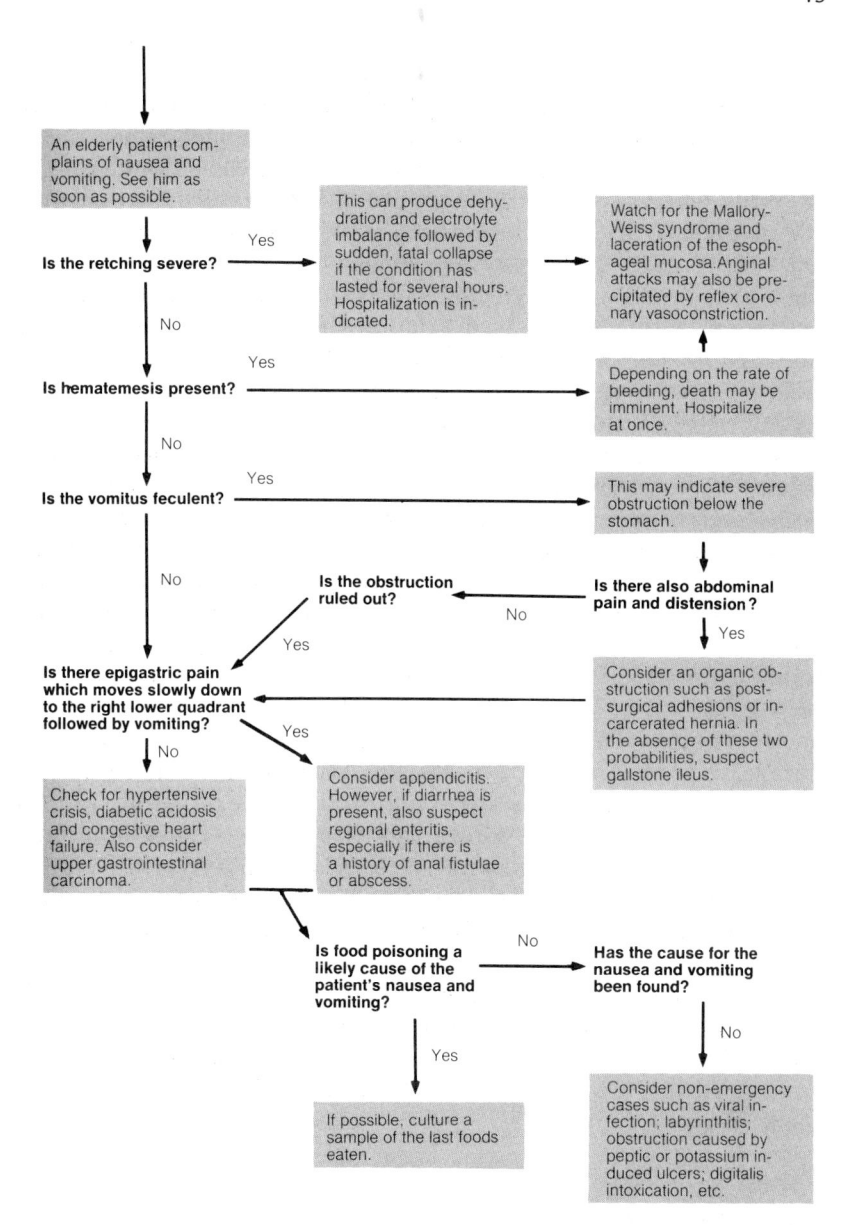

Figure 3-9 Diagnosing nausea and vomiting in the elderly. From P.P. Lamy et al. *The Aging Gut.* Princeton, N.J.: E.R. Squibb & Sons, 1977. Reprinted with permission.

not as frequent as might be expected as the thyroid has a large reserve capacity. There is a 65% decrease in anabolic steroids but only a 20%

decrease in adrenal steroids, shifting the balance in favor of the catabolic activity of the adrenal steroids.

Loss of reproductive capability may result from an increasing deficiency of certain biogenic amines in the hypothalamic region of the brain. Production of epinephrine and L-dopamine slows with age, and changing levels of luteinizing hormone (LH) and follicle stimulating hormone (FSH) affect estrogen and testosterone production.

The female In the aging woman the mucosal lining of the vagina becomes thinner. Vaginal length and width are shortened and expansive ability is decreased. Clitoral response seems to continue until age 70. The cervix and uterus are reduced in size, responding to reduced sex-steroid stimulation. Postmenopausal women lose 75% to 85% of estrogen and progesterone production compared with the level of steroid secretion in their reproductive years. Estrogen decline results in changes in the uterus, cervix, vaginal lining, glandular breast tissue, and the rate of bone loss (Longcope 1978). Many of these conditions can produce undesirable symptoms. Steroid replacement therapy has often been used, but its place in therapy is by no means secure. Hot flashes can be treated with hormones, but only in low doses and with periodic reviews. For atrophic vaginitis, local estrogen preparations have proven beneficial, but again, treatment must be periodic and not prolonged.

The male FSH and LH levels begin to rise in men in the fourth decade, and increase rapidly in later life. Estradiol levels do not change in the man, but there is a sharp fall in plasma testosterone in men around the sixth decade (Greenblatt et al 1976). Testosterone not bound to protein (approximately 1% to 2%) falls more markedly in old age, because there is a concomitant rise in sex hormone-binding globulin (SHBG). The mean unbound testosterone in extreme old age is about one-third that of young men.

The testes become smaller in old age, and spermatogenesis diminishes, as does the total Leydig cell mass after the age of 40, most likely because of vascular degeneration. Male sexual activity varies from individual to individual. Health, desire, and sociosexual environment influence activity.

Hemopoietic System

The elderly hemopoietic system is at risk because many drugs prescribed for the elderly in their chronic care can adversely affect this system. Chloramphenicol and phenylbutazone, among others, can cause aplastic anemia; alpha-methyldopa, nitrofurantoins, sulfonamides, and others have been implicated in hemolytic anemia;

and the chlorothiazides, phenylbutazone, quinidine, and the sulfonylureas have been associated with thrombocytopenic purpura (Pisciotta 1974).

Immune System

The immune system may have a primary role in the control of aging (Buckley and Roseman 1976; Burnett 1973). The immune system consists of bone marrow, spleen, and lymph nodes (Makinodan 1976). The function of the immune system is to protect an individual from external (infectious bacteria and viruses) and internal (cancer cells) antigens. The elderly are very sensitive to pathogenic invasion. This increased sensitivity may result from increased use of immunosuppressive drugs or a cumulative destruction of the immune system by ionizing radiation (Heidrick and Makinodan 1972). However, in most instances increased sensivitity to infectious diseases is related to a decline in both the humoral and cell-mediated response. This decline in turn is generally related to an increase in the frequency of autoimmune and immune complex diseases, cancer, and viral and fungal infections. It is possible that arthritis and diabetes mellitus may result from a breakdown of the body's immune defense mechanism.

The weight of the spleen begins to decrease in the sixth decade, which is one reason for the diminished activity of the immune system. The reticuloendothelial system is also thought to be involved in diminished antibody response. There is an acceleration in the rate of accumulation of gamma globulin accompanied by an acceleration in the rate of decrease of other serum-globulin fractions. Altered immunologic responses appear with relative hypoglobulinemia in apparently healthy older individuals (Buckley and Dorsey 1970).

Most often, aging of the thymus immunity system is correlated with an increased disease incidence in old age. The normal immune response in humans is mediated by the interaction of mononuclear phagocytes, T-lymphocytes, and B-lymphocytes. The thymus, especially the cortex, involutes progressively with age (Fernandez and Schwartz 1976). T-cells are depleted and the proportion of B-cells increases. While both T- and B-cell functions decline with age, T-cell activity declines more sharply. The capacity to synthesize IgG decreases more sharply than the capacity to synthesize IgM and the inability to sustain IgG antibody production is probably responsible for the decline in the effectiveness of the immune system. Thymosin may increase T-cell production, which may build immune defenses and decrease tumor growth and progress. This concept is being pursued in several clinical trials.

Musculoskeletal System

Many clinicians associate muscular weakness with aging. Atrophy, however, does not necessarily indicate disuse. It is doubtful that group atrophy of muscle fibers is pathognomonic of denervated skeletal muscle. Lack of vitamin D, simple disuse, decrease of neurotrophic agents such as ACh, or a decrease of hormonal control (Kochakian 1956) are among the divergent factors that may cause muscular atrophy. There is a loss of mass and strength in the striped muscle. Red muscles decrease in number and white muscle fibers decrease primarily in volume. Nonmuscular scar tissue replaces lost muscle fibers. Ultimately, rapid voluntary movement is less easy (Rockstein 1968).

Aging affects collagen and elastin, the major components of connective tissue. Collagen is the force-resistant component of connective tissue and seems most elastic between the ages of 20 and 40 years. With age, collagen acquires increased crystalline orientation, decreased water content, greater tensile strength, increased stiffness, and increased thermal contractility (Lamy 1973).

The metabolic diseases of the skeleton severely affect the elderly. Osteoporosis is one of these metabolic diseases. It has been defined as a reduction in bone mass below that which normally characterizes the skeleton for age, sex, and race of an individual. In osteoporosis, there is decreased bone density without a change in chemical composition of bone (Albanese et al 1975).

Maximum skeletal maturity is less in white women than in white men and black men. Black women and Italian women seem to suffer least from osteoporosis. Net skeletal mass is lowest in postmenopausal white women. With aging, bone resorption tends to outpace new bone formation, gradually leading to a decrease in bone density throughout the body. Bone loss begins earlier in females, particularly those with an early menopause, than in males, and taller subjects lose bone less rapidly in both sexes. Menopause appears to accelerate bone loss but not all menopausal women develop osteoporosis (Leeming 1973; Ingham 1974; *Medical Letter* 1976; Avioli 1976). In general, bone loss does not increase with age but represents a linear fall throughout an individual's life span. There is about an 8% decrease per decade in women and a 3% decrease per decade in men. In well-nourished individuals, the decrease in bone mass is unrelated to calcium intake.

Immobilization can cause osteoporosis at any age. Weight-bearing is important in mineralization of bone. Exercise and physical therapy can help prevent progression of the disease in menopausal or elderly patients. Conversely, diminished exercise is associated with increased bone loss. Osteoporosis, with a liability for fractures, affects 25% of women over the age of 65 and about 6% of men over 65 years of age.

After age 45, the incidence of fractures in the neck of the femur doubles with each five years of age and, by the age of 80, a woman has a 20% chance to sustain a fractured hip and an equal chance to suffer vertebral compression. Usually, there are no overt signs and symptoms of osteoporosis until structural failure occurs.

Much literature is devoted to possible treatments of osteoporosis. Most often disputed is the use of estrogens, and it is probably still the consensus that estrogens should not be used for long-term prophylaxis or treatment. An initial favorable response may be lost to a secondary decrease in bone formation. Based on a negative calcium balance often observed in patients with osteoporosis, treatment with calcium and/or vitamin D is suggested, but there is no clear-cut evidence that this is helpful. Elderly patients may require supplementary vitamin D if their dietary calcium intake is low and exposure to sunlight is reduced. There have been preliminary and apparently favorable reports of treatment with calcitonin, a peptide hormone, for periods ranging up to 29 months; suppression of bone resorption has been reported. Overall, there is still no drug that has been shown to be safe and effective for the prevention or treatment of osteoporosis, although it has been claimed that a daily intake of at least one gram of calcium, and perhaps more, throughout life is needed to maintain normal bone density (Albanese 1975).

Osteomalacia, also called adult rickets, occurs most often in women. It is assumed that about 3% of women over the age of 65 suffer from osteomalacia, which is characterized by failure of newly formed bone to calcify. In osteomalacia, decreased bone density, mainly caused by a loss of calcium content of bone matrix, occurs when there is a lack of vitamin D to use calcium in bone formation. Difficulty in walking or inability to walk are the major symptoms. Bone pain is usually present. Calciferol 1.25 mg daily for two weeks followed by calcium and vitamin D therapy can cure osteomalacia. However, therapy with calciferol should not be prolonged as hypercalcemia followed by renal failure can result.

Finally, a 6% incidence of Paget disease has been reported for those more than 65 years of age. This disease affects the pelvis, lumbar spine, femur, tibia, skull, and clavicle. Simple, symptomatic measures are usually used. Preliminary reports on the use of calcitonin seem to indicate that it is effective in bringing relief from pain and the improvement of the bony appearances.

Other problems As previously noted, the elderly are increasingly subject to falls; women are more susceptible than men (Gryfe et al 1977). The increased incidence in falls has been correlated with a change in gait; the elderly do not lift their feet as high as do younger persons and are more likely to stumble. Furthermore, sway is significantly increased in the elderly, suggesting a physiologic decline in postural control. In addition, the elderly cannot correct their balance once they have stumbled (Overstall et al 1977).

Mobility, essential to the quality of life, is also often hindered by foot problems which neither the elderly person nor family members often feel important enough for treatment. Almost all diabetic patients and at least 50% of patients with circulatory problems must be assumed to have foot problems (Schank 1977).

Renal System

It is well established that renal function declines with age (Friedman et al 1972; Rowe et al 1976), even in the absence of disease. The changes probably occur because of vascular insufficiency.

Kidney Combined kidney weight is less than 1% of body weight, but the normal kidneys receive 20% of the cardiac output and the nephrons process more than 170 liters of glomerular filtrate each day. The kidney has considerable functional reserve. Therefore, the aging kidney is most often not responsible for clinically significant symptomatology; however, concomitant illness and other stress may create demands which cannot be met adequately (Rosen 1976). Furthermore, the effect of aging on the kidney, one of the major excretory organs, may have profound effects on the therapeutic management of elderly patients. (See Chapter 13.)

Structural age-related changes are manifested by a weight loss. Between the fourth and eighth decades, the kidneys lose approximately one-fifth of their weight, more weight being lost from the cortex than from the medulla (McLachlan 1978). This weight loss is ascribed to a loss in number and size of excretory units. The number of nephrons decreases by 50% between the fourth and seventh decades. The surviving units, however, make an increasing contribution toward maintenance of homeostasis (Bricker 1972). The epithelial cells in the kidney, as well as kidney size, glomeruli, and tubule cells may decrease (Rockstein 1968). Glomeruli tend to be fewer with age, but there is a wide individual difference. Degenerative changes in the tubules, especially the proximal convoluted tubules, are observed. Interstitial fibrosis becomes pronounced after the seventh decade, as do fibrotic changes in the glomeruli. Vascular alterations take place even in the absence of hypertension. Vascular changes in normotensive patients over 70 years of age are similar to those observed in younger, hypertensive patients.

The two excretory functions of the kidney, to preserve the volume of body fluids and to maintain composition of those fluids, are affected by aging (Figure 3-10) (Lamy et al 1977d). Functional changes in the kidney of even healthy older individuals are the rule rather than the exception; major changes begin in the fourth decade. The formation rate of glomerular filtrate, effective renal plasma flow, and tubular

Glomerular filtration rate decreases over 40% in a lifetime.

Tubular function decreases over 40% in a lifetime.

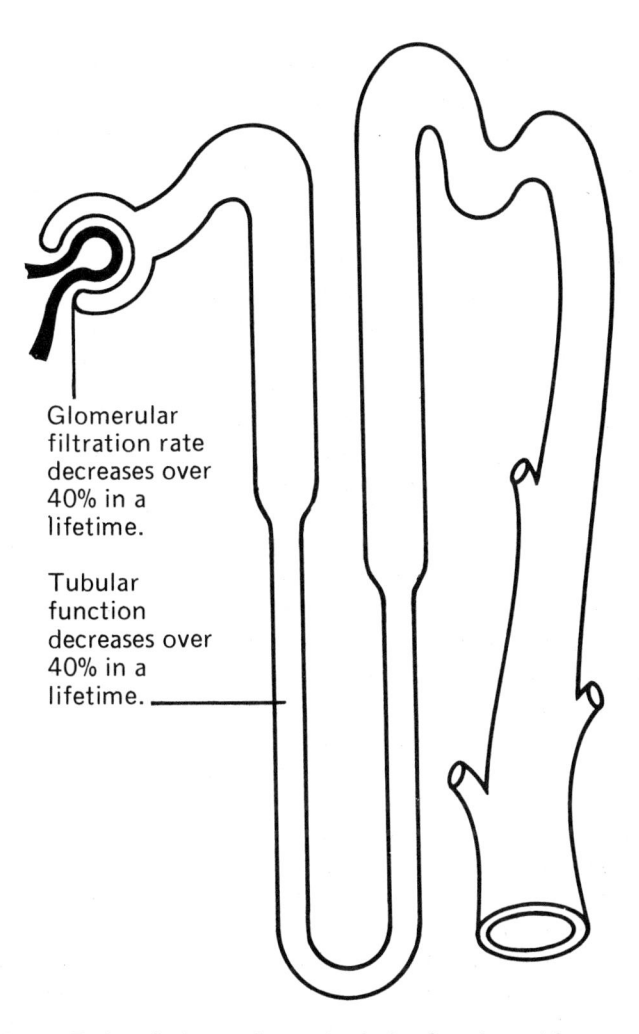

Figure 3-10 Reduced glomerular and tubular function with age. From P.P. Lamy et al. *The Aging Kidney*. Princeton, N.J.: E.R. Squibb & Sons, 1977. Reprinted with permission.

excretory capacity all decrease by more than 40% between the ages of 20 and 90. As glomerular and tubular function decline in a similar fashion, the balance between the two remains unaltered.

Blood urea nitrogen at maturity averages 12.9 mg% and rises to 21.1 mg% at age 70. Decrements in tubular function are characterized by a reduced concentrating ability. There is also loss of the normal diurnal excretory patterns and the development of nocturia. However, it should be noted that one-third of all patients over the age of 65 have normal glomerular and tubular function and more than two-thirds have normal glomerular function. A reduced glomerular filtration rate is not only a function of the glomeruli but is also caused by changes in cardiac output. The renal fraction of cardiac output is reduced. In healthy but aging kidneys, the essential pH regulation of body fluids continues. The rate at which the acid-based balance is regulated slows, but remains effective.

Renal function loss tends to be somewhat greater than the proportional loss of lean body mass. For this reason, the renal function can be estimated by measuring first urinary creatinine levels and then serum creatinine levels to calculate creatinine clearance.

Altered age-related kidney function actually depends upon a number of factors. Arteriosclerosis and infections frequently cause reduced kidney function, and changes due to hypertension and diabetes are common. Apparently, renal arteriosclerosis develops independently of hypertension, and the degree of vasodilation induced by acetylcholine or sodium loading is reduced by age. Kidney stones are a frequent cause of morbidity, possibly presenting as renal insufficiency without pain. Pyelonephritis is probably the most common renal disease in the aged man, usually stemming from obstruction caused by bladder neck pathology. Pyelonephritis is often responsible for acute failure in chronic renal disease.

Only a few individuals who live past the age of 60 remain free from renal or vascular pathology (Dontas 1969). As the kidney is the primary route of excretion for most drugs and their metabolites, it is important to assess the remaining renal excretory capacity carefully and individually to prevent drug accumulation and possible toxicity.

Urinary tract Age changes take place in the urinary bladder, but the exact nature of these changes is still speculative. Changes probably occur in the elastic tissue surrounding the bladder neck and the glands or ducts which are sometimes called the female prostate. Prostatic enlargement is common, but incidence reports are conflicting. Some enlargement is probably present in 30% of those 60 years and older; gross prostatic enlargement may range from 30% to 50% in males over 60 years of age, and figures as high as 75% have been cited. Patients who have no apparent symptoms relating to prostatism are said to suffer from silent prostatism (Finestone and Rosenthal 1971). An association between cardiovascular disease and prostatic enlargement has been suggested (Dietze 1969).

In any case, benign prostatic hypertrophy and adenocarcinoma of the prostate are the most characteristic, urologic problems of the aging male (Basso 1977). An annual checkup that includes a rectal examination and a complete urinalysis is recommended.

With aging, there is an increased likelihood of obstruction in the lower urinary tract coupled with an increased susceptibility of the urogenital system to infection. Urinary tract infection is second only to pulmonary disease as the most frequent cause of febrile episodes in the elderly.

Electrolyte balance Water and electrolyte imbalance can occur easily in the elderly, and can just as easily be ignored (Dietze 1969). Compensatory renal, pulmonary, endocrine, and buffer mechanisms are limited, and even slight changes in water electrolyte balance can cause severe damage.

Hyponatremia is a common disorder of fluid and electrolyte balance. Dilutional hyponatremia occurs most often, particularly in patients with cardiac decompensation or decreased intravascular volume, which can be caused by diuretics. Patients with uncomplicated dilutional hyponatremia have very low urine sodium concentrations (less than 20 mEq/liter). Depletional hyponatremia, which is much less common, is caused by total body sodium depletion, leaving patients dehydrated, with orthostatic hypotension and tachycardia (Krumlovsky 1975). Therapy for hyponatremia depends upon its etiology. For example, a patient with congestive heart failure and hepatic cirrhosis will most likely have an excess of total body sodium and water; the patient will be hypervolemic and edematous, and urinary sodium will be low and probably be treated with water restriction.

The patient with uncomplicated dilutional hyponatremia is most often treated by restricting sodium intake to 500 mg/24 hrs. Treatment of depletional hyponatremia consists of salt replacement.

Drugs and the renal system The renal system is particularly susceptible to drug toxicity (Roxe 1975). Various drugs can produce nephrotoxic reactions which could present clinically as acute or chronic renal failure, systemic lupus erythematosus, nephrotic syndrome, and renal tubular syndromes. Some drugs may also cause disturbances of the fluid and electrolyte balance and metabolism (Curtis 1977). Drugs may affect the arteries, glomeruli, tubules, and the interstitium of the kidneys (Table 3-5). The elderly man is further at risk for the cumulative effect of drugs that can cause acute urinary retention, which can be both painful and frightening. Urinary retention can be precipitated by drugs that increase bladder neck tone, such as the decongestants found in many nonprescription common cold

Table 3-5
Some Nephrotoxic Drugs

Drugs	Disease State
Gold salts, phenytoin, propylthiouracil, sulfonamides, thiazides	Arteritis
Hydralazine, phenylbutazone, sulfonamides	Glomerular changes
Acetaminophen, aminoglycosides, ferrous sulfate, penicillin, quinine, salicylates	Acute tubular necrosis
Ampicillin, methicillin, phenindione, rifampin, sulfonamides and other	Interstitial nephritis

preparations, or those that decrease the detrusor tone, such as the anticholinergics and certain psychotropic drugs.

Respiratory System

Lung perfusion in elderly normal subjects resembles that in young normal subjects. While some nonuniformity of lung perfusion might be expected as part of the normal aging process, perfusion defects present as pulmonary abnormalities. Age-associated changes in the lung resemble emphysema. Muscular strength declines. The chest wall stiffens and becomes progressively harder (Campbell and Lefrak 1978). There is loss of elastic tissue surrounding the alveoli and alveolar ducts, the chest will have an increased anteroposterior diameter due to rib and vertebral decalcification, and there will be weakening of the respiratory muscles (Dhar et al 1976). These changes lead to decreased lung efficiency.

Forced vital capacity and forced expiratory volume diminish as early as age 25. The mean rate of decline is approximately 32 ml per year for men and 25 ml per year for women. By age 60 maximum breathing capacity will have decreased by 50%. Loss of elastic recoil is responsible for increases in residual volume and increases in compliance and closing volume (Friedman et al 1976; Kent 1978). Arterial oxygen tension declines linearly with age. This decreased efficiency results in a decreased functional reserve of the lung. Even minor, pathologic disorders can overburden the respiratory system and lead to a severe decrease in arterial oxygen content. The elderly are prone to develop respiratory diseases. There seems to be an inverse relationship between vital capacity and morbidity and mortality, and a direct relationship between diminished vital capacity and the likelihood of myocardial infarction (Dhar et al 1976).

Emphysema is common. Changes in lung connective tissue are thought to lead to emphysema (Smith 1971), but a genetic deficiency in alpha-1-antitrypsin has been advanced as a possible causative factor. Smoking, of course, increases the rate of emphysema.

Chronic obstructive lung disease accelerates greatly the age-related loss of pulmonary function. Patients must be kept well hydrated, which is especially difficult in patients using diuretics who may also have an impaired thirst mechanism. The elderly tolerate poorly the effects of pneumonia. Even healthy elderly may have poor muscle tone that might impair their ability to clear the tracheobronchial secretions. Retained excretions enhance bacterial growth. Altered immunity may also play a role in predisposing the elderly to pneumonia. Secretory immunoglobulin (IgA) of the nasal and respiratory mucosal surfaces, which deters viral infections, decreases with advancing age. Lipid pneumonia still occurs as a consequence of the use of mineral oil as a laxative. The presence of reactivated tuberculosis should always be considered in aged persons with pulmonary symptoms and abnormal x-ray findings (DuBrow 1976). It is estimated that 1.8% of the population over the age of 70 may have tuberculosis (Geboes and Bossaert 1977b).

Drugs and the lungs The lungs perform metabolic transformation of some drugs, although only to a small extent. On the other hand, drugs may precipitate acute or chronic pulmonary toxicity. This is particularly true when more aggressive drug treatment of the elderly is proposed for many diseases formerly left untreated. A number of drugs used frequently by the elderly may sensitize the lungs to potentially adverse reactions that could ultimately result in congestive heart failure or respiratory insufficiency. Some drugs such as penicillin, streptomycin, and tetracycline may cause allergic asthma; the beta-blocking agents can cause bronchoconstriction; and nitrofurantoin can cause a syndrome of dyspnea, fever, pulmonary infiltration, and eosinophilia. Long-term use of corticosteroids can lead to opportunistic infections, and gold therapy may cause chronic bronchitis (Rosenow 1978; *British Medical Journal* 1976; Kursh et al 1975).

Sensorium

A well-functioning sensorium enables a person to use data received from the sense organs. A decrement in this function can lead to a person's inability to participate even adequately in daily activities, severe psychiatric problems in some patients, and to social isolation in many. Thus, while a certain decrement with age is probably inevitable, it is disturbing to note that corrective actions, where they are possible, are often not undertaken as the decrement is "simply a symptom of old age." Yet, elderly people report that hearing and vision are of prime importance for a healthy old age (Rupp 1970).

Among the common impairments of patients admitted to long-term care facilities, those involving the sensorium occupy a prominent place (Table 3-6).

**Table 3-6
Most Common Impairments on Admission
to Long-Term Care Facilities***

Impairment	Percentage
Impaired vision	68
Hearing loss	33
Speech impairments	32
Loss of some or all teeth	92
Lack compensating restoration	38
Confusion	54

*Long-Term Care Facility Improvement Study, Introd. Report Office of Nursing Home Affairs, DHEW Publ. No. (OS) 76-50021, Rockville, Md., 1975.

Vision Some decrease in visual acuity must be expected with aging. General medical conditions can also have harmful effects on vision. However, failing eyesight is not a natural and inescapable concomitant to aging (Kornzweig 1977) and in many patients vision can be corrected to an acceptable level. Visual impairment is sometimes accepted as something about which nothing can be done. Alternatively, the elderly may seek self-prescribed palliative treatment rather than corrective action (Buseck 1976). It must be stressed that even in persons 90 years of age, at least 40% have useful to good vision, and another 30% have fair to adequate vision. Figure 3-11 and Table 3-7 depict the extent of visual impairment among the elderly. Most optical difficulties are caused by changes in the refraction of the eye. A certain amount of discomfort in bright light is common in old age, and even a healthy eye requires two-thirds more light to perform the same function at 60 years of age that it needed at 20 years of age. Structural and functional changes of the eye have been divided into two categories (Bell 1969).

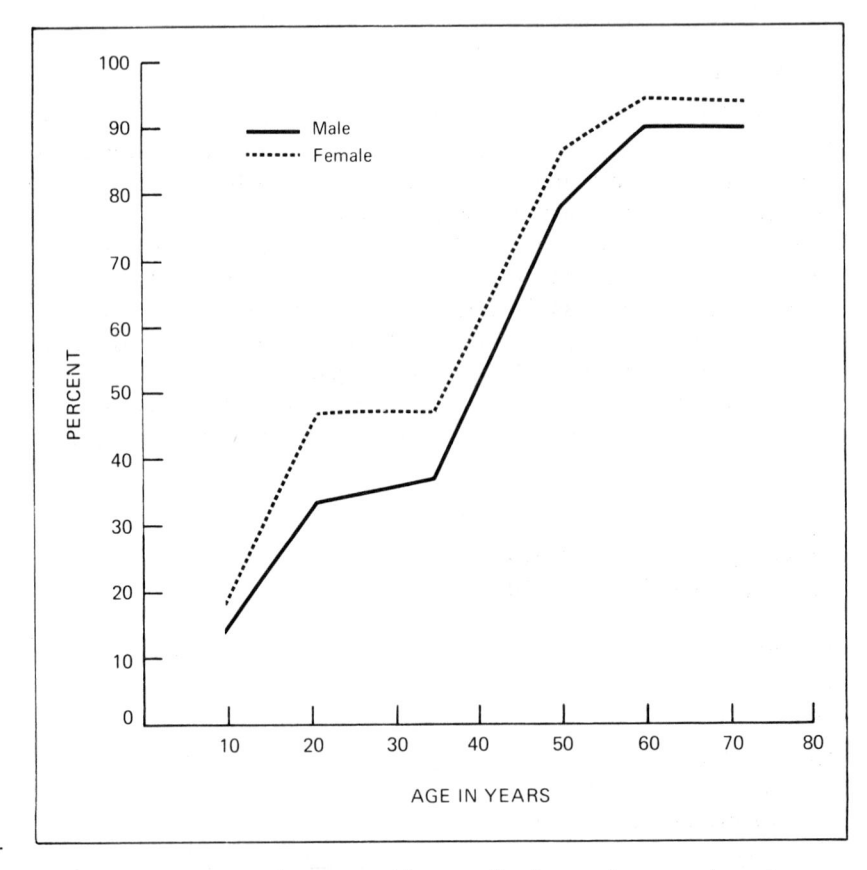

Figure 3-11 Percent of persons with corrective lenses, by age and sex. Source: National Center for Health Statistics.

Table 3-7
Prevalence of Visual Impairments*

	Male		Female	
Age	General	Severe	General	Severe
All ages	51	5	44	8
45–64	74	6	53	7
65 and over	183	38	220	53

*Per 1000 persons.
Source: *Prevalence of Selected Impairments, U.S., 1971.* DHEW Publ. No. (HRA) 75-1526. Rockville, Md.: National Center for Health Statistics, 1975.

First, there are changes involving the mechanical aspects of the lens, which usually begin at age 40 and revolve around physical changes of the dioptric media. They lead to decreased accommodation, glare tolerance, and transmission of light. Second, there are retinal or metabolic changes. These begin usually in the sixth decade and revolve around decreased oxygen supply, neuronal death, or both. They lead to shrinkage of the visual field, delayed dark adaption, and other conditions. Specifically, then, there is a gradual loss of accommodation, development of senile miosis, increased lens opacity, decreased peripheral vision, and senile yellowing of the lens. Less light reaches the eye in senile miosis. Therefore, the elderly will need more light to perform daily activities. More time is also required for the eye to adjust when a person moves from a light to a dark area. Therefore, it is important for elderly persons, particularly those living alone, to use night lights in order to prevent accidents.

Increased lens opacity causes light to scatter, leaving the elderly more sensitive to glare. One way to ameliorate this problem is to use several sources of lesser intensity rather than one strong light source. In addition, the senile lens yellows. There is an age-related production of a high-molecular weight, yellow, insoluble substance in the inner region of the lens (Garcia-Castineiras et al 1978). This yellowing of the lens leads to inability to distinguish blue and green colors; thus, these colors should not be used to color-code anything that should be brought to an elderly person's attention. In contrast, the elderly will be able to distinguish red, yellow, and orange colors, which can be used to locate objects.

Finally, decreased peripheral vision can limit perception and ambulation. An unsteady gait may result, especially if vision impairment is accompanied by decreased hearing acuity. In addition to these impairments, some elderly persons develop dyslexia (inability to read) and dysgraphia (inability to write) although their vision may be nearly perfect.

Speech and hearing Changes affecting the speech and hearing of the elderly involve all parts of the auditory system. Verbal communication tends to deteriorate, regardless of the physical and mental health (von Leden 1977). Thirty percent to 50% of the elderly will have impaired hearing, and voice changes are inevitable. All efforts possible must be made to deal with these changes as communication is vital to the ability of a person to function and to perform daily tasks of living adequately.

The rate of speech, its quality and its vitality will probably change with age. Vocal intensity will be sharply reduced, as will the ability to sustain sound. Atrophic changes, such as muscle atrophy, reduced vocal fold thickness, and increased vocal fold stiffness, can shift the vocal range to higher pitch levels (Meyerson 1976). On the other hand, hormonal influences and thickening of the vocal cord can at times shift the vocal range to lower frequencies. In general, quavering appears and the voice sometimes becomes monotonous, high-pitched, and nasal (Lamy 1973).

Some elderly may develop aphasia. They lose the capacity to use words as symbols. Blocking of the cerebral arteries is most often cited as the cause of this impairment. Others may develop dysphasia, ie, difficulty in speaking or understanding the spoken language (Rockstein 1968).

Dysarthria, a condition in which speech sound production is sometimes impaired, is caused by lesions of the central or peripheral nervous systems. Auditory dysfunction is a major health problem for people over 65 years of age. Impaired hearing may be associated with primary aging, ototoxicity of drugs, environmental noises, or diseases affecting the sense of audition. The Committee on Aging of the United States Senate has conservatively estimated that impaired hearing restricts 30% to 50% of the elderly, which means that between 10 and 15 million elderly may be affected (Tables 3-8 and 3-9). The data in these tables indicate that a great many elderly develop some hearing deficiency that interferes with good communication. Impaired hearing may then prevent the elderly from seeking social contacts, and the quality of their lives may be severely restricted. Those with severe hearing impairment are often despondent, hopeless, bitter, apathetic, and listless. Hearing loss can lead to decreased awareness of the environment in depth, which in turn causes isolation, maladjustment, confusion, anxiety, and depression.

The most common sensorineural hearing loss is presbycusis. Over 2 million people, most older than 45 years of age, are affected by this disorder. Although it is considered a consequence of aging, it occurs more often in industrialized nations, suggesting that noise may play a part in its development. Two pathologic changes are apparently responsible for presbycusis. Epithelial atrophy begins in middle age

Table 3-8
Prevalence of Hearing Impairment*

Age	Male	Female
All ages	81	63
46–64	140	91
65–74	278	194
75 and over	449	366

*Per 1000 persons.
Source: *Prevalence of Selected Impairments, US., 1971.* DHEW Publ. No. (HRA) 75-1526. Rockville, Md.: National Center for Health Statistics, 1975.

Table 3-9
Bilateral Hearing Loss

Age	% U.S. population	Persons with hearing loss (%)
3–14	25.0	5.3
15–44	43.2	13.7
45–64	21.8	28.8
65 and over	10.1	52.2

Source: *Persons with Impaired Hearing, U.S., 1971,* DHEW Publ. No. (HRA) 76-1528. Rockville, Md.: National Center for Health Statistics, 1975.

and is characterized by a progressive degeneration of sensory hair cells, supporting cells, and the stria vascularis of the cochlea.

Neural atrophy begins later in life. It is associated with degeneration of the cells of the spiral ganglion and the neurons of the cochlear nerves and high auditory pathways. Presbycusis may be related to a number of problems or medical conditions, such as prolonged tension or emotional disorders and cardiovascular disease. The development of presbycusis is depicted in Table 3-10. In patients so afflicted, speech will be audible but not understandable. In the neural type of presbycusis, speech discrimination is 30%, which means that the patient can hear only every third word and, of course, does not understand what is being said. Individuals will be particularly affected by the high tone loss and may not hear doorbells or the telephone, both of which are usually high-pitched (Belal 1975; Cooper 1976; Hull and Traynor 1977; Lehman and Miller 1970).

Table 3-10
Development of Presbycusis

Age	Effect
Fifth decade	Mild high tone loss, mainly consonants
Sixth decade	Progressive loss, mainly in high frequency tones
Seventh decade	Loss involves entire auditory spectrum
Eighth decade	Greater degree of cochlear loss with degeneration of auditory part

No treatment for this condition is available, but experimentally, high doses of vitamin A are used in combination with cortisone and papaverine. In communicating with a patient afflicted with presbycusis, the use of a loud voice is not helpful. As the patient cannot distinguish and understand the spoken word, a person should face this patient, speak slowly, and give the patient an opportunity to observe lip movement.

Drugs and the auditory system   Hearing loss should not simply be ascribed to old age or presbycusis. Ototoxicity from drugs is not uncommon and can lead to both reversible and irreversible sensorineural hearing loss (Table 3-11) (Meyerhoff and Paparella 1978).

Table 3-11
Drugs Associated with Hearing Loss

Aminoglycosides	Ethacrynic acid
Amikacin	Fenoprofen
Gentamicin	Furosemide
Kanamycin	Indomethacin
Neomycin	Mechlorethamine
Paromomycin	Quinine
Streptomycin	Salicylates
Tobramycin	Vancomycin
Chloroquine	Viomycin

Skin

Aging of the skin is accompanied by thinning and atrophy of the epidermis, by decreased secretion of sebum, and by increased dryness of the skin. Both the sweat glands and the sebaceous glands apparently decrease in size and number. The skin gradually becomes dry, yellow, and wrinkled. Yellowing and thickening are particularly observed in areas exposed to the sun (Cripps 1977).

The total lipid content of the dermis does not appear to change, while both the trypsin and gelatin fractions decrease with age. There is a progressive decline in the collagen content of the dermis. The cellular content of the dermis decreases and the average elastin content increases nearly threefold between the ages of 20 and 80 (Pearce and Grimmer 1972). The external appearance of the skin is determined by the horny layer, the sebum, and the cutaneous fat film which is decreased with advancing age. Changes of the collagen fibers, decrease of the acid mucopolysaccharides, and a fall in the water content of the skin combine to cause a relaxation of the aging skin (Zesch 1974). There is no question that sunlight is the major cause of skin cancer and skin aging (Howell 1960).

Body Temperature and Thermoregulation

Perspiration volume is considerably diminished in the elderly, who also experience difficulty in maintaining constant body temperature. Rectal temperature of very old people can vary between 21° and 32°C (Rockstein 1968) and oral temperatures between 33° and 37°C. Unquestionably, elderly persons have lower body temperatures. Many of the elderly with low oral temperatures do not appear ill and many do not feel cold. Apparently, they have lower warmth and cold thresholds (Fox et al 1973). There is also a progressive thermoregulatory impairment. People at risk for developing hypothermia also seem to have a low resting peripheral blood flow, a nonconstrictor pattern of vasomotor response to cold, and a higher incidence of orthostatic hypotension (Collins et al 1977).

Spontaneous hypothermia can occur among apparently healthy, elderly people. Many drugs can interfere with the thermoregulatory mechanism. Their effect on body temperature depends upon the ambient temperature (Higgins et al 1964; Impallomeni and Ezzat 1976). Metabolic disorders also occasionally impair thermoregulation; myxedema is often cited (Hedley 1975).

Older persons, especially women, do not perspire as much as do younger persons and do not start to perspire until higher body temperatures are reached. Heat applications, particularly to large body areas, may then provoke hyperthermia. Both dehydration and hyperthermia may result in acute organic brain syndrome. Before an elderly patient receives heat treatment, the patient's temperature sensation should be tested. The elderly often fail to feel burning, especially in the legs. Deep heat by ultrasound or shortwave must be used cautiously. Low intensity heat from a warm bath or moist packs are often used in treatment.

REFERENCES

Albanese, A.A., Edelson, H., Lorenze, E.J. et al. Problems of bone health in elderly: ten-year study. *NY State J Med.* 75:308, 1975.

American Thoracic Society. Preventive therapy of tuberculosis infection. *Am Rev Respir Dis.* 110(3):1, 1974.

Atkinson, L., Gibson, I.I.J.M., and Andrews, J. The difficulties of old people taking drugs. *Age Ageing.* 6:144, 1977.

Avioli, L.V., McDonald, J.E., and Lee, S.W. The influence of age on the intestinal absorption of 47-Ca absorption in post-menopausal osteoporosis. *J Clin Invest.* 44:1960, 1965.

Avioli, L.V. Senile and postmenopausal osteoporosis. *Adv Intern Med.* 21:391, 1976.

Ball, M.J. Neuronal loss, neurofibrillary tangles and granulovacuolar degeneration of the hippocampus with ageing and dementia. *Acta Neuropathol.* (Berlin) 37:111, 1977.

Barrett, J.H. *Gerontological Psychology.* Springfield, Ill.: Charles C Thomas Co., 1972.

Barron, S.A., Jacobs, L., and Kinkel, W.E. Changes in size of normal lateral ventricles during aging determined by computerized tomography. *Neurology* 26:1011, 1976.

Barton, E.M., Plemons, J.K., Willis, S.L. et al. Recent findings on adult and gerontological intelligence. *Am Behav Sci.* 19:224, 1975.

Basso, A. The prostate in the elderly male. *Hosp Practice.* 12(10):117, 1977.

Bayley, N., and Oden, M.H. Maintenance of intellectual ability in gifted adults. *J Gerontol.* 10:91, 1955.

Belal, A. Presbycusis: psychological or pathological. *J Laryngol Otol.* 89:1011, 1975.

Bell, B. The longitudinal approach to aging studies in visual function. Proceedings of the Eighth International Congress of Gerontology, Vol. I. Washington, D.C., 1969.

Bender, A.D. The effect of increasing age on the distribution of peripheral blood flow in man. *J Am Geriatr Soc.* 13:192, 1965.

Berman, P.M., and Kirsner, J.B. The aging gut. II. Diseases of the colon, pancreas, liver, and gallbladder, functional bowel disease and iatrogenic disease. *Geriatrics* 27:117, 1972.

Berman, P.M., and Kirsner, J.B. Recognizing and avoiding adverse gastrointestinal effects of drugs. *Geriatrics* 29:59, 1974.

Blum, J.E., and Jarvick, L.F. Intellectual performance of octogenarians as a function of education and initial ability. *Hum Dev.* 17:364, 1975.

Blumenthal, H.T. Aging: biologic or pathologic? *Hosp Practice.* 13(4):127, 1978.

Bokey, L., and Hugh, T.B. Oesophageal ulceration associated with doxycycline therapy. *Med J Aust.* 1:236, 1975.

Brandfonbrenner, M., Landowne, M., and Shock, N.W. Changes in cardiac output with age. *Circulation.* 12:557, 1955.

Bricker, N.S. On the pathogenesis of the uremic state. *N Engl J Med.* 286:1093, 1972.

British Medical Journal. Editorial. Drug reactions and the lung. 2:1030, 1976.

Brizzee, K.R. Gross morphometric analyses and quantitative histology of the aging brain. Edited by J.M. Ordy, and K.R. Brizzee. In *Neurobiology of Aging.* New York: Plenum Press, 1975.

Buckley, C.E., and Dorsey, F.C. The effect of aging on human serum immunoglobulin concentrations. *J Immunol.* 105:964, 1970.

Buckley, C.E., and Roseman, J.M. Immunity and survival. *J Am Geriatr Soc.* 24:241, 1976.

Burnett, F.M. A genetic interpretation of aging. *Lancet* 2:480, 1973.

Buseck, S.A. Visual status of the elderly. *J Gerontol Nurs.* 2(5):34, 1976.

Busse, E.W. The clinical implications of brain wave changes over time. Presented at the 25th Annual Meeting of the Gerontological Society. Puerto Rico, 1972.

Campbell, E.J., and Lefrak, S.S. How aging affects the structure and function of the respiratory system. *Geriatrics* 33(6):68, 1978.

Chaitin, H. Clinical patterns of acute diverticulitis. *J Am Geriatr Soc.* 14:871, 1966.

Colin-Jones, D.G. Problems of peptic ulceration in the elderly. *Postgrad Med.* 51(5)suppl:41, 1975.

Collins, K.J., Dore, C., Exton-Smith, A.N. et al. Accidental hypothermia and impaired temperature homeostasis in the elderly. *Br Med J.* 1:353, 1977.

Cooper, A.F. Deafness and psychiatric illness. *Br J Psychiatry.* 129:216, 1976.

Cragg, B.G. The density of synapses and neurons in normal, mentally defective and aging brains. *Brain* 98:81, 1975.

Cripps, D.J. Skin care and problems in the aged. *Hosp Practice.* 12(4):119, 1977.

Crosby, W.H. Senile freckles. *J Am Hosp Assoc.* 234:1059, 1975.

Crowson, T.D., Head, L.H., and Ferrante, W.A. Esophageal ulcers associated with tetracycline therapy. *J Am Hosp Assoc.* 235:2747, 1976.

Curtis, J.R. Diseases of the urinary system. *Br Med J.* 2:242, 1977.

DeCarlo, T.J. Recreation participation patterns and successful aging. *J Gerontol.* 29:416, 1974.

Diamond, M.C. The aging brain: some enlightening and optimistic results. *Am Sci.* 66:66, 1978.

Dietze, F. Geriatrische Aspekte des Wasser und Elektrolythaushaltes. *Z Alternsforsch.* 22:265, 1969.

Dhar, A., Shastri, S.R., and Lenora, R.A.K. Aging and the respiratory system. *Med Clin North Am.* 6:1121, 1976.

Domonkos, A.N. The aging skin. *Cutis* 4(5):539, 1968.

Dontas, A.S. Renal disease in old age. Proceedings of the Eighth International Congress of Gerontology, Vol. 1. Washington, D.C., 1969.

DuBrow, E.L. Reactivation of tuberculosis: a problem of aging. *J Am Geriatr Soc.* 24:481, 1976.

Eddy, D.E., and Harman, D. Rat brain fatty acid composition: effect of dietary fat and age. *J Gerontol.* 30:647, 1977.

Evans, K.T., and Roberts, G.M. Where do all the tablets go? *Lancet* 2:1237, 1976.

Feinberg, I. Changes in sleep cycle patterns with age. *J Psychiatr Res.* 10:283, 1974.

Fernandez, G., and Schwartz, J.M. Immune responsiveness and hematologic malignancy in the elderly. *Med Clin North Am.* 60:1253, 1976.

Finch, C., and Hayflick, L. *The Biology of Aging.* New York: Van Nostrand Reinhold Co., 1977.

Finestone, A.J., and Rosenthal, R.S. Silent prostatism. *Geriatrics* 26:89, 1971.

Ford, J.M., and Roth, W.T. Do cognitive abilities decline with age? *Geriatrics* 32:59, 1977.

Fox, R.H., MacGibbon, R.D., Davies, L. et al. Problem of the old and the cold. *Br Med J.* 1:21, 1973.

Friedman, G.D., Klatsky, A.L., and Siegelaub, A.B. Lung infection and risk of myocardial infarction and sudden death. *N Engl J Med.* 294:1071, 1976.

Friedman, S.A., Raizner, A.E., Rosen, H. et al. Functional defects in the aging kidney. *Ann Intern Med.* 76:41, 1972.

Frolkis, V.V. *Practical Geriatrics.* Basel: S. Karger, 1975.

Garbus, S.B., and Lamy, P.P. *Managing the Aging Hypertensive.* Darien, Conn.: Patient Care, 1976.

Garcia-Castineiras, S., Dillon, J., and Spector, A. Detection of tyrosine in cataractous human lens protein. *Science* 199:897, 1978.

Garth, S.N., and Young, R.W. Concurrent fat loss and fat gain. *Am J Phys Anthropol.* 14:497, 1956.

Geboes, K., and Bossaert, H. Gastrointestinal disorders in old age. *Age Ageing.* 6:197, 1977a.

Geboes, K., and Bossaert, H. Reactivation of tuberculosis in old age. *J Am Geriatr Soc.* 25:318, 1977b.

Geokas, M.C., and Haverback, B.J. The aging gastrointestinal tract. *Am J Surg.* 117:881, 1969.

Granick, S., and Patterson, R.D. (Eds.). *Human Aging II. An Eleven-Year Follow-Up Biomedical and Behavioral Study.* DHEW Publ. No. (HSM) 71-9037. Washington, D.C.: U.S. Government Printing Office, 1971.

Greenberg, B. Reaction time in the elderly. *Am J Nurs.* 73:2056, 1973.

Greenblatt, R.B., Oettinger, M., and Bohler, C.S.S. Estrogen-androgen levels in aging men and women: therapeutic considerations. *J Am Geriatr Soc.* 24:173, 1976.

Grollman, A., and Grollman, E.F. *Pharmacology and Therapeutics.* Philadelphia: Lea and Febiger, 1960.

Gruebl, M., Klein, K., and Siedeck, H. Zur Koronartherapie in der Geriatrie. *Wiener Med Wochenschr.* 123:1, 1973.

Grunstein, J.A.H. The problem of postural hypotension. *Gerontol Clin.* 16:171, 1974.

Gryfe, C.I., Amies, A., and Ashley, M.J. A longitudinal study of falls in an elderly population. I. Incidence and morbidity. *Age Ageing.* 6:201, 1977.

Hayflick, L. The cell biology of human aging. *N Engl J Med.* 295:1302, 1976.

Hedley, D.W. Cold and old. *Update* 11:115, 1975.

Heidrick, M.L., and Makinodan, T. Nature of cellular deficiencies in age-related decline of the immune system. *Gerontologia* 18:305, 1972.

Higgins, E.A., Iampietro, P.P., Adams, T. et al. Effects of a tranquilizer on body temperature. *Proc Soc Exp Biol Med.* 115:1017, 1964.

Howell, J.B. The sunlight factor in aging and skin cancer. *Arch Dermatol.* 82:865, 1960.

Hull, R.H., and Traynor, R.M. Hearing impairment among aging persons in the health care facility, their diagnosis and rehabilitation. *J Am Health Care Assoc.* 3(1):14, 1977.

Impallomeni, M., and Ezzat, R. Hypothermia associated with nitrazepam administration. *Br Med J.* 1:223, 1976.

Ingham, J. Osteoporosis: diagnosis and treatment. *Drugs* 8:290, 1974.

Jarvick, M.E., Gritz, E.R., and Schneider, N.G. Drugs and memory disorders in human aging. *Behav Biol.* 7:643, 1972.

Kahn, R.L., Zarit, S.H., Hilbert, N.M. et al. Memory complaint and impairment in the aged. *Arch Gen Psychiatry.* 32:1569, 1975.

Kent, S. The aging lung. I. Loss of elasticity. *Geriatrics* 33(2):124, 1978.

Keys, A., Taylor, H.L., and Grande, F. Basal metabolism and age of adult man. *Metabolism* 22:579, 1973.

Kochakian, D.D. Effect of castration on weight and composition of muscles of guinea pig. *Endocrinology* 58:315, 1956.

Kohn, R.R. Human aging and disease. *J Chronic Dis.* 16:5, 1963.

Kornzweig, A.L. Visual loss in the elderly. *Hosp Practice.* 12(7):51, 1977.

Kronenberg, R.S., and Drage, C.W. Attenuation of the ventilatory heart rate responses to hypoxia and hypercapnia with aging in normal men. *J Clin Invest.* 52:1812, 1973.

Krumlovsky, F.A. Hyponatremia. *Ration Drug Ther.* 9(5):1, 1975.

Kursh, E.D., Mostyn, E.M., and Persky, L. Nitrofurantoin pulmonary complications. *J Urol.* 113:392, 1975.

Labouvie-Vief, G., and Gonda, J.N. Cognitive strategy training and intellectual performance in the elderly. *J Gerontol.* 31:327, 1976.

Ladislas, R. New directions in research on arterial diseases. *CNRS Res.* 5:12, 1977.

Lamy, P.P. Physiological changes in late life. Edited by E.W. Busse. In *Theory and Therapeutics of Aging.* New York: MedCom, Inc., 1973.

Lamy, P.P. Therapeutics and the elderly. *Addict Dis.* 3(3):311, 1978.

Lamy, P.P., and Kitler, M.E. The geriatric patient: age-dependent physiologic and pathologic changes. *J Am Geriatr Soc.* 19:871, 1971.

Lamy, P.P., and Vestal, R.E. Drug prescribing for the elderly. *Hosp Practice.* 11(11):111, 1976.

Lamy, P.P., Filiatrault, L., Harris, R. et al. *The Aging Cardiovascular System.* Princeton, N.J.: E.R. Squibb & Sons, 1977a.

Lamy, P.P., Eisdorfer, C., Kassel, V. et al. *The Aging Brain.* Princeton, N.J.: E.R. Squibb & Sons, 1977b.

Lamy, P.P., Cummins, B., Kassel, V. et al. *The Aging Gut.* Princeton, N.J.: E.R. Squibb & Sons, 1977c.

Lamy, P.P., Kassel, V., Lane, W. et al. *The Aging Kidney.* Princeton, N.J.: E.R. Squibb & Sons, 1977d.

Leeming, J.T. Skeletal disease in the elderly. *Br Med J.* 4:472, 1973.

Lehman, R.H., and Miller, A.L. Presbycusis. *J Am Geriatr Soc.* 18:486, 1970.

Linzback, A.J. The pathogenesis of cardiac insufficiency in hypertension. *Triangle* 14(1):17, 1975.

Longcope, C. Hormones: beneficial or dangerous to the aged? *J Am Geriatr Soc.* 26:145, 1978.

Louria, D.B., Joselow, M.M., and Browder, A.A. The human toxicity of certain trace elements. *Ann Intern Med.* 76:307, 1972.

Maddox, G.L. Activity and morale. *Soc Forces.* 42:195, 1963.

Makinodan, T. Immunobiology of aging. *J Am Geriatr Soc.* 24:249, 1976.

McLachlan, M.S.F. The ageing kidney. *Lancet* 2:143, 1978.

Medical Letter. Osteoporosis. 18:99, 1976.

Meyerhoff, W.L., and Paparella, M.M. Diagnosing the cause of hearing loss. *Geriatrics* 33(2):95, 1978.

Meyerson, M.D. The effects of aging on communication. *J Gerontol.* 31(1):29, 1976.

Miller, N.E., and Dworkin, B.R. Effects of learning on visceral functions–biofeedback. *N Engl J Med.* 296:1274, 1977.

Nandy, K. Neuroanatomical changes in the aging brain. Presented at the Symposium of Biomedical Aspects of Senile Dementia and Related Disorders. St. Louis, Mo., 1978.

Nejat, J., and Greif, E. The aging heart: a clinical review. *Med Clin North Am.* 60:1059, 1976.

Ordy, J.M. Principles of mammalian aging. Edited by J.M. Ordy, and K.R. Brizzee. In *Neurobiology of Aging.* New York: Plenum Press, 1975.

Ordy, J.M., and Kaak, B. Neurochemical changes in composition, metabolism and neurotransmitters in the human brain with age. Edited by J.M. Ordy, and K.R. Brizzee. In *Neurobiology of Aging.* New York: Plenum Press, 1975.

Overstall, P.W., Exton-Smith, A.N., Imms, F.J. et al. Falls in the elderly related to postural imbalance. *Br Med J.* 1:261, 1977.

Painter, N.S. Diet and disease: dietary fibre. Diverticular disease of the colon: the effect of the high fibre diet. *R Soc Health J.* 95:194, 1975.

Palmore, E. Facts on aging: a short quiz. *Gerontologist* 17:316, 1977.

Parker, J.C. The old age syndrome: subtle cerebral degeneration bronchopneumonia. *Geriatrics* 27:94, 1972.

Pearce, R.H., and Grimmer, B.J. Age and the chemical constitution of normal human dermis. *J Invest Dermatol.* 58:347, 1972.

Pemberton, J. Oesophageal obstruction and ulceration caused by oral potassium therapy. *Br Heart J.* 32:267, 1970.

Pisciotta, A.V. Idiosyncratic hematologic reactions to drugs. *Postgrad Med.* 55(5):105, 1974.

Polland, W.S. Histamine test meals: analysis of 988 consecutive tests. *Arch Intern Med.* 51:903, 1933.

Post, J., and Hoffman, J. Cell renewal patterns. *N Engl J Med.* 279:248, 1968.

Riccitelli, M.L. Vitamin C therapy in geriatric patients. *J Am Geriatr Soc.* 20:34, 1972.

Roberts, W.C., and Perloff, J.K. Mitral valvular disease: a clinicopathologic survey of the conditions causing the mitral valve to function abnormally. *Ann Intern Med.* 77:939, 1972.

Rockstein, M. The biological aspects of aging. *Gerontologist* 8:124, 1968.

Rodstein, M. *Accidents and Aging People, Working with Older People: A Guide to Practice,* Vol. 3. The Aging Person: Needs and Services, PHS Publ. No. 1459. Washington, D.C.: U.S. Government Printing Office, 1970.

Rosen, H. Renal disease in the elderly. *Med Clin North Am.* 6:1105, 1976.

Rosenow, E.C. Drugs that may induce pulmonary disease. *Geriatrics* 33(1):64, 1978.

Rossman, I. The anatomy of aging. Edited by I. Rossman. In *Clinical Geriatrics.* Philadelphia: J.B. Lippincott, 1971.

Rowe, J.W., Andres, R., Tobin, J.D. et al. Age-adjusted standards for creatinine clearance. *Ann Intern Med.* 84:567, 1976.

Roxe, D.M. Toxic nephropathy due to drugs. *Ration Drug Ther.* 9(12):1, 1975.

Rupp, R.R. Understanding the problems of presbycusis. *Geriatrics* 25:100, 1970.

Samorajski, T. Age-related changes in brain biogenic amines. Edited by H. Brody, D. Harman, and J.M. Ordy. In *Aging,* Vol. 1. New York: Raven Press, 1975.

Sandberg, L.B. Elastin structure in health and disease. *Int Rev Connect Tissue Res.* 7:159, 1976.

Schank, M.J. A survey of the well elderly: their foot problems, practices, and needs. *J Gerontol Nurs.* 3(6):10, 1977.

Shklar, G. The effects of aging upon the oral mucosa. *J Invest Dermatol.* 47:115, 1966.

Shock, N.W., and Yiengst, M.J. Age changes in basal respiratory measurements and metabolism in males. *J Gerontol.* 10:31, 1955.

Shock, N.W. Physiological aspects of aging in man. *Ann Rev Physiol.* 23:97, 1961.

Shuster, M.M. Disorders of the aging GI system. *Hosp Practice.* 11(9):95, 1976.

Sklar, M. Functional bowel distress and constipation in the aged. *Geriatrics* 27:79, 1972.

Smith, A.D. Aging and interference with memory. *J Gerontol.* 30:319, 1977.

Smith, B.H., and Sethi, P.K. Aging and the nervous system. *Geriatrics* 30:109, 1975.

Smith, B.S. Connective tissue in chronic obstructive airways diseases. *Geriatrics* 26:146, 1971.

Sokoloff, L. Cerebral circulation and metabolism in the aged. Edited by S. Gershon, and A. Raskin. In *Aging,* Vol. 2. New York: Raven Press, 1975.

Spirduso, W.W. Reaction and movement time as a function of age and physical acitivity level. *J Gerontol.* 30:435, 1975.

Stare, F.J. Three score and ten plus more. *J Am Geriatr Soc.* 25:529, 1977.

Starr, P. Thyroxine therapy in preventive geriatrics. *J Am Geriatr Soc.* 3:217, 1955.

Steinheber, F.U. Interpretation of gastrointestinal symptoms in the elderly. *Med Clin North Am.* 6:1141, 1976.

Stoermer, A. Das Herz im Alter. *Munch Med Wochenschr.* 109:1157, 1967.

Stumpf, W.E., Sar, M., and Aumueller, G. The heart: a target organ for estradiol. *Science* 196:319, 1977.

Turnbull, A.R., and Isaacson, P. Ischaemic colitis and drug abuse. *Br Med J.* 2:1000, 1977.

von Leden, H. Speech and hearing problems in the geriatric patient. *J Am Geriatr Soc.* 25:422, 1977.

Wallace, D.J. The biology of aging: 1976, an overview. *J Am Geriatr Soc.* 25:104, 1977.

Weinberg, J. Environment, its language and the aging. *J Am Geriatr Soc.* 18:681, 1970.

Zesch, A. Pharmakologische and Kosmetische Beeinflussung der Altershaut. *Z Geront.* 7:422, 1974.

4 Sociogenic Aging

Stereotypic perceptions all too often still determine the level and extent of care given to the elderly. Outcome of specific therapeutic regimens is thought of negatively, as the elderly may be viewed as poor medical risks. Thus, an intimate knowledge of the elderly is necessary for those who are involved in geriatrics.

SOME FACTS

With advancing age, most persons face a change in their economic and possibly their social status. Income is most likely fixed and far less than that enjoyed during peak productive years. Lessened economic and social status, in turn, may lead to a perceived feeling of uselessness and to withdrawal. There is an excess amount of leisure time and an inability to use it effectively. This, coupled with a narrowed interest range and social isolation, can be the basis of depression, which is then often treated with drugs.

Loss of economic independence may lead to neglect in obtaining dentures, spectacles, or hearing aids, thus depriving a person of sensory input. This, in turn, may lead to deterioration of spirit and intellect and to further social isolation and depression (Nicholson 1974).

The elderly face a high level of psychosocial and physical stress. Sudden lifestyle changes can result in agitated or depressed behavior. These changes include multiple life problems, such as loss of family, a job, friends, or health, and even such often overlooked factors as loss of access to cherished ethnic foods and beverages (Sherr 1976). To cope successfully with the demands of these changes, an increasing level of psychologic reaction is needed as well as a high degree of adaptation, at a time when capacities for these functions diminish and when society is least supportive.

Furthermore, interdependence of physical and mental illness becomes more prominent at these age levels. It is often difficult to determine whether behavioral disturbances are a sign of somatic disease or a response to changed environmental factors (Eisdorfer 1975). Changed behavioral patterns could become important risk factors in certain conditions like coronary artery disease. Among coping mechanisms observed among the elderly is an increased alcohol consumption. The typical elderly drinker is between 55 and 69 years of age, widowed, divorced, or separated, unemployed, and living in an apartment or boarding house (Lamy 1978).

HOW OTHERS VIEW THE ELDERLY

The old are the newest underprivileged minority (Fischer 1977). They are viewed as inferior and they are therefore accorded little status (McTavish 1971). Gerontophobia or gerophobia is widespread and is responsible for the fact that most people believe that the vast majority of the elderly are senile, in a chronic care facility, homebound or bedbound, or unable to perform even normal daily activities. Gerontophobia may be a rejection by younger people of the thought that they, too, are growing old.

Change in public attitude toward the elderly is intimately intertwined with societal changes. Formerly, the old were venerated but not necessarily admired or liked. They possessed money and power. Today, each decade brings about major changes, which render many skills obsolete. Thus, underlying social conditions are frequently related to both physical and mental status. Sociogenic aging has no physical basis, it stems from folklore and prejudice. Prejudice and discrimination against aged people have been termed ageism (Butler and Lewis 1977).

Many stereotypes of the elderly abound (Bennett and Eckman 1973). Attitudes are negative (Peterson and Eden 1977); the most negative attitudes are probably exhibited by adolescents. Children as young as five years old can differentiate between adults and older persons. Young children view the elderly as warm, permissive, and helpful. Thus, children have a positive feeling of affection but a stereotypic or negative attitude toward the physical aspects of aging (Seefeldt et al 1977). Teenagers see old age as a time of lost identity and disorientation, while adults view it as a threat to financial and physical independence.

Often, the elderly are patronized and arbitrarily excluded from any significant social roles and/or active participation in the establishment and continuum of their therapeutic regimen. The "big brother syndrome" is still rampant in medicine; too often, the provider "knows" what is best and tries to impose this regimen. Rarely are elderly patients asked what they want; if they then disagree, they are classified as irritable, unable to accept change, and uncooperative. Yet active cooperation of patient and primary care provider is essential for a favorable therapy result. It makes no sense to prescribe a special therapy or diet, for example, if it is clear that the patient will not cooperate. The patient's outlook must be accepted and the physician must work around it.

To be able to participate in this important process, the patient must retain cognitive ability which, in the absence of disease, depends on the level of patient activity. Yet, the patient perceives negative feelings. It would seem that most mental and attitudinal changes seen in old people are not biologic effects of aging, but are the results of role-playing with the individual acting on society's dictum that the elderly are supposed to be physically and mentally infirm (Comfort 1976). This role-playing may exaggerate the effects of decreased physiologic functions.

Even in institutions designed specifically to care for the elderly, it is possible to encounter negative attitudes toward the aging among the staff (Knopf 1972). A nursing home environment does not demand intellectual involvement of the patients. Nursing homes and other institutions actually project a totalitarian image; regimentation is achieved through pressure. Individualism is not encouraged, and the patient learns that to be popular and even to get help, there must be compliance with rules and regulations. A pervasive institutional idiom reinforces that loss of individuality. Patients are often addressed like children and, too often, explanations of procedures and therapy are not given (Toynbee 1977). Thus, lack of stimulation and boredom may lead to anxiety, depression, and apparent intellectual impairment.

Similar difficulties are encountered by the ambulatory elderly patient. In general, Americans still suffer from a personal and institutionalized prejudice against older people. "Gallows" humor regarding the elderly is often used, and epithets such as "crock," have become synonymous with the older person (Butler 1976).

This type of prejudice or ageism can prevent the elderly patient from active participation in a care program. For any successful treatment plan, the patient should be forced to remain in a decision-making role. Yet, medicine has viewed the elderly as sickly, depressed, and depressing (Butler and Lewis 1977). Medical problems are thought to be intractable and, therefore, an elderly person gains little from medical attention.

Many health professionals do not like to work with elderly patients (Carmichael and Linn 1974) and their negative feelings relate to impatience and boredom with the elderly and resentment of their physical and mental deterioration (Cyrus-Lutz and Gaitz 1972). Given a choice, the majority of health professionals rank the aged last among preferred clients (Gunter 1971). This type of feeling may have found its apex in the prediction of a British physician, Dr John Goundry, that a "death pill" or "demise pill" will be available and possibly obligatory by the end of the century, as the economics of geriatrics are devastating and more potentially dangerous than nuclear war.

Attitudes are triggers for behavior, and the two do not always match. Nurses manifest a stereotypic attitude toward the aged (Campbell 1971; Gillis 1973). They seem to prefer patients who are neat, appreciative, conforming, yet communicating and socially active. Special care is often extended to persons of high social status, but patients who place extra demands on the system are not valued (White 1977).

A recent physician survey demonstrated generalized medical disinterest in the care of the aged (Miller et al 1976). Most physicians feel competent to manage the elderly, although, in this survey, 50% had had no significant exposure to geriatric medicine in their medical education. Forty percent of the physicians interviewed felt that the nursing home was a place to die, and only 21% felt that they continued to be in charge of their patient after the patient had been placed in a nursing home.

This feeling of competence is not necessarily matched by fact. In another study, the primary diagnosis for 100 patients admitted to a nursing home was inaccurate or noninformative in 64 cases, and the secondary diagnosis was lacking or inaccurate in 84 cases (Miller and Elliot 1976).

Fortunately, attitudes are changing. Older workers have a more positive attitude toward the elderly (because they are closer to older age?), and social workers who chose to work with older patients had the most positive attitudes. Among younger professionals, nurses had the most positive attitude (Wolk and Wolk 1971).

HOW THE ELDERLY VIEW THEMSELVES

Many elderly do not identify themselves with others their age. Those over 65 years of age often place themselves at middle age, particularly if they are active and relatively healthy (Jeffers et al 1962; Kastenbaum and Durkee 1964). Many elderly claim to have experienced little or no personal rejection because of their age (Kahana et al 1977), but this may simply be a reluctance to complain, and, thus, be in danger of stereotypic classification (Kahana and Coe 1975). The elderly do not necessarily fear death, but, not surprisingly, they view illness as a significant impediment to a meaningful existence (Ninivaggi and Harris 1976). More than anything, they fear disease which may incapacitate them (Savitz 1976). They also dread the loss of significance and independence, and they fear abandonment, suffering, and pain.

Their most frequent complaint is weakness, followed by complaints about loss of memory and hearing deterioration, although the latter may be, in fact, a decline in the effort to listen.

On the other hand, the elderly are more mature and have learned to adapt to many situations. Maturity and judgment increase with age, as does tolerance with fewer illusions. An aged person, in fact, becomes a mature person and not an old person. The elderly are most concerned with others, especially a spouse or children. The elderly do tend to be more rigid in their attitudes and personalities. They are more cautious, being aware of their diminished capacity to control the environment (Brink 1978). In general, geriatric rigidity is usually well correlated with poor adjustment. In most cases they are very considerate and tolerant (Lawson 1977). They also have expectations on how they should act or are expected to act. They tend to assume a behavior they think is appropriate for their chronologic age (Neugarten et al 1968).

The elderly have themselves a negative attitude toward old age and they devalue their own roles and social positions (Kahana 1970). A recent Harris poll, sponsored by the National Council on Aging, tried to elicit attitudes toward aging, including perceptions of problems, perceptions of personality and attitudes, feelings toward growing old, and perceptions of the treatment of the old (Henretta et al 1977). The results of the poll indicate that the old, like the young, have accepted the negative images of old age, apparently assuming that life is tough for most people over the age of 65 years. Interestingly, many individuals felt that they were the exception to the rule. All were afraid that being older would mean not being needed (Harris et al 1975).

Older people may panic when there is danger of being separated from their family. They would like to live separately, but close to the family.

Elderly people do not want to overwhelm the physician with their problems and are reluctant to seek help. They may be ill and suffer considerable disability without complaining or without contacting a physician. The reasons for this behavior include acceptance of disabilities as natural and inevitable, a more stoic attitude, a reluctance to trouble the doctor, fear of being viewed in stereotypic terms, and such factors as difficulty in making an appointment or traveling to the physician's office (Brocklehurst et al 1978).

However, even in an environment in which economics and transportation are not tangible barriers, the elderly still do not use physician services extravagantly. They do not complain unnecessarily and their complaints may not be a reasonable interpretation of the problems. They often conceal complaints for fear of being identified as old and useless (Eckstein 1976).

It is important to realize that age and adaptation are related and severity of a disease may be a more critical factor in determining adaptation to illness than chronologic age (Zarit and Kahn 1977). Finally, the elderly may be reluctant to see a physician because of fear of bad news or fear of appearing unrealistic about seeking help.

Thus, it seems clear that the elderly at times may have to play a sick role to receive positive social rewards and that elderly patients may be thrust into patterns of negative health behavior by the behavior of others toward them.

WHAT NEEDS TO BE DONE?

In the past, the care of geriatric patients has been marked by terms such as "clinical undertaking" and "predeath care." An active approach is needed that will yield positive results (Hodkinson and Jefferys 1972). Attitudes of caregivers are directly related to the quality of care. Therefore, if old people are viewed as competent, functional, and capable individuals, health care will aim at preserving these attributes (Solomon and Vickers 1977).

Physicians, and presumably all health care providers, must express a genuine interest and concern for the geriatric patient and his/her problems (Harris 1975). It is imperative to preserve the patient's identity within the health care delivery system; which can be accomplished by explaining the meaning of any medical problem to the patient, keeping in mind the patient's age, self-respect, dignity, and understanding. Often, the health professional will have to change and adapt, as cultural, ethnic, and religious backgrounds may be very strongly ingrained in the elderly and this may prevent the elderly from adapting. There must be improved education of medical students and physicians, as well as other health care providers in the care of the elderly (Leaf 1977).

REFERENCES

Bennett, R., and Eckman, J. Attitudes toward aging: a critical examination of recent literature and implications for future research. Edited by C. Eisdorfer, and M.P. Lawson. In *The Psychology of Adult Development and Aging.* Washington, D.C.: American Psychological Association, 1973.

Brink, T.L. Geriatric rigidity and its psychotherapeutic implications. *J Am Geriatr Soc.* 26:274, 1978.

Brocklehurst, J.C., Leeming, J.T., Carty, M.H. et al. Medical screening of old people accepted for residential care. *Lancet* 2:141, 1978.

Butler, R.N. *Medicine and Aging.* Washington, D.C.: National Institute on Aging, 1976.

Butler, R.N., and Lewis, M.I. *Aging and Mental Health: Positive Psychosocial Approaches.* St. Louis: C.V. Mosby Co., 1977.

Campbell, M. Study of the attitudes of nursing personnel toward the geriatric patient. *Nurs Res.* 20:147, 1971.

Carmichael, J., and Linn, M. Functioning of the elderly patient in relation to the physician's diagnosis of organic brain syndrome. *J Am Geriatr Soc.* 22:217, 1974.

Comfort, A. *A Good Age.* New York: Crown Publishers, 1976.

Cyrus-Lutz, C., and Gaitz, C. Psychiatrists' attitudes toward the aged and aging. *Gerontologist* 12:163, 1972.

Eckstein, D. Common complaints of the elderly. *Hosp Practice.* 11(4):67, 1976.

Eisdorfer, C. Observations on the psychopharmacology of the aged. *J Am Geriatr Soc.* 23:53, 1975.

Fischer, D.H. *Growing Old in America.* New York: Oxford University Press, 1977.

Gillis, S.M. Attitudes of nursing personnel toward the aged. *Nurs Res.* 22:517, 1973.

Gunter, L.M. Students' attitudes toward geriatric nursing. *Nurs Outlook.* 19(7):466, 1971.

Harris, L. et al. *The Myth of Reality of Aging in America.* Washington, D.C.: National Council on Aging, Inc., 1975.

Harris, R. Maintaining the geriatric patient's identity. *Geriatrics* 75:1252, 1975.

Henretta, J.C., Campbell, R.T., and Gardocki, G. Survey research in aging: an evaluation of the Harris survey. *Gerontologist* 17:160, 1977.

Hodkinson, H.M., and Jefferys, P.M. Making hospital geriatrics work. *Br Med J.* 4:536, 1972.

Jeffers, F.C., Eisdorfer, C., and Busse, E.W. Measurement of aged identification: a methodological note. *J Gerontol.* 17:437, 1962.

Kahana, E. Different generations view each other. *Geriatr Focus.* 9:10, 1970.

Kahana, E., and Coe, R. Alternatives in long-term care. Edited by S. Sherwood. In *Long-Term Care: A Handbook for Researchers, Planners, and Providers.* New York: Spectrum Publications, Inc., 1975.

Kahana, E., Liang, J., Felton, B. et al. Perspectives of aged on victimization, "ageing," and their problems in urban society. *Gerontologist* 17:121, 1977.

Kastenbaum, R., and Durkee, N. Young people view old age. Edited by R. Kastenbaum. In *New Thoughts on Old Age.* New York: Springer Publishing Co., Inc., 1964.

Knopf, O. Aging. *Mt Sinai J Med.* 39:356, 1972.

Lamy, P.P. Therapeutics and the elderly. *Addict Dis.* 3(3):311, 1978.

Lawson, I. Three myths about the aged. In *The Medical Director in the Long-Term Care Facility.* Chicago: American Medical Association, 1977.

Leaf, A. Medicine and the aged. *N Engl J Med.* 297:887, 1977.

McTavish, D.G. Perceptions of old people: a review of research methodologies and findings. *Gerontologist* 11:90, 1971.

Miller, D.B., Lowenstein, R., and Winston, R. Physicians' attitudes toward the ill aged and nursing homes. *J Am Geriatr Soc.* 24:498, 1976.

Miller, M.B., and Elliot, D.F. Errors and omissions in diagnostic records on admission of patients to a nursing home. *J Am Geriatr Soc.* 24:108, 1976.

Neugarten, B.L., Moore, J.W., and Lowe, J.C. Age norms, age constraints, and adult socialization. Edited by B.L. Neugarten. In *Middle Age and Aging.* Chicago: The University of Chicago Press, 1968.

Nicholson, W.J. Disturbances of the special senses and other functions. *Br Med J.* 1:33, 1974.

Ninivaggi, F.J., and Harris, R. Attitudes toward living and death. *Geriatrics* 76:1493, 1976.

Peterson, D.A., and Eden, D.Z. Teenagers and aging: adolescent literature as an attitude source. *Educ Gerontol.* 2:311, 1977.

Savitz, H.A. Mental hygiene for the aged. *Geriatrics* 76:1850, 1976.

Seefeldt, C., Jantz, R.K., Galper, A. et al. Children's attitudes toward the elderly: educational implications. *Educ Gerontol.* 2:301, 1977.

Sherr, V.T. Benjamin Franklin and geropsychiatry: vignettes for the bicentennial year. *J Am Geriatr Soc.* 24:447, 1976.

Solomon, K., and Vickers, R. Attitudes of health workers toward old people. Presented at the 30th Annual Meeting of the American Gerontological Society. San Francisco, 1977.

Toynbee, P. *Patients.* New York: Harcourt Brace Jovanovich, 1977.

White, C.M. The nurse-patient encounter: attitudes and behaviors in action. *J Gerontol Nurs.* 3(3):16, 1977.

Wolk, R.L., and Wolk, R.B. Professional workers' attitudes toward the aged. *J Am Geriatr Soc.* 19:624, 1971.

Zarit, S.H., and Kahn, R.L. Aging and adaptation to illness. *J Gerontol.* 30:o7, 1977.

5 Can Aging Be Decelerated?

The dream of eternal youth pursued by people throughout the ages continues—still unsuccessfully. Historically, many diverse "cures" for aging have been tried. King David tried to stave off aging by sleeping with young virgins, later people tried eating the marrow of young bears, and testicles of tigers were eaten in India.

POTIONS AND CURES

The snake oil dispenser at the turn of the century was preceded by others, often cloaked in the mantle of science. Possibly only the efforts to create gold from lead in the Middle Ages have created similar passions and hopes. The snake oil dispenser is still here. At the turn of the century, fermented milk was ingested fervently, and today we hear marvelous claims for yogurt. Transplantation of animal gonads to humans occurred in the 1920s. Dr Paul Niehans in Switzerland suggested the injection of cells of unborn lambs and black sheep. In luxurious clinics still operating today, such world-renowned personages as Pope Pius XII, Charlie Chaplin, and Winston Churchill are said to have been treated.

In France, Dr Saint Pierre touted the injection of blood serum into older men and women. Aromatotherapy, offered by Ivan Popov in France, was rather expensive but was probably less harmful than the use of cytotoxic serums during the 1940s.

Now there is KH3, Gerovital, or Gerovital H-3, created by Dr Anna Aslan, a director of the Rumanian Institute of Geriatrics in Bucharest. It is sold in many European countries (in some without a prescription). For many years, Dr Aslan has reported unusual results with procaine injections, suggesting "cures" for complaints such as senescence, arthritis, arteriosclerosis, high blood pressure, eczema, wrinkled skin, skin blotches and depigmentation, baldness or gray hair, deafness, neuritis, neuralgia, Parkinson disease, a host of psychiatric disorders, and of course, impotence. In the 1950s, it was claimed that repeated injections of procaine hydrochloride could rejuvenate aged and debilitated persons and reduce the biologic age of an individual below the chronologic age (LaBalla 1972). Nikita Khrushchev and Ho Chi Minh have long been rumored to have benefitted from these treatments, although it was most likely a powerful placebo effect that helped them.

Gerovital H-3 appears to be a simple solution of procaine hydrochloride which also contains, for pharmaceutical but not medical reasons, benzoic acid and potassium metabisulfite. Many trials with this substance have been reported (Berryman et al 1961; Fee and Clark 1961; Hirsh 1961; Isaacs 1962; Kent 1976). Recently, data from 285 articles and books, describing treatment in more than 100 thousand patients in the past 25 years, have been reviewed (Ostfeld et al 1977). It was concluded that Gerovital seems to have no ameliorative effect on either psychologic or physiologic functions, but may have a possible transient and beneficial effect on depressive symptomatology, similar to a monoamine oxidase inhibitory effect.

Yet, even though there are no convincing reports of the effectiveness of this substance in the treatment of diseases in elderly people, a company in Nevada manufactures it for in-state use only.

SOME EXPERIMENTAL EFFORTS

More serious efforts aimed at delaying or even preventing the process of aging have been reported. Estrogen and estrogen-progesterone combinations have been used to halt or at least influence beneficially age-associated changes of the skin, the cardiovascular system, the urogenital tract, the nervous system, and the skeleton. Steroid therapy has been used in perimenopausal women and has also been used in insomnia, irritability, melancholia, and waning libido. Substances are being investigated which are thought to modify the rate of aging (see Table 5-1).

Table 5-1
Substances That Might Modify the Rate of Aging

Substance	Theoretical basis
Antioxidants	Scavenge free radicals; improve stability of information systems
Radioprotectants	Assume aging similar in nature to radiation damage
Protein synthesis inhibitors	Break "vicious circle" perpetuating transcription errors
Lysosome stabilizers	Prevent escape of enzymes including lysosome DNAse
Immunosuppression	Abolish aging effects due to autoimmune reaction
Anti-cross-linking agents	Aging due to cross-links in long-term molecules
Hormonal agents	Retard senescent program:
Anabolic	Prevent decline in protein storage and muscle strength
Somatotrophin	Maintain young pattern of protein synthesis
Prednisolone	Anti-autoimmune? Slow synthesis of nonsense proteins (auto-antigens)
17-ketosteroids	Decline most closely parallels human senescence
Antimetabolic drugs	Delay synthesis of nonsense proteins, simulate caloric restriction

Source: A.B. Chinn. Working with older people, Vol. 4, PHS Publ. No. 1459, *Clinical Aspects of Aging.* Washington, D.C.: US Government Printing Office, 1971.

The most noteworthy of these substances involves the use of antioxidants which are thought to complex free-circulating radicals, thus reducing their age-accelerating effect. The increased use of vitamin C (ascorbic acid) and vitamin E are probably related to this theory. There does seem to be evidence that vitamin E protects an individual to some degree from the effects of pollution.

In other experiments, the lives of insects have been extended by decreasing their body temperature. After the temperature regulatory nuclei in the hypothalamus were medicated, the body temperatures were reduced from normal to 86°F. Extrapolation of these results predicts that the human life span could be extended to 200 years.

However, even a reduction of two to three degrees in human body temperature would slow human physiology to an unacceptable level. Similarly, another approach which has been termed the most practical so far, revolves around a very low caloric intake. In Japan, it was found that mice severely restricted in their caloric intake, which resulted in a 10% underweight, would show an increase in life span of 30%. Concern has been expressed that at this level of caloric intake humans would simply not have enough energy to pursue even simple tasks of daily living.

EXERCISE

Much has also been written about the value of physical fitness and exercise in the aging population. Data are presented in Tables 5-2 and 5-3, but definitive conclusions are still not possible until a sufficient number of longitudinal studies are performed.

Table 5-2
Comparison of the Effects of Aging and Physical Conditioning on the Cardiovascular System

Variable	Effect of aging	Effect of physical conditioning
A. Submaximal exercise		
1. Heart rate at standard work	Little or no change	Decrease
2. Recovery time for heart rate	Increase	Decrease
3. Systolic blood pressure at standard work load	Increase	Decrease
4. Pulmonary ventilation per liter of oxygen consumed	Increase	Decrease
5. Blood lactate concentration at standard work load	Increase	Decrease
B. Maximal exercise		
1. Oxygen consumption		
a. ml/kg/min	Decrease	Increase
b. ml/kgLBM/min	Decrease	Increase
2. Heart rate	Decrease	Little or no change or slight decrease
3. Stroke volume	Slight decrease	Increase
4. Cardiac output	Slight decrease	Slight increase
5. Blood lactate concentration	Decrease	Increase

Source: J.S. Skinner. Exercise, aging and longevity. Proceedings of 8th International Congress of Gerontology. Washington, D.C., 1969, p. 48. Reprinted with permission.

Table 5-3
Comparison of the Effects of Aging and Physical Conditioning on Body Composition and Motor Performance

Variable	Effect of aging	Effect of physical conditioning
A. Body composition		
1. Weight	Increase (to age 60, then decrease)	Decrease or no change (after 60?)
2. Fat	Increase (to age 60, then decrease)	Decrease (after 60?)
3. Fat-free weight	Decrease	Increase (after 60?)
4. Total body water	Decrease	Increase*
5. Intracellular water	Decrease	Increase*
B. Motor performance		
1. Strength	Decrease	Increase
2. Muscular endurance	Decrease	Increase
3. Speed	Decrease	Increase
4. Power	Decrease	Increase
5. Balance	Decrease	Increase or no change
6. Muscular efficiency	Slight decrease	Slight increase or no change
7. Neuromuscular co-ordination		
a. fine motor skills	No change	No change
b. gross motor skills	Decrease	Increase

*Proportional to change in fat-free weight.
Source: J.S. Skinner. Exercise, aging and longevity. In Proceedings of 8th International Congress of Gerontology. Washington, D.C., 1969, p. 48. Reprinted with permission.

Degenerative changes that can result from prolonged inactivity, either forced or elective, have been documented based on data obtained from American astronauts. Specifically, for the elderly, many complications of inactivity and bed rest are well known. Cardiovascular deconditioning is probably one of the most important complications of inactivity. Quite a number of other negative effects can be listed, including a negative nitrogen balance, decreased resting pulse rate, weight loss, muscle weakness, bowel and bladder dysfunction, ankylosis, respiratory deconditioning, inappropriate secretion of antidiuretic hormone, and overgrowth of opportunistic organism (Oster 1976; Goldman 1977). Among the chief factors leading to emotional sterility, depression, and anxiety with associated agitation are a decline in sensory function and locomotor function (Dénes 1976). Ineffectual behavior and abnormalities in reflex time responses are associated frequently with inactivity in the elderly.

Inactivity and bed rest may also adversely affect drug metabolism and produce unanticipated drug effects. There are, in fact, no criteria for the need for bed rest and no measure for its adequacy. Bed rest may, indeed, be unwise in some circumstances and should not be suggested routinely. Conversely, there is evidence that work and activity contribute positively to well-being. Those who keep active and/or work after retirement are more likely than nonactive or nonworking people to describe themselves as being in good health. It has been stated that the cardiopulmonary system of former "minor" athletes is likely to be younger than it would appear otherwise and that these people are likely to live longer than the general population.

The term *gerokinesiatrics* denotes the prevention and/or management of physical problems of the elderly by means of gymnastics or muscular action. Ludotherapy (treatment by games) brings withdrawn elderly patients into contact with other people, which improves their physical health. The increase in cerebral blood flow and circulation and the greater feeling of well-being observed in elderly persons participating in this type therapy often are the reasons for striking changes in ability to cope with stress.

Exercise is an important part of the management of the elderly individual. It promotes cardiovascular fitness, muscle tone, and increased vitality. In some cases, it may even delay the noticeable signs of aging. Elderly persons should promote physical fitness through exercise, but the activity should not exceed the capacity of the aged cardiovascular, musculoskeletal, and respiratory systems (Schmidt 1974). Rhythmic exercises are very suitable for older persons, as they place minimum stress on the heart. Walking is very beneficial.

Sometimes, it is best not to use the term *exercise* as an elderly person may feel unable to cope with an exercise program. The term *physically active* can evoke a better response. In some instances, activity should start with short walks, first covering only a few blocks. Later, perhaps, walks can be extended to a quarter mile and the distance can be gradually increased to one mile. Then the patient might be encouraged to decrease gradually the time it takes to walk that mile. This activity improves musculoskeletal function and the mental outlook of the patient. Physical conditioning, of course, also directly benefits the cardiovascular system.

Specific exercise programs can produce specific, physiologic improvements in the elderly and exercise therapy has been positively correlated with cognition (DeCarlo et al 1977). In general, patients participating in an exercise program have significantly better health ratings than those who do not participate (Frekany and Leslie 1975; Powell 1974). Participation in endurance-type exercise between the ages of 20 and 70 years improves maximum work capacity (Hodgson and Buskirk 1977). The greater vulnerability of the elderly to higher temperatures and higher humidities must be taken into consideration. The elderly most likely suffer from a reduced efficiency of temperature regulation; drug therapy can further jeopardize temperature regulation, and as the elderly perspire less, they benefit less from evaporative cooling.

As far as the cardiovascular system is concerned, it has been suggested that fit and active people are spared the complications of atherosclerosis (Morris and Crawford 1958; Mann et al 1972), and that exercise even enlarges atherosclerotic vessels so that the capacity of coronary vessels increases, despite the presence of atherosclerosis (Karvonen et al 1961). Activity exerts a sparing effect on coronary heart disease (Paffenbarger et al 1977; Keys 1970) and there is evidence of a threshold for the intensity of activity needed to protect against coronary heart disease (Morris et al 1973). A graduated exercise program can be beneficial in increasing collateral circulation in arteriosclerosis obliterans, leading to a significant return of ambulation with exercise (Moylan 1975).

The musculoskeletal system benefits from exercise that stresses relaxation and stretching of tight muscles as well as strengthening of weak muscles, even in patients with advanced osteoarthritic changes (Kraus 1978). Improvement of mobility of the spinal and lower limb joints by systematic exercise can be achieved even in patients over 70 years of age (Gore 1972).

Finally, protection against senile involution of brain cells can be achieved by physical exercise, which stimulates metabolism, respiration, blood circulation, and digestion (Spirduso 1977).

REFERENCES

Berryman, J.A.W., Forbes, H.A.W., and Simpson-White, R. Trial of procaine in old age and degenerative disorders. *Br Med J.* 2:1683, 1961.

DeCarlo, T.J., Castiglione, L.V., and Cavusoglu, M. A program of balanced physical fitness in the preventive care of elderly ambulatory patients. *J Am Geriatr Soc.* 25:331, 1977.

Dénes, Z. Old-age emotions. *J Am Geriatr Soc.* 24:465, 1976.

Fee, S.R., and Clark, A.N.C. Trial of procaine in the aged. *Br Med J.* 2:1680, 1961.

Frekany, G., and Leslie, D. Effects of an exercise program on selected flexibility measurements of senior citizens. *Gerontologist* 15:182, 1975.

Goldman, R. Rest: its use and abuse in the aged. *J Am Geriatr Soc.* 25:433, 1977.

Gore, I.Y. Physical activity and ageing—a survey of Soviet literature. *Gerontol Clin.* 14:65, 1972.

Hirsh, J. Clinical trial of procaine hydrochloride. *Br Med J.* 2:1684, 1961.

Hodgson, J.L., and Buskirk, E.R. Physical fitness and age, with emphasis on cardiovascular function in the elderly. *J Am Geriatr Soc.* 25:385, 1977.

Isaacs, B. Trials of procaine in aged patients. *Br Med J.* 1:188, 1962.

Karvonen, M.J., Rautaharju, P.M., Orma, E. et al. Cardiovascular studies on lumberjacks. *J Occup Med.* 3:49, 1961.

Kent, S. A look at Gerovital—the "youth" drug. *Geriatrics* 31:95, 1976.

Keys, A. Coronary heart disease in seven countries. *Circulation* 41 (suppl 1):I-1–I-211, 1970.

Kraus, H. Reconditioning aging muscles. *Geriatrics* 33(6):93, 1978.

LaBalla, F.S. Pharmacolongevity: control of aging by drugs. Edited by A.A. Rubin, In *Search for New Drugs*. New York: Marcel Dekker, 1972.

Mann, G.V., Spoerry, A., Gray, M. et al. Atherosclerosis in the Masai. *Am J Epidemiol.* 95:26, 1972.

Morris, J.N., and Crawford, M.D. Coronary heart disease and physical activity of work: evidence of a national necropsy study. *Br Med J.* 2:1485, 1958.

Morris, J.N., Chave, S.P.W., Adam, C. et al. Vigorous exercise in leisure time and the incidence of coronary heart disease. *Lancet* 1:333, 1973.

Moylan, J.A. Problems of aging: diagnosing and treating leg pain due to arteriosclerosis obliterans. *Postgrad Med.* 58(4):135, 1975.

Oster, C. Sensory deprivation in geriatric patients. *J Am Geriatr Soc.* 24:461, 1976.

Ostfeld, A., Smith, C.M., and Stotsky, B.A. The systemic use of procaine in the treatment of the elderly: a review. *J Am Geriatr Soc.* 25:1, 1977.

Paffenbarger, R.S., Hale, W.E., Brand, R.J. et al. Work energy level: personal characteristics and fatal heart attack: a British cohort effect. *Am J Epidemiol.* 105:200, 1977.

Powell, R. Psychological effects of exercise therapy upon institutionalized geriatric mental patients. *J Gerontol.* 29:157, 1974.

Schmidt, J. Bedingungen fuer Sport im Alter. *Med Klin.* 69:371, 1974.

Spirduso, W.W. Reaction and movement time as a function of age and physical activity level. *J Gerontol.* 30:435, 1977.

6 Health Care Expenditures and Drugs

NATIONAL HEALTH CARE EXPENDITURES

Depending on the source, data on health care expenditures may differ slightly. The overall impression derived from all data, regardless of source, is one of galloping increases and exceedingly large outlays. The United States spent approximately $139.3 billion dollars for health care in the year ending 30 June 1976. This was a 14% increase compared to the previous year. Both the total amount and the rate of increase continue to grow substantially. In fiscal year 1977, it is estimated that expenditures reached $162.5 billion, an increase of more than 16% over 1976 (Tables 6-1 and 6-2). This annual growth in national health expenditures exceeds the growth in expenditures for any other goods or services. As a result, the health care portion of the Gross National Product (GNP) increased from 8.4% in 1975 to 8.6% in 1976 (Figure 6-1). These increases in expenditures and percent of GNP continue a trend. In 1950, health care outlays accounted for 4.5% of the GNP. By 1970, that portion had increased to 7.2%. The recent, accelerated rate of growth has been explained on the basis of the high inflationary rate in medical care prices, as well as technologic advances and other quality changes, population growth, and increased utilization of health care services and facilities.

The major share of national health expenditures pays for hospital care (Figure 6-2). In 1950, hospital care cost $3.7 billion, or 31% of total

Table 6-1
Health Care Expenditures, USA

	Billion of dollars			Percentage of Gross National Product		
	1950	*1965*	*1975*	*1950*	*1965*	*1975*
Hospitals	3.7	13.2	46.6	1.4	2.0	3.3
Physicians	2.7	8.4	22.1	1.0	1.3	1.6
Drugs	1.6	4.6	10.6	0.6	0.7	0.7
Nursing homes	0.2	1.3	9.0	0.1	0.2	0.6

Source: Social Security Administration, 1975.
Total in 1975: $142.4 billion and 8.3% of GNP.

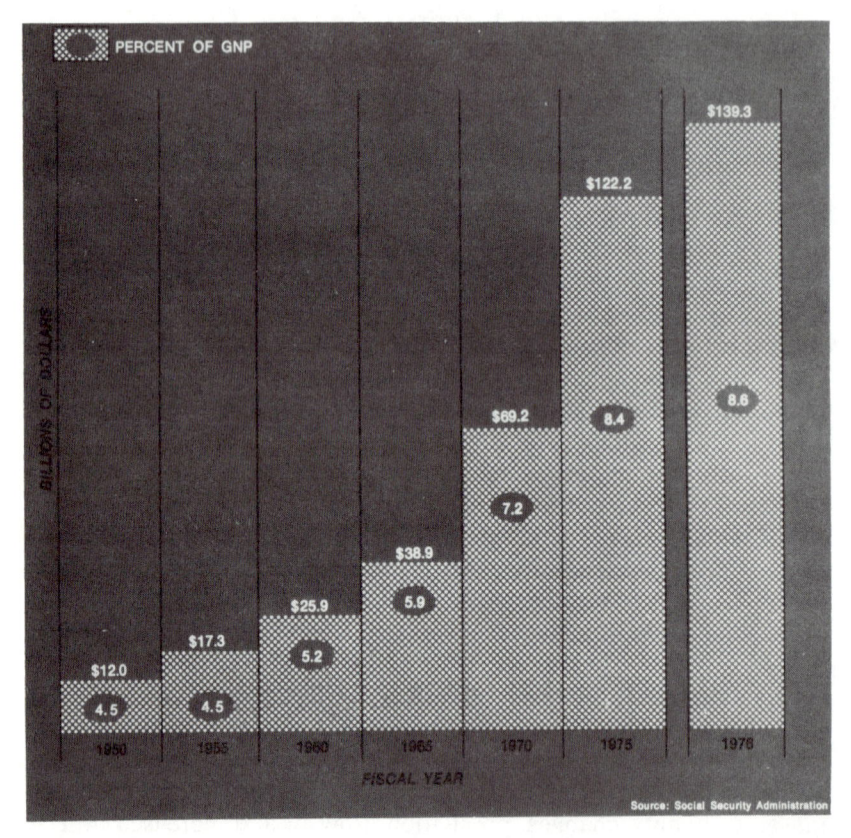

Figure 6-1 National health expenditures and percent of GNP—selected fiscal years 1950–1976.

Table 6-2
Health Care Expenditures, Fiscal Year 1977

Type	Expenditure ($)*	Percent of total
Hospitals	65.5	40.0
Physicians	32.2	20.0
Nursing homes	12.6	8.0
Drugs	12.5	8.0
Administrative expenses and public health programs	11.3	7.0
Dentists	10.0	6.0
Other	9.6	6.0
Construction	5.1	3.1
Research	3.7	2.3

*In billions of dollars.

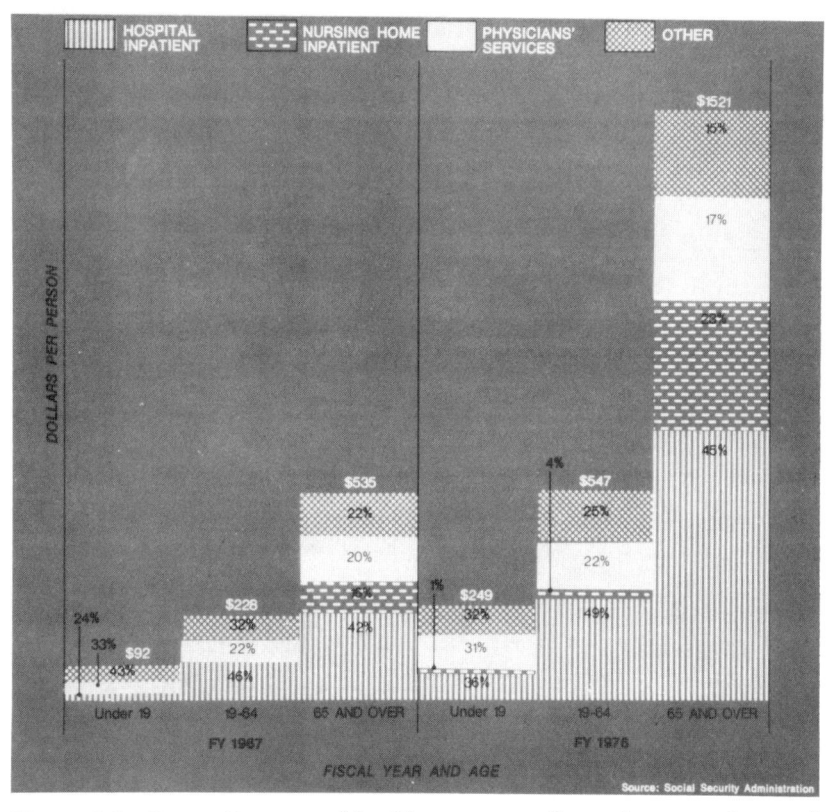

Figure 6-2 Per capita personal health care expenditures by age and type of expenditure—fiscal years 1967 and 1976.

health care spending. In 1970, it took $25.9 billion, or 37%. By 1976, hospital costs amounted to more than $55.4 billion, or 40% of the total. This growth is partly attributed to an increase in the population and an aging of the population. Expenditures for nursing home care are rising most rapidly, having increased from $3.8 billion, or 6% of the total in 1970 to $10.6 billion, or 8% of the total health care bill in 1976. As the number of old people increases, this component of health care expenditures will probably increase too. The proportionate shares of the health care dollar are depicted in Figure 6-3 for 1974.

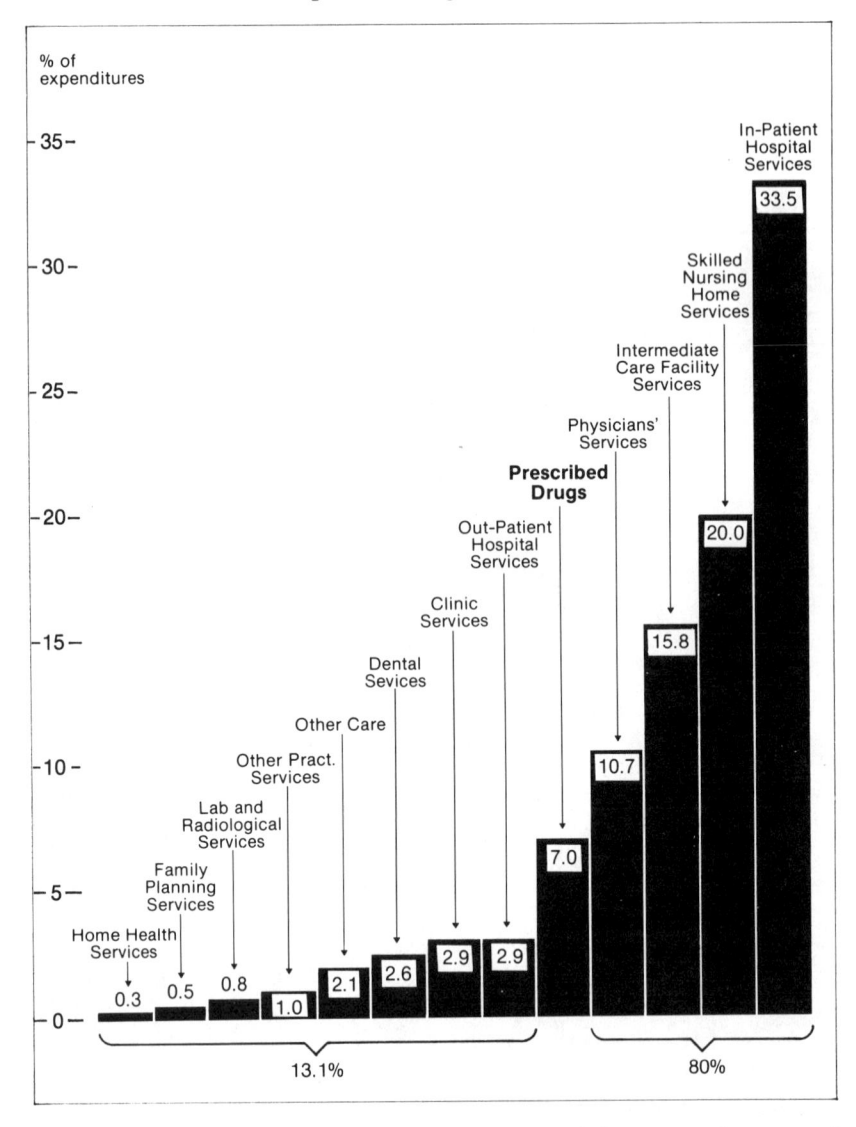

Figure 6-3 The distribution of the health care dollar: apportionment of medical care expenditures under public assistance programs, 1974.

As the share for hospital care and nursing home care increases, the share for other health care services declines proportionally. Physicians' services declined to 19% from 22% in 1950, dentists' services from 8% to 6%, and payments for drugs and drug sundries from 14% to 8%. Part of the latter decrease may be related to new regulations that no longer permit reimbursement for nonprescription drugs.

HEALTH CARE COSTS OF THE ELDERLY

Although they comprise only approximately 10% of the population of the United States, the elderly use more than 27% of the health care dollar. They comprise 30% of the adult patients in the general medical and surgical units of hospitals and the majority of residents in nursing homes are elderly (Somers and Somers 1967; Cantor and Mayer 1972). Similar statistics have been published in England (Hunt 1973). Regardless of income, disability is a prevalent characteristic of the elderly. In 1972, more than 40% of noninstitutionalized elderly (compared to 13% of the general population) had some limitations of normal activity because of a chronic condition. Limitations tend to occur more frequently in elderly with low incomes. Although only 5% of the older American population is institutionalized at a given time, 25% of the elderly are institutionalized at some time in their older years. Elderly persons, regardless of the type of illness or injury, tend to be confined to bed and to be restricted in activity longer than any other persons. Seventeen percent of those 65 years and older are admitted to hospitals for acute care at least once a year, for a total of 33.3 admissions per 100 population. The average length of stay is approximately 12.2 days (all diagnoses), resulting in 4077 days/1000 population, 65 years and over/year of acute hospital care generated. The hospital stay of the elderly is two to three times longer compared with that of middle-aged persons with similar diseases. Thus, older people spend more time as inpatients. For example, in 1974, children aged 5 to 12 years spent less than one-half day per year in a hospital and adults between the ages of 55 and 64 years spent two days per year. In contrast, people between 65 and 74 years spent 3.3 days/year and those older than 75 years of age averaged 5.6 days per year (US Department of Health, Education and Welfare 1978).

The increase with age in nursing home time is even more dramatic. Young people do not spend time in nursing homes; even those between the ages of 55 and 64 years average less than one-half day per year. This increases to 4.4 days/year for those between 65 and 74 years, to 21.5 days for those between 75 and 84 years, and those over 85 years, spend an average of 86.4 days per year in a nursing home (Figure 6-4). The elderly spent more time in nursing homes than in hospitals. Those over 75 years of age spent six times as much time in nursing homes as in hospitals. Thus, it is not at all surprising that health care costs increase with age (Figure 6-5).

The Department of Health, Education and Welfare reported to the Congress of the United States that health care costs for the elderly had risen from $8.2 billion in fiscal year 1966 to $34.9 billion in fiscal year 1976. Health care costs of the elderly increased at an annual rate of 15.5% in that decade, as compared to 11.8% for those under 65 years of age. Per capita expenditures for the elderly in 1976 ($1521) were almost three times greater than those for persons 19 to 64 years of age ($547), and more than six times higher than those for persons under the age of 19 years. Although out-of-pocket health expenses increase in almost all categories with age (Table 6-3), more than two-thirds of the money spent on the personal health care of individuals older than 65

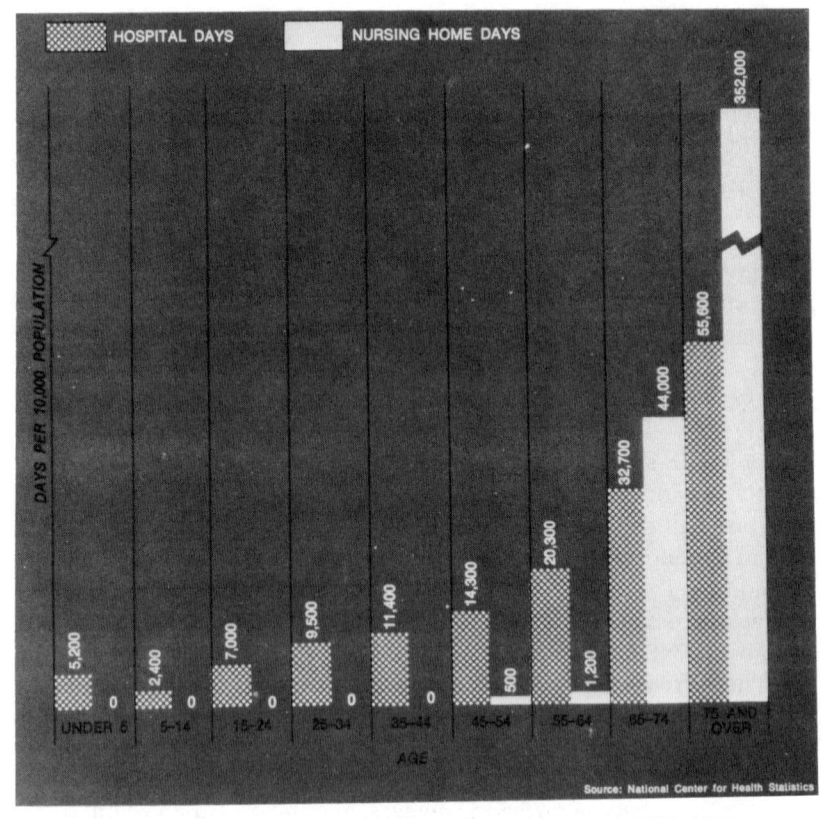

Figure 6-4 Days in hospitals and nursing homes by age—1973–1974.

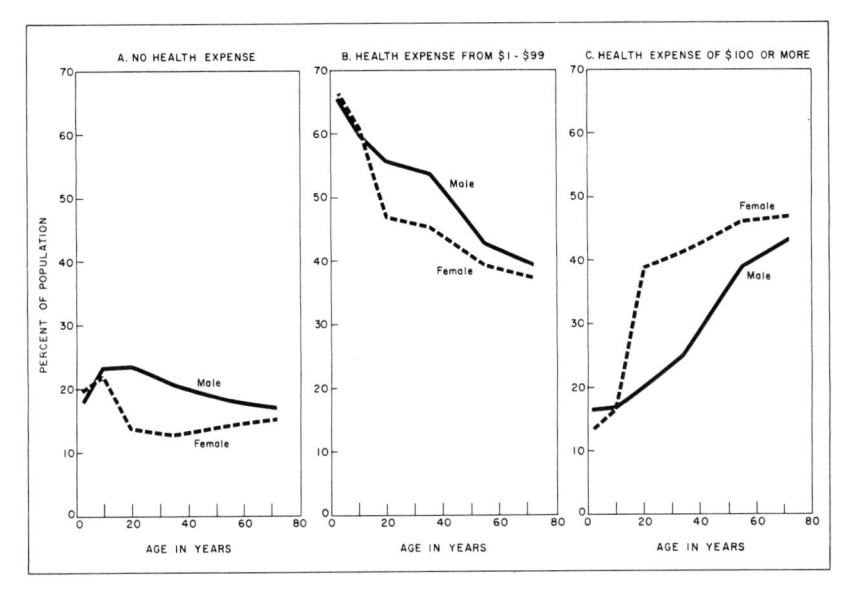

Figure 6-5 Percent of population, by amount of health expenditures per year according to sex and age.

Table 6-3
Average Out-of-Pocket Health Expenses $/Year

	Years of Age			
Expenses	<17	17–44	45–64	65+
All	152	246	386	425
Hospital	99	195	352	293
Doctor	55	99	128	143
Dental	75	95	125	105
R Drugs	28	41	83	109
Optical	51	65	64	62
Health insurance	64	84	130	138
Other	79	135	127	259

Source: Current estimates. From the Health Interview Survey, U.S. 1975, DHEW Publ. No. (HRA) 77-1543. Rockville, Md.: National Center for Health Statistics, 1977.

years is for hospital care and nursing homes, and only 17% is spent for physicians' services. In contrast, less than two-fifths of the expenditures for people under age 19 years is spent for hospitals and nursing homes (almost all of it is spent for hospitals), but almost 33% is used to reimburse for physician services. For people aged 19 to 64 years, about one-half of the expenditures are for hospital and nursing home care and 20% for physician services.

Differences in expenditures probably reflect differences in the types of illnesses experienced by different age groups and the types of services used to manage those illnesses. The national average for nursing home care exceeds $7000 per year and skilled nursing care can cost more than $10,000 per year per resident. The frail elderly, living alone, enter institutions at an earlier stage of debility and remain institutionalized longer than others (Weissert 1978). In Connecticut, an average length of stay in nursing homes of more than 600 days has been postulated; and in southern Massachusetts, it has been suggested that the cost for 8000 nursing home residents ($3.6 million per month) could be reduced to $672,000 per month if these people could be managed in the community (Morris and Harris 1972).

The cost to the elderly of health care services is high and continues to rise disproportionately. Public and private third-party payments for medical care increased from 30% in 1966 to 68% in 1976, still leaving a large share of the total health care cost uncovered. The Senate Special Committee on Aging, in a report issued in July 1975, noted that health care costs for senior citizens are three times higher than for younger persons, with Medicare covering only 38% of the costs. The committee, therefore, strongly urged reimbursement for eyeglasses, hearing aids, dentures, and outpatient prescriptions.

DRUGS AND THE ELDERLY

The increased incidence of disease with advancing age is reflected by an increased drug use by the elderly and increased prescribing of drugs for the elderly. The most serious health problems are encountered among the old-old group. The healing process is impaired and even minor problems, if not treated and permitted to linger, can develop into major problems (Kovar 1977). There are not yet any systematic epidemiologic studies on drug use, misuse, and abuse on large populations of elderly persons (Bozzetti and MacMurray 1977), and it is frequently not realized that the use of drugs in geriatric patients has the potential to reduce the patient's quality of life. Nearly all drugs pose, potentially, special problems in geriatric medicine, but certain drugs deserve special attention because of their increased use or because they may pose particular challenges to the prescriber. Anticoagulants, anticonvulsants, antihypertensives, antibiotics, antineoplastic agents, cardiac drugs, and psychotropic drugs cause severe adverse effects with increasing frequency in the elderly (Wallace and Watanabe 1977). Even less frequently recognized, quite possibly, is the fact that nonprescription drugs too can cause potential problems, particularly in the elderly. Ten percent of more than 4000 studies between 1962 and 1975 on drug abuse in the elderly deal with the possible adverse pathologic and physiologic effects on the elderly caused by nonprescription drugs (Basen 1977). For example, bromide intoxication was, at one time, not infrequent (Carney 1971; Stewart 1973) and antihistamines, anticholinergics, and aspirin have all been associated with severe adverse effects in the elderly (Morrant 1975; Bengstson et al 1975; George 1972; Murray et al 1971).

Exemplifying the problem is the case of an 80-year-old woman with high blood pressure, congestive heart failure, diabetes, ankle edema, and obesity. Her physician prescribed a regimen including an oral hypoglycemic agent, a reducing diet, a long-acting oral nitrate, nitroglycerin, a thiazide diuretic, and antacids. Periodically, she also takes a blood thinner. The patient takes the diuretic only when she has a headache. Despite the label instructions, she takes two or three at a time. Once, in order not to forget, she took the oral hypoglycemic, to be taken twice a day, in the morning at short intervals. She keeps all drugs in the refrigerator in the belief that this will preserve them, while in reality the condensation that occurs when the containers are taken from the refrigerator may cause deterioration and inactivation of the drugs.

Probably, only two of the drugs in her regimen are justified. The diuretic is appropriate therapy for her congestive heart failure and hypertension, but may make treatment of her diabetes more difficult. If diabetic control is significantly impaired by the thiazide diuretic, consideration should be given to the substitution of insulin for the oral hypoglycemic agent, although it is not clear whether the patient needs any hypoglycemic agent. If diabetic control is still needed, her physician might try another antihypertensive agent and discontinue the diuretic. In addition, the patient probably would benefit from carefully monitored digitalis therapy for congestive heart failure. If digitalis is added to her regimen, she should be encouraged to follow directions carefully for potassium supplements if needed.

Unfortunately, the patient does not understand the dietary instructions and does not follow them. She overeats. Her physician treats her gastric symptoms with antacids. The vasodilators were prescribed only because of vague complaints of chest pain. In 10 years, the physician has not changed the regimen, even though lack of success should have prompted review and change. It would have been far better for the physician to have taken the time to explain the need for adherence to the diet, to make sure that the diuretic was taken as directed, and to consider whether or not the chest pains merited any drug therapy at all.

Thus, despite the need for special care in prescribing drugs for the elderly, they receive an extraordinary number of drugs. It has been reported that more than 85% of elderly ambulatory patients and almost 95% of elderly institutionalized patients receive drugs (Laventurier and Talley 1977; Law and Chalmers 1976), 25% of which may be ineffective or unneeded (Bergman 1975). In the early part of this decade, Americans 65 years of age and over received approximately 22% of all prescriptions, even though at that time they accounted only for 9% of the total population. The mean number of prescriptions received per family increases consistently with the age of the head of the household. In general, individuals over 65 years of age receive more prescription medications than does any other age group. The average number of new prescriptions and refills for those 65 years and older is more than twice that for the total population, and nearly three times that for those under 65 years of age (National Center for Health Statistics 1967).

Drug use is age-specific and reflects patient risk to various types of diseases. Drugs prescribed for regular (chronic) use are more frequently prescribed for the elderly, while drug use intended for occasional use does not change with age (Sotaniemi and Palva 1972). This confirms simply that in chronic medical conditions, reliance on associated drug therapy tends to increase with age (National Center for Health Statistics 1967). While it was predicted in the early 1970s that the annual prescription demand for the aged through 1980 would be 9.3 per man and 13.1 per woman (Froh 1971), the elderly already averaged more than 13 prescriptions per year in 1974 (Lamy and Vestal 1976). (Specific data are presented in Figure 6-6.) In one study, about one-half of 127 randomly selected patients over 70 years of age were on long-term therapy, using drugs associated with heart disease, depression, or anxiety (Shaw and Opit 1976). In general, studies have shown that cardiovascular drugs account for 25% of the 100 most frequently prescribed drugs for those 65 years and older, diuretics for approximately 15%, and analgesics for approximately 13%. In addition, it is safe to assume that the elderly, similar to the younger age groups, use nonprescription drugs, mainly analgesics, antacids, laxatives, and vitamins.

A study of day treatment center patients confirmed the belief that there is a direct association among chronic illness, limitation of activity, and number of drugs prescribed and/or used (Boykin et al 1978). Although the total number of drugs prescribed and/or used bears little

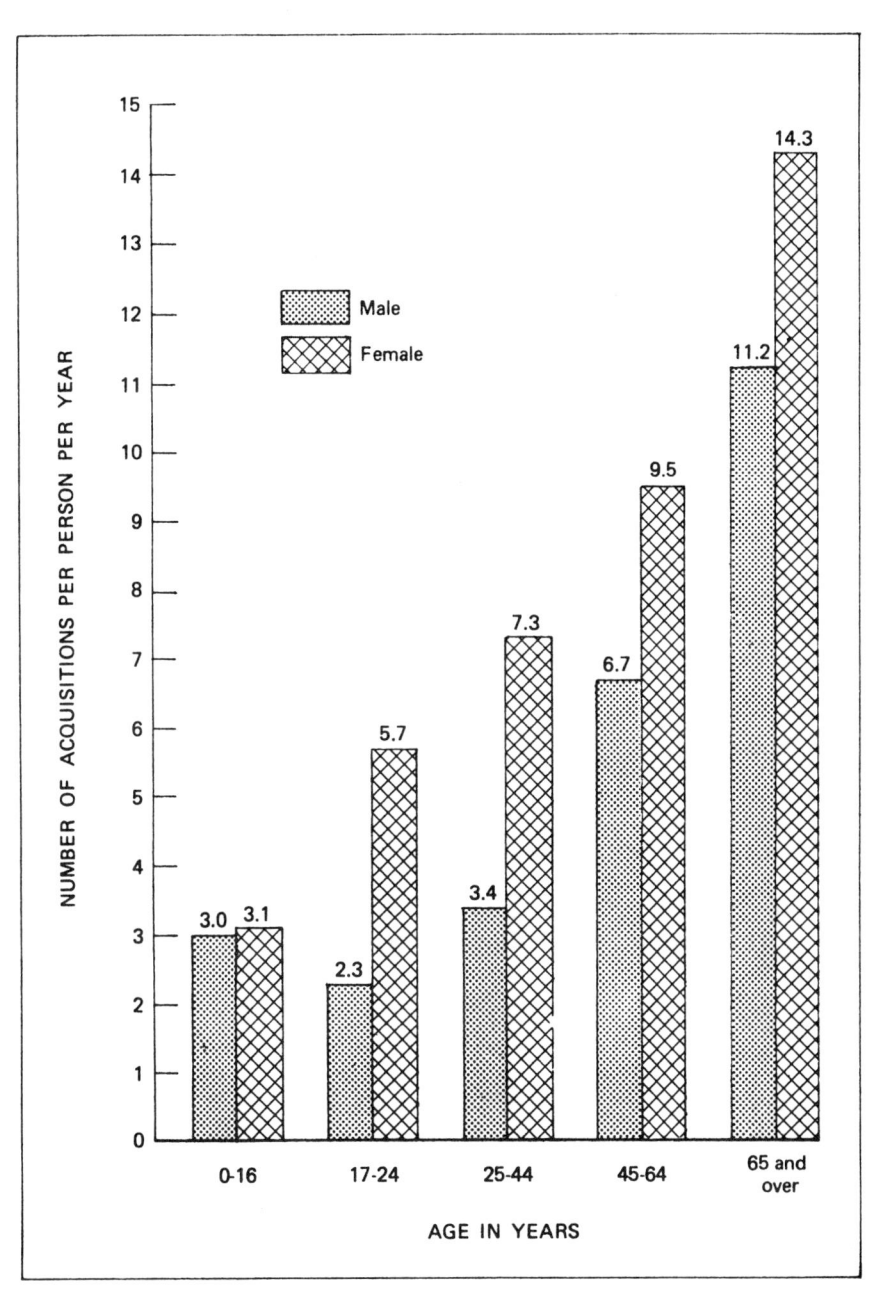

Figure 6-6 Number of acquisitions of prescribed medicine per person per year, by sex and age.

relation to the number of diagnoses (Table 6-4), it is clear that patients use a large number of nonprescription drugs (Table 6-5), and that a very large number of drugs are ordered "as needed" (Table 6-6), which tends to increase the average number of drugs and administered doses (Ingman et al 1975).

Somewhat different statistics are documented for institutionalized elderly. The number of prescription drugs per patient in an institution has been variously estimated as between five and 12. In 1971, the average hospitalized Medicare patient received about 10 drugs (Nithman et al 1971). Recently, it was shown that the leading drugs for institutionalized elderly patients were the tranquilizers, which in one study constituted almost 20% of all drug use. An audit of drugs used in

Table 6-4
Diagnoses and Drug Use in a Day Treatment Center Population

No. of diagnoses	Total no. of drugs
1	5
2	11
3	11
4	15
5	13
6	16
7	9

Source: Boykin, S.P., Burkhart, V.P., and Lamy, P.P. Drug use in a day treatment center. *Am J Hosp Pharm.* 35:155, 1978.

Table 6-5
Nonprescription Drug Utilization by a Day Treatment Center Population

Category	Prescribed	Actually used
Anti-infective agents	3	4
CNS drugs	21	33
Cough and cold	--	7
EENT	2	21
Gastrointestinal drugs	23	61
Skin preparations	4	58

Source: Boykin, S.P., Burkhart, V.P., and Lamy, P.P. Drug use in a day treatment center. *Am J Hosp Pharm.* 35: 155, 1978.

nursing homes in New Jersey, Illinois, and Ohio (Table 6-7) showed that of the 12 most frequently used drugs, four were tranquilizers, four were sedatives, and four were analgesics (*Nursing Home Care* 1975). (Other drug use data, collected by different government agencies, are presented in Tables 6-8–6-11.)

Table 6-6
Drugs Ordered on a PRN Basis for Day Treatment Center Patients

Category	Percent of drugs PRN
Antihistamines	50
Autonomic agents	25
Cardiovascular drugs	17
CNS drugs	47
Cough and cold	95
Gastrointestinal	100
Skin preparations	100

Source: Boykin, S.P., Burkhart, V.P., and Lamy, P.P. Drug use in a day treatment center. *Am J Hosp Pharm.* 35:155, 1978.

Table 6-7
Most Prescribed Drugs by Number of Prescriptions

1. Thorazine (T)	23,126
2. Darvon compound (A)	21,436
3. Mellaril (T)	17,977
4. Phenobarbital (S)	9,663
5. Chloral hydrate (S)	8,264
6. Doriden (S)	7,802
7. Librium (T)	7,259
8. Aspirin and Bufferin (A)	6,875
9. Nembutal (S)	6,133
10. Valium (T)	5,308
11. Darvon (T)	4,681
12. Indocin (A)	4,477

Key: T = Tranquilizer, A = Analgesic, S = Sedative.
Source: 14-Month study. Drugs paid for by Medicaid in Illinois, New Jersey, and Ohio nursing homes. Subcommittee on Long-Term Care, Special Committee on Aging, U.S. Senate, Nursing home care in the United States: failure in public policy, Supporting Paper No. 2, Drugs in nursing homes: misuse, high costs, and kickbacks. Washington, D.C.: U.S. Government Printing Office, 1975.

Table 6-8
Range in Percent of Prescriptions Per Patient in Skilled Nursing Facilities

Number of prescriptions	Percent of patients
None	0.1
One	3.8
Two	6.3
Three	10.9
Four	11.9
Five	12.9
Six	12.7
Seven	10.0
Eight	9.4
Nine	6.4
Ten	4.9
Eleven	3.2
Twelve	2.6
Thirteen	1.8
Fourteen	1.3
Fifteen or more	1.8

Source: Long-term care facility improvement campaign. Monograph No. 2, Physicians' drug prescribing patterns in skilled nursing facilities, U.S. DHEW, PHS, Office of Long Term Care, DHEW Publ. No. (OS) 76-50050, Washington, D.C.: U.S. Government Printing Office, 1976.

Table 6-9
Most Frequently Used Drugs in Skilled Nursing Facilities

Drug category	Percent patients receiving
Cathartics	53.3
Analgesics and antipyretics	47.7
Tranquilizers	44.8
Diuretics	33.8
Vitamins	33.3
Sedatives and hypnotics	33.2
Cardiac drugs	28.9
Skin and mucous membrane	17.7
Anti-infectives	16.9
Antacids and absorbents	14.2
Antihistamines	13.8
Hypotensives	12.4
Eye, ear, nose, and throat	11.8
Spasmolytics	11.4
Insulin and antidiabetic agents	11.1
Electrolyte replacements	9.9

Table 6-9 *(continued)*

Drug category	Percent patients receiving
Vasodilating agents	8.6
Antidepressants	8.4
Anticonvulsants	7.4
Estrogens/androgens	3.5
Thyroid replacements and antithyroid agents	2.5
Adrenals	2.2
Anticoagulants	1.0

Source: Long-term care facility improvement study, Introductory Report, Office of Nursing Home Affairs, DHEW Publ. No. (OS) 76-50021, Rockville, Md., 1975.

Table 6-10
Twenty Most Frequently Prescribed Drugs for Patients in Skilled Nursing Facilities in Rank Order

Drug
Aspirin*
Magnesium hydroxide*
Multivitamins*
Digoxin
Propoxyphene
Thioridazine
Furosemide
Chloral hydrate and chloral betaine
Dioctyl sodium sulfosuccinate*
Chlorpromazine
Aluminum hydroxide and/or magnesium hydroxide*
Diazepam
Potassium
Bisacodyl
Ferrous (iron) preparations*
Diphenylhydantoin
Hydrochlorothiazide
Diphenoxylate
Insulin
Diphenhydramine

*Nonprescription drug
Source: Long-term care facility improvement campaign. Monograph No. 2, Physicians' drug prescribing patterns in skilled nursing facilities. U.S. DHEW, PHS, Office of Long Term Care, DHEW Publ. No. (OS) 76-50050, Washington, D.C.: U.S. Government Printing Office, 1976.

Table 6-11
Prescription Drug Use in Skilled Nursing Facilities

Drug	Percent of patients
Psychotropic	51.3
Cardiac, antihypertensives, diuretics	13.0
Vasodilators	11.5
Insulin	10.5
Antidepressants	8.6
Estrogens	4.4

No. of Patients: 283,915
No. of Prescription Drugs: 1,731,360
Av. No. of Rx Drugs/Patient: 6.1
Source: Long-term care facility improvement campaign. Monograph No. 2, Physicians' drug prescribing patterns in skilled nursing facilities. U.S. DHEW, PHS, Office of Long Term Care, DHEW Publ. No. (OS) 76-50050, Washington, D.C.: U.S. Government Printing Office, 1976.

Drug Costs

In prescribing for the elderly, one must carefully consider the patient's ability to meet the economic demands of medical care. Only 60% of physician cost is paid from public funds and, more importantly, only 13% of drug cost is so paid.

It has been estimated that 20% of the elderly's out-of-pocket expenditures are for medicine (National Council on Aging 1970). (Actual expenditures are presented in Table 6-12 and Figure 6-7.) This is a significant expenditure when one considers that the elderly are on fixed incomes and are, in most instances, no longer wage earners (Ching-Piao et al 1978). (More data on prescribed medicines and their cost are documented in Table 6-13 and Figure 6-8.) Table 6-14 depicts the conditions for which drugs are most frequently prescribed and specific costs of prescriptions. Prescription costs also tend to rise with an increase in major activity limitation (Table 6-15).

Table 6-12
Out-of-Pocket Expense for Medicines*

	Male	Female
All ages	$18.60	$28.60
45–64 years	32.30	43.70
65 years and over	54.60	66.30

*Per person per year
Source: Out-of-pocket cost and acquisition of prescribed medicines, U.S. 1973. DHEW Publ. No. (HRA) 77-1542, Rockville, Md.: National Center for Health Statistics, 1977.

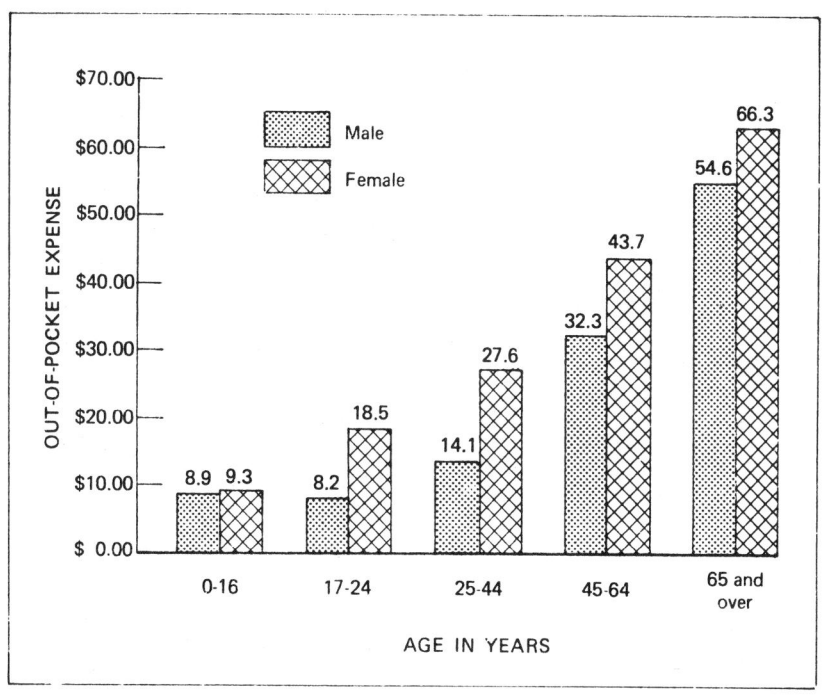

Figure 6-7 Out-of-pocket prescription medicine expense per person per year, by age and sex.

Table 6-13
Prescribed Medicines

	All ages	45–64 years	65 years and over
Percent of population	100	21	9.8
Percent of R acquired	100	29	22
Percent of R paid for by patient or family	74.1	73.6	75.7
No. of R obtained per person/year	5.8	8.2	13.2
Av. cost/purchase	$4.80	$5.40	$5.40

Source: Out-of-pocket cost and acquisition of prescribed medicines, U.S. 1973. DHEW Publ. No. (HRA) 77-1542, Rockville, Md.: National Center for Health Statistics, 1977.

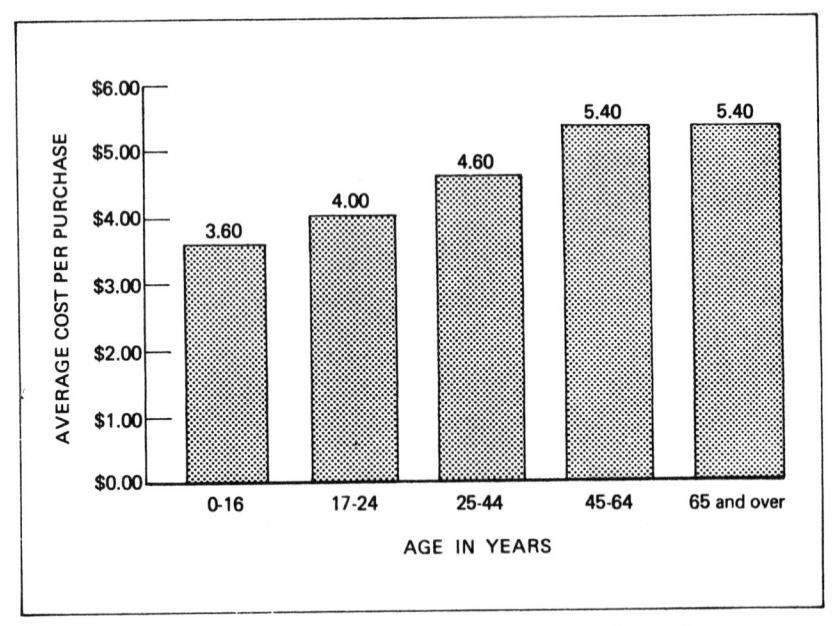

Figure 6-8 Average cost per purchase of prescribed medicine, by age.

Table 6-14
Conditions for Which Drugs Were Most Frequently Prescribed

Condition	All ages	45–64 years	65 years and over
High blood pressure	6.8	10.9	13.2*(5.80)†
Heart conditions	5.4	7.8	12.4 (5.20)
Arthritis and disorders of bones and joints	3.8	5.4	7.5 (6.40)
Mental and nervous conditions	7.5	10.3	7.1 (5.20)
Other digestive system conditions	4.5	4.8	5.3 (4.40)
Other disorders of circulatory system	1.9	1.9	4.7 (6.90)
Diabetes	2.8	4.4	4.6 (6.30)
Eye or ear conditions	3.9	2.4	3.4 (4.60)

*Percent Distribution.
†Av. cost per prescription in 1973.
Source: Out-of-pocket cost and acquisition of prescribed medicines, U.S. 1973. DHEW Publ. No. (HRA) 77-1542, Rockville, Md.: National Center for Health Statistics, 1977.

Table 6-15
Major Activity Limitation and Cost of Prescribed Medicine*

Status	All ages	45–64 years	65 years and over
Limitation but not in M.A.	$ 45.50	62.30	57.00
Limitation in amount or kind of M.A.	$ 76.90	87.70	91.10
Unable to perform M.A.	$100.00	103.00	111.50

*Per Person Per Year.
M.A.: Major activity, ie, work, keep house, school activity
Source: Out-of-pocket cost and acquisition of prescribed medicine, U.S. 1973. DHEW Publ. No. (HRA) 77-1542, Rockville, Md., National Center for Health Statistics, 1977.

These figures and data become more meaningful when the so-called "gray area" population is considered. These people do not qualify for medical assistance, but have an income near the poverty level, and may be unable to meet even normal medical expenses. In large metropolitan areas, one-fifth to one-quarter of the elderly population may fall into this category. Thus, it is likely that many elderly, upon receiving a prescription, may not obtain the prescribed drug for lack of funds.

Medication costs are an important factor in health expenditures for the elderly. Yet, they actually represent a small proportion of total health care expenditures. In selecting a medication, particularly for the elderly, the emphasis should not be on cost but rather on the efficacy (Weintraub 1976).

REFERENCES

Basen, M.M. The elderly and drugs—problem overview and program strategy. *Public Health Report.* 92(1):43, 1977.

Bengstson, U., Angervall, L., and Johansson, L. Phenacetin abuse and renal pelvic carcinoma. *Int J Clin Pharmacol.* 12:290, 1975.

Bergman, H.D. Prescribing drugs in a nursing home. *Drug Intell Clin Pharm.* 9:365, 1975.

Boykin, S.P., Burkhart, V.P., and Lamy, P.P. Drug use in a day treatment center. *Am J Hosp Pharm.* 35:155, 1978.

Bozzetti, L.P., and MacMurray, J.P. Drug misuse among the elderly: a hidden menace. *Psychiatr Ann.* 7:155, 1977.

Cantor, M. and Mayer, M. *Health Crisis for the Older New Yorkers, Facts for Action Series.* New York: Office for the Aging, 1972.

Carney, M.W.P. Five cases of bromism. *Lancet* 2:523, 1971.

Ching-Piao, C., Townsend, E.J., and Ross-Townsend, A. Substance use and abuse among community elderly: the medical aspect. *Add Dis.* 3:357, 1978.

Froh, R.B. Supply and demand of prescription drugs—1970–1980. *J Am Pharm Assoc.* 11:534, 1971.

George, A. A survey of drug use in a Sydney suburb. *Med J Aust.* 2:233, 1972.

Hunt, L.B. The elderly in hospital: recent trends in use of medical resources. *Br Med J.* 4(suppl):83, 1973.

Ingman, S.R., Lawson, I.R., and Pierpaoli, P.G. et al. A survey of the prescribing and administration of drugs in long-term care institutions for the elderly. *J Am Geriatr Soc.* 23:309, 1975.

Kovar, M.G. Health of the elderly and use of health services. *Public Health Rep.* 92:9, 1977.

Lamy, P.P., and Vestal, R.E. Drug prescribing for the elderly. *Hosp Practice.* 11(1):111, 1976.

Laventurier, M.F., and Talley, R.B. The incidence of drug-drug interactions in a Medi-Cal population. *Cal Pharm.* 20:18, 1977.

Law, R., and Chalmers, C. Medicines and elderly people: a general practice survey. *Br Med J.* 1:565, 1976.

Morrant, J.C.A. Medicines and mental illness in old age. *Can Psychiatr Assoc J.* 20:309, 1975.

Morris, R., and Harris, E. Home health services in Massachusetts: their role in the care of the long-term sick. *Am J Public Health.* 62:1088, 1972.

Murray, R.M., Adams, J.H., and Greene, J.G. Analgesic abuse and dementia. *Lancet* 2:242, 1971.

National Center for Health Statistics. *Prescribed and Non-Prescribed Medicines—Types and Use of Medicines.* DHEW Publ. No. 1000, Ser. 10, No. 39. Rockville, Md., 1967.

National Council on Aging. *The Golden Years: A Tarnished Myth.* Washington, D.C., 1970.

Nithman, C.J., Parkhurst, Y.E., and Sommers, E.B. Physicians' prescribing habits: effects of Medicare. *JAMA.* 217:585, 1971.

Shaw, S.M., and Opit, L.J. Need for supervision in the elderly receiving long-term prescribed medication. *Br Med J.* 1:505, 1976.

Somers, H.M., and Somers, A.R. *Medicare and the Hospitals.* Washington, D.C.: Brookings Institute, 1967.

Sotaniemi, E., and Palva, I.P. The use of polypharmaceutical drug therapy in a medical ward. *Ann Clin Res.* 4:158, 1972.

Special Committee on Aging, United States Senate. Nursing home care in the United States: failure in public policy. Supporting Paper No. 2: *Drugs in Nursing Homes: Misuse, High Costs, and Kickbacks.* Washington, D.C.: U.S. Government Printing Office, 1975.

Stewart, R.B. Bromide intoxication from a nonprescription medication. *Am J Hosp Pharm.* 30:95, 1973.

U.S. Dept. of Health, Education and Welfare. *Health, United States, 1976–1977,* DHEW Publ. No. (HRA) 77-1233. Hyattsville, Md.: National Center for Health Services Research, 1978.

Wallace, D.E., and Watanabe, A.S. Drug effects in geriatric patients. *Drug Intell Clin Pharm.* 11:597, 1977.

Weintraub, M. Medication costs in perspective. *Drug Ther.* 6(9):178, 1976.

Weissert, W.G. Cost of adult day care: a comparison to nursing homes. *Inquiry* 15:10, 1978.

7 The Health Status of the Elderly

The term "aging" is often used synonymously with "illness," although there is no correlation between the two terms. The synonymous use of them probably arises from the fact that, in evaluating the health status of elderly persons, health standards developed for young adults are used as criteria. It is not possible to apply the term "well" equally to both a young and an elderly person.

An understanding of the elderly person's health status and outlook is vital to the successful medical management of older patients, as many misconceptions have developed (Palmore 1977):

1. Approximately 80% of all elderly are healthy enough to engage in normal activities.
2. Only about 5% of those over 65 years of age are residents of long-term care institutions. Only about 9% of those over 75 years of age are institutionalized.
3. Of those elderly living in the community, only about 5% are house- or bedbound.
4. Most elderly are not senile.

Up to the age of 75 years, most people are self-sustaining and functioning, and it is only after age 75 that intractable problems of ill health and dependency become more prevalent (Anderson 1977). Most of the elderly do not consider themselves to be in poor health (Table 7-1). Two-thirds of the noninstitutionalized elderly report that, compared with other people their age, their health is good or excellent. Only 9% report their health as poor (Table 7-2). Men report five times as frequently as women that they cannot pursue their major activity; the difference is large even after age 75. About 82% of the noninstitutionalized elderly report that they have no limitations of mobility and need no help. The old-old (Neugarten's classification) ambulatory patients have more heart and genitourinary problems, while the young-old are more often treated for anxiety, hypertension, ulcers, musculoskeletal, skin, and psychiatric problems. The old-old receive more medications, and are considered to be in poorer health by the primary care provider

Table 7-1
Health Status of Noninstitutionalized Elderly: A Self Rating*

Sex and Age	Excellent	Good	Fair	Poor
Male				
65–74	28.5	39.8	21.5	9.3
75 and over	27.5	40.3	21.3	9.8
Female				
65–74	29.2	41.4	21.5	7.2
75 and over	28.6	39.3	21.8	9.4

*U.S. 1975
Data are based on household interviews of a sample of the civilian noninstitutionalized population.
Source: Division of Health Interview Statistics, National Center for Health Statistics, Data from the Health Interview Survey, 1977.

Table 7-2
Noninstitutionalized Elderly in Poor Health or Unable to Carry on Major Activity

Age group (years)	Reporting Poor Health (%) Both sexes	Men	Women
65–74	8.1	9.3	7.2
75 and over	9.5	9.8	9.4

	Unable to Carry on Major Activity (%)		
65–74	14.0	25.5	5.2
75 and over	22.9	36.8	14.5

Source: National Center for Health Statistics, 1977.

(Linn et al 1977). The perception of their health status by the elderly is illustrated by a case report:

Mr and Mrs Smith, members of a senior citizens center, have been married six months. It is the second marriage for both. Mr Smith is a 71-year-old black, retired musician with a fifth-grade education. He lives with Mrs Smith in a one-bedroom apartment in the inner city. The apartment is definitely overpriced; it is roach-infested, has inadequate plumbing, and is generally in poor condition. Despite these conditions, Mr and Mrs Smith are reluctant to move as they have signed a lease and fear the loss of their security deposit. The apartment is within walking distance of the church, grocery store, and drugstore.

Mr Smith had a stroke three years ago, but is ambulatory and in general good condition. He takes medication for hypertension, but asserts that he has never been told that he has high blood pressure. Mr Smith also takes aspirin, vitamins, antacid, laxatives, and quinidine on a regular basis.

Because of his age and the stroke, Mr Smith retired three years ago. His monthly social security check of $129.80 is his total income. He feels that amount gives him "just enough to get by on," though he admits they could use more money for food and clothes. All of Mr Smith's income is used to pay the rent on the apartment.

Aside from financial need, Mr Smith would like to work, just to have "something to fill up time." For this reason, he has made application to become a Foster Grandparent. If accepted in the program, he would have a little more income and believes that "working will make him happier." Mr Smith has a good appetite, but often has difficulty eating because of poorly fitting dentures. However, Mr Smith does not see a dentist because of the cost. In general, Mr Smith believes himself "happy" and to be "better off than most."

Mrs Smith is a 69-year-old black, retired laundress with an eighth-grade education. She has a multitude of physical problems: heart condition, hypertension, obesity, and arthritis. She is taking several medications on a regular basis, including digitalis, diuretics, and antihypertensives.

Mrs Smith is the "manager" of the family. She takes care of Mr Smith, does the shopping, washing, cleaning, and cooking. Her daughter, who lives nearby, is 52 years old but, because of illness, is unable to assist her.

Some time ago, Mrs Smith was examined by her private physician and was told that she had a lump in her left breast. Subsequently, Mrs Smith was seen at a nearby hospital, but has not kept a second appointment. Her physician believes that she has breast cancer.

Mrs Smith has also applied to be a Foster Grandparent, but was told that she was ineligible as her monthly income was too high. She receives $316 per month from her first husband's social security account. She is not sure that she can continue to collect this money since she has remarried. She worries about losing the little income she has. Mrs Smith's teeth are in poor condition. Overall, Mrs Smith feels that she has it better than most people her age.

The elderly frequently face illness. They are more prone to chronic diseases and they are at risk for iatrogenic illness from drug actions.

Interference with key enzyme systems and breakdown of homeostatic mechanisms are the underlying causes of many of these diseases (Adelman 1975). It is important to recognize that old age is physiologic, not pathologic, and many "old age diseases" can be avoided or arrested if diagnosed and treated in time (Vinogradov and Revutskaya 1972). There is no presentation of illness unique to the elderly, as multiple pathology is not uncommon at earlier ages (Leonard 1976). The elderly face problems that are common to patients of all ages, such as diabetes, depression, and fevers, but these may have special manifestations in later life. Some problems are more or less unique to the elderly, such as chronic lymphatic leukemia, polymyalgia rheumatica, multiple myeloma, and senile dementia. Life changes, which the elderly encounter with increasing frequency, are met with efforts of readjustment. The psychophysiologic activation secondary to this readjustment can impact negatively on a person's illness susceptibility (Rahe et al 1974).

On the positive side, certain qualities of the elderly can support treatment. Fears of dependency, abandonment, suffering, and pain may be present, but the elderly patient has a high state of maturity and has adapted to many situations. While there may be diminished resistance and speed of adjustment to stress, there is an adaptive flexibility for survival. Acknowledgement of these patient characteristics, as well as knowledge of the unmet needs of the elderly (Table 7-3) (which, if allowed to remain can interfere with stated treatment regimens) are basic to successful medical management.

Table 7-3
Unmet Needs of Noninstitutionalized Elderly

Need	Elderly in need (%)
Transportation	7
Food shopping	7
Personal care	6
Social contacts	5
Food preparation	5
Housekeeping	5
Emergency assistance	3
Social interaction	1
Medical or paramedical assistance	1

Source: The Survey Research Program, University of Massachusetts at Boston, and the Joint Center for Urban Studies, Massachusetts Institute of Technology, and Harvard University, 1976.

CHRONIC DISEASES AND DISABILITIES

Statistics show that approximately 80% of the elderly, as compared with 40% of those younger than 65 years of age, have one or more chronic diseases (Task Force on Prescription Drugs 1968). Six of seven noninstitutionalized persons 65 years and older have at least one chronic condition (Vital and Health Statistics 1973, 1974). Untreated illnesses and disabilities are believed to exist in disturbing proportions among the elderly (Anderson 1960). One study in England showed patients between 70 and 72 years of age to have 3.2 diseases or disabilities, of which more than 20% were unknown to the primary physician (Currie et al 1974). It has been said that if less than three important disorders are found in an elderly patient, at least one important diagnosis has been missed. The elderly suffer from many degenerative changes, which tend to interact with multiple disease states, complicating their health status. Accumulation of diseases and interactions among chronic processes would seem to be the rule in geriatric patients. The prevalence of some chronic conditions is shown in Table 7-4, and the prevalence of selected chronic circulatory conditions is depicted in Figure 7-1. Among one group of 200 geriatric patients, an average of six diseases was found, which was very similar to the five to six diagnoses per patient among 250 elderly in a later study (Rosin 1975). Diagnosis is usually difficult. Environmental and interpersonal factors contribute to disease multiplicity, but the complaints of the elderly are often less well defined than those of younger patients. The most common complaints of the elderly are listed in Table 7-5, but, in general, self-reporting of illness by older persons is unsatisfactory for

Table 7-4
Prevalence of Some Chronic Conditions*

Condition	All ages (A)	65 years and over (B)	B/A
Neuralgia + neuritis			
specified	1.9	9.0	4.7
unspecified	8.2	33.5	4.1
Diabetes	20.4	78.5	3.8
Sciatica	4.3	11.9	2.7
Diseases of urinary system	28.0	60.7	2.2
Diseases of kidney and ureter	6.5	10.0	1.5
Anemias	14.5	20.9	1.4
Thyroid conditions	13.9	19.7	1.4
Migraine	21.8	14.7	0.7

*Rate per 100 persons
Source: DHEW Publ. No. (HRA) 77-1536. Rockville, Md.: National Center for Health Statistics, 1977.

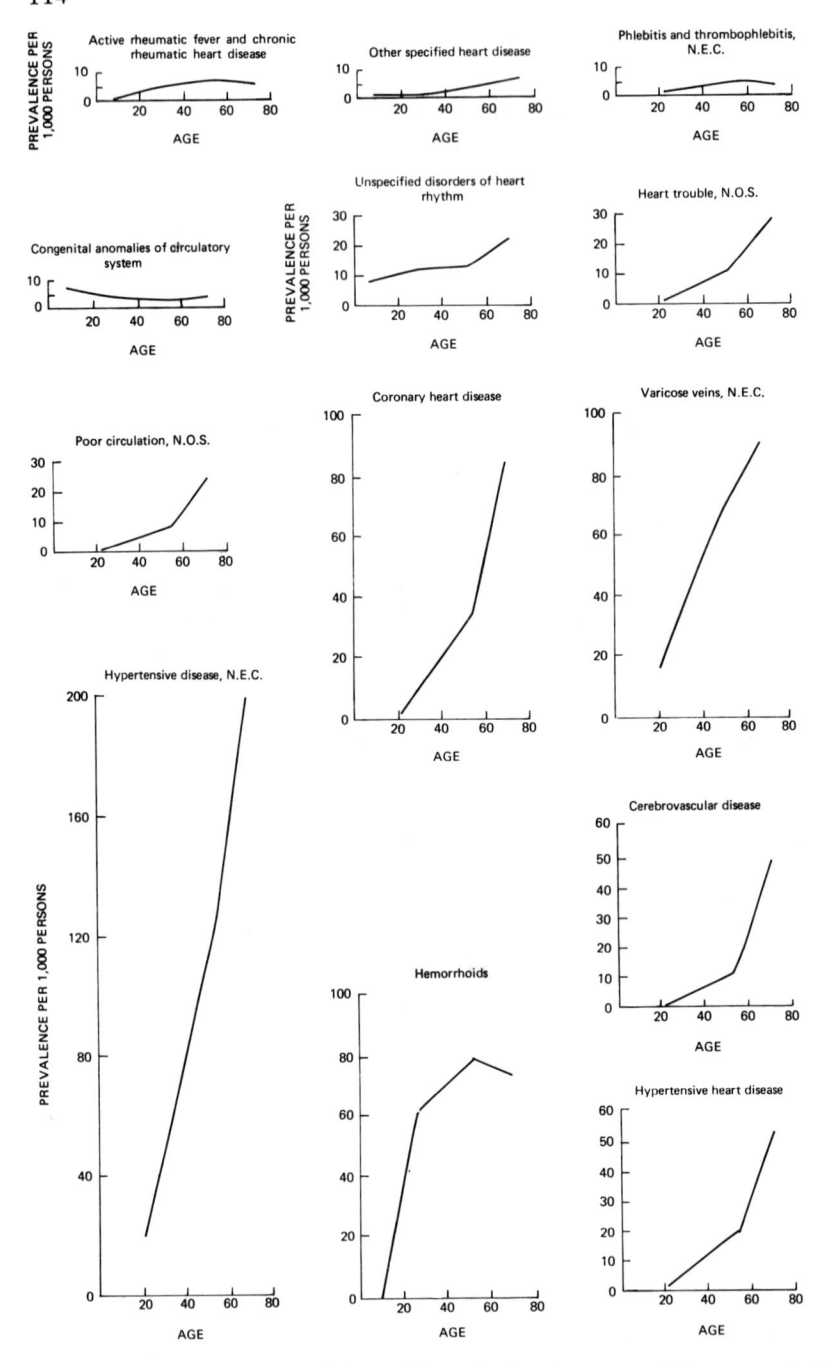

Figure 7-1 Prevalence of selected chronic circulatory conditions reported in health interviews per 1000 persons, by age. Source: Health Resources Administration. Prevalence of chronic circulatory conditions, United States, 1972. U.S. DHEW, Publ. No. (HRA) 75-1521, Series 10, No. 94. Washington, D.C.: U.S. Government Printing Office, 1974.

Table 7-5
Most Common Complaints of the Elderly

Complaint/Disease	Percent of total
Emotional problems	20.0
Cardiovascular	13.0
Muscles, tendons, joints, bones	11.0
Gastrointestinal	10.0
Urinary tract infection	8.5
Vision and hearing	5.0
Respiratory	5.0

Source: D. Eckstein. Common complaints of the elderly. *Hosp Practice.* 11(4):67, 1976.

the detection of disease. Postmortem examinations have revealed as many as 15 clinical or pathologic conditions, some of which may have been asymptomatic (Reichel 1976).

Polypathology in the elderly is the rule, rather than the exception. What has not been readily accepted is the fact that most diseases of the elderly are not age-specific. In 1968, the most frequently observed diseases in the elderly were listed as arthritis and rheumatism, hearing impairment, heart disease and cardiovascular conditions, high blood pressure, visual impairment, gastrointestinal disorders, chronic sinusitis, mental and nervous diseases, and genitourinary problems. A similar list (Eckstein 1976) cited heart problems, hypertension, arthritis, mental and nervous diseases, gastrointestinal disorders, genitourinary problems, diabetes, respiratory problems, circulatory and related foot conditions, and chronic skin disorders. These are not age-specific diseases, but, as previously mentioned, they may have special manifestations in the elderly person, as they may often occur simultaneously. Obesity and foot problems are often disregarded, which can lead to impaired locomotor function and, thus, poorer health status.

In addition, degenerative diseases and multiple pathology can lead to physical limitations among the elderly. In 1971, 16.9% of all Americans over the age of 65 years were unable to carry on major activities because of some chronic condition; the figure for all ages was only 2.9% (Supreme Court 1976). Serious consequences can result; elderly with three or more disabilities are more than twice as likely to be bedridden than those with fewer than three (Shanas 1977). Activity and mobility limitations increase sharply with advancing age (Figures 7-2 and 7-3); only slightly more than 54% of those over 65 years of age have no activity limitations due to chronic disease (Table 7-6), and almost 83% have no mobility limitation due to chronic disease (Table 7-7). Many of the chronic diseases affecting the elderly patient are responsible for these limitations (Table 7-8).

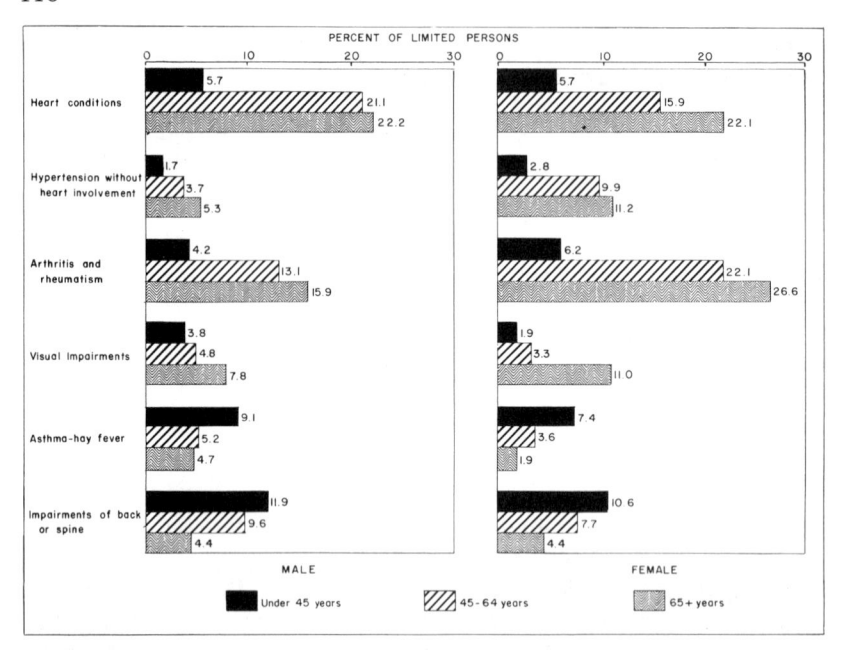

Figure 7-2 Percent of persons with activity limitations who reported selected chronic conditions as a cause of their limitation, by sex and age. Source: Health Services and Mental Health Administration. Chronic conditions causing activity limitations, United States, July 1963–June 1965. PHS Publ. No. 1000, Series 10, No. 51. Washington, D.C.: U.S. Government Printing Office, 1969.

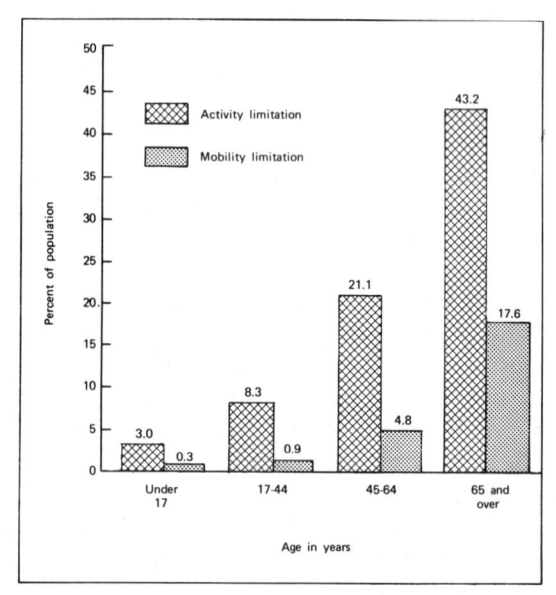

Figure 7-3 Percent of population with limitation of activity or mobility due to chronic conditions, by age. Source: Health Resources Administration. Limitations of activity and mobility due to chronic conditions, United States, 1972. DHEW Publ. No. (HRA) 75-1523, Series 10, No. 96. Washington, D.C.: U.S. Government Printing Office, 1974.

Table 7-6
Activity Limitation
(Due to Chronic Condition)

	1972 All ages	1972 65 years and over	1977 All ages	1977 65 years and over
No limitation	87.3	56.8	85.9	54.1
Some limitation	3.1	5.3	3.5	6.6
Limitation in major activity*	6.6	21.6	7.3	22.1
Unable to perform major activity	3.0	16.3	3.3	17.1

*Ability to work, keep house, engage in school activity.
Source: Limitation of activity and mobility due to chronic conditions, U.S. 1972. DHEW Publ. No. (HRA) 75-1523. Rockville, Md.: National Center for Health Statistics, 1974.

Table 7-7
Mobility Limitation
(Due to Chronic Condition)

	All ages	65 years and over
No limitation	96.8	82.4
Trouble getting around alone	1.3	5.8
Needs help in getting around alone	1.0	6.7
Confined to house	0.9	5.2

Source: Limitation of activity and mobility due to chronic conditions, U.S. 1972. DHEW Publ. No. (HRA) 75-1523. Rockville, Md.: National Center for Health Statistics, 1974.

Table 7-8
The Ten Leading Causes for Activity Limitation in the Elderly

Cause	Affected (%)
Heart condition	23.5
Arthritis and rheumatism	23.2
Visual impairment	9.8
Hypertension without heart involvement	8.7
Diabetes	6.8
Impairment* of lower extremities and hip	6.0
Other conditions of circulatory system	5.9
Cerebrovascular disease	4.9
Emphysema	4.4

*Except paralysis and absence.
Source: Limitation of activity due to chronic conditions, U.S. 1974. DHEW Publ. No. (HRA) 77-1537. Rockville, Md.: National Center for Health Statistics, 1977.

ACUTE CONDITIONS

The elderly succumb to fewer acute illnesses than does the general population. A person over 65 years of age has an average of 1.3 acute illnesses per year, as compared to 2.1 per year for all ages (Comfort 1976). Figure 7-4 shows a steady decrease in the incidence of acute conditions with age; most of the attacks occur between October and December (Table 7-9). However, elderly people, whether or not they were limited in activity or mobility by chronic conditions, were forced to restrict their usual activities an average of 5½ weeks per person in 1975. One-third of that time resulted from acute illness or injury. Although the elderly suffer from fewer acute conditions than do younger people, acute conditions cause an increased number of days of restricted activity, underscoring the increased vulnerability of the elderly (Table 7-10).

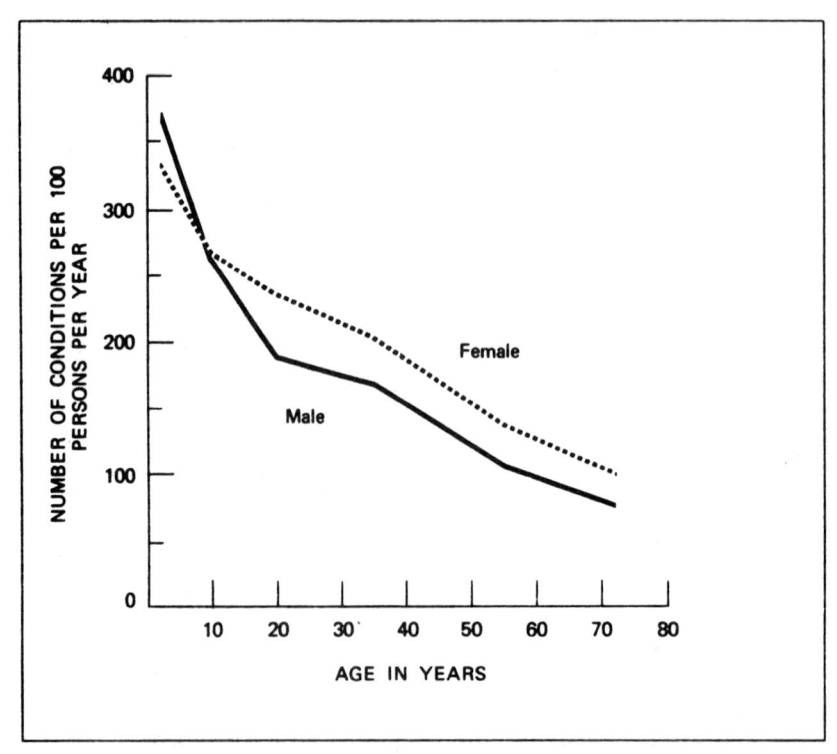

Figure 7-4 Incidence of acute conditions per 100 persons per year by sex and age. Source: Health Resources Administration. Acute conditions. Incidence and associated disability, United States, July 1974–June 1975. DHEW Publ. No. (HRA) 77-1541, Series 10, No. 114. Rockville, Md.: National Center for Health Statistics, 1977.

Table 7-9
Days of Bed Disability due to Acute Conditions*

Quarter	All ages M	All ages F	45–64 years M	45–64 years F	65 years and over M	65 years and over F
July–Sept	67	84	53	76	85	88
Oct–Dec	97	21	117	97	127	206
Jan–March	127	192	118	189	153	173
April–June	70	84	77	76	70	124

*Per 100 Persons.
Source: Acute conditions, incidence and associated disability, U.S., 1974–1975. DHEW Publ. No. (HRA) 77-1541. Rockville, Md.: National Center for Health Statistics, 1977.

Table 7-10
Acute Conditions

Per 100 Persons	All ages	65 years and over
Number of acute conditions	198	196
Days of restricted activity	917	1084
Days of bed disability	397	433

Patients not institutionalized.
Source: Acute conditions, incidence and associated disabilities, U.S., 7/1972–6/1973. DHEW Publ. No. (HRA) 75-1525. Rockville, Md.: National Center for Health Statistics, 1975.

PHYSICIAN VISITS

The elderly are the least likely of all adults to use hospital outpatient clinics and less than 10% of their contact with the medical care system occurs at such clinics. More than two-thirds of the elderly are under the care of either a family practitioner or an internist. The bulk of ambulatory care for the elderly revolves around follow-up and continuing care, which is exemplified by the fact that one-fourth of physician visits are for diseases of the circulatory system (Kovar 1977). Office visits per year increase in direct parallel to advancing age (Figure 7-5) and they occur more often for a serious reason than among younger people (Figure 7-6). The rate of visits to physicians for persons aged 65 and over is more than double the rate for those 15 years or younger, and for all ages visits by females occur more frequently than males (Koch and Dennison 1977).

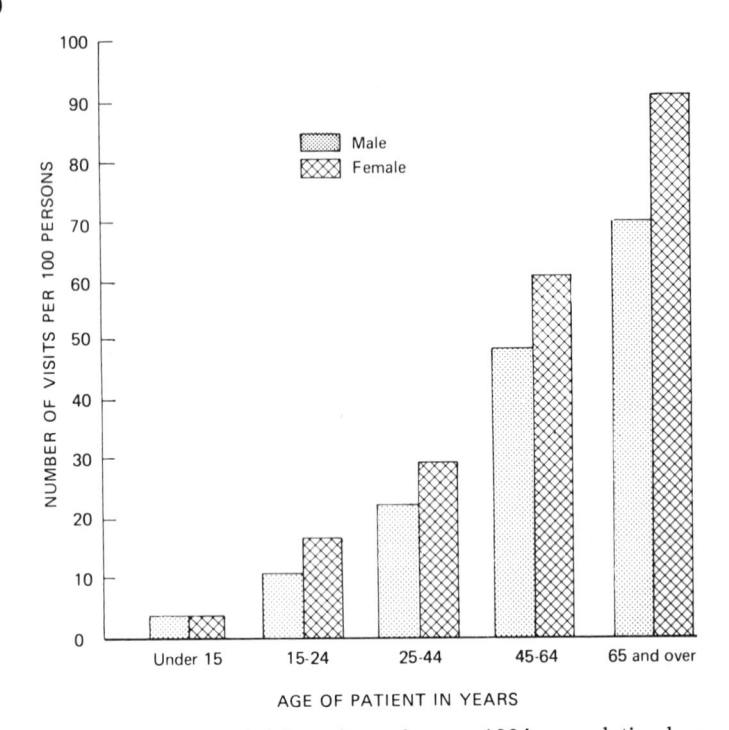

Figure 7-5 Annual rate of visits to internists per 100 in population by sex and age of patient: United States, January–December 1975. Source: Cypress, B.K., Office Visits to Internists: National Ambulatory Medical Care Survey, United States, 1975, *Adv Data.* 16:1, 1978.

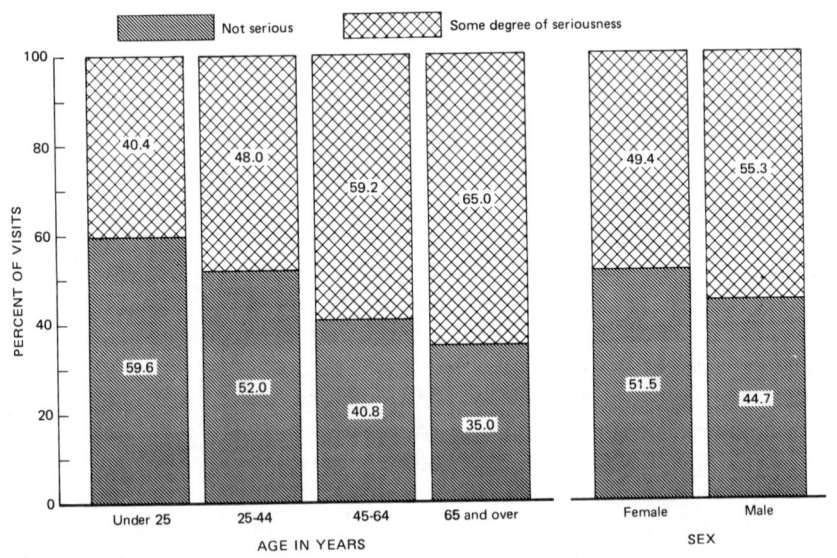

Figure 7-6 Percent of office visits by degree of seriousness of patient's problem, by patient's age and sex: United States, January–December 1975. Source: Koch, H.K., and Dennison, N.J. Ambulatory medical care rendered in physicians' offices: United States, 1975. *Adv Data.* 12:1, 1977.

THE HOMEBOUND

Aged homebound are among the medically unreached (Brickner et al 1975). Several studies have shown that between 15% and 20% of elderly persons living in the community have three or more debilities. Although a majority of the frail elderly are white, black elderly are proportionately more often frail, black males being frail four times as frequently as white males (Shanas 1977). Based on 1975 population figures, and assuming that 15% of the elderly living in the country need help and cannot be left alone, there may be as many as 2,400,000 bed- or housebound elderly in the country (Shanas 1961; Anderson 1977). Approximately 25% of the elderly in private homes are thought to need medical services (Shanas 1974) and 40% of the noninstitutionalized elderly may have disabilities that interfere to a greater or lesser extent with their major work or recreational activities (National Center for Health Statistics 1971). The proportion of the population receiving treatment at home rises chronologically (Figure 7-7). At age 60, one in ten persons receives home treatment; at age 70, one in five; at 75, one in three; and at age 80, 50% receive home treatment (Vinogradov and Revutskaya 1972). Those caring for elderly living in the community must take into account the effect of maintaining frail and debilitated elderly at home. In Britain, the physical health of the closest relative was impaired in 58% of the cases. In 12%, employment of the closest relative was affected, and in 14% of families, there was an income loss (Sainsbury and de Alarcon 1969).

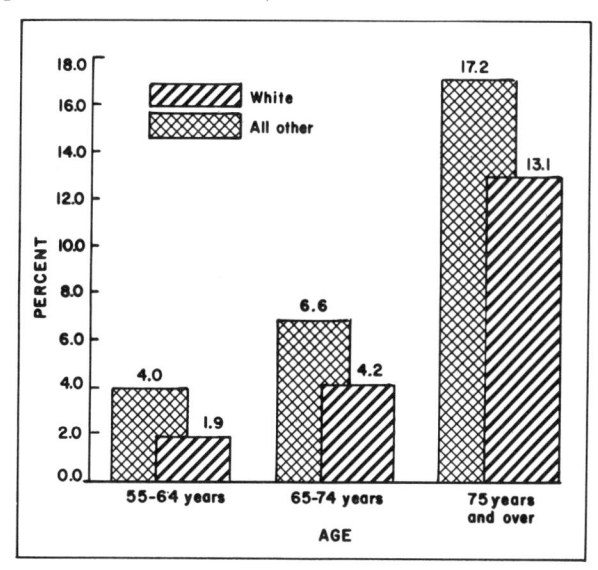

Figure 7-7 Percent of persons receiving home care, by age and race. Source: Health Services and Mental Health Administration. Home care for persons 55 years and over, United States, July 1966–June 1968. DHEW Publ. No. (HSM) 72-1062. Rockville, Md.: National Center for Health Statistics, 1972.

HOSPITALIZATION

Although the elderly do not actively seek institutionalization, admissions increase with age. In 1973, the admission rate among Medicare patients was 320 per 1000 population, while the rate for the entire population was 140. Among the elderly institutionalized patients, 45% are occasionally or usually incontinent, 49% are occasionally or usually confused, and 59% are unable to manage finances. There has been a steady increase in the incidence of hospitalization of the elderly (Table 7-11). In 1974, when the elderly constituted 11.4% of the population, they accounted for 20% of all hospitalizations and incurred one-third of all hospital charges, mainly for chronic diseases (Jones et al 1975). Between 1964 and 1972, there was almost a 50% increase in the incidence of hospitalization of patients 75 years and older (Table 7-12). In general, the days spent per hospitalization increases greatly with age (Table 7-13) as does the average length of stay (Table 7-14).

Table 7-11
Population with at Least One Short-Stay Hospitalization

Age	7/60–6/62	7/65–6/66	1968	1972
All ages	9.3	10.0	9.6	10.6
Under 15 years	5.0	5.6	5.1	5.7
15–44 years	12.3	12.4	11.3	11.7
45–64 years	9.5	10.9	10.2	11.9
65 years and over	11.2	13.0	15.5	16.7

Source: Persons hospitalized by number of episodes and days hospitalized in a year, U.S. 1972. DHEW Publ. No. (HRA) 77-1544. Hyattsville, Md.: National Center for Health Statistics, 1977.

Table 7-12
Patients Discharged from Short-Stay Hospitals*

Age	7/63–6/64	1972	Increase (%)
All	107.6	124.2	15.4
Under 5	94.3	105.2	11.6
5–14	53.1	56.5	6.5
15–24	83.5	86.2	3.2
25–34	104.3	114.4	9.7
35–44	116.7	141.4	21.2

Table 7-12 *(continued)*

Age	7/63–6/64	1972	Increase (%)
45–54	142.3	151.0	6.1
55–64	151.3	171.1	13.1
65–74	181.2	236.2	30.4
75 and over	206.7	306.3	48.2

*Per 1000 persons, excluding hospitalization for delivery.
Source: Hospital discharges and length of stay: short-stay hospitals, U.S. 1972. DHEW Publ. No. (HRA) 77-1534. Rockville, Md.: National Center for Health Statistics, 1976.

Table 7-13
Hospital Days

	Number of Hospital Days*			
Age	1–7	8–14	15–30	31 and over
All ages	64.6	18.4	11.2	5.8
Under 17	81.5	10.5	5.4	2.6
17–44	75.9	14.6	6.6	2.9
45–64	49.6	25.6	16.5	8.2
65 and over	36.3	26.9	22.9	13.8

*Short-stay hospital. Percent of persons hospitalized.
Source: Persons hospitalized by number of episodes and days hospitalized in a year, U.S. 1972. DHEW Publ. No. (HRA) 77-1544. Hyattsville, Md.: National Center for Health Statistics, 1977.

Table 7-14
Average Length of Stay (Days)

	All ages	65 years and over
7/62–6/63	8.4	14.1
7/63–6/64	8.1	12.1
7/65–6/66	8.1	12.7
7/66–6/67	8.6	13.8
1967	8.5	13.5
1968	9.2	15.8
1969	9.0	14.9
1970	8.6	13.1
1971	8.5	12.7
1972	8.4	12.9
1973	8.1	12.2
1974	8.4	11.7

Source: Hospital discharges and length of stay: short-stay hospital, U.S. 1972. DHEW Publ. No. (HRA) 77-1534. Rockville, Md.: National Center for Health Statistics, 1976.

NURSING HOMES

Nursing homes are an outgrowth of the old, often municipally operated almshouses and church-operated facilities. The number of nursing home beds available increased by almost 131% between 1963 and 1974 (Figure 7-8). The term nursing home covers a multitude of care facilities, including extended care facilities, skilled nursing facilities, and intermediate care facilities. Lately, hospices have demanded more attention and that concept, as well as the concept of day treatment centers may be expanded in the future.

The 1965 Social Security Amendments define extended care as short, posthospital care financed by Medicare. Skilled nursing care was defined as care provided under supervision of a physician to Medicaid patients in a licensed facility. In 1968, Social Security Amendments added the concept of intermediate care, ie, care beyond room and board, but not care requiring the levels specified for extended or skilled care.

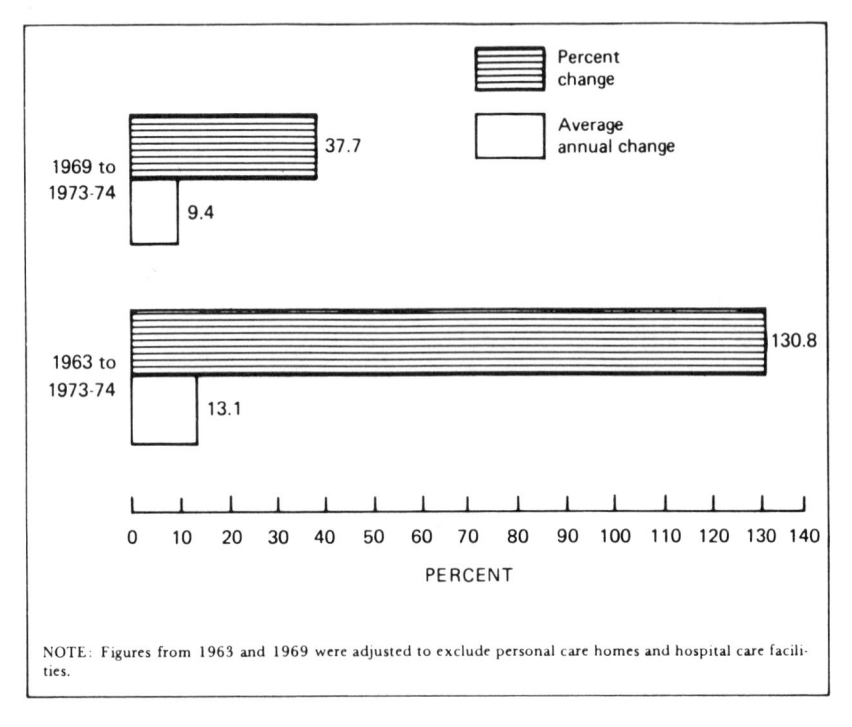

NOTE: Figures from 1963 and 1969 were adjusted to exclude personal care homes and hospital care facilities.

Figure 7-8 Percent change in the number of nursing home beds and the average annual change for 1963, 1969, and August 1973–April 1974, United States. Source: Health Resources Administration. Utilization of nursing homes, United States: National nursing home survey, August 1973–April 1974. DHEW Publ. No. (HRA) 77-1779. Hyattsville, Md.: National Center for Health Statistics, 1977.

It is interesting to note that federal legislation thus distinguished extended care chiefly by the emphasis on nursing care, yet only somewhat less than 10% of the over 800,000 employed registered nurses are employed in these facilities, most in administrative capacities (Wolfe 1977). This is important because nursing home care differs substantially from hospital care. The primary physician is required to see the resident at least once every month or two months; the main responsibility for care rests with other health professionals. Only approximately 20% of physicians believe that they retain complete control of the patient, once the patient has been admitted to the long-term care facility.

By law, every licensed facility must now employ a licensed medical director and the Patient's Bill of Rights attempts to set ground rules for proper care (Appendix 7-A). Generally, patients are referred to as residents and not patients.

Nursing home care has been viewed synonymously with long-term care, but it must be emphasized that it is only one alternative to long-term care (although other alternatives have been sadly neglected). There is undue reliance on this type of facility, probably because of Medicaid provisions. There are now almost 1,330,000 beds in the 23,000 nursing homes compared to approximately 1,050,000 beds in short-stay hospitals. In 1973, the admission rate to nursing homes was 19 per 1000 Medicaid population.

Although Medicaid reimburses on a flat daily rate, a rate which has been judged inappropriate by many in the nursing home industry, overall cost is exceedingly high. If one assumes a cost of about $30 per patient per day, the annual cost per patient would be approximately $11,000. This is approximately 70% of the median family income in the United States (Health Resources Administration 1977). At the beginning of 1974, about 4% of the elderly were nursing home residents. They are, on the average, older than elderly people in the community. Almost 83% were 75 years of age and older, in contrast with 36% of the noninstitutionalized elderly. Implications for medical care and drug therapy are staggering. Demographic characteristics of elderly in nursing homes are given in Figures 7-9 and 7-10. Table 7-15 presents a detailed breakdown. In view of the fact that females, on the average, are more sensitive to adverse drug reactions and are, in general, more vulnerable to drug therapy, it is noteworthy that almost three-quarters of elderly residents in nursing homes are females.

There is a high correlation between the physical and mental status of residents in nursing homes. Poor physical status almost always is correlated with poor mental functioning (Goldfarb 1962, 1974). Sixty-three percent of nursing home residents are classified as senile, 31% are bedfast or chairfast, and 35% are incontinent. Almost 50% cannot

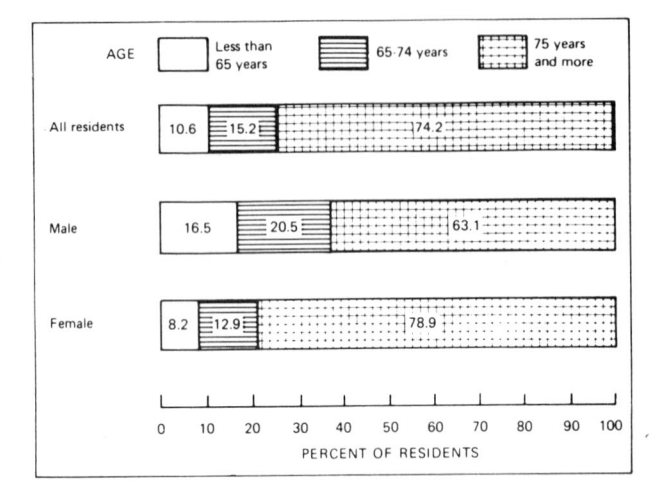

```
                    ┌─────────┐ Less than      ┌─────────┐ 65-74 years    ┌─────────┐ 75 years
            AGE     │         │ 65 years       │ ≡≡≡≡≡≡≡ │                │ ░░░░░░░ │ and more
                    └─────────┘                └─────────┘                └─────────┘

All residents   10.6 │ 15.2 │                       74.2

Male            16.5 │  20.5  │                   63.1

Female          8.2 │12.9│                      78.9

                0    10   20   30   40   50   60   70   80   90   100
                              PERCENT OF RESIDENTS
```

Figure 7-9 Percent distribution of residents by sex and age: United States, August 1973–August 1974. Source: Health Resources Administration. Utilization of nursing homes, United States: National nursing home survey, August 1973–April 1974. DHEW Publ. No. (HRA) 77-1779. Hyattsville, Md.: National Center for Health Statistics, 1977.

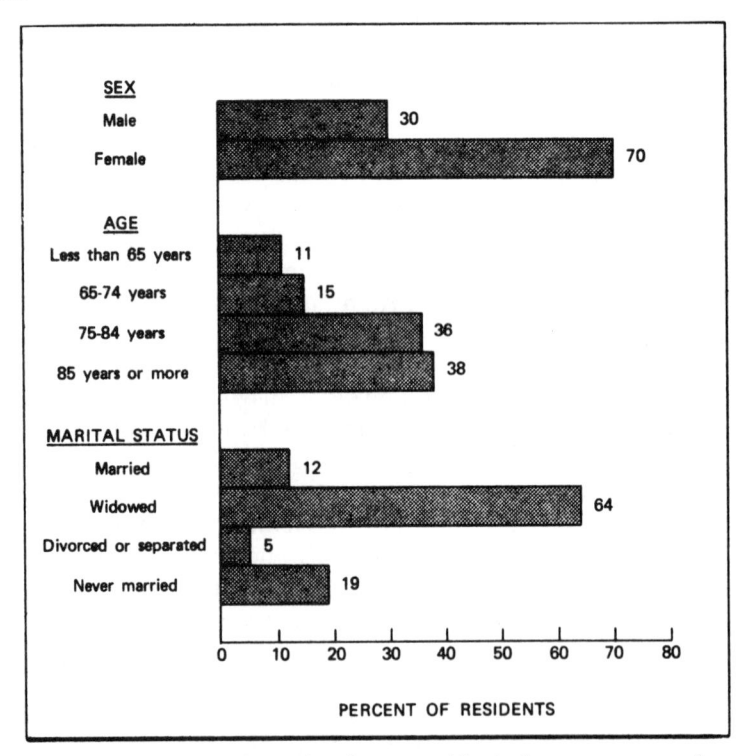

```
SEX
  Male                                30
  Female                                                      70

AGE
  Less than 65 years        11
  65-74 years               15
  75-84 years                              36
  85 years or more                          38

MARITAL STATUS
  Married                   12
  Widowed                                              64
  Divorced or separated   5
  Never married             19

         0    10   20   30   40   50   60   70   80
                   PERCENT OF RESIDENTS
```

Figure 7-10 Percent of nursing home residents by sex, age, and marital status: United States, 1973–1974. Source: Health Resources Administration. Characteristics, social contacts, and activities of nursing home residents, United States, 1973–74: National nursing home survey. DHEW Publ. No. (HRA) 77-1778. Rockville, Md.: National Center for Health Statistics, 1977.

Table 7-15
Patient Distribution in Skilled Nursing Facilities

Age	Percent
Under 20	1.7
20–64	20.4
65–69	5.3
70–74	10.0
75–79	12.7
80–84	18.7
85–89	20.0
90 and over	11.2
Males	27.1%
Females	72.9%

Source: Long-term care facility improvement study, introductory report. Office of Nursing Home Affairs. DHEW Publ. No. (OS) 76-50021, Rockville, Md., 1975.

see well enough to read, even with glasses, 35% cannot hear an ordinary telephone conversation, and 24% suffer from a speech impairment. Specific findings are presented in Tables 7-16–7-21. These elderly, plagued by multiple pathology and physical impairments, are most at risk to unpredictable drug action. Yet, they are also the group who receive most drugs, and thus must be carefully monitored.

Table 7-16
Diagnostic Admission Profile for Patients in Skilled Nursing Facilities*

Diagnosis	Percent
Heart disease	43.1
Chronic brain disease	32.7
Arteriosclerosis and hypertension	24.9
Musculoskeletal system diseases	21.4
Stroke	19.1
Fractures	18.0
Diabetes	14.9
Digestive system disease	11.5
Genitourinary disease	10.4
Neuroses and psychoses	10.1

*65 years and over.
Source: Long-term care facility improvement study, introductory report. Office of Nursing Home Affairs. DHEW Publ. No. (OS) 76-50021, Rockville, Md., 1975.

Table 7-17
The Leading Primary Admission Diagnoses for Skilled Nursing Facility Patients*

Diagnosis	Percent
Heart disease	18.0
Chronic brain disease	15.2
Stroke	11.3
Fractures	9.9
Arteriosclerosis and hypertension	6.9
Diabetes	5.4
Musculoskeletal system diseases	4.9
Neurological disease	4.1
Neuroses and psychoses	4.1
Mental retardation	2.8

*65 years and over.
Source: Long-term care facility improvement study, introductory report. Office of Nursing Home Affairs. DHEW Publ. No. (OS) 76-50021, Rockville, Md., 1975.

Table 7-18
Heart Diseases in Patients in Skilled Nursing Facilities*

Disease	Percent of population
Hypertension	14.2
Congestive heart failure	12.9
Cardiac arrhythmias	9.0

Source: Long-term care facility improvement study, introductory report. Office of Nursing Home Affairs. DHEW Publ. No. (OS) 76-50021, Rockville, Md., 1975.

Table 7-19
Leading Postadmission Diagnoses for Skilled Nursing Facility Patients*

Diagnostic Groups	Percent
Genitourinary system disease	13.1
Eye and ear diseases	10.6
Decubitus ulcer and other skin conditions	9.3
Musculoskeletal system diseases	8.5
Heart disease	8.1
Fractures	7.3
Digestive system diseases	6.2
Respiratory system diseases	5.8

*65 years and over.
Source: Long-term care facility improvement study, introductory report. Office of Nursing Home Affairs. DHEW Publ. No. (OS) 76-50021, Rockville, Md., 1975.

Table 7-20
Medically Defined Conditions of Patients in Skilled Nursing Facilities

Medically defined condition	Percent
Neurological disorders	33.6
Arthritis	18.1
Diabetes mellitus	15.7
Hypertension (essential)	14.2
Congestive heart failure	12.9
Mental illness	10.4
Cardiac arrhythmias	9.0
Urinary tract infections	8.6
Respiratory disease	7.3
Malignancy	5.8
Angina and/or myocardial infarction	5.2
Anemia	4.6
Alcoholism	2.2
Drug abuse	0.1

Source: U.S. Department of Health, Education and Welfare, 1976.

Table 7-21
Health Status of Patients in Skilled Nursing Facility

Function	Percent
Bathes without help	6.6
Dresses without help	16.2
Eats without help	47.0
Uses toilet without help	25.7
No bladder function problem	39.6
No bowel function problem	49.1
No orientation problem (time, place, person)	45.8
Appropriate behavior	58.4
No hearing impairment	67.1
Normal speech	68.0
No visual impairment	29.6

Source: Long-term care facility improvement study, introductory report. Office of Nursing Home Affairs. DHEW Publ. No. (OS) 76-50021, Rockville, Md., 1975.

MORTALITY

Diseases that commonly lead to death have been correlated with aging in three ways (Kohn 1963). First, there is the aging process. Under the usual conditions, this process is irreversible. Arteriosclerosis might be one of these diseases; everyone has it and would eventually die from it. There are certain diseases that do not afflict all members of the population, but their incidence increases with advancing age. Cancer of the colon is an example, but incidence of lung or kidney cancer decreases in the very old. Finally, there are diseases that neither occur in all people nor show age-related patterns, but their manifestations are more serious in advanced age, such as pneumonia, hernias, and intestinal obstructions.

As expected, most deaths occur in people over 65 years of age (Table 7-22). Nevertheless, the death rate for those older than 65 years has declined appreciably. From 1950 to 1975, mortality rates for the elderly declined 13%. In 1965, there were 6118 deaths per 100,000 people 65 years and over, and in 1975 there were 5432. From 1965 to 1975, mortality rates declined by 16% for people aged 65 to 74 years, by 10% for those between 75 and 84 years of age, and by 25% for those 85 years and older.

The ten leading causes of death by age and sex are given in Table 7-23, and the specific death rates by disease in Tables 7-24 and 7-25. The leading cause of death among the elderly is heart disease, which is responsible for almost 50% of all deaths among those 65 years and older. Malignant neoplasms and cerebrovascular diseases, in combination with heart disease, account for 75% of all deaths among the elderly. The same three disease states account for 53% of all deaths among people under 65 years of age.

Substantial declines in two of the three leading causes of death, heart disease and cerebrovascular disease, account for the mortality decrease in the elderly. In contrast, the death rate from cancer continues to increase.

According to the National Center for Health Statistics, deaths from major cardiovascular diseases have fallen below one million for the first time in nine years (Table 7-26). Since 1950, the mortality rate from stroke fell by 39% and from rheumatic fever and rheumatic heart disease by 66%. Since 1970, the death rate from hypertension and hypertensive heart disease declined by 28%. The rate for coronary heart disease and its complications, heart attack and sudden death, has dropped 7% since 1970.

Table 7-22
Mortality in the United States, 1975

Total number of deaths			1.9 million
Over 65 years — total			1.2 million
	65–74	0.1	
	75–84	0.8	
	85 and over	0.3	

Source: Health, United States, 1975–1976. U.S. DHEW, PHS, Health Resources Administration. Hyattsville, Md., 1976.

Table 7-23
Mortality, Ten Leading Causes of Death, Age Group and Sex, 1974

	All ages Male	All ages Female	Ages 35–54 Male	Ages 35–54 Female	Ages 55–74 Male	Ages 55–74 Female	Age 75+ Male	Age 75+ Female
1.	Heart diseases 411,492	Heart diseases 326,679	Heart diseases 49,066	Cancer 28,961	Heart diseases 199,960	Heart diseases 104,867	Heart diseases 159,182	Heart diseases 204,900
2.	Cancer 196,746	Cancer 163,726	Cancer 27,330	Heart diseases 14,923	Cancer 109,548	Cancer 80,553	Cancer 54,415	Stroke 80,024
3.	Stroke 90,394	Stroke 117,030	Accidents 14,697	Stroke 5618	Stroke 34,351	Stroke 30,349	Stroke 49,129	Cancer 49,571
4.	Accidents 73,209	Accidents 31,413	Cirrhosis of liver 8738	Accidents 4767	Accidents 12,884	Diabetes 9737	Pneumonia, influenza 15,076	Arterio-sclerosis 16,535
5.	Pneumonia, influenza 29,787	Pneumonia, influenza 24,990	Stroke 5824	Cirrhosis of liver 4704	Cirrhosis of liver 10,795	Accidents 6420	Arterio-sclerosis 9967	Pneumonia, influenza 15,940
6.	Cirrhosis of liver 21,806	Diabetes 22,193	Suicide 5588	Suicide 2892	Pneumonia, influenza 9336	Cirrhosis of liver 5339	Accidents 7095	Diabetes 10,210
7.	Suicide 18,595	Arterio-sclerosis 19,010	Homicide 5262	Diabetes 1809	Emphysema 9184	Pneumonia, influenza 5167	Emphysema 5684	Accidents 8672
8.	Homicide 16,747	Diseases of infancy 12,069	Pneumonia, influenza 2497	Pneumonia, influenza 1605	Diabetes 7496	Arterio-sclerosis 2361	Diabetes 5364	Hernia and intestinal obstruction 2077

Table 7-23 *(continued)*

	All ages		Ages 35–54		Ages 55–74		Age 75+	
	Male	Female	Male	Female	Male	Female	Male	Female
9.	Diseases of infancy 16,717	Cirrhosis of liver 11,513	Diabetes 1864	Homicide 1267	Suicide 4723	Emphysema 2361	Hypertension 1740	Hypertension 2040
10.	Emphysema 15,794	Suicide 7088	Emphysema 884	Nephritis 550	Arteriosclerosis 3063	Suicide 1670	Nephritis 1578	Gastritis 2002

Data based on the National Vital Registration System. National Center for Health Statistics, Health Resources Administration, DHEW (in preparation).

Table 7-24
Death Rate for the Leading Causes of Death Among Persons 65 Years and Over*

	Deaths per 100,000 persons			
Cause of Death	1950	1965	Male 1975	Female 1975
Heart disease	2861	2824	2933	2037
Malignant neoplasm	857	901	1301	725
Cerebrovascular disease	924	901	741	722
Influenza, pneumonia	191	214	239	151
Arteriosclerosis	—	—	120	125
Diabetes mellitus	121	123	103	120
Bronchitis, emphysema, asthma	—	—	153	31
Cirrhosis of liver	35	35	58	22

Source: Health, United States, 1976-1977. U.S. DHEW, PHS, Health Resources Administration 1977. DHEW Publ. No. (HRA) 77-1232.

Table 7-25
Mortality, Morbidity and Disability Rates

	Age (years)		
	17-44	45-64	65 and over
Death rate*	2.3	12.0	50.0
Heart disease†	1.0	2.5	9.0
Arthritis†	0.3	5.5	26.0
Disability rate‡	1.5	5.0	21.0

*Deaths per thousand per year
†Cases per 100 noninstitutionalized persons
‡Percent population unable to carry out major activity of daily living
Source: National Center for Health Statistics, 1970.

Table 7-26
Percent Decline in Death Rates for Selected
Cardiovascular Conditions by Age: United States 1970–1975

	Condition		
Age	Hypertensive disease	Stroke	Coronary heart disease
15–24	0	12.5	33.3
25–34	55.6	22.2	28.6
35–44	55.6	25.0	19.3
45–54	43.4	22.6	13.8
55–64	32.7	20.8	14.3
65–74	31.1	21.1	16.4
75–84	32.4	14.2	12.0
85+	29.3	11.9	8.4
All	35.4	17.8	14.0

Source: National Center for Health Statistics, 1977.

Undoubtedly, modern chemotherapy can claim much credit for this decline (Figure 7-11). However, over-reliance on drugs will not lead to further declines unless it is matched with other health care measures. Public health measures were responsible for a large decline in the death rate from tuberculosis by the time the first effective, antituberculosis agents were introduced. Chlorination of water led to a drastic decrease in typhoid; and the infant mortality rate decreased because of a reduction in diarrhea and pneumonia, resulting from social changes rather than from medical breakthroughs.

Because elderly females react differently than do males to certain drugs (Liddell et al 1975) and in view of the fact that the white, elderly woman has the greatest risk for adverse drug reactions, it should be reiterated that the death rate for men age 65 years and older was 6% higher in 1900 and the gap has widened considerably (Table 7-27).

Table 7-27
Death Rate*

Year	Male/Female
1900	106/100
1950	127/100
1965	141/100
1975	147/100

*For persons over 65 years of age.

Leading Causes of Death—1900 and 1970

1900 Rank	1900 Death Rate/ 100,000	Cause of Death	1970 Rank	1970 Death Rate/ 100,000
1	202.2	Influenza & pneumonia	5	30.5
2	194.4	Tuberculosis	—	—
3	142.7	Gastroenteritis	—	—
4	137.4	Diseases of the heart	1	360.3
5	106.9	Cerebral hemorrhages & vascular lesions affecting CNS	3	101.7
6	81.0	Chronic nephritis	—	—
7	72.3	All accidents	4	54.2
8	64.0	Cancer & other malignant neoplasms	2	162.0
9	62.6	Certain diseases of early infancy	6	20.9
10	40.3	Diphtheria	—	—

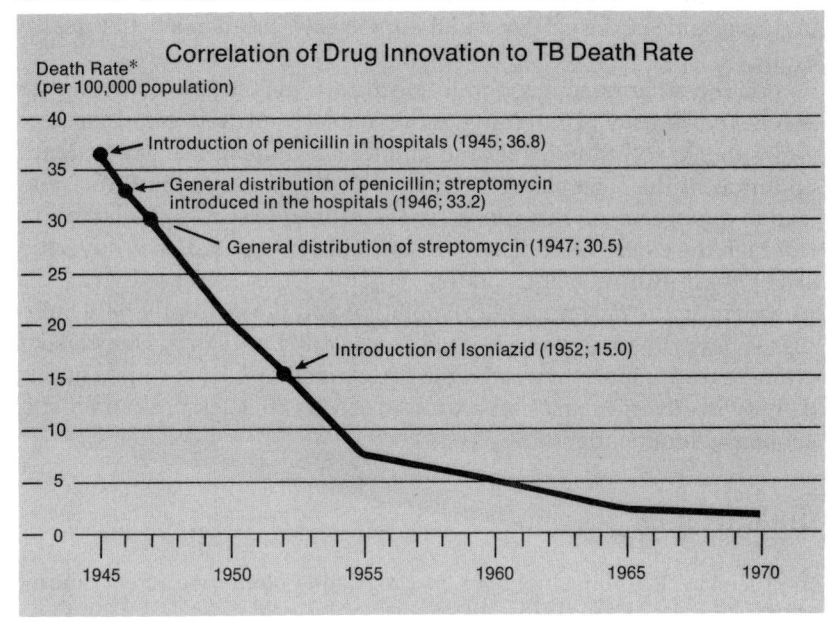

Correlation of Drug Innovation to TB Death Rate

Death Rate* (per 100,000 population)

- Introduction of penicillin in hospitals (1945; 36.8)
- General distribution of penicillin; streptomycin introduced in the hospitals (1946; 33.2)
- General distribution of streptomycin (1947; 30.5)
- Introduction of Isoniazid (1952; 15.0)

* "Death Rates" refer to crude death rates, — unadjusted for age and sex of the population.
Adapted from: Fact Book, Pharmaceutical Manufacturers Association, Washington, D.C., 1973, p. 52, 53.

Figure 7-11 Correlation of drug innovations to death rates from tuberculosis. Reprinted with permission, Roche Laboratories, Nutley, N.J.

Among people 65 years and older, there are only 69 men for every 100 women, the ratio decreasing from 77 per 100 between 65 and 74 years to 48 per 100 at 85 years and over. One reason for this increasing divergence is the fact that life expectancy for women has increased substantially. Therefore, the clinician prescribing for the elderly must consider yet another variable in drug action, as most of the elderly patients are female.

FUTURE HEALTH STATUS

Current knowledge of diseases and their effect on the elderly may not be applicable to future geriatric populations. On one hand, it might be expected that the elderly will have an enhanced health status. Better dietary habits, such as restricted salt and sugar intake, reduction of fat and cholesterol consumption, and increased physical activity may cause changes. Environmental manipulation, leading to greater social involvement and less social isolation, more productivity and fewer economic constraints may also help. Higher educational levels in the current adult population may influence the mental acuity of future generations, and thus their health status. Technical developments, such as the greater availability of better prostheses and safer and more sophisticated surgical and diagnostic procedures may also contribute to an enhanced health status for the future elderly. Again, a better understanding of the elderly and their needs will lead to a better quality of life.

On the other hand, economic constraints may lead to consumption of cheaper meats, containing more cholesterol and fat. Increased atmospheric pollution levels and an increased incidence of accidental pollution of the food chain, such as with Kepone and the PBCs, may lead to a more negative outlook for the future. Diseases of adaptation, to which the elderly urban poor are particularly exposed, may adversely affect their future health status. Possibly, the increased drug use prevalent in the current adult population and the currently held belief that social problems can be treated successfully with drugs may lead to an increased incidence in adverse drug reactions. Lack of productive activity in advanced age can lead to a feeling of uselessness and loss of economic independence.

REFERENCES

Adelman, R.C. Impaired hormonal regulation of enzyme activity during aging. *Fed Proc.* 34:179, 1975.

Anderson, O.W. Reflections on the sick aged and the helping systems. *J Gerontol Nurs.* 3(2):14, 1977.

Anderson, W.F. An approach to preventive geriatric medicine. *Gerontol Clin.* 2:55, 1960.

Brickner, P.W., Duque, T., and Kaufman, A. The homebound aged, a medically unreached group. *Ann Intern Med.* 82:1, 1975.

Comfort, A. *A Good Age.* New York: Crown Publishers, 1976.

Currie, C., MacNeill, R.M., Walker, J.G. et al. Medical social screening of patients aged 70 to 72 by an urban general practice health team. *Br Med J.* 2:108, 1974.

Eckstein, D. Common complaints of the elderly. *Hosp Practice.* 11(4):67, 1976.

Goldfarb, A.I. Prevalence of psychiatric disorders in metropolitan old age and nursing homes. *J Am Geriatr Soc.* 10:77, 1962.

Goldfarb, A.I. *Aging and Organic Brain Syndrome.* Ft. Washington, Pa.: McNeil Laboratories, 1974.

Health Resources Administration. *Health, United States, 1976-1977.* DHEW Publ. No. (HRA) 77-1232. Hyattsville, Md., 1977.

Jones, S., Carr, J., and Hauk, W.W. *Medicare Impact on Hospital Utilization, A Report to the Social Security Administration.* Boston: Department of Preventive and Social Medicine, Harvard Medical School, 1975.

Koch, H.K., and Dennison, N.J. Ambulatory medical care rendered in physicians' offices: United States, 1975. *Adv Data.* 14:1, 1977.

Kohn, R.R. Human aging and disease. *J Chronic Dis.* 16:5, 1963.

Kovar, M.G. Health of the elderly and use of health services. *Public Health Rep.* 92:9, 1977.

Leonard, J.C. Can geriatrics survive? *Br Med J.* 1:1335, 1976.

Liddell, D.E., Williams, F.M., and Briant, R.H. Phenazone (Antipyrine) metabolism and distribution in young and elderly adults. *Clin Exp Pharmacol Physiol.* 2:481, 1975.

Linn, B.S., Linn, N.W., and Knopka, F. The very old patient in ambulatory care. Presented at the 30th Annual Meeting of the Gerontology Society. San Francisco, 1977.

National Center for Health Statistics. *Health for the Later Years of Life.* Rockville, Md., 1971.

Palmore, E. Facts on aging. *Gerontologist* 17:315, 1977.

Rahe, R.H., Romo, M., Bennett, L. et al. Recent life changes, myocardial infarction, and abrupt coronary death. *Arch Intern Med.* 133:221, 1974.

Reichel, W. Multiple problems in the elderly. *Hosp Practice.* 11(3):103, 1976.

Rosin, A.J. How a geriatric outpatient clinic can assist the family physician. *Geriatrics* 30(11):67, 1975.

Sainsbury, P., and de Alarcon, J.G. The psychiatrist and the geriatric patient: the effects of community care on the family of the geriatric patient. Proceedings of the Annual Spring Scientific Colloquium, Northern New England Branch, American Psychiatric Association, 1969.

Shanas, E. *The Health of Older People: A Social Survey.* Cambridge: Harvard University Press, 1961.

Shanas, E. Health status of older people. Cross-national implications. *Am J Public Health.* 64:261, 1974.

Shanas, E. Living arrangements and housing of old people. Edited by E.W. Busse, and E. Pfeiffer. In *Behavior and Adaptation in Late Life.* Boston: Little, Brown and Co., 1977.

Supreme Court of the United States: Virginia State Board of Pharmacy et al. vs Virginia Citizens Consumer Council, Inc., et al. No. 74-895. May 24, 1976.

Task Force on Prescription Drugs, Department of Health, Education and Welfare. *The Drug Users.* Washington, D.C.: U.S. Government Printing Office, 1968.

Vinogradov, N.A., and Revutskaya, R.M. Geriatric care oriented to preventive medicine. *Geriatric Focus* 11(2):1, 1972.

Vital and Health Statistics. Data from the National Survey, Series 12, No. 22. *Chronic Conditions and Impairments of Nursing Home Residents, U.S. 1969.* DHEW Publ. No. (HRA) 74-1707. Washington, D.C., 1973.

Vital and Health Statistics. Data from the National Survey, Series 12, No. 24. *Measures of Chronic Illness Among Residents of Nursing and Personal Care Homes, U.S. June-August 1969.* DHEW Publ. No. (HRA) 74-1709. Washington, D.C., 1974.

Wolfe, M. Toward quality health care for the aged: education, legislation, and service. *J Gerontol Nurs.* 3(2):12, 1977.

APPENDIX A

ARTICLE 43, § 565C ANNOTATED CODE OF MARYLAND

§ 565C. Rights of Patients in Skilled Nursing Facilities and Intermediate Care Facilities. *(Effective January 1, 1976)*

(a) *Declaration of patient's rights.*—It is the intent of the General Assembly and the purpose of this section to promote the interests and well-being of the patients and residents of skilled nursing facilities and intermediate care facilities. It is declared to be the public policy of this State that the interests of the patient be protected by a declaration of a patient's bill of rights and by requiring that the facilities treat their patients in accordance with the provisions of this bill of rights, which shall include, but not be limited to, the following:

(1) Every patient and resident shall be treated with consideration, respect, and full recognition of their dignity and individuality;

(2) Every patient and resident shall receive care, treatment and services which are adequate, appropriate, and in compliance with relevant federal and State law and regulations;

(3) Every patient and resident, prior to or at the time of admission and during stay, shall receive a written statement of the services provided by the facility, including those required to be offered on an as-needed basis, and of related charges including any charges for services not covered under medicare or medicaid, or not covered by the facility's basic per diem rate. Upon receiving such statement, the patient shall sign a written receipt which must be retained by the facility in its files;

(4) Every patient shall receive from his attending physician or the resident physician of the facility complete and current information concerning his diagnosis, treatment and prognosis in terms and language the patient can reasonably be expected to understand, unless medically inadvisable. The patient and resident shall participate in the planning of his medical treatment, may refuse medication and treatment and know the medical consequences of such actions, and shall give prior informed consent to participation in experimental research. Written evidence of compliance with this last provision, including signed acknowledgments by the patient, shall be retained by the facility in its files;

(5) Every patient and resident shall have placed at his/her bedside by the facility the name, address and telephone number of the physician responsible for his care;

(6) Every patient and resident shall receive respect and privacy in his medical care program. Case discussion, consultation, examination, and treatment are confidential and should be conducted discreetly. Those not directly involved in the patient's care must have the permission of the patient to be present. Personal and medical records shall be treated confidentially and the consent of the patient or resident shall be obtained for their release to any individual outside the facility, except as needed in case of the patient's transfer to another health care institution or as required by law or third party payment contract, or to any individual inside the facility who has no demonstrable need for such records;

(7) Every patient and resident has the right to be free from mental and physical abuse, and free from chemical and physical restraints except as authorized by a physician according to clear and indicated medical need;

(8) Every patient and resident shall receive from the administrator or staff of the facility a reasonable response to his requests;

(9) Every patient and resident shall be provided with information as to any relationship of the facility to other health care and related institutions insofar as the patient's care is concerned;

(10) Every patient and resident shall receive reasonable continuity of care which shall include, but not be limited to, what appointment times and physicians are available;

(11) Every patient and resident may associate and communicate privately and without restriction with persons and groups of his choice on his own or their initiative at any reasonable hour; may send and shall receive mail promptly and unopened; shall have access at any reasonable hour to a telephone where he may speak privately; and shall have access to writing instruments, stationery, and postage;

(12) Every patient and resident has the right to manage his own financial affairs. If, at the patient's written request, the facility manages the patient's financial affairs, it shall have available for inspection a monthly accounting and shall furnish the patient with a quarterly statement of the patient's account. The patient and resident shall have unrestricted access to such account at reasonable hours;

(13) If married, every patient and resident shall enjoy privacy in visits by his/her spouse and, if both are inpatients of the facility, they shall be afforded the opportunity where feasible to share a room, unless medically contraindicated;

(14) Every patient and resident shall enjoy privacy in his/her room, and facility personnel shall respect this right by knocking on the door before entering a patient's room except when the patient or resident is asleep;

(15) Every patient and resident has the right, personally or through other persons or in combination with others, to present

grievances and recommend changes in policies and services on behalf of himself or others to the facility's staff or administrator, the State Office on Aging, or other persons or groups without fear of reprisal, restraint, interference, coercion, or discrimination;

(16) A patient or resident may not be required to perform services for the facility without his/her consent and the written approval of the attending physician;

(17) Every patient and resident has the right to retain and use his/her personal clothing and possessions where reasonable, and the right to security in their storage and use;

(18) A patient or resident may not be transferred or discharged from a skilled nursing facility or intermediate care facility except for medical reasons, the patient's own or other patient's welfare, or non-payment for the stay. If such cause is reasonably believed to exist, the patient or resident shall be given at least thirty (30) days advance notice of the proposed action together with the reasons for the decision and an opportunity for an impartial hearing to challenge such action if the patient so wishes. In emergencies such notice need not be give [given].

(b) *Devolving of rights.*—Where consistent with the nature of the right, all of the above rights, particularly as they pertain to a person adjudicated incompetent in accordance with State law, or a patient who is found medically incapable by his attending physician, or a patient who is unable to communicate with others, shall devolve upon the patient's guardian, next of kin, sponsoring agency, or representative payee (except when the facility itself is representative payee) selected pursuant to § 205 (j) of the Social Security Act.

8 Diagnosis

Early diagnosis is of major importance when dealing with the elderly, as they are less able than younger people to cope with their illnesses, both mentally and physically. Even minor disease states, if allowed to remain undiagnosed and to linger, may lead to major clinical consequences. Health, according to the World Health Organization is a "state of complete physical, mental, and social well-being and not merely the absence of disease or infirmity." This ideal cannot easily be applied to the elderly, as the concept of "being well" may differ substantially between younger and older people; the older person is often forced to accept and adapt to the effects of age decrements. However, the definition does serve to highlight the need not to restrict the diagnostic process to medical problems only but to expand it to include an evaluation of the patient's social and economic status as well.

Diagnosis is often less a matter of finding what changes or disorders are present than to determine what stage they may have reached. The diagnostic process may be directed primarily toward finding ways to minimize the effects of a patient's infirmities, which can be one of the most gratifying experiences for a geriatrician.

Prevailing stereotypes still cause many treatable problems to remain unidentified, unacknowledged, and untreated. Too often, many problems are still dismissed as inevitable concomitants of aging (Cohen 1977). A case history serves to illustrate the difficulties that may be encountered and the ease with which problems could be ascribed to aging:

> An elderly patient presents with nocturnal paresthesia of hands and fingers, edema of hands and fingers, incomplete flexion of fingers, weakness of handgrip, morning stiffness and pain, painful shoulders, nocturnal muscle spasms in extremities, impaired tactile sensation, pain and stiffness in knees, transitory nocturnal paralysis of entire arm, edema in feet and ankles, painful elbow, and paresthesia of facial cheeks.

A considerable amount of medical sleuthing led to the conclusion that these were not symptoms of aging but that the patient suffered from a vitamin B-6 deficiency. Treatment with pyridoxine was clinically beneficial (Folkers et al 1977).

Diagnostic failure may begin with a failure to establish the patient's correct age (Hunter et al 1978) and may also rest with the patient's reluctance or inability to provide a detailed history. The patient may present only the chief complaint, neglecting to mention other acute or chronic symptoms. This has been referred to as a "hoarding of illness" (Anderson 1966). It is not unusual for elderly persons to accept physical limitations as a normal concomitant of aging, undeserving of medical attention. Furthermore, they may be reluctant to "bother the busy physician." Under-reporting of disease is particularly prevalent among anxious persons.

Confusion, possibly caused by drug overuse or an adverse response to the usual drug dosage, may make it impossible to obtain a detailed history. Family and friends, though, cannot necessarily be relied on for information. They may overstate a patient's condition, possibly for the purpose of having the patient institutionalized; on the other hand, they may understate problems in order to keep the patient out of an institution.

The difficulties of diagnosis or the lack of perseverance on the part of the clinician are attested to by the fact that large numbers of elderly persons have significant medical problems or mental disorders which remain unrecognized (Schuckit et al 1977; Agate 1970). Most commonly, anemia, cardiac failure, failing eyesight, deafness, and urinary symptoms are overlooked. Above all, though, the most serious problem is the exceeding difficulty of distinguishing between "normal" age-related changes and disease changes. Nomograms to measure the patient's physiologic performance against age-adjusted standards are still being developed and are not yet available.

CLINICAL PRESENTATION

Diagnostic difficulties are compounded by the absence of classical signs and symptoms and difficulty in physical examination:

- The patient may present with painless myocardial infarction.
- There may be sepsis without fever.
- Pneumonia may present as confusion.
- There may be nonbreathless pulmonary edema.

"Failure to thrive" may be indicative of chronic illness, combining anxiety, depression, weight loss, refusal to eat, incontinence, and mental failure. Malignant diseases, chronic infections, rheumatic diseases, severe anemia, chronic constipation, hyponatremia, or hypokalemia could all be responsible for failure to thrive.

Weakness is a common complaint (Andriola 1978); 75% of people over 75 years of age will complain of weakness, fatigue, and dizziness. There may be tiredness, lack of energy, or a specific weakness when walking or climbing stairs. Parkinson disease or depression could well be the cause of this.

Pain perception and recognition may be strikingly abnormal. Acute pain does not seem to be as sharply perceived, or reacted to, but chronic pain seems to be worse (Hunt 1976). Pain may be absent in myocardial infarction or ruptured appendix (Reichel 1976). This abnormal response may result from the aging process in the nervous tissue, diminishing the intensity of pain signals reaching the brain. On the other hand, heightened pain reaction is likely in patients with pressure sores, rheumatoid arthritis, and malignant disease.

Instead of experiencing pain, a patient may react to an inflamed, thrombosed external hemorrhoid or to myocardial infarction with a sudden onset of agitated behavior and confusion.

Referred pain appears to dominate pain of local origin. This is not only important in diagnosis, but also in rehabilitative procedures. For example, soft tissue may be overstretched in an attempt to establish range of motion without any protest from a patient insensitive to pain. Chronic pain may present as depression. If a patient seems to rationalize functional impairment as pain, this possibility should be suspected (Indeck 1978). Functional impairment may include loss of short-term memory, motor function, or sensory perception.

Angina pectoris is more likely to have atypical features in the elderly than in younger persons. Instead of chest pain, there may be dyspnea. Patients may also have an atypical distribution of pain that simulates other medical entities. As previously noted, no significant chest pain may be present in acute myocardial infarction, but radiation of pain may be prominent and extend to the abdomen. The patient may present with shortness of breath, secondary to acute left heart failure. Headache may be minor in subdural hematoma, and, in meningitis, there is sometimes little fever and neck stiffness.

The incidence of thyrotoxicosis is greater in older than in younger persons. Almost one-half of the patients may have an unusual thyrotoxic syndrome complex. Typical symptoms are likely to be less pronounced or they may be almost totally absent. The patient may not appear hyperkinetic, and prominent eyes, tremor, tachycardia, hypertension, or excessive sweating may be absent. Thyrotoxicosis may instead present as a nonspecific clinical picture of depression and apathy with weight loss, constipation, and anorexia. Anxiety and irritability will most likely be absent. The course of disease may be dominated by cardiac decompensation, gastrointestinal symptoms, abnormalities of the calcium metabolism, osteoporosis, or confusion(Rønnov-Jessen and Kirkegaards 1973).

Hypothyroidism is most often seen as fatigue, sluggishness, withdrawal behavior, and senile atrophic skin changes, all of which can easily be attributed to signs of old age (Morrow 1978).

An age-related decrement of brain function can be responsible for confusion and disorientation as a first sign of infection, pneumonia, cardiac failure, coronary occlusion, electrolyte imbalance, anemia, or dehydration. Lethargy, dehydration, and constipation may be age-related symptoms, but they may also result from potassium depletion caused by diuretic therapy. Depression, frequently encountered, may be the result of social isolation or may have been caused by drugs such as reserpine, methyldopa, digitalis, propranolol, procainamide, or phenobarbital (Waal 1976). Thus, the abnormality of clinical presentation may make diagnosis complex and difficult.

LABORATORY TEST VALUES

The problem of diagnosis is made still more difficult by the fact that some test norms change and some do not. Values for albumin, calcium, cholesterol, glucose, alkaline phosphatase, urea, and uric acid tend to change with age (Bender and Grams 1975; Caird 1973). Other tests, such as urinalysis or serum electrolytes, do not change with age, although there is an age-related increase in the frequency of hyponatremia (Weissman et al 1971).

The question facing the clinician is a difficult one to answer. Does an abnormal laboratory test result indicate a disease state or does a normal value indicate absence of disease? Consideration must be given to the fact that many test values have been established in normal, younger persons and increased values may well be normal for the patient's age. For example, a normal serum creatinine value in an elderly person is not proof of a normal glomerular filtration rate, as decreased production of creatinine will cause normal values despite decreased glomerular filtration (Perrier and Gibaldi 1973; Kristensen et al 1974). Some age- and sex-related changes are well known, such as changes in the systolic and diastolic blood pressures (Table 8-1) and the reduction of glucose tolerance with age. Decreased glucose tolerance, though, is not universal and in the nondiabetic population may be caused by diabetes-related genes, insulin antagonism, or vascular disease. However, faced with reduced glucose tolerance, the physician must decide whether this is a normal, age-related change or a pathologic change. If the clinician were to accept normative standards, then most elderly persons, based on glucose tolerance decline, would be diagnosed as diabetics (Andres 1971). Incidentally, in elderly diabetic women, the frequency of cystopyelonephritis may occur in up to 60% of all patients, but frequently there is a complete lack of characteristic symptoms (Koenigstein and Hirn 1975).

Table 8-1
Age- and Sex-related Changes in Systolic and Diastolic Blood Pressure

Age (yrs)	Systolic (Mean)	Diastolic (Mean)
Males		
20	122.9	76.0
30	126.1	78.5
40	129.0	81.2
50	134.5	83.4
60	141.8	84.5
Females		
20	115.7	71.7
30	119.8	74.9
40	127.0	79.5
50	137.3	83.5
60	144.0	85.0

Adapted from: A.M. Master, L.I. Dublin, and H.H. Marks. The normal blood pressure range and its clinical implications. *JAMA.* 143(17):1464, 1950.

There is a consistently wider spread of hematology values. Erythrocyte and hematocrit values are lower than standard adult values and wider levels are seen with hemoglobin levels, the leukocyte count, and the differential count (Earney and Earney 1972). The sedimentation rate tends to be elevated in anemia.

When using diagnostic tests, the clinician must consider the altered physiologic state. It has been suggested that larger than usual test doses of tuberculin may be required to elicit allergy in older people (Myers and Hartig 1959), but not all elderly people show decreased sensitivity (Woodruff and Chapman 1971). In studying the influence of aging on skin reactivity, it has been found that the incidence of positive skin reactions to food allergens is highest in the first decade of life, decreases slightly to age 50, and then declines sharply. Skin tests with histamine show the same decrease in sensitivity (Tuft et al 1955). Failure to demonstrate a positive reaction may be due to loss in skin reactivity rather than lack of specific sensitivity.

A large number of the elderly show evidence of liver dysfunction when the usual standard value for a number of liver tests is applied. Although these changes usually indicate organ changes, the functional capacity of the liver may be adequate and the changes may also be compatible with normalcy for this particular age group (Means and Lamy 1974).

OTHER DIAGNOSTIC PROBLEMS

In several disease states of the elderly, metabolic activities of the nerve cells in the cerebral cortex are affected. This can result in reduced cerebral blood flow and a clouding of consciousness. Vitamin B-12 deficiency, pyridoxine deficiency, hypokalemia, alkalosis, hyperthermia, and hypothermia caused by drug therapy could all be responsible.

Aphasia may interfere with diagnosis. To differentiate the etiology of coma in the elderly, the following mnemonic (Rein 1978) has been suggested:

AEIOU plus TIPPS

Alcoholism	Trauma
Epilepsy	Infection
Insulin (increase or decrease)	Poison
Opium	Psychogenic
Uremia	Shock

It must also be remembered that diagnostic test procedures, per se, can cause anxiety and confusion. Some present potential hazards, such as the barium enema. The cleansing of the colon prior to the test is still too often performed with an oral dose of castor oil. While this is well tolerated by younger patients, the resulting diarrhea can cause severe fluid and electrolyte disturbances in the older patient, resulting in hypotension and shock.

Fever of unknown origin may be caused by drugs, such as aspirin and other headache remedies, antimicrobials, barbiturates, isoniazid, methyldopa, nonprescription decongestants, and quinidine. Fever may also be related to the use of indwelling urethral catheters or an endotracheal tube (Jacoby and Swartz 1973), but there may not be an elevated white blood count in bacterial infections (Wolff et al 1975).

It is well recognized that many drugs can interfere with laboratory test values. The elderly, for whom polypharmacy is often a way of life, are therefore particularly susceptible to such interference (Dunderman 1970; Christian 1970). For example, when a patient is asked to determine urine glucose, one must remember that Clinitest action is susceptible to interference from such drugs as ampicillin and furosemide.

REFERENCES

Agate, J.D. *The Practice of Geriatrics.* Springfield, Ill.: Charles C Thomas, 1970.

Anderson, W.F. *The Prevention of Illness in the Elderly: The Rutherglen Experiment in Medicine in Old Age.* London: Sir Isaac Pitman and Sons, Ltd., 1966.

Andres, R. Aging and diabetes. *Med Clin North Am.* 55:835, 1971.

Andriola, M.J. When an elderly patient complains of weakness. *Geriatrics* 33(6):79, 1978.

Bender, K.J., and Grams, R.R. Monitoring the geriatric patient. *J Am Pharm Assoc.* NS15:21, 1975.

Caird, F.I. Problems of interpretation of laboratory test values in the old. *Br Med J.* 4:348, 1973.

Cohen, G.D. Approach to the geriatric patient. *Med Clin North Am.* 61:855, 1977.

Earney, W.W., and Earney, A.J. Geriatric hematology. *J Am Geriatr Soc.* 20:174, 1972.

Folkers, K., Saji, S., Kaji, M. et al. Biochemical evidence for a deficiency of vitamin B-6 in the carpal tunnel syndrome. *Acta Pharm Svec.* 14(suppl):38, 1977.

Hunt, T.E. Management of chronic non-rheumatic pain in the elderly. *J Am Geriatr Soc.* 24:402, 1976.

Hunter, K.I., Linn, M.W., and Linn, B.S. Misperceiving the age of the sick elderly patient. *Geriatrics* 33(5):88, 1978.

Indeck, W. Evaluating and managing chronic pain. *Geriatrics* 33(5):59, 1978.

Koenigstein, R.P., and Hirn, S. Zur Pathologie and Therapie der Chronischen Cystopyelonephritis bei der Altersdiabetikerin. *Aktuel Gerontol.* 5:329, 1975.

Kristensen, M., Molholm Hansen, J., Kampman, J. et al. Drug elimination and renal function. *J Clin Pharmacol.* 14:307, 1974.

Means, B.J., and Lamy, P.P. Diagnostic tests, drugs, and the geriatric patient. *J Am Geriatr Soc.* 22:258, 1974.

Morrow, L.B. How thyroid disease presents in the elderly. *Geriatrics* 33(4):42, 1978.

Myers, A.J., and Hartig, H. Tuberculosis lingers as the life span lengthens. II. *Geriatrics* 14:801, 1959.

Perrier, D., and Gibaldi, M. Estimation of drug elimination in renal failure. *J Clin Pharmacol.* 13:458, 1973.

Reichel, W. Multiple problems in the elderly. *Hosp Practice.* 11(3):103, 1976.

Rein, T. Approaching the comatose geriatric patient. *Patient Care* 12(13):249, 1978.

Rønnov-Jessen, V., and Kirkegaards, C. Hyperthyroidism—a disease of old age. *Br Med J.* 1:41, 1973.

Schuckit, M.A., Miller, P.L., and Hahlbohm, D. Unrecognized psychiatric illness in elderly medical-surgical patients. *J Gerontol.* 30:655, 1977.

Tuft, L., Heck, V.M., and Gregory, D.C. Studies on sensitization as applied to skin test reactions. III. Influence of age upon skin reactivity. *J Allerg.* 26:359, 1955.

Waal, H.J. Propranolol-induced depression. *Br Med J.* 2:50, 1976.

Weissman, P.N., Shenkman, L., and Gregerman, R.I. Chlorpropamide hyponatremia: drug-induced inappropriate antidiuretic-hormone activity. *N Engl J Med.* 284:65, 1971.

Woodruff, C.E., and Chapman, P.T. Tuberculin sensitivity in elderly patients. *Am Rev Respir Dis.* 104:261, 1971.

9 Some Patient Factors Governing Responses to Drugs

A great number of factors combine to determine the outcome of a specific drug regimen. In the elderly, these factors multiply to yield a less predictable response to drugs. Some of these are apparent, such as the morbidity and mortality from diseases, (which affect the elderly differently than they do younger persons [Table 9-1]), and the changing male/female ratio among elderly patients; the male death rate is higher throughout every decade of life (Table 9-2). Drug use differs with the sex of the patient. Women, for example, report a higher number of psychiatric disturbances than men. Most likely, though, they do not as a group experience a greater incidence of mental illness, but sociocultural patterns permit a greater expression of emotion by women and physicians seem to expect that women require more mood-modifying drugs than men. It seems more acceptable for women to be expressive about difficulties (Phillips and Segal 1969; Cooperstock 1971).

Table 9-1
Mortality, Morbidity, and Disability Rates*

	Age (years)		
	17-44	45-64	65 and over
Death rate†	2.3	12.0	50.0
Heart disease‡	1.0	2.5	9.0
Arthritis‡	0.3	5.5	26.0
Disability rate§	1.5	5.0	21.0

*US, 1970
†Deaths per thousand per year
‡Cases per 100 noninstitutionalized persons
§Percent population unable to carry out major activity of daily living

Table 9-2
Deaths by Sex and Age — 1972

Age	Male	Female
All ages	1,095,310	866,640
Less than 1	34,290	25,920
1-4	6220	4820
5-14	9570	6500
15-24	36,130	12,810
25-34	28,870	13,790
35-44	42,890	25,400
45-54	107,540	60,820
55-59	86,240	46,030
60-64	113,760	61,830
65-69	133,180	82,110
70-74	138,820	124,320
75-79	133,280	101,990
80-84	113,250	131,620
85 +	104,550	167,290
Unaccountable	1740	1400

Other factors may not be as apparent, or may not be taken into consideration, yet they can seriously alter a patient's response to a particular drug. Among these are certain genetic or biologic factors and several environmental factors.

GENETIC OR BIOLOGIC FACTORS

Inherited traits are not peculiar to the elderly, but the elderly may lack sufficient reserve capacity and the influence of these factors may therefore be more devastating. Inherited factors may change the absorption, metabolism, distribution, and excretion of a drug and thus the magnitude of response. They may also alter tissue sensitivity.

Patients may be slow or fast acetylators of certain drugs. Acetylator phenotype influences the therapeutic effects and toxicity of several drugs (Drayer and Reidenberg 1977). The variable metabolism of isoniazid is probably the best-known example of genetic influence on drug metabolism. Mongoloid populations are primarily rapid acetylators, while among the Israeli Baghdad Jewish population only 25% are rapid acetylators (Table 9-3). Slow acetylators are apt to develop high and longer-lasting blood levels of isoniazid (Evans 1971). Even if these patients receive the "usual" dose of isoniazid, drug accumulation will occur. This, in turn, interferes with vitamin B-6 (pyridoxine) metabolism and results in peripheral neuropathy. This undesirable effect can be overcome by administration of pyridoxine. Slow acetylators receiving phenytoin concurrently with isoniazid often exhibit signs of phenytoin toxicity; accumulated isoniazid interferes with the metabolism of phenytoin. On the other hand, rapid acetylators are more likely to develop hepatitis when given isoniazid (LaDu and Kalow 1968; Goldman 1974).

The lupus-like syndrome induced by procainamide occurs more frequently in slow acetylators (Woosley et al 1978). Other drugs affected include hydralazine, phenelzine, and sulfapyridine.

In some individuals, a prolonged period of apnea can follow administration of succinylcholine if their plasma contains an abnormal

Table 9-3
Prevalence of Rapid Acetylators

Origin	Percentage prevalence
Eskimos	95
Korea	89
Japan	88
Norway	80
Vietnam	72
Brazil	67
North America	
Indians	79
Blacks	48
Whites	45
Baltic region	39
India	39
Sweden	32

Adapted from: M.D. Rawlins. Variability in response to drugs. *Br Med J.* 4:91, 1974.

variant of pseudocholinesterase (Kalow 1962). Certain drug-induced glaucomas are also related to inherited abnormalities, as is an unusual resistance to coumarin-type anticoagulants.

Among the inherited traits that can lead to altered tissue sensitivity is the so-called primaquine sensitivity. Sardinians, other males of Mediterranean origin, Sephardic Jews, Greeks, Iranians, Orientals, and, to a somewhat lesser extent, American blacks may have a congenital glucose-6-phosphate dehydrogenase (G-6-PD) deficiency, which may be activated to hemolytic anemia by primaquine and similar drugs (Table 9-4). About 11% of American blacks are thought to be G-6-PD deficient, but hemolytic reactions are more common and severe in patients of Mediterranean origin than they are in blacks (Beutler 1971; *Medical Letter* 1975). Recently, it has been reported that the combination of sulfamethoxazole and trimethoprim, used frequently to treat urinary tract infections in the elderly, can cause hemolytic anemia in G-6-PD deficient individuals and that megadoses of ascorbic acid (vitamin C), acting as a strong reducing agent, can also lead to hemolytic anemia in patients deficient in G-6-PD (Campbell et al 1975).

Table 9-4
Drugs Implicated in Causing Hemolysis in G-6-PD Deficiency

Analgesics:
  Acetanilid
  Acetophenetidin
  Acetylsalicylic acid*
  Antipyrine

Sulfonamides and sulfones:
  Diaphenylsulfone
  Salicylazosulfapyridine
  Sulfacetamide
  Sulfamethoxypyridazine
  Sulfanilamide
  Sulfapyridine
  Sulfisoxazole*
  Sulfoxone*
  Thiazosulfone

Antimalarials:
  Pamaquine
  Pentaquine
  Primaquine
  Quinacrine
  Quinocide

Nonsulfonamide antibacterial agents:
  Chloramphenicol†
  Furazolidone
  Furmethonol
  Neoarsphenamine

Table 9-4 *(continued)*

    Nitrofurantoin
    Nitrofurazone
    Para-aminosalicylic acid

Miscellaneous:
    Ascorbic acid
    Dimercaprol (BAL)*
    Isoniazid
    Mestranol
    Methyldopa
    Methylene blue*
    Nalidixic acid
    Naphthalene
    Phenylhydrazine
    Piperazine
    Quinidine‡
    Quinine‡
    Tolbutamide
    Trinitrotoluene
    Vitamin K water soluble analogues*

*Slightly hemolytic in blacks, or only in very large doses.
†Possibly hemolytic in Caucasians, but not in blacks or Orientals.
‡Hemolytic in Caucasians, but not in blacks.

ENVIRONMENTAL FACTORS

Diverse societal factors such as race, religion, ethnic background, folklore, and diet can influence a patient's response to a particular therapeutic regimen or a patient's entire health behavior. Cultural patterns also influence the use of health resources (Mechanic 1976). Illness perception can create barriers to treatment based on cultural concepts (Scott 1973). For example, guilt tends to be a symptom of depression only in Westernized populations; depressive illness in terms of Western symptomatology is almost unknown among natives in equatorial Africa (Bazzoni 1970). Among elderly of different cultural backgrounds, there may be different concepts of illness, and disease may be thought of as an embarrassing handicap rather than a biologic change (Merskey 1978). Many of these traits may not necessarily be found only among the elderly, but they occur more frequently and severely in the elderly as exaggerated deep-seated mental and behavioral characteristics of childhood and early life (Sadowski and Weinsaft 1975). In elderly people, there is usually an exaggeration of previous personality traits that may have been culturally influenced in early age. These early traits often surface as aging progresses and become cumulatively stronger.

The influence of ethnic groups on the health status of individual members is important. The smaller an ethnic group in relation to the total population, the higher the diagnosed rate of mental illness; presumably the small group canot give sufficient social support. This has been documented for Chinese in Canada, Italians in Boston, and blacks and whites in various parts of Baltimore (Rabkin and Struening 1976). Actually, very little is known about different reactions to drug therapy among ethnic groups. In German subjects, the diuretic and natriuretic response to two diuretics was greater and potassium excretion less than in English subjects, but the discrepancy was ascribed to differences in dietary intake (Branch et al 1976). Jamaicans have shown little or no response to propranolol, but the reason has not yet been determined. It is thought that some etiologic factor may determine the effectiveness of beta blockers (Humphreys and Delvin 1968). Black patients respond more quickly to tricyclics than white patients. This might be explained by the slower metabolism of the tricyclics by blacks, which leads to higher blood levels earlier in the treatment cycle. However, this can also lead to increased adverse effects and treatment failure if the therapeutic plasma range is exceeded (Overall et al 1969; Raskin and Crook 1975; Ziegler and Biggs 1977).

At one time, it had been thought that pernicious anemia affected primarily elderly, northern Europeans (Carmel and Johnson 1978). However, it does not seem to be as rare in American blacks or Indians as once assumed. Indeed, its incidence in blacks may equal or even exceed that in whites of all origins (Hart and McCurdy 1971), and it may develop earlier in black women and possibly in Latin American women.

It may not be ethnic differences that determine drug use at all, but rather fashion in drug use, leading to apparent differences in disease prevalence in different countries. A comparative study of tranquilizer use in the United States and some European countries found that antianxiety drugs were used by 7% of men in Spain, but 12% in Belgium; while the percentage of women ranged from 12% in Spain to 21% in France. It was suggested that sociocultural determinants influenced antianxiety drug use (Balter et al 1974). The need for antianxiety drugs may change with the differing coping mechanisms of various ethnic groups. Cultural differences may also influence disease presentation. For example, alcoholism and its morbidity is influenced by culturally determined behaviors and attitudes. On the other hand, the physician's cultural background and beliefs may be the determining factors. Schizophrenia is much more readily and frequently diagnosed by American than by British physicians (Blackwell 1976). American schizophrenics are said to display more bizarre ideas, the Japanese are more assaultive, and Eskimos are more catatonic.

Differences in drug use in different countries may also be due to variations in recognition of disease entities, and differences in local practices. A disease called "hepatic insufficiency" is recognized in Latin countries (Cedillos 1976), while in Eastern Europe, the "low blood pressure syndrome" is well known and is considered a treatable disease. This syndrome involves headaches and occasional visual disturbance and sufferers seem unable to work (Stolley 1976).

Thus, based on a patient's cultural background, coping mechanism, and genetic make-up, and the physician's cultural background and beliefs, it is reasonable to expect that disease presentation and drug action may differ in patients of different ethnic groups.

There is then no question that sensitivity to cultural differences and understanding of their meanings are prerequisites to successful therapy and treatment of the elderly (Mostwin 1972).

In the United States, there is an increasing interest in the health characteristics of minority groups. Differences among the elderly minorities are exemplified by the fact that whites, in general, consider themselves old at age 75, blacks at 65, and Hispanic-Americans at age 55. However, it is extremely difficult to arrive at valid conclusions about the aged minorities. Difficulties rest with the fact that more than 40% of Hispanic-Americans are under 17 years of age; 37% of the black population is under 17 years of age, compared to only 29% of the general population (Moy and Wilder 1978).

Those planning for health services for elderly minority members must address within-culture differences (Orleans and Kurowski 1977). Some may be apparent. For example, one would expect solar degeneration of the skin much more frequently in fair-haired blue-eyed Scandinavians than in people with a Mediterranean background or in blacks (Cripps 1977), but it may be difficult to relate patterns of segregation found in retirement places to subcultural differences in religion and food preferences (Quadagno et al 1977). Also, there is almost no research being conducted on elderly American Indians because so few survive into old age, especially those living on reservations. The life expectancy among American Indians is only 45 years.

Almost all minorities in the United States are more at risk to morbidity and mortality than whites. This is caused by a number of complex factors in addition to ethnic backgrounds. Important factors include economic status and nutrition.

There is no question that the patient's economic status can importantly influence disease presentation and drug response, either directly or indirectly. Aging poverty in urban areas is significantly compounded by membership in a minority ethnic group (Kim and Wellons 1977). The Pennsylvania Department of Public Welfare selected five criteria to determine the elderly most at risk, including minority status. It is not unusual to hear of double, triple, and even quadruple jeopardy in regard to the elderly, depending on age, domicile, sex, and minority status.

Elderly, economically disadvantaged persons who do not qualify for reimbursement for drugs, may choose to select herbs and other folklore medications. Home remedies may often serve well as placebos, but cannot take the place of a needed drug.

Actually, some "cures" are neither expensive nor harmful. They may help by filling some psychological or cultural need. Some cultures seem to benefit greatly from herb remedies, and some arthritic patients have been convinced that the copper bracelet is helpful. The primary provider must recognize unorthodox approaches to health care, and should not totally discourage or ridicule those that are neither expensive nor harmful (National Commission on Arthritis 1976). The indirect effect of the patient's economic status should not be discounted, either. For example, patients of low socioeconomic status seem to prefer the more sedative effect of barbiturates to the antianxiety agents for alleviation of anxiety symptoms (Rickels 1968). The sedative effect presumably helps obliterate the boredom and threat of daily living. But the major effect of a disadvantaged economic status may be on nutritional habits and thus the health status.

Nutritional and caloric needs are determined by cultural as well as economic influences. The cultural behavior is most powerful in old age and these behavioral patterns may well antagonize medical needs (Haydu 1975). The special nutritional needs of the elderly blacks, Asian-Americans, American Indians, and Hispanic-Americans have been recognized (White House Conference on Aging 1971). Yet, accomplishments in this area are still few. The First Health and Nutrition Examination Survey (HANES) has shown that among the elderly, white men tend to be more obese than black men. Protein deficiencies occur somewhat more frequently among blacks of lower income groups than whites. Thiamine deficiency is seen most often in blacks over 60 years of age.

Among people with incomes below the poverty level, 21% of whites, as opposed to 36% of blacks, had food intakes of less than 1000 calories per day. Older blacks also have somewhat lower vitamin C levels than whites in the same age group; and almost 30% of blacks over 60 years of age showed low hemoglobin levels and almost 42% had low hematocrits.

Hispanics and Hispanic-Americans often adhere to a diet heavy in saturated fats. Transients may find adherence to a dietary regimen almost impossible, particularly if they eat in restaurants that serve heavily salted foods. Thus, environmental and cultural influences and lack of skills make it very difficult to change eating habits, even though medically this may not only be desirable but necessary.

HEALTH STATUS OF THE ETHNIC ELDERLY

Definite differences in the health status of ethnic elderly have been documented. For example, the elderly black incur somewhat fewer short-stay hospital episodes than do other ethnic groups, but they suffer somewhat more from activity limitations because of chronic conditions (Tables 9-5 and 9-6).

Table 9-5
Selected Health Characteristics–All Ages

	Total population	Spanish origin	Black	Other
Activity limitation (chronic condition)	14.3	13.5	17.4	14.0
Doctor visits	75.5	70.4	74.2	76.2
Short-stay hospital episode	10.6	10.4	10.6	10.6
Restricted activity (days/year)	18.2	20.3	23.3	17.6
Bed disability (days/year)	7.1	9.3	9.9	6.6
Days lost from work	5.3	5.0	7.4	5.1

Source: C.S. Moy, and C.S. Wilder. Health characteristics of minority groups, United States, 1976. *Adv Data.* 27:1, 1978.

Table 9-6
Selected Health Characteristics–Persons 65 Years and Over

	Total population	Spanish origin	Black	Other
Activity limitation (chronic condition)	45.4	45.9	52.8	44.6
Doctor visits	80.0	79.4	78.8	80.2
Short-stay hospital episode	18.3	17.1	12.9	18.8
Days restricted activity (days/year)	40.0	53.1	52.5	38.4
Bed disability (days/year)	15.1	20.5	18.5	14.6

Source: C.S. Moy, and C.S. Wilder. Health characteristics of minority groups, United States, 1976. *Adv Data.* 27:1, 1978.

THE USE OF HEALTH FACILITIES
BY THE ETHNIC ELDERLY

Only a very small percentage of the one million nursing home patients are members of minority groups, even though their health needs are proportionally greater (Table 9-7). Discrimination is one factor, particularly in regard to black patients (Butler 1975), but language barriers (Asian-Americans and Spanish-speaking Americans) and cultural problems (American Indians) also play a role (Special Committee on Aging 1975). In comparison to white residents, a greater proportion of Spanish Americans have been in nursing homes for only a short time. In 1977, about 56% of the Spanish Americans in nursing homes had been residents of nursing homes for less than one year (Zappolo 1977). The elderly minority members may be at a particular disadvantage as the nonaffluent patients seem to be placed into nursing homes lacking treatment resources (Kosberg 1973).

Table 9-7
Number and Percent of Nursing Home Residents by Race or Ethnicity: United States, 1973–1974

Race or Ethnicity	Number	Percent
All residents	1,075,900	100.0
White*	1,010,400	93.9
Black	49,300	4.6
Spanish American	12,000	1.1
Other	4200	0.4

*Excludes Spanish American
Source: Characteristics, social contacts, and activities of nursing home residents, United States, 1973-74. National Nursing Home Survey, U.S. DHEW, PHS, Health Resources Administration, DHEW Publ. No. (HRA) 77-1778, Rockville, Md.: National Center for Health Statistics, 1977.

There may be other reasons for the apparent underutilization of long-term care facilities by the elderly. In general, it is the accepted belief that racial minorities have more extended family resources and, therefore, elderly family members are less likely to be placed into a nursing home. On the other hand, whites may often feel guilty about sending a family member to a nursing home, while rural blacks in the South may consider it an achievement to get a family member admitted to a nursing home where there is hot and cold running water, heat, and cleanliness. Culture may play an important part in the significant underutilization of nursing care facilities by older Mexican-Americans. If at all possible, Hispanic-American families try to keep an elderly family member out of a nursing home, viewing nursing homes not as a viable alternative to care but as a last resort (Eribes and Bradley-Rawls 1978).

Sociocultural factors may have a profound effect on the decision to seek treatment and on the response to disease symptoms. For example, requests for antianxiety drugs may differ with the coping mechanism exhibited by various ethnic groups. Similar conclusions can be drawn for analgesics. For many ethnics, it may be deflating and disillusioning to require medication. In general, there is little variation in pain threshold among different people. It is the psychologic response to pain that varies greatly among individuals and in the same individual under different circumstances and in different settings. Social factors, cultural and family response patterns may determine whether or not a particular experience is painful and whether treatment must be sought (Koldomy and McLoughlin 1966; Melzack 1973). The need to know and understand a person's cultural background in response to pain has been clearly demonstrated (Zborowski 1952, 1959). The Irish and "old Americans" seem to differ greatly in their response to pain from Italians and Jews. An Italian in pain is mainly concerned with the analgesic effect of the drug. Once helped, the Italian will most likely forget the episode of pain. On the other hand, a Jewish patient often is reluctant to accept a drug because of an unstated fear and apprehension of its possible habit-forming effect. Moreover, the Jewish patient might be concerned that the analgesic effect achieved was only temporary and that the underlying problem may not have been solved.

Religion can influence response to disease and drug treatment. Truly religious patients are helped by their faith (Kubler-Ross 1974), and with advancing age more people view religion as very important in their life. Only 49% of the total population view religion as very important, while 71% of those over 65 years of age are strongly religious (Harris et al 1975). Thus, it is not surprising that church programs for the elderly had the highest percent of satisfied users among the many programs offered (Guttman 1977). Polish and Italian families preferred church-operated services to government-operated services. Catholic church-operated long-term care facilities were preferred by 57% of a study population, followed by services operated by local ethnic organizations (Fandetti and Gelfand 1974). The introduction of Hebrew chants lessened the use of tranquilizers in one institution (Lissitz 1969; Dominick and Stotsky 1969).

On the other hand, strong religious beliefs, if unrecognized, may have deleterious effects on health status. Jewish patients, on religious grounds, may refuse all medications during Yom Kippur, although the Talmud specifically exempts life-saving and necessary medications under the principle that mandates that a Jewish person should live for tradition. (This is only a 28-hour period and adverse medical effects probably would not result.) Strongly orthodox Jewish patients may refuse pork-based insulin and medications packaged in gelatin capsules, which are also derived from pork, and the assistance of a rabbi may be necessary to convince these patients that they do not contravene the teachings of the Talmud by accepting these medications. While elderly patients in general often accept the disabilities of old age, cultural influences of Oriental Jews may encourage a strong, fatalistic acceptance of disability of old age (Galinsky et al 1978). One question has not yet been satisfactorily answered concerning the use of kosher meats by hypertensive patients. Does this kind of meat contain too much salt to be part of a low sodium diet or is most of it washed off in preparation?

In the therapeutic management of Spanish-speaking elderly persons, it is necessary to understand that even those who may speak English may hesitate to do so, as Spanish is a symbol of their cultural tradition and of their existence as a social group. Older Mexican-Americans are particularly vulnerable compared to other elderly persons. They probably have the most negative perception, compared to blacks and whites, in terms of feelings of sadness and worry that life is not worth living (Streib 1976). In general, older Mexican-Americans are poor and undereducated. Socioeconomic conditions and negative perceptions are strong environmental barriers that preclude them from seeking help (Torres-Gil and Becerra 1977). Yet little is known or published about their health needs (Delgado and Finley 1978). Some clinicians estimate that about 50% of Spanish-speaking patients consult a curer-herbalist before consulting a physician (Clark 1970), others strongly dispute the extensive use of folk strategies (Orleans et al 1977), and still others feel that their ethnic diet, rich in large amounts of spices, salt, and other condiments, is of value to respiratory patients (Ziment 1975).

In terms of illness and health behavior and the influence of racial minority status on these behavioral indices, most is known through studies of black and white populations. The aged blacks have approximately twice the number of health problems as the white aged (Shanas 1977), and it is a well-known fact that hypertension is a threat to black men at an early age (Curry 1977). For those delivering health care, it is important to realize that the incidence of frail health among black males is four times that of white males. Because of differential mortality rates, more whites than blacks reach the age of 75 and over. Of the noninstitutionalized elderly, black women report the greatest restricted mobility. Black women are more than twice as likely as white women to be functionally incapacitated. Eighteen percent of all blacks and 13% of all whites are restricted in their physical mobility. Among black women, 25% are restricted, being either bedfast, housebound or unable to go outdoors without difficulty (Shanas 1977; Ostfeld and Gibson 1972; Shanas 1974; Shanas and Hauser 1974). Black women are the most incapacitated group among noninstitutionalized, elderly persons and are most in need of help in self-care. Capacity for self-care among blacks is less than among whites, and blacks are twice as likely to report difficulties with common tasks. Therefore, blacks report more time spent ill in bed, and they also report more physician contacts. The health perception of blacks is also poorer than that of whites; blacks more often judge their health to be poor and are less likely to report good health.

The elderly have often been described as "health optimists." But there is a sharp difference between aged blacks and aged whites. Only one-third of all black aged probably judge their health to be good, while at least one-half of aged white feel in good health. Conversely, blacks report their health as poor twice as often as whites.

Many of the black elderly delay seeking medical and dental care; lack of money is cited as the major reason for these delays. Seven percent of the elderly blacks who perceive the need for either an eye examination or corrective glasses delay obtaining either, as opposed to only 2% of white elderly persons. Other reasons for not seeking care include dislike for the primary provider, dislike for long waiting periods, a feeling of hopelessness and helplessness, and a pronounced conviction that a particular illness or disorder is not severe (Shanas 1977).

Widowed white elderly are much more likely to live alone than are blacks, but they are more likely than blacks to live close to a child. Fewer black elderly than whites enjoy some aspect of retirement. For all, government benefits are the main source of income, but multiple income sources are the rule among elderly rather than the exception. In rural areas, whites have significantly poorer social resources than blacks. On the other hand, blacks in rural areas tend to be poorer in physical and dental health than whites. They often lack access to transportation and live in poorer housing. In a crisis, both blacks and whites will turn to their families for help, but blacks are more likely to also turn to social agencies (Rosen 1977).

In general, in rural communities, blacks use health services less frequently than whites. Differences in prescribing of pain relievers, tranquilizers, and vitamins/minerals for members of the two races exist, but not for antihypertensives (Salber et al 1976; Greene et al 1978; Salber et al 1979). In general, whether in urban or rural setting, whites receive more prescribed medicines (49%) than blacks (36%). Blacks are also less likely to use nonprescribed medications, regardless of social status (National Center for Health Statistics 1977; Andersen et al 1970; Rabin and Bush 1975). It has been suggested, in an effort to elucidate the reason for these differences, that it may be more difficult to terminate a physician-patient encounter with whites than with blacks. The writing of a prescription, for whites, would be considered one effective way to terminate the visit.

It is quite clear that those rendering health services to the elderly must be familiar with and must take into consideration the influence on health behavior, disease presentation, and drug response to such varied factors as inherited traits, sociocultural factors, racial and ethnic differences among patients, and economic constraints.

ADDENDUM

Most studies investigating variations of drug-metabolizing ability in different patient groups have been performed with Caucasian subjects. Only one study has investigated non-Caucasian subjects, who had a slightly longer antipyrine half-life (Fraser et al 1976). In a more recent study, Sudanese subjects exhibited a significantly lower mean antipyrine clearance and higher volume of distribution than a group of English people. Interestingly, comparable values for Sudanese living in England fell somewhere between the values obtained for the Sudanese and English subjects.

Different populations can have differences in drug disposition, but environmental factors seem to predominate over ethnic differences caused by genetic variation (Branch et al 1978).

REFERENCES

Andersen, R., Smedby, B., and Anderson, O.W. *Medical Care Use in Sweden and the United States–A Comparative Analysis of Systems and Behavior.* Chicago, Ill.: Center for Health Administration Studies, 1970.

Balter, M.B., Levine, J., and Manheimer, D.I. Cross-national study of the extent of anti-anxiety/sedative drug use. *N Engl J Med.* 290:769, 1974.

Bazzoni, W. Affective disorders in Iraq. *Br J Psychiatry.* 117:195, 1970.

Beutler, E. Hexose monophosphate shunt. *Semin Hematol.* 8:311, 1971.

Blackwell, B. Culture, morbidity, and the effects of drugs. *Clin Pharmacol Ther.* 19:668, 1976.

Branch, R.A., Read, P.R., Levine, D. et al. Furosemide and bumetanide: a study of responses in normal English and German subjects. *Clin Pharmacol Ther.* 19:538, 1976.

Branch, R.A., Salih, S.Y., and Homeida, M. Racial differences in drug metabolizing ability: a study with antipyrine in Sudan. *Clin Pharmacol Ther.* 24:283, 1978.

Butler, R.N. *Why Survive? Being Old in America.* New York: Harper and Row, 1975.

Campbell, G.D., Steinberg, M.H., and Bower, J.D. Ascorbic acid-induced hemolysis in G-6-PD deficiency. *Ann Intern Med.* 82:810, 1975.

Carmel, R., and Johnson, C.S. Racial patterns in pernicious anemia. *N Engl J Med.* 298:647, 1978.

Cedillos, R.A. Variations in disease prevalence in the Americas. *Clin Pharmacol Ther.* 19:675, 1976.

Clark, M. *Health in the Mexican-American Culture.* Berkeley, Calif.: University of California Press, 1970.

Cooperstock, R. Sex differences in the use of mood-modifying drugs: an explanatory model. *J Health Soc Behav.* 12:238, 1971.

Cripps, D.J. Skin care and problems in the aged. *Hosp Practice.* 12(4):119, 1977.

Curry, C.L. Hypertension in black men. *Drug Ther.* 7(5):28, 1977.

Delgado, M., and Finley, G.E. The Spanish-speaking elderly: a bibliography. *Gerontologist* 18:387, 1978.

Dominick, J.R., and Stotsky, B.A. Mental patients in nursing homes. IV. Ethnic influences. *J Am Geriatr Soc.* 17:63, 1969.

Drayer, D.E., and Reidenberg, M.M. Clinical consequences of polymorphic acetylation of basic drugs. *Clin Pharmacol Ther.* 22:251, 1977.

Eribes, R.A., and Bradley-Rawls, M. The underutilization of nursing home facilities by Mexican-American elderly in the Southwest. *Gerontologist* 18:363, 1978.

Evans, D.A. Inter-individual differences in metabolism of drugs: the role of genetic factors. *Acta Pharmacol Toxicol.* 29(suppl 3):256, 1971.

Fandetti, D.V., and Gelfand, D.E. Care of the aged: attitudes of white ethnic families. *J Gerontol.* 20:684, 1974.

Fraser, H.S., Bulpitt, C.J., Kahn, C. et al. Factors affecting antipyrine metabolism in West African villagers. *Clin Pharmacol Ther.* 20:369, 1976.

Galinsky, D., Herschkoren, H., Kaplan, M. et al. The need for a new approach to neglected elderly patients. *Geriatrics* 33(1):109, 1978.

Goldman, P. Patient factors governing responses to drugs. *Drug Ther.* 4(4):50, 1974.

Greene, S.B., Salber, E.J., and Feldman, J.J. Distribution of illness and its implications in a southern rural community. *Med Care.* 16:863, 1978.

Guttman, D. (Ed.). The impact of needs, knowledge, ability, and living arrangements on decision-making of the elderly. Final report. AOA Grant 90-A-522, 1977.

Harris, L. et al. *The Myth and Reality of Aging in America.* Washington, D.C.: National Council on the Aging, Inc., 1975.

Hart, R.J., and McCurdy, P. Pernicious anemia in Negroes. *Ann Intern Med.* 74:448, 1971.

Haydu, G.G. Aging and experience forms. *Geriatrics* 75:1556, 1975.

Humphreys, G.S., and Delvin, D.G. Ineffectiveness of propranolol in hypertensive Jamaicans. *Br Med J.* 2:601, 1968.

Kalow, W. *Pharmacogenetics, Heredity and the Response to Drugs.* Philadelphia: W.B. Saunders Co., 1962.

Kim, P.K.H., and Wellons, K.W. Quadruple jeopardy: to be old, poor, and black in an urban area. Presented at the 39th Annual Meeting of the Gerontology Society. San Francisco, 1977.

Koldomy, A.L., and McLoughlin, P. *Comprehensive Approach to the Theory of Pain.* Springfield, Ill.: Charles C Thomas, 1966.

Kosberg, J.I. Differences in proprietary institutions caring for affluent and nonaffluent elderly. *Gerontologist* 13:299, 1973.

Kubler-Ross, E. *On Death and Dying.* New York: MacMillan Co., 1974.

LaDu, B., and Kalow, W. Pharmacogenetics. *Ann NY Acad Sci.* 151:691, 1968.

Lissitz, S. The challenge of the senile aged. *Gerontologist* 9(2):114, 1969.

Mechanic, D. Stress, illness, and illness behavior. *J Hum Stress.* 2(2):2, 1976.

Medical Letter. Glucose-6-phosphate dehydrogenase deficiency. 17:3, 1975.

Melzack, R. *The Puzzle of Pain.* New York: Penguin Books, 1973.

Merskey, H. Diagnosis of the patient with chronic pain. *J Hum Stress.* 4(2):3, 1978.

Mostwin, D. In search of ethnic identity. *Soc Casework.* 53:1, 1972.

Moy, C.S., and Wilder, C.S. Health characteristics of minority groups, United States, 1976. *Adv Data.* 27:1, 1978.

National Center for Health Statistics. *Out-of-Pocket Cost and Acquisition of Prescribed Medicines, US, 1973.* DHEW Publ. No. (HRA) 77-1542. Rockville, Md., 1977.

National Commission on Arthritis and Related Musculoskeletal Diseases. *Report to the Congress of the United States, Volume I: The Arthritis Plan.* DHEW Publ. No. (NIH) 76-1150. Washington, D.C.: National Institutes of Health, 1976.

Orleans, M., Kurowski, B. Health need assessment of Mexican-American elderly: a report of available opportunities for meeting differential demands. Presented at the 30th Annual Meeting of the Gerontology Society. San Francisco, 1977.

Orleans, M., Kurowski, B., and Clayton, C. The diversity of health perceptions among populations of Mexican-American elderly: implications for clinical practice. Presented at the 30th Annual Meeting of the Gerontology Society. San Francisco, 1977.

Ostfeld, A.M., and Gibson, D.C. (Eds.). *Epidemiology of Aging.* DHEW Publ. No. (NIH) 75-711. Washington, D.C.: U.S. Government Printing Office, 1972.

Overall, J.E., Hollister, L.E., and Kimbell, I. Extrinsic factors influencing responses to psychotherapeutic drugs. *Arch Gen Psychiatry.* 21:89, 1969.

Phillips, D., and Segal, B. Sexual status and psychiatric symptoms. *Am Sociol Rev.* 34:58, 1969.

Quadagno, J., Kuhar, R., and Peterson, W. Race relations in a public housing retirement community. Presented at the 30th Annual Meeting of the Gerontology Society. San Francisco, 1977.

Rabin, D.L., and Bush, P.J. Who's using medicines? *J Community Health.* 1:106, 1975.

Rabkin, J.G., and Struening, E.L. Life events, stress, and illness. *Science* 199:194, 1976.

Raskin, A., and Crook, T.H. Antidepressants in black and white inpatients. *Arch Gen Psychiatry.* 32:643, 1975.

Rickels, J. *Psychopharmacology: A Review of Progress 1952-1967.* PHS Publ. No. 1836. Washington, D.C.: U.S. Government Printing Office, 1968.

Rosen, C.E. A comparison of black and white rural elderly. Presented at the 30th Annual Meeting of the Gerontology Society. San Francisco, 1977.

Sadowski, A., and Weinsaft, P. Behavioral disorders in the elderly. *J Am Geriatr Soc.* 23:86, 1975.

Salber, E.J., Greene, S.B., Feldman, J.J. et al. Access to health care in a southern rural community. *Med Care.* 14:971, 1976.

Salber, E.J., Greene, S.B., Gagnon, J.P. et al. Black/white differentials in medication use: a study of drug use in rural North Carolina. *Contemp Pharm Practice.* 2(1):4, 1979.

Scott, R.D. The treatment barrier. *Br J Med Psychol.* 46:45, 1973.

Shanas, E. Health status of older people, cross-national implications. *Am J Public Health.* 64:261, 1974.

Shanas, E. *National Survey of the Black Aged, Final Report.* Washington, D.C.: Social Security Administration, 1977.

Shanas, E., and Hauser, P.M. Zero population growth and the family life of old people. *J Soc Issues.* 30:79, 1974.

Special Committee on Aging, U.S. Senate. *Nursing Home Care in the United States: Failure in Public Policy.* Supporting Paper No. 8, Access to nursing homes by U.S. minorities. Washington, D.C.: U.S. Government Printing Office, 1975.

Stolley, P.D. How study of geographic epidemiology of disease can help in detection of adverse drug reactions. *Clin Pharmacol Ther.* 19:679, 1976.

Streib, G.F. Social stratification and aging. Edited by R.H. Binstock, and E. Shanas. In *Handbook of Aging and the Social Sciences.* New York: Van Norstrand Reinhold Co., 1976.

Torres-Gil, F., and Becerra, R.M. The political behavior of the Mexican-American elderly. *Gerontologist* 17:392, 1977.

White House Conference on Aging, 1st Reader. DHEW Publ. No. (AOA) 147. Washington, D.C., 1971.

Woosley, R.L., Drayer, D.E., Reidenberg, M.M. et al. Effect of acetylator phenotype on the rate at which procainamide induces antinuclear antibodies and the lupus syndrome. *N Engl J Med.* 298:1157, 1978.

Zappolo, A. *Characteristics, Social Contacts, and Activities of Nursing Home Residents, US: 1973–1974.* National Nursing Home Survey, Vital and Health Statistics, Series 13, No. 27. DHEW Publ. No. (HRA) 77-1778. Rockville, Md.: National Center for Health Statistics, 1977.

Zborowski, M.M. Cultural components in response to pain. *J Soc Sci.* 8:16, 1952.

Zborowski, M.M. Cultural components in response to pain. Edited by H.D. Stein, and R.A. Cloward. In *Social Perspectives on Human Behavior.* New York: The Free Press, 1959.

Ziegler, V.E., and Biggs, J.T. Tricyclic plasma levels. *JAMA.* 238:2167, 1977.

Ziment, I. Why folk remedies for bronchitis persist. *Patient Care* 9(14):25, 1975.

10 Some Considerations Before Prescribing

TO TREAT OR NOT TO TREAT

Polypathology can easily lead to polypharmacy. It has been strongly suggested that not all patient complaints should be answered with a prescription, that convenience drugs should be eliminated, and that drug use should be kept to a minimum (Rossman 1971; Brocklehurst 1973; Hodkinson 1975; Anderson 1974; Forbes 1974; Gibson 1974). It should also be kept in mind that the placebo is a potent therapeutic agent (Benson and Epstein 1975).

In some instances it is not clear whether an elderly patient should be treated. For example, there is a predictable age-related decline in glucose tolerance. Yet it is uncertain whether this age-related change is pathologic or normal, and the clinical implications have not been ascertained; thus, the need for treatment is not clear (Andres 1971).

Hypertension

Raised diastolic and systolic pressures are common in old age, yet hypertension in the elderly is difficult to define (Jackson et al 1976).

Systolic levels of up to 220 mm Hg have been found in healthy old people. It has been suggested that diastolic pressures of up to 120 mm Hg in symptomless elderly do not indicate therapy. On the other hand, in the Veterans Administration study, patients aged 60 or older with systolic pressures of 90 mm Hg or higher were routinely treated to reduce the risk of cardiovascular morbidity. This morbidity included stroke arising from aneurysms that may occur in small blood vessels, congestive heart failure caused by left ventricular hypertrophy, or progressive renal failure caused by plaques in large vessels. The Veterans Administration study showed clearly that the risk of congestive heart failure and cerebrovascular accident in men over 60 years of age can be reduced by treatment of hypertension, while the risk of coronary artery disease was not reduced.

Still, it has been questioned whether antihypertensive therapy will reduce mortality in persons over 60 years of age (Jackson et al 1976). Caution has been advised in the treatment of the elderly for hypertension as in the presence of decreased vessel elasticity, a large reduction in blood pressure may critically decrease cerebral blood flow. Confusion, drowsiness, fainting attacks, collapse, visual disturbances, and convulsions have all occurred when symptomless elderly hypertensive patients were treated. Therefore, it has been suggested that accelerated-phase hypertension, angina, heart failure, transient cerebral ischemia, and decreasing renal function are strong indicators for therapy, while in milder, asymptomatic cases, a therapeutic goal should first be carefully established (Briant 1977). Treatment may lower blood pressure but may result in drug-induced morbidity.

It would appear, therefore, that until more information becomes available, which permits the development of a clearer picture of hypertension in the elderly, some patients will suffer from neglect and others from drug therapy.

When treatment of hypertension is instituted, it is necessary to recognize that chronic care management of hypertension changes. Modification must be expected and the patient must be closely monitored. For example, the patient may develop a tolerance to a particular drug, thus necessitating increased dosage levels and possibly an increased incidence of side effects. Gout and/or diabetes may also necessitate changes in an established regimen.

SELECTION OF PROPER DOSE

The absence of a comprehensive body of knowledge on drugs and aging poses a serious problem, as physicians have no prescription guidelines on which to rely (National Institute on Aging 1977). Package inserts more often than not give an innocuous and not very helpful statement such as, "In the elderly, the dosage should be limited to the smallest effective amount." This, of course, demands monitoring that is not always possible with ambulant patients. Specific recommendations, such as those put forward by the FDA concerning the cautious use of neuroleptic drugs in order to reduce the risk of producing tardive dyskinesia, are rare. In that instance, the FDA recommends drug holidays (*FDA Drug Bulletin* 1973). Drugs should probably be administered according to the principle that enough drug is given to achieve the desired therapeutic response with minimal untoward effects. In all cases, the impaired capacity of the elderly patient to tolerate complex drug regimens should be kept in mind, as should be the fact that aging alters drug effects, which alter senescent functions. Failure to quantitate the reactive capacities of aging body resources should be avoided, and the prescriber must be familiar with confirmed pharmacologic data regarding the elderly.

Recommended dosage levels can and should be used only as a rough guide, a starting point in the search for the applicable dose for a particular patient. As in the elderly, in general, smaller dosage levels are required to achieve the desired therapeutic results, one-half to one-third of the usual adult dosage is often recommended as a starting dose. A useful rule of thumb is that in a patient over 70 years of age the dose employed should be one-third of that used for a subject of the same weight who is half the patient's age (Powell 1977). Body weight alone is of little help in determining the correct dose (Lamy and Kitler 1971).

When dealing with drugs whose action is purely substitutive, ie, vitamin or trace elements, the dosage level should probably remain the same, regardless of age. This is also true of chemotherapeutic agents and antibiotics; their intended target organisms are bacteria, which are not affected by human aging. It has been suggested that all drugs intended to treat exogenous diseases should be given at the usual dose, regardless of age. However, the patient's disease state or greater sensitivity to side effects may make application of this rule impossible (Lamy 1974).

Other guidelines have been suggested. One is that at age 65 drug doses should be reduced by about 10% from the standard doses for ages 20 through 60, by 20% at age 75, and by 30% at age 85. Another suggestion is that the drug dose should be reduced by 1% after age 50, 20% by age 65, and 30% by age 80 (Blancke 1976). More specific recommendations are available for drug administration to patients with impaired renal function. Validated nomograms are available, but individualization of the dose is still mandatory. When a decreased dose is necessary to prevent accumulation and toxicity in the patient with renal insufficiency, the clinician may choose either a variable dosage regimen or a variable frequency regimen. In the former, smaller doses are administered at the same intervals as the usual dose (Brater 1976). Most often, the latter approach is recommended (Bennett et al 1974). Thus, it is clear that in the elderly, more so than in the adult patient, the dose of the appropriate drug must be regulated with regard to diagnosis, sex, height, weight, age, general physical condition, mental outlook, environmental situation, and other medications in use (Weg 1973).

Multiple Medications

A knowledge of other medications being taken by the patient is essential, as many times drugs may lead to adverse effects (Table 10-1) which can be fatal (Table 10-2) and as sometimes the name of the drug may be misleading to the patient. The trade name of a drug product may not indicate, for example, that the patient is using salicylates (Table 10-3), which may interfere with other drugs or diagnostic procedures.

Table 10-1
Adverse Drug Effects in Older Persons*

Drug	Patients Affected (%)
Antibiotics	30.5
Anticoagulants	15.1
Antirheumatics	13.1
Psychotropics	10.1
Sera, Vaccines	9.1
Corticosteroids	4.6
Cardiovascular drugs	3.4

*Total of 1000 cases.
Adapted from: H. Kaiser. Spezielle Therapie im Alter. 6th Europ Congr Clin Gerontology, Bern, 1971.

Table 10-2
Fatal Adverse Reactions in Older Persons*

Drug	Patients Affected (%)
Anticoagulants	52.6
Antibiotics	10.5
Sera, Vaccines	7.0
Corticosteroids	5.3
Psychotropics	5.3
Antirheumatics	3.5
Cardiovascular drugs	3.5

*Based on 57 cases.
Adapted from: H. Kaiser. Spezielle Therapie im Alter. 6th Europ Congr Clin Gerontology, Bern, 1971.

Table 10-3
Some Nonprescription Drugs Containing Salicylates

Drug	Aspirin or equivalent (mg)
Alka-Seltzer	324
Anacin	400
Arthropan	648
BC powder	648
Calurin	300
Dolor	230
Duradyne	230
Fizrin	324
Liquiprin	325
Measurin	660
P-A-C	228
Stanback	324
Vanquish	227

Drug Hazard

A better means of selecting the correct dose may be an assessment of a drug's projected hazard to the individual patient. The antiarrhythmics, antimicrobials, digitalis, diuretics, and quinidine are drugs that are most often cited as potentially hazardous (Cluff et al 1975).

These drugs have a narrow therapeutic index (Melmon 1978). The elderly for whom these drugs are prescribed are, therefore, at high risk for three reasons. First, their disease state is severe. Second, the narrow therapeutic index demands precise prescribing. Finally, the elderly have reduced capabilities to handle drugs and their effects. Thus, it must be the major goal of the prescriber to manipulate the dosage regimen in such a fashion as to minimize to the best degree possible the hazard of drugs. This is difficult even with well-established drugs and could be viewed as a nearly impossible task with newly marketed drugs.

Quite likely, only long-term use of a particular drug with a large number of patients will elicit the appearance and incidence of certain side effects. In addition, most drugs have not been tested for particular effects in the elderly. The FDA does not require that the factor of aging be considered when new drugs are tested for psychoactivity. Therefore, it has been suggested that all studies of drug metabolism, pharmacokinetics, and efficacy include a reasonably sized sample of elderly subjects (Philipson 1976).

VACCINES

Elderly patients have lower hemagglutination-inhibiting antibody levels and poorer serologic response to vaccination than younger persons. Based on these considerations and poor experiences with smallpox vaccinations in the elderly, it is thought that the elderly should not be vaccinated. Reinforcing this view is the fact that the elderly may suffer from immune deficiency states and/or receive immunosuppressive drugs.

On the other hand, some elderly may never have been vaccinated for certain diseases, and others most likely will not have kept up their tetanus protection.

Thus, while it seems undesirable to use multiple inoculations for the elderly, advancing age coupled with multiple pathology, is a strong indication for several vaccinations. This is especially true now because of frequent travel to foreign countries.

Mortality from epidemic influenza is usually substantial among the elderly (Howells et al 1975). Therefore, the Bureau of Biologics of the Food and Drug Administration recommends influenza vaccination for all people over the age of 65 years.

REFERENCES

Anderson, W.F. Administration, labeling, and general principles of drug prescription in the elderly. *Gerontol Clin.* 16:4, 1974.

Andres, R. Aging and diabetes. *Med Clin North Am.* 55:835, 1971.

Bennett, W.M., Singer, I., and Coggins, C.J. A guide to drug therapy in renal failure. *JAMA.* 230:1544, 1974.

Benson, H., and Epstein, L. The placebo effect. A neglected asset in the care of patients. *JAMA.* 232:1225, 1975.

Blancke, F.W. Geriatrics and gerontology: two rapidly advancing fields. In *Geriatric Considerations in Drug Therapy.* Madison, Wisc.: Center for Health Science, University of Wisconsin, 1976.

Brater, D.C. Renal insufficiency. *Drug Ther.* 6(10):191, 1976.

Briant, R.H. Drug treatment in the elderly: problems and prescribing rules. *Drugs* 13:225, 1977.

Brocklehurst, J.C. (Ed.). *Testbook of Geriatric Medicine and Gerontology.* Edinburgh: Churchill Livingstone, 1973.

Cluff, L.E., Caranasos, G.J., and Stewart, R.B. Clinical problems with drugs. Edited by L.H. Smith. In *Major Problems in Internal Medicine.* Philadelphia: W.B. Saunders Co., 1975.

FDA Drug Bulletin. Tardive dyskinesia associated with antipsychotic drugs. May 2, 1973.

Forbes, J.A. Prescribing for the elderly in general practice and the problem of record keeping. *Gerontol Clin.* 16:14, 1974.

Gibson, I.I.J.M. Hospital drugs in the home. *Gerontol Clin.* 16:10, 1974.

Hodkinson, H.M. *An Outline of Geriatrics.* London: Academic Press, 1975.

Howells, C.H.L., Vesselinova-Jenkins, C.K., Evans, A.D. et al. Influenza vaccination and mortality from bronchopneumonia in the elderly. *Lancet* 1:381, 1975.

Jackson, G. Mahon, W., Pierscianowski, T.A. et al. Inappropriate antihypertensive therapy in the elderly. *Lancet* 2:1317, 1976.

Lamy, P.P., and Kitler, M.E. Drugs and the geriatric patient. *J Am Geriatr Soc.* 19:23, 1971.

Lamy, P.P. Geriatric drug therapy. *Clin Med.* 81(5):52, 1974.

Melmon, K.L. The challenge to widen the therapeutic index of hazardous drugs. *Hosp Formulary.* 13(1):33, 1978.

Philipson, R. Drugs and the aged: policy issues and utilization of research findings. Presented at the Annual Meeting, American Association for the Advancement of Science. Boston, 1976.

Powell, C. Brain failure in old age. *Age Ageing.* 6(suppl):83, 1977.

Rossman, I. (Ed.) *Clinical Geriatrics.* Philadelphia: J.B. Lippincott Co., 1971.

Weg, R. Drug interaction with the changing physiology of the aged: practice and potential. Edited by R.H. Davis, and W.K. Smith. In *Drugs and the Elderly.* Los Angeles: Ethel Percy Andrus Gerontology Center, University of Southern California, 1973.

11 The Little White Pill

Confusion reigns supreme. The clinician has just completed a thorough drug history and has elicited the fact that the patient apparently takes a number of little white pills, an equal number of big white pills, and a few yellow pills. Could the little white pill be Lanoxin, Lasix, Oretic, Serpasil, or Zyloprim? Among the big white pills might be aspirin, Diamox, Diuril, Gantrisin, Ismelin, or Orinase. The little yellow pills might be Elavil, Esidrix, or Valium, or they could also be Chlor-Trimeton. This confectionary of big and little pills, indistinguishable by color, may lead to inadvertent, incorrect use and serious clinical consequences if the patient remembers only that a little white pill must be taken once a day—or was that three times a day?

NONPHARMACOLOGIC BASIS OF THERAPEUTICS

Imagine an elderly hypertensive patient with congestive heart failure, diabetes mellitus, glaucoma, a urinary tract infection, and other complaints. This patient may receive Lanoxin, Oretic, and Serpasil, all little white pills. It is very doubtful that he or she, likely suffering from impaired vision, can differentiate among them on the basis of tablet imprints or by the fact that some might be scored and others not. This patient may have also been prescribed Diuril, Diamox, and Gantrisin, being forced to select carefully at the correct time from three little white pills and three big white pills (Figure 11-1). If the condition of the patient does indeed demand this polypharmacy, then the physician can possibly lessen the chance of mistake by applying the principles of the "nonpharmacologic basis of therapeutics" (Mazzullo 1972). Can Edecrin be used instead of Oretic? It has a distinctive green color and an oblong shape. Instead of Serpasil, can Raudixin be used, which is a distinctive red, sugar-coated tablet? By using this principle, the patient now has one little white pill, a green oblong pill, and a small red one. Confusion is reduced. But what about the big white pills? Can Azo Gantrisin be used instead of Gantrisin? It has a deep purple color, but it will also color the urine red. Instead of Orinase, the clinician may use Diabinese, which is blue and has a distinctive shape. Thus, as Figure 11-2 shows, the patient may be helped considerably by careful selection of drugs based on their physical appearance.

The nontherapeutic basis of therapeutics is an often-overlooked reason for patients noncompliance. The total number of tablets prescribed, their size, shape, and color are all important. The patient's appreciation of the relative importance of each medication will most likely influence the outcome of the treatment plan.

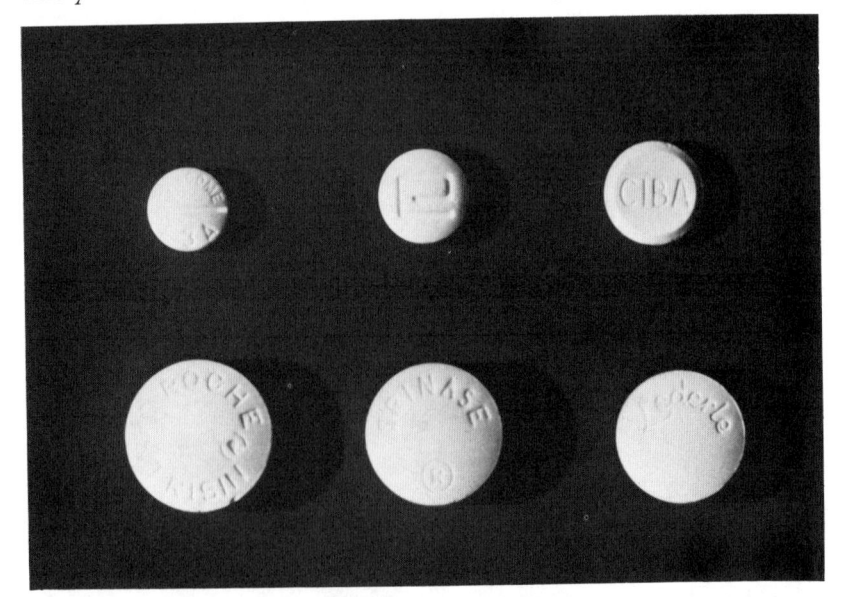

Figure 11-1 A typical but possibly confusing regimen for an elderly patient. Adapted from: J.M. Mazzullo. The non-pharmacologic basis of therapeutics. *Clin Pharmacol Ther.* 13:157, 1972.

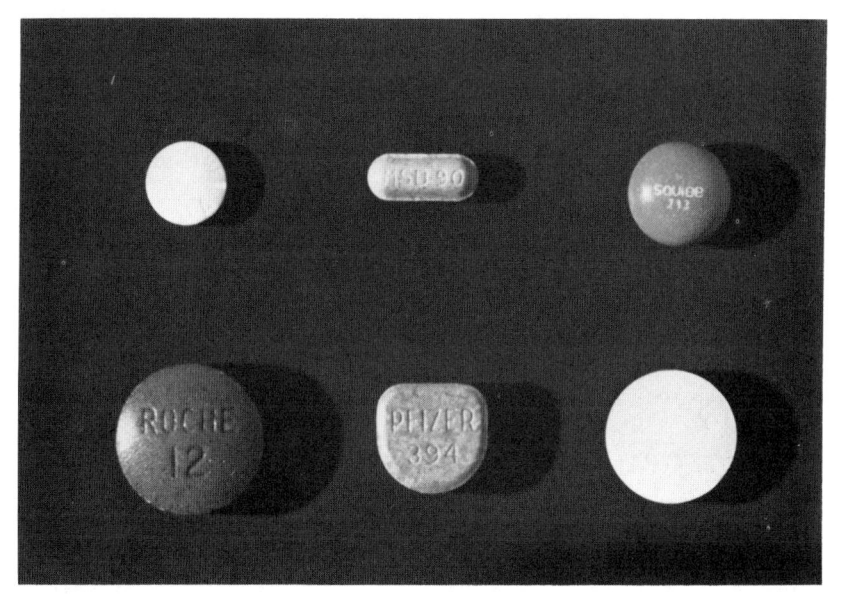

Figure 11-2 Less confusing regimen. Adapted from: J.M. Mazzullo. The non-pharmacologic basis of therapeutics. *Clin Pharmacol Ther.* 13:157, 1972.

Color

Elderly patients may react in a different way to colors than do younger people. For example, quite some time ago a strychnine preparation, colored green, was marketed for stimulation of appetite. The elderly may still associate this green color with the poisonous ingredient and fail to take green preparations.

The use of colors in pharmaceutical preparations has a long history, possibly dating back to the Chinese physician-priests and the ancient Egyptians. Numerous studies have now shown that color (and/or order of administration) can affect responses to various drugs, such as sleep medication, antianxiety drugs, and analgesics (Cattanea et al 1970; Hare 1955; Exton-Smith et al 1963; Sunshine et al 1964; Kantor et al 1966; Shapira et al 1970; Huskisson 1974). A recent study has demonstrated that a hypnotic colored blue was more effective than one colored orange (Lucchelli et al 1978).

Odor and Taste

Similarly, the use of medicinal odors has been associated with the practice of medicine and pharmacy since the beginning of recorded history. This may have particularly important implications for the elderly. These patients, of course, most likely suffer from reduced taste and olfactory sensations. More importantly, they grew up in a time when a medicine smelled and tasted "like medicine." More than likely medicines were simple extractions of natural products, often marketed with little effort to create a pleasant flavor or odor. Thus, the elderly may simply not accept modern pharmaceutical formulations as effective.

A medication that tastes bad can also negate the best developed treatment plan. For example, calcium tablets may be unacceptable to the patient, but the liquid dosage form of calcium may prevent this problem. Drug default by schizophrenic patients could be alleviated by using chlorpromazine syrup instead of tablets (Wilson and Enoch 1967).

DOSAGE FORM

Liquid dosage forms are often recommended for the elderly who may have problems swallowing tablets. As a matter of fact, the FDA continues to certify certain tetracycline suspensions and syrups as they may be needed for geriatric patients. On the other hand, tremor may make it impossible for the patient to measure the correct dose volume, and a solid form may be indicated.

Tablets are marketed so that the patient can "easily" break them in half. It is doubtful that the elderly can always do that. In addition, this may lead the patient to believe that it can be done with all tablets. If not cautioned, the patient may well break an extended-dose tablet in half, completely negating its effect.

Indiscriminate substitution of one dosage form for another can lead to problems. Important differences in clinical response can result when a particular drug is administered as a solution, suspension, tablet, or capsule. This has been demonstrated, for example, for digoxin preparations (Huffman and Azarnoff 1972; Shaw et al 1973). Lithium capsules are said to produce a more predictable serum level than do lithium tablets (Vickers and Solomon 1975). Differences in inert ingredients may be responsible for different therapeutic outcomes (Boman et al 1971).

Antacids present a particular problem. Marketed in suspension form, they must be well shaken before the dose is measured. Elderly patients, unable to do so, may switch to chewable tablets. However, the large surface area needed for a good effect cannot be attained even with prolonged chewing of tablets. The patient may report that the antacid has "lost its effectiveness" and a different therapeutic approach may be selected by the physician, who is unaware of the substitution (Brody and Bachrach 1959; Piper and Fenton 1964).

The selected dosage form must be reviewed in terms of the patient's disease state. Dysphagic patients should receive methenamine mandelate tablets in the form of crushed tablets with semisolid food, as the suspension has caused lipid pneumonia in senile individuals with dysphagia (Timmerman and Schroer 1973).

Finally, the alkaloids may present a problem. Alkaloidal salts cannot be used interchangeably. For example, quinidine gluconate contains 62% of the alkaloids, while quinidine sulfate contains 82% alkaloid (Aviado and Salem 1975).

From the few examples cited, it is clear than an intimate knowledge of the nonpharmacologic principles of therapeutics is not only helpful, but is necessary to achieve patient cooperation and the desired therapeutic outcome (Arthur 1974).

REFERENCES

Arthur, M.D. Formulation of drugs for the elderly. *Gerontol Clin.* 16:25, 1974.

Aviado, D.M., and Salem, H. Drug action, reaction, and interaction. I. Quinidine for cardiac arrhythmias. *J Clin Pharmacol.* 15:477, 1975.

Boman, G., Hanngren, A., Malmborg, A.S. et al. Drug interaction: decreased serum concentrations of rifampin when given with PAS. *Lancet* 1:800, 1971.

Brody, M., and Bachrach, W.H. Comparative biochemical and economic considerations. *Am J Dig Dis.* 4:435, 1959.

Cattanea, A.D., Lucchelli, P.E., and Filippucci, G. Sedative effects of placebo treatment. *Eur J Clin Pharmacol.* 3:43, 1970.

Exton-Smith, A.N., Hodkinson, H.M., and Cronmie, B.W. Controlled comparison of four sedative drugs in elderly patients. *Br Med J.* 2:1037, 1963.

Hare, E.H. Comparative efficacy of hypnotics, a self-controlled, self-recorded clinical trial in neurotic patients. *Br J Prev Soc Med.* 9:140, 1955.

Huffman, D.H., and Azarnoff, D.L. Absorption of orally given digoxin preparations. *JAMA.* 222:957, 1972.

Huskisson, E.C. Simple analgesics for arthritis. *Br Med J.* 2:196, 1974.

Kantor, T.G., Sunshine, A., Laska, E. et al. Oral analgesic studies: pentazocine hydrochloride, codeine, aspirin, and placebo and their influence on response to placebo. *Clin Pharmacol Ther.* 7:447, 1966.

Lucchelli, P.E., Cattanea, A.D., and Zattoni, J. Effect of capsule color and order of administration of hypnotic treatment. *Eur J Clin Pharmacol.* 13:153, 1978.

Mazzullo, J.M. The non-pharmacologic basis of therapeutics. *Clin Pharmacol Ther.* 13:157, 1972.

Piper, D.W., and Fenton, B.H. An evaluation of antacids in vitro, Part II. *Gut* 5:585, 1964.

Shapira, K., McClelland, H.A., Griffiths, N.R. et al. Study on the effects of tablet colour in the treatment of anxiety states. *Br Med J.* 2:446, 1970.

Shaw, T.R.D., Raymond, K., Howard, M.R. et al. Therapeutic non-equivalence of digoxin tablets in the United Kingdom: correlation with tablet dissolution rate. *Br Med J.* 4:763, 1973.

Sunshine, A., Laska, E., Meisner, M. et al. Analgesic studies of indomethacin as analyzed by computer techniques. *Clin Pharmacol Ther.* 5:699, 1964.

Timmerman, R.J., and Schroer, J.A. Lipoid pneumonia caused by methenamine mandelate suspension. *JAMA.* 225:1524, 1973.

Vickers, R., and Solomon, K. Geriatric doses. *JAMA.* 233:22, 1975.

Wilson, J.D., and Enoch, M.D. Estimation of drug rejection by schizophrenic in-patients, with analysis of clinical factors. *Br J Psychiatry.* 113:209, 1967.

12 Nutrition and Drug-Food Interactions

A number of basic processes of digestion and absorption of nutrients are impaired by the aging process. Psychosocial and economic problems may exacerbate nutritional problems, and dietary imbalances and deficiencies can adversely affect the health status of the elderly (Alfin-Slater et al 1978a). There is considerable evidence that in cases of malnutrition, protein and amino acid deficiency should be suspected, as well as vitamin deficiencies (Brock 1975). Malnutrition plays a critical role in the morbidity and mortality of the very old. It decreases significantly human immunocompetence, making the patient more susceptible to infections. Undernutrition also increases the susceptibility of the patient to non-healing decubitus ulcers, and is frequently a contributing factor in the mortality of the very old.

There have been many reports on the effects of malnutrition on the absorption, tissue uptake, tissue response, and rate of elimination of drugs (Campbell and Hayes 1974) reducing the effectiveness of drugs.

On the other hand, chronic drug administration often can lead to nutritional deficiencies in the elderly. Diuretics, for example, may increase the need for potassium as well as magnesium and zinc. A large intake of aspirin (needed in rheumatoid arthritis) increases the need for vitamin C.

In addition, polypathology in the elderly may lead to nutritional deficiencies. A mild heart condition, impaired digestion, dietary restrictions caused by diabetes, and poor dentition may reduce the patient's nutritional status. The patient's medical problems, therefore, serve as a subset to nutritional problems.

The elderly must have a sufficient intake of foods rich in essential nutrients and avoid nutritional depletion (Harper 1978). While it has been recommended that the federal government assume the responsibility for making adequate nutrition available to all elderly persons (White House Conference on Aging 1971), actions are still needed to improve such programs.

A poor nutritional state can have serious sequelae in the aging person, including osteomalacia and permanent damage to both fibrous tissue and collagen formation (Garbus and Lamy 1976). A good nutritional state, on the other hand, in combination with a healthy environment and absence of disease, opposes marked brain deterioration with age (Diamond 1978). Yet, with increasing age, diets tend to become poorer, particularly deficient in ascorbic acid, calcium, and iron and can be characterized by protein-caloric malnutrition (PCM) (LeBovit 1965; Fry et al 1963; Johnson and Feniak 1965). It appears that the elderly are the most vulnerable of any groups to nutrient deficiencies (Nutrition Canada 1973) and yet the knowledge of nutritional requirements for those over 65 years is still insubstantial and fragmentary (Kelly 1978).

However, it is being recognized increasingly that nutrition is a major factor affecting life and health and that an adequate intake of essential nutrients is a basic requirement for good health. Senator George McGovern, as head of the Senate Agriculture Subcommittee on Nutrition, urged the National Commission on Digestive Diseases (March 2, 1978) to recommend "the absolutely necessary increases for... nutrition research" and called the maintenance of a healthful diet "the most basic health-promoting action each of us can undertake." The senator suggested that good nutrition is the most basic form of preventive medicine.

THE AMERICAN DIET

In 1977, the United States Senate Select Committee on Nutrition and Human Needs (the McGovern Committee) released new dietary goals for the United States (Table 12-1). The committee noted the increasingly sedentary life of Americans and estimated that obesity, a type of malnourishment, ranges from 20% to 50% of the population. Overconsumption of fats, specifically saturated fats, as well as cholesterol, sugar, salt, and alcohol were linked to six of the ten leading causes of death: heart disease, cancer, stroke, diabetes, arteriosclerosis, and cirrhosis of the liver.

Difficulty in obtaining good nutritional information is highlighted by the recent admonition to regard the diet-heart era as ended (Mann 1977) and the immediate and intense dispute arising from that suggestion.

The McGovern Committee expressed concern that the proportion of calories from two of the three basic sources of food energy has shifted significantly in this century. Since 1909, fat consumption has increased approximately 25%, and fat accounts for almost 42% of current caloric intake. Caloric intake based on carbohydrates has diminished from more than 55% to 46%, and much of this is now supplied by the empty calories of sugar and alcohol. Fats, sugar, and alcohol are relatively low in vitamins and minerals and overconsumption can, therefore, lead to vitamin and mineral deficiencies (Kelly 1978).

The McGovern Committee has suggested that cholesterol consumption be decreased to 300 mg per day (somewhat difficult as one egg contains approximately 300 mg). In a revision, the Committee modified its original recommendations to reduce the consumption of meat and eggs.

Table 12-1
US Dietary Goals

	Percentage	
	Current diet	Dietary goals
Fats	42	30
Saturated	16	10
Unsaturated	26	20
Protein	12	12
Carbohydrates	46	58
Complex	22	43
Simple sugar	24	15

Salt consumption should be reduced between 50% and 85% to approximately three grams per day (two hot dogs may contain almost that amount) (Alfin-Slater et al 1978b). No one would argue with the suggestion that there should be an increased consumption in fruits and vegetables, although caution is indicated with the consumption of organic health foods (Alfin-Slater et al 1978c). The decreased consumption suggested for meat will most likely not find ready acceptance; as would its replacement by poultry and fish. This would demand a drastic change in ingrained dietary patterns. The substitution of nonfat milk for whole milk has been advocated for some time, but it must be kept in mind that low-fat milk contains a higher amount of sodium than whole milk.

The American Dietetic Association and the American Heart Association have endorsed the report with reservation, while the American Medical Association has strongly criticized it saying there is "insufficient evidence...to support the need for, or the benefit from, major changes in the national diet as proposed." The report can be used as a general guideline even though the exact amounts suggested are questionable (Alfin-Slater et al 1978c). In suggesting a diet for a patient, individual and ethnic backgrounds have to be considered.

Finally, the distribution of caloric intake is important. Caloric intake should be spaced evenly throughout the day or undesirable effects may occur. For example, a person who does not eat breakfast and very little lunch, can gain weight. An evening meal of predominantly carbohydrates, even though relatively low in calories, can lead to malabsorption, as many of the carbohydrate calories cannot be converted to energy at one time and will, instead, be converted in the liver to fat.

NUTRITIONAL NEEDS OF THE ELDERLY

The nutritional needs of the elderly are not age-specific. They are intimately related to nutritional balance, which is not simply a reflection of a balanced intake, particularly in the elderly (Howell and Loeb 1969). Nutrient requirements of the elderly are usually decreased because of lower basal metabolism and decreased physical activity (National Center for Health Statistics 1974; 1975). There is also decreased caloric intake with increasing age. Others suggest that reduced caloric intake is reflected in diminished basal metabolism and diminished energy expenditure (McGandy et al 1966). Others feel that the most important reason for lowered intake is the rising incidence of disease and physical disability in the old-old or frail-old, which in turn can lead to reduced appetite (Exton-Smith 1975). In any case, physiologic requirements change with age because of various factors. Nutritional intake, though, must still meet two major demands, ie, requirements for growth and repair of normal structure, and those for the production of energy to provide for functional needs. The growth and repair of normal structure are met by sufficient intake of protein and amino acids, while energy needs are met by caloric intake. Most foods consumed are used to meet the body's energy needs, including the fats, carbohydrates, and proteins not needed for structural upkeep.

Few data are available to document decreased needs in the elderly. It has been shown that a 75-year-old man has a metabolic rate approximately 15% lower than a 30-year-old man and that total body water in that time span decreased by 18%. The proportion of body fat to body weight may increase with age, and the increase of body fat with a proportionate decrease of lean body mass is undesirable. For men, energy expenditure expressed in calories per day decreases 21% between the ages of 20 years and 74 years, and a further 31% between 75 years and 99 years (Hughes 1969). Thus, the National Research Council has suggested that caloric intake be reduced by 5% between the ages of 22 years and 35 years, and by 3% per decade between the ages of 35 and 55 years, and by another 5% per decade after the age of 55 years.

In assessing nutritional needs for a particular elderly person, age, sex, metabolism, size, occupation, environment, hormonal balance, and physical activity must all be taken into consideration. Decline of health and a multitude of subclinical or frank diseases may alter drastically the nutritional needs of the elderly (Exton-Smith 1975).

MALNUTRITION

Two types of malnutrition could be encountered among the elderly. Primary malnutrition is caused by deficient or excess intake of food, while secondary malnutrition is caused by faulty utilization of nutrients (National Center for Health Statistics 1975). The greater vulnerability of the elderly to nutritional deficiencies is caused by factors responsible for either or both of these malnutritional states.

Factors in Primary Malnutrition

Many factors have been identified which, singly or combined, can lead to deficient or excess food intake by the elderly. Older people, particularly the old-old, may be less conscious of hunger because of a reduced sense of taste and smell, and possibly reduced stomach activity. A reduced sense of taste is related to a reduction in the number of taste buds, which can amount to about 60% between the ages of 30 years and 75 years (Chinn 1971; Hughes 1969).

Eating can also be influenced by loss of teeth. This can lead to reduced food intake or to increased intake of those foods, mainly carbohydrates, which can be chewed without teeth. Mandibular atrophy and atrophic changes in the tongue can be contributing factors. Failing physical and mental health can also alter established dietary patterns, and improvement in those conditions can lead to better nutritional health (United States Department of Agriculture 1975; Anderson 1971; Rao 1973; Sevringhaus 1972; Mayer 1972).

Visible body changes are often not comfortably accepted by the elderly (Goffman 1959) and they may respond to physiologic and psychologic stress with a depressive state (Stenback 1965). Depression is often related to poor nutritional intake as is the so-called age-appropriate behavior frequently assumed by the elderly (Neugarten et al 1968). Poor dietary intake or eating habits then can lead to further decreased physical and mental vigor, which results in worse eating habits. Depression can also be caused by apparently good nutritional management of an elderly person with a particular disease, such as hypertension. Low caloric food, a low fat, low cholesterol, and low salt diet, combined with admonition of no alcohol intake and the prohibition of smoking can lead to a depressive state and poor nutritional intake. The patient may also make a conscientious effort to respond to a particular disability, such as incontinence, by reducing fluid intake arbitrarily and severely, which could lead to constipation.

Vulnerability to malnutrition or nutritional deficiencies in the elderly depends on socioeconomic factors and well-established dietary patterns. This includes food shopping problems and the degree of interest in food preparation, as well as the capability and availability of facilities to prepare foods.

It has long been assumed that a substantial number of elderly citizens do not have the economic resources to achieve a good dietary intake (Goldstein 1968), that the quality of dietary intake is closely related to income (United States Department of Agriculture 1957), and that those living in urban areas, particularly the poorer, central urban areas, may have to shop in stores with a limited food choice, and the prices there may be higher than in other areas (United States Senate 1968; United States Department of Labor 1966). Almost 25% of one city population was designated "gray area" people, ie, people who have an income level that does not permit the support of their medical needs, yet their income is insufficient to meet even normal medical needs (Central Maryland Health Systems Agency 1978). Presumably, a similar pattern holds for nutritional needs. While difficulties in obtaining and preparing food, changed economic status, and social isolation and depression have been cited for deficient nutrient intake (Exton-Smith 1975), low income also often leads to high fat, high sugar diets in older people (Kelly 1978) as these foods presumably counteract hunger well and may not be too expensive. However, they are, as previously noted, of poor nutritional quality, leading to vitamin, mineral, and possibly protein deficiencies.

In addressing the problem of primary malnutrition or nutritional deficiencies, one must also take into account food-use patterns. These are established early in life and are usually set in middle age. They are bound to culture and ethnicity (Howell and Loeb 1969). Thus, changes suggested, even if necessary, may be contraindicated psychologically.

It is known that older men tend to define their status in terms of food and drink, which can be important cures of possible discontent and depression (Goffman 1961). Older men, living alone, eat more breakfast cereals and bread, while single women eat more crackers, cake, and pie (Howell and Loeb 1969).

Finally, it has been suggested that particularly the older poor may exhibit a decided lack of knowledge of what constitutes a desirable diet (National Center for Health Statistics 1975). In response to primary nutritional deficiencies, a complex set of factors must be addressed, which requires a sufficient knowledge of nutrition as well as the attributes and attitudes of the elderly and their environment.

Factors in Secondary Malnutrition

While proper dietary intake is one major requirement for a good nutritional status, proper utilization of nutrients under physiologic conditions through ingestion, digestion, absorption, metabolism, and excretion is the second major requirement (National Center for Health Statistics 1975). Interference with any of these functions should be suspected in the elderly. Both endogenous and exogenous factors can influence the chain of proper utilization of nutrients.

a) Interference with intake: Certain disorders of the esophagus are prevalent among the elderly, including spasms, cancer, hiatus hernia, or diverticulosis, which can retard food passage to the stomach (Howell and Loeb 1969), leading to subclinical malnutrition.

b) Interference with digestion: The processes of primary and secondary aging contribute to poor digestive processes. Hypo- and achlorhydria are not uncommon (Lamy and Kitler 1971; Lamy 1973) and the elderly suffer frequently from hypermotility of the stomach and intestinal hypomotility. Digestive processes may be impaired through atrophy of the salivary glands and a corresponding loss of the relevant digestive enzymes. Digestive enzyme activity may also be reduced in the stomach, pancreas, and small intestine. There may be diminished production of bile from the liver and the biliary system.

c) Interference with absorption: Atrophy of mucous membranes and decreased vascularity may interfere with absorption of nutrients. The number of absorbing cells in the intestine may be reduced.

d) Interference with distribution: There is an age-specific reduction in the efficiency of the vascular system, and a redirection of cardiac output (Lamy and Kitler 1971; Lamy 1973). This may lead to less efficient delivery of nutrients to target organs, a process that could be exacerbated by diseases such as atherosclerosis and other circulatory diseases.

e) Interference with storage and utilization: There may be a loss of cells involved in the utilization and storage of nutrients, as well as of those cells in structural units that produce the enzymes for these processes (Howell and Loeb 1969).

f) Interference with metabolism: Mineral and electrolyte metabolism may be changed by tissue changes. Diminished metabolic rate and endocrine function may lead to reduced metabolism.

g) Increased excretion: Kidney function is reduced with age (Lamy and Kitler 1971; Lamy 1973) and possibly further reduced by disease states. With advancing age, there is also a general loss of muscle (protein) mass; the combination of these factors may increase urinary loss of protein.

In addition, it has been established that drugs can cause loss of appetite, gastrointestinal irritation, and malabsorption (Alfin-Slater 1978c). In assessing possible causes of nutritional deficiencies, drug intake should be carefully checked.

EVALUATION OF NUTRITIONAL STATUS

In the absence of severe malnutrition, evaluation of the nutritional status of an elderly person is difficult (Weit and Houser 1963). It is often assumed that the nutritional status must be good if a person apparently consumes the correct core foods in the correct amounts and if the weight is appropriate. Among factors commonly considered in assessing an individual's nutritional needs are age, body size, previous and current nutrient intake, and presence of disease or pathologic states that affect nutrient metabolism. The Health and Nutrition Examination Survey (HANES)* (National Center for Health Statistics 1974; National Center for Health Statistics 1975) tested for malnutrition by obtaining information on a person's dietary intake, both qualitatively and quantitatively, and using biochemical tests of blood and urine. This was followed by clinical examinations, ie, the observation of visible signs and symptoms, and by various body measurements. It must be noted, though, that dietary information is obtained on a 24-hour recall basis, and many older people can probably not cooperate sufficiently in such detail because of mental deterioration or communication difficulties (Exton-Smith 1968). The intake and laboratory information is compared to the Recommended Dietary Allowances (RDA) (Food and Nutrition Board of the National Academy of Sciences 1974) for vitamins and minerals (Table 12-2) to the suggested intake of proteins, fats, and carbohydrates, and to normal values of nutrition-related blood tests (Alfin-Slater 1978a) (Table 12-3).

---

*As HANES evaluated only noninstitutionalized persons between one and 74 years old, there are still no data on the nutritional status of elderly 75 years and older and the approximately one million elderly residents in nursing homes.

Table 12-2
RDA of Vitamins and Minerals*

Nutrient	Infants and Children To 7 years	Infants and Children 7-10 years	Adults Male	Adults Female	Adults Pregnant	Adults Lactating	Principal food sources
Fat-soluble vitamins							
Vitamin A	1400-2500 IU	3300 IU	5000 IU	4000 IU	5000 IU	6000 IU	Butter, yellow vegetables, liver, egg yolk
Vitamin D	400 IU	400 IU	400 IU	400 IU	400 IU	400 IU	Butter, egg yolk, ultraviolet radiation, fortified milk
Vitamin E (tocopherols)	4-9 IU	10 IU	15 IU	12 IU	15 IU	15 IU	Vegetable oils, cereals, eggs, green leafy vegetables
Vitamin K	—	—	—	—	—	—	Turnip greens, broccoli, lettuce
Water-soluble vitamins							
Vitamin C (ascorbic acid)	35-40 mg	40 mg	45 mg	45 mg	60 mg	80 mg	Citrus fruits, tomatoes, cabbage, green peppers
Folacin	0.05-0.2 mg	0.3 mg	0.4 mg	0.4 mg	0.8 mg	0.6 mg	Green vegetables, nuts, liver
Niacin	5-12 mg	16 mg	18 mg	16 mg	18 mg	20 mg	Enriched bread and cereals, liver, meat, fish, nuts
Vitamin B_1 (thiamine)	0.3-0.9 mg	1.2 mg	1.4 mg	1.2 mg	1.5 mg	1.5 mg	Wheat germ, enriched bread and cereals, grains, pork, nuts, legumes
Vitamin B_2 (riboflavin)	0.4-1.1 mg	1.2 mg	1.5 mg	1.4 mg	1.7 mg	1.9 mg	Milk, liver, cooked spinach and other green leafy vegetables, enriched bread and cereals

Table 12-2 *(continued)*
*RDA of Vitamins and Minerals**

	Infants and Children		Adults					
Nutrient	To 7 years	7-10 years	Male	Female	Pregnant	Lactating	Principal food sources
Vitamin B_6 (pyridoxine)	0.3–0.9 mg	1.2 mg	2.0 mg	2.0 mg	2.5 mg	2.5 mg	Organ meats, fish, cereals, legumes
Vitamin B_{12}	0.3–1.5 µg	2.0 µg	3.0 µg	3.0 µg	4.0 µg	4.0 µg	Only foods from animal sources
Minerals							
Calcium	360–800 mg	800 mg	800 mg (1200 mg, ages 11–18)	800 mg (1200 mg, ages 11–18)	1200 mg	1200 mg	Milk, turnip greens, soybeans
Phosphorus	240–800 mg	800 mg	800 mg (1200 mg, ages 11–18)	800 mg (1200 mg, ages 11–18)	1200 mg	1200 mg	Liver, wheat germ, meat
Iodine	35–80 µg	110 µg	130 µg	100 µg	125 µg	150 µg	Iodized salt, ocean fish, seafood
Iron	10–15 mg	10 mg	10 mg	18 mg	18 mg	18 mg	Liver, meat, eggs, wheat germ, enriched bread and cereals
Magnesium	60–200 mg	250 mg	350 mg	300 mg	450 mg	450 mg	Nuts, soybeans, green leafy vegetables
Zinc	3–10 mg	10 mg	15 mg	15 mg	20 mg	25 mg	Nuts, green leafy vegetables
Potassium	—	—	—	—	—	—	Cantaloupe, bananas, oranges, apricots, watermelon

*To this date, no RDAs for elderly persons have been developed; and all recommendations regarding "proper" food intake for and by the elderly are based on the "usual" adult RDAs.
Food and Nutrition Board, National Research Council. *Recommended Dietary Allowances*, 8th ed. Washington, D.C.: National Academy of Sciences, 1974. Reprinted with permission.

Table 12-3
Approximate Nutrient Content of Foods*

			Vitamins					Minerals				
		Protein	A	B_1	B_2	Niacin	C	Fe	Ca	P	K	Na
Average prepared portion	Calories	gm	IU	mg	mg	mg	mg	mg	mg	mg	mg	mg
MEAT, FISH, POULTRY, EGGS												
Beef												
Hamburger, 3 oz	245	21	20	—	—	5.3	—	2.7	9	145	320	100
Roast beef, 3 oz	390	16	60	—	—	3.0	—	2.1	7	105	350	60
Sirloin, 6 oz broiled	660	40	100	—	—	8.0	—	5.0	16	300	640	120
Corned beef, 3 oz	185	22	20	—	0.2	2.9	—	3.7	17	100	60	1200
Chicken												
6 oz broiled	370	46	520	—	0.2	14.0	—	2.8	20	500	700	100
6 oz fried	490	50	400	—	0.2	10.0	—	3.6	25	430	640	100
Chile with beans, 1 cup	325	19	100	—	0.2	3.5	—	4.2	100	360	500	1060
Clams, 6 oz steamed	175	24	200	—	—	1.8	—	11.0	150	220	460	350
Cod, 4 oz broiled	200	32	200	—	0.1	3.0	—	1.0	35	300	450	120
Crabmeat, 3 oz	90	14	—	—	—	2.1	—	0.8	38	170	100	900
Egg, 1 whole	75	6	590	—	0.15	—	—	1.2	27	103	60	61
Flounder, 4 oz baked	230	35	—	—	—	3.0	—	1.6	25	400	650	260
Gelatin, 1 cup	155	4	—	—	—	—	—	—	—	—	—	125
Halibut, 4 oz broiled	200	30	500	—	—	11.0	—	0.9	16	300	600	65
Lamb												
Chop, 6 oz broiled	720	36	—	0.15	0.3	7.0	—	4.5	15	200	400	120
Leg, 6 oz roasted	630	40	—	0.2	0.4	10.0	—	5.5	18	400	500	150

193

Table 12-3 *(continued)*

		Protein	Vitamins						Minerals				
Average prepared portion	Calories	gm	A IU	B_1 mg	B_2 mg	Niacin mg	C mg	Fe mg	Ca mg	P mg	K mg	Na mg
Liver												
Chicken, 3 medium	140	22	32,200	0.2	2.4	11.8	20	7.4	16	240	160	51
Calf, 3 oz	225	25	30,000	0.2	3.6	14.0	32	12.2	11	460	480	100
Lobster in shell, 1 lb	200	40	—	0.2	—	4.0	—	1.2	130	400	375	430
Luncheon meats												
Bologna, 2 oz	125	7	—	—	—	1.3	—	1.2	4	54	110	550
Frankfurter, 1 large	250	14	—	0.1	0.2	2.5	—	1.2	6	50	215	1200
Ham, 3 oz	250	20	—	0.3	0.15	2.5	—	2.2	7	250	370	1000
Oysters, ½ cup raw	85	8	320	0.2	0.2	3.3	—	6.6	113	150	120	80
Pork												
Bacon, 2 slices crisp	95	4	—	—	—	0.8	—	0.5	2	42	65	600
Chops, 4 oz broiled	230	18	—	0.7	0.2	4.3	—	2.5	9	280	450	35
Salt pork, 2 oz	470	3	—	—	—	—	—	0.4	19	—	—	1350
Salmon, 3 oz canned	120	17	60	—	0.2	6.8	—	0.7	160	280	340	600
Swordfish, 4 oz broiled	180	27	2000	—	—	10.5	—	1.1	20	250	780	50
Tuna, 3 oz canned	170	25	70	—	0.1	11.0	—	1.2	7	300	240	700
Turkey, 6 oz roasted	500	50	—	—	0.2	15.0	—	6.0	40	600	600	100
BREADS AND CEREALS												
Biscuit, 1	130	3	—	—	—	0.7	—	0.7	61	58	40	200

Bread										
Wheat, 1 slice	55	2	—	—	—	0.7	—	0.5	23	54	40	140
Enriched white, 1 slice	65	2	—	—	—	0.5	—	0.5	15	30	35	130
Cereals										
Cornflakes, 1 cup enriched	110	2	—	0.1	—	0.6	—	1.2	6	15	40	165
Oatmeal, 1 cup	150	5	—	0.2	—	0.4	—	1.7	21	140	142	200
Wheat germ, ½ cup	125	8	—	0.7	0.3	1.5	—	2.7	30	370	270	2
Doughnut, 1	135	2	40	—	—	0.4	—	0.4	23	63	26	80
Nuts and seeds										
Cashews, ½ cup	400	12	70	0.3	0.1	1.2	—	2.9	30	245	325	40
Peanuts, ⅓ cup	290	13	—	0.2	0.1	8.6	—	1.0	37	200	340	2
Peanut butter, ⅓ cup	300	12	—	0.3	0.1	6.2	—	0.9	29	154	310	300
Sesame seeds, ½ cup	280	9	15	0.4	0.1	2.7	—	5.2	580	300	360	30
Sunflower seeds, ½ cup	280	12	—	1.8	0.2	13.6	—	3.5	60	420	460	15
Pies										
Apple, 1 slice	330	3	220	—	—	0.3	1	0.5	9	30	100	400
Pumpkin, 1 slice	265	5	2500	—	0.1	0.4	8	1.0	70	95	220	285
Rice										
Brown, 1 cup	250	5	—	0.2	—	3.0	—	1.3	26	200	100	6
Enriched white, 1 cup	23	4	—	—	—	0.4	—	0.5	15	75	80	2
Sugars										
White, 1 tbsp	50	—	—	—	—	—	—	0.5	25	—	—	—
Brown, 1 tbsp	53	—	—	—	—	—	1	0.2	1	7	50	5
Honey, 1 tbsp	60	—	—	—	—	—	1	0.3	9	1	2	2
Maple syrup, 1 tbsp	50	—	—	—	—	—	—	0.3	9	2	1	3

Table 12-3 *(continued)*

		Protein	Vitamins A	B₁	B₂	Niacin	C	Minerals Fe	Ca	P	K	Na
Average prepared portion	Calories	gm	IU	mg	mg	mg	mg	mg	mg	mg	mg	mg
DAIRY PRODUCTS												
Butter, 1 tbsp	100	—	460	—	—	—	—	—	3	—	4	120
Cheddar cheese, 1 oz	100	4	230	—	0.1	—	—	0.1	135	130	30	180
Cottage cheese, 1 cup	195	38	20	0.1	0.6	0.1	—	0.9	200	380	180	600
Ice cream, 1 cup	300	6	740	—	0.3	0.1	—	0.1	175	150	170	140
Milk												
Skim, 1 cup	90	9	—	0.1	0.4	0.2	1.5	0.1	300	235	54	19
Whole, 1 cup	165	8	390	0.4	0.4	0.2	1.5	0.1	285	230	52	19
Yogurt, 1 cup	120	8	170	0.1	0.4	0.2	—	0.1	300	270	50	19
FRUITS AND VEGETABLES												
Apple, 1	70	—	50	—	—	—	3.0	0.4	8	13	130	1
Apricots, ½ cup dried	220	4	8000	—	—	3.0	9.0	4.0	50	75	780	20
Banana, 1	85	1	190	—	—	0.7	10.0	0.7	8	44	390	1
Broccoli, 1 cup	45	5	5000	—	0.2	1.2	105.0	2.0	190	100	400	15
Cabbage, 1 cup	40	2	150	—	—	0.3	55.0	0.8	80	50	240	25
Cantaloupe, ½	40	1	6000	—	—	1.0	65.0	0.8	33	65	900	40
Carrot, 1	20	—	5000	—	—	0.3	3.0	0.4	20	20	200	25
Collard greens, 1 cup	50	5	12,000	—	0.2	1.6	75.0	1.2	280	75	400	40
Corn, 1 cup	170	5	520	—	0.1	2.4	14.0	1.3	10	102	400	5

197

Food												
Dates, ½ cup dried	250	2	50	0.05	0.1	2.0	—	2.8	50	55	650	1
Grapefruit, ½ cup	50	1	10	—	—	0.3	72.0	0.5	20	54	290	4
Kale, 1 cup	45	4	8000	—	0.2	0.8	60.0	1.3	130	57	260	30
Lemon juice, ½ cup	30	—	20	—	—	0.1	50.0	0.2	8	13	80	4
Orange, 1	60	2	240	1	—	0.3	75.0	0.5	50	40	300	—
Peas and beans (dried)												
Kidney beans, 1 cup	230	15	—	0.1	0.1	1.5	—	4.6	74	350	750	6
Lentils, 1 cup	210	15	40	—	—	1.2	—	4.1	50	240	500	15
Lima beans, 1 cup	260	16	—	0.3	0.1	1.3	—	1.5	15	75	300	1
Split peas, 1 cup	230	16	80	0.4	—	1.8	—	3.4	22	180	500	30
Potato, 1 baked	100	2	10	0.1	—	1.2	15	0.7	13	65	500	4
Prunes, 1 cup	300	3	1800	—	0.2	1.8	3	4.5	60	100	800	10
Raisins, ½ cup	230	2	15	0.1	—	0.4	—	2.8	50	110	575	19
Spinach, 1 cup	25	3	12,000	0.1	0.2	0.6	30	0.2	125	33	470	75
Tomato, 1	30	1	2600	—	—	0.8	35	0.9	16	40	360	5
Watermelon, 1 wedge	120	2	520	—	—	0.2	6	1.2	63	100	600	2

*Commercially prepared foods vary somewhat in nutritional content.
R. Alfin-Slater, J.J.B. Anderson, R.C. Bozian, et al. Nutrition in everyday practice. *Patient Care* 12(4):February 28, 1978. Reprinted with permission.

In weight assessment, standard weight-height tables are not necessarily applicable (Alfin-Slater et al. 1978a), and it is probably better to compare the weight with the correct weight for the age range of 25 to 29 years (Weit and Houser 1963). Particular attention should be paid to vegetarians. Vegetarian diets may be based only on plant food sources (total vegetarians or vegans), plant foods plus dairy products (lactovegetarians), or plant foods plus dairy products and eggs (lacto-ovovegetarians) (National Academy of Sciences 1975). Complete vegans, who do not eat any animal protein, are subject to vitamin B-12 deficiency and possible iron deficiency. Increased consumption of fibrous foods containing phytates may also decrease mineral absorption (Alfin-Slater et al. 1978c).

CORE FOODS

Protein, carbohydrates, and fat provide the energy needs for all activities. Protein and carbohydrates supply four calories per gram, while fat supplies nine calories per gram. Alcohol, supplying empty calories, provides seven calories per gram.

Proteins

Many studies have been performed in order to elicit protein and amino acids requirements for the elderly. Results do not agree. However, there seems to be little protein deficiency in elderly persons, perhaps because there is a decreased protein requirement with advancing age. Possibly, this is related to the decrease of skeletal muscles with advancing age. This significant portion of total body protein decreases from 45% of body weight in the young to approximately half that in persons 70 years of age and older.

However, the elderly may, in fact, need a higher proportion of protein than younger people, as they often suffer from hypochlorhydria, which might diminish the absorption of nutrients from food (Alfin-Slater et al. 1978b). In general, the need for protein is increased by stress caused by fever, for example, or by underlying diseases that may impair the digestion, absorption, and metabolism of some nutrients. These effects would be magnified in the elderly who often have limited nutritional reserves.

Based on the belief that the minimum requirements for total protein do not change significantly with age, it is recommended that healthy elderly males consume at least 56 gm/day and females 46 gm/day (Winick 1977). Eggs are an inexpensive source of protein and those over 65 years of age should not fear hypercholesterolemia.

Protein is needed to provide nitrogen and amino acids for muscle and tissue and other nitrogen-containing substances. Dietary proteins also act to provide essential and nonessential amino acids, which serve as precursors for neurotransmitters (Young 1978). Older people probably do better and have fewer and less severe complications from acute and chronic illnesses when they ingest an adequate protein diet (Howell and Loeb 1969). Protein deficiency has been correlated with poor mental and emotional function, such as apathy, irritability, suspiciousness, and depression (Howell and Loeb 1969). While self-selected diets of the elderly may often be deficient in protein, elderly persons can use effectively dietary protein for protein synthesis and accumulation of protein reserves (Watkins 1966). The proteins of cereals and vegetables in general have a lower nutritional quality than those of animal origin, which contain higher concentrations of essential amino acids (Butterworth 1974).

There is sharp disagreement, however, on the required amount of protein. It has been suggested that 0.5 gm/kg of body weight is sufficient, with perhaps increased intake of lysine and methionine (Howell and Loeb 1969). The need for methionine and leucine, essential amino acids, rises sharply after age 50 (McLeod et al 1974a). Thus, an intake of at least six ounces of lean meat or its equivalent* per day has been recommended. It has also been recommended that two glasses of whole or skimmed milk and an average portion of meat per day would provide 0.9 gm/kg of body weight and that this is the minimum essential intake (Watkins 1966). Protein needs have also been pegged at approximately 1.0 gm/kg of body weight per day (Young 1978), and it has been suggested that there is no difference in the requirement between young and old in the branch-chained amino acids, leucine, isoleucine, and valine. When dietary intake of leucine declines, production of isoleucine and valine increases (Young 1978). Higher mandatory intakes have been suggested, eg, 1.5 to 2.0 gm/kg of body weight (Rao 1973).

There is, however, agreement that the diet must contain a sufficient amount of protein, which must contain all amino acids needed for tissue maintenance. While there is still no agreement as to what constitutes "sufficient," there is agreement that meat, fish, poultry, eggs, and cheese are important because they supply all essential amino acids. Vegetables, cereals, bread, and gelatin are incomplete proteins because they do not contain all essential amino acids.

There is further agreement that in case of disease, protein intake should be increased with caution, as excess intake may be contraindicated in kidney or liver disease.

---

*One egg or 1 oz of cheese = 1 oz lean meat. One pint of milk = 2 oz of lean meat.

Carbohydrates

Normally, carbohydrates should provide about 58% of the total energy content of a diet, but as previously noted, the contribution of carbohydrates in the American diet has decreased since the turn of the century in favor of increased fat consumption. Generally, with increasing age, carbohydrate intake should constrict, but insufficient intake can cause loss of tissue protein to equalize the caloric deficit, can mobilize fat with a concurrent rise in blood cholesterol, and can lead to increased sodium and water excretion, which results in electrolyte imbalance and lack of energy. Insufficient carbohydrate intake can also result in inadequate intake of bulk and fiber, which in turn can lead to constipation and other disturbances.

The dietary goals for the United States suggest that the intake of complex carbohydrates, ie, such substances as bread and cereals, be almost doubled. In contrast, the intake of simple carbohydrates like sugar, should be drastically curtailed. They provide only empty calories, devoid of essential minerals and vitamins. The elderly lean toward excessive carbohydrate intake. These foods usually require little or no preparation and are less expensive than proteins. Finally, there have been suggestions that carbohydrate intake be spaced evenly throughout the day to stimulate insulin secretion (Howell and Loeb 1969).

Fats

Fat consumption in the United States is higher than in most other countries. While it has been estimated as high as 50% of total energy needs, the McGovern Committee estimated a somewhat lower total of 42%, an increase of 25% since 1909. Fats are necessary as a vehicle for the fat-soluble vitamins A, D, E, and K. They are popular, as they enhance the flavor and taste of foods. Among the poor, fats are popular as they most easily appease hunger, by reducing stomach acidity and motility (Howell and Loeb 1969).

A reduction in fat intake will not necessarily lead to weight loss. Along with a fat reduction, there must be a proportional reduction in total caloric intake. A reduction in both is necessary in order to restrict the energy value of the dietary intake of elderly persons. This can be achieved by substituting fish and poultry for meats, dairy products, and eggs.

A major medical and epidemiologic controversy has arisen around the role of fats in atherosclerotic and blood cholesterol levels, and considerations of arteriosclerosis are now dominated by controversy about dietary fat and cholesterol (Kaunitz 1975). Cholesterol is a necessary component of the digestive process. It is absorbed roughly proportional to the amount ingested (Myrant 1975). It is converted to bile salts and, thus, has a basic function in the absorption of fat, vitamins, and minerals (Flynn 1978). A report in 1970 stated that populations with high average cholesterol levels and high atherosclerotic disease rates have diets high in total calories and saturated fats (Keys 1970). Preventive strategy, including a nutritional strategy, was strongly recommended (Inter-Society Commission on Heart Disease 1970). In industrialized countries, the average cholesterol level continues to rise to age 50 to 55 years in men and 60 to 65 years in women. Reduction of fat and cholesterol intake would be desirable in those individuals whose average serum cholesterol values fall in the upper half of their population group (National Heart and Lung Institute 1971). Elevated blood lipid levels were identified as causative factors of atherosclerosis (Blackburn 1978) and dietary control is the therapy of choice for elevations of cholesterol and triglycerides (Coronary Drug Project Research Group 1975). Treatment includes overall caloric restriction with carbohydrate control and fat restriction. (Coronary Drug Project Research Group 1975). Cardiovascular health can be promoted by restricting cholesterol and saturated fat intake, as well as that of simple carbohydrates (Civin et al 1976). A population diet high in saturated fats and cholesterol leads to mass hyperlipidemia and atherosclerotic coronary heart disease (Blackburn 1977).

Despite this evidence, it has been said that it is not yet proven that dietary modification can prevent atherosclerosis and heart disease in man (Ahrens 1976). Despite dietary manipulation and increased intake of low cholesterol diets and polyunsaturated fats, the cholesteremia of the US population has remained unchanged, and research into the dietary prevention of atherosclerosis has been unconvincing (Mann 1977). Reduced dietary cholesterol intake, as well as the decreased intake of total fats and increased intake of polyunsaturated fatty acids, suggested by the McGovern Committee are not warranted for many, including the aged (Olson 1977).

Trace Elements and Minerals

The Recommended Dietary Allowances lists the essential minerals (National Academy of Sciences 1974). Minimum needs have been established for those with well-defined human requirements (Mann 1977). Minerals fulfill various roles in the human body. They may act to catalyze biochemical reactions, form the structural center of enzymes or vitamins, or activate hormones, as is the case with iodine for thyroid and chromium for insulin.

Quality, quantity, and balance of intake all play a role in determining adequacy of intake. The interdependence of these substances is illustrated by the equilibrium of sodium, potassium, and chloride. Calcium may decrease the availability of many trace elements and can thus increase dietary requirements (Mertz 1978; Prasad 1976; Davies 1972; WHO Expert Committee 1973; Underwood 1977). Copper requirements depend on sulfur and molybdenum, and iron adequacy depends on meat intake or vitamin C. Dietary fiber can decrease the availability of calcium, magnesium, and zinc, and protein increases calcium needs. The availability of several trace elements can be significantly decreased by phosphates, phytates, coffee, and tea. Thus, a varied diet is necessary to meet all human needs. Deprivation of essential trace elements can shorten the life span, but excessive accumulation can be toxic. Metal concentrations in tissue, serum, and urine are often altered by infections, stress, drug use, and disease states (Ulmer 1977).

Supplemental trace elements should be given with caution, as toxicity of metals is cumulative and as trace metals can be potent modifiers of the oxidative drug-metabolism activity of the microsomal enzyme system. The effect of metals on the heart and kidney could bring about acute and possibly irreversible damage. In toxic levels, metals can depress cellular respiratory functions (Maines and Kappas 1977).

Three catagories of trace elements are listed, including those with well defined human requirements like iron, zinc, and iodine. A second category includes those for which a human need is known to exist, but that need has not yet been quantified. Chromium, manganese, copper, selenium, and molybdenum fall into this category. Finally, there are trace elements required by animals, but no need has been demonstrated for them for humans. Arsenic, cadmium, fluorine, nickel, silicone, tin, and vanadium are among those (Mertz 1978). Possible intake needs have been estimated for some of these (Mertz 1978):

Chromium	50-200 mcg/day
Copper	2 mg/day
Manganese	2.5 mg/day
Molybdenum	150 mcg/day
Selenium	75 mcg/day

In older people, calcium and iron either are or are viewed generally as specifically important.

Calcium Calcium is necessary to maintain normal bone matrix. Data on calcium and changes in calcium balance with aging are confusing and not definitive. Calcium balance tends to become negative with aging, and there are many elderly with osteoporosis who are in negative calcium balance (Whedon 1959). It has been suggested that adults who have symptoms of osteoporosis receive at least 1 gm/day of calcium, either in the gluconate form as a tablet or through dietary sources. Risk is minimal, and though a positive effect has not been demonstrated, there may be a beneficial effect in preventing further bone loss (Albanese 1977; Winick 1977).

Calcium deficiency may result from any of several factors:

a) Diminished calcium absorption
b) Impaired ability to reabsorb calcium through the kidneys
c) Decreased physical activity that may promote increased excretion of calcium

While it is recognized that concurrent low intake of calcium and vitamin D in combination with malabsorption of vitamin D can lead to osteomalacia, a low calcium balance need not necessarily be a cause. However, in the differential diagnosis of bone pain, especially backache, in the elderly, osteomalacia should always be suspected (Aaron 1974). As there is universal bone loss with aging (Nordin et al 1962), a relationship was suggested between calcium intake and calcium loss (Garn 1975), which is greater when a patient is confined to bed.

In women between the ages of 35 years and 50 years, skeletal loss is about 5% to 10% per decade (Hearney et al 1977). In a study involving about 130 of these women, those on higher self-selected calcium intake had a more positive calcium balance than those with lower intakes. On average, these women had a negative balance of about 0.03 gm/day. A daily intake of 1.2 gm was suggested, which is in excess of the current RDA for calcium.

Others question the absolute relationship of a low calcium balance with bone loss. It has been shown that balance can be maintained with an intake of as little as 0.2 to 0.4 gm/day. Elderly often do not use milk or dairy products in sufficient amounts, and those foods supply calcium most easily. Therefore, it has been suggested that daily intake should comprise about 0.8 to 1.0 gm (Whedon 1959), which is still 20% higher than the RDA for calcium, even though current literature suggests that dietary intake of calcium, vitamin D, or fluoride does not seem to inhibit further bone loss (Wylie 1977).

Iron Iron is necessary to prevent hypochromic anemia. It plays an important physiologic role, particularly in the synthesis of hemoglobin and myoglobin (Beal 1971). A clear understanding of the effect and toxicity of iron is necessary in view of the seemingly popular view that iron is a pep pill which can cure apathy and listlessness, particularly in old age.

The average human absorbs about 10% of the dietary iron intake. When iron stores are diminished, an adaptive process is activated, so that up to 20% to 30% is absorbed in iron-deficient persons. The type iron administered is important. Ferrous iron is absorbed more efficiently than ferric iron, and 25% of an inorganic iron salt is absorbed in people with normal levels, while iron-deficient people absorb up to 60% of inorganic iron salts. Ascorbic acid seems to increase the amount of iron absorbed, as does the presence of meat in an iron-containing meal. The mode of action of this so-called "meat-factor" is still unknown (Mertz 1978). All sources of animal protein are not equivalent in their effect on nonheme iron absorption. Beef, lamb, pork, liver, fish, and chicken increase iron absorption two to four times, but no increase is seen with milk, cheese, or eggs (Cook and Monsen 1976). The best sources of dietary iron are fish and meat. Eggs, spinach, and some other vegetables contain a high iron content, but these form insoluble salts with phosphates and phytates, making the iron unavailable for absorption (*Medical Letter* 1978).

Excess iron is stored in ferritin, which contains 20% its weight in iron. Ferritin can be stored by any cell. If additional iron, which is unneeded, is given, iron storage disease develops. In that case, hemosiderin is formed, which is a storage form of excess iron in the liver. Excess accumulation can lead to liver destruction. Elderly men, in particular, can be seen with hemochromatosis, which is caused by excessive iron intake and is characterized by hemosiderin deposits in the liver, pancreas, and other organs. This condition is often associated with cirrhosis and glycosuria. The rate of iron accumulation in people with hemochromatosis can most likely be increased by an increased dietary iron load (Finch and Monsen 1972).

The relatively high degree of interest in iron and iron supplementation revolves around the fact that it has been suggested that iron deficiency appears to be common in many communities, that anemia occurs in about 5% to 20% of the elderly (Ehtisham and Cape 1977), that about 5% of American women have mild iron-deficiency anemia (National Center for Health Statistics 1974), and that iron-deficiency anemia is not uncommon in the elderly (Morgan 1967). Iron therapy should not be instituted unless the deficiency state has been identified. In the subclinical stage, body iron is depleted, which is followed by depletion of the iron storage sites and, finally, in the third stage, the circulating hemoglobin iron pool is reduced (Savin 1977).

The prevalence of anemia, which must be viewed not as a disease but as a symptom of some other condition, is much disputed and depends on the definitions used. Iron-deficiency anemia is most often defined in terms of an arbitrarily selected level of hemoglobin (Crosby 1977). This will yield varied results (Ehtisham and Cape 1977), and completely different statistics can develop when the criterion selected is the disability caused by anemia, and not the hemoglobin level. Using this as a index, iron-deficiency anemia would not be clinically significant until the level of hemoglobin reaches the 8 gm range (Elwood and Hughes 1970). Low hemoglobin values and the dislike for iron-rich foods in addition to limited intake of vitamin C are not necessarily related to the aging process, but are often related to psychosocial and physiologic factors often encountered in the elderly (Boykin 1976).

Anemia is not a cohort of the aging process. Elderly persons living alone, suffering from apathy or depression, having diminished mobility and, particularly, those over 75 years of age are most at risk of developing anemia (Thomas 1973). Increased incidence of anemia has been shown among patients in the poorer health groups (Williams and Nixon 1974).

Anemia is more common in those who require hospitalization. Its presence suggests other disorders (Ehtisham and Cape 1977). It may be caused by a diet poor in iron content, and the core city poor, originally from rural areas, may be most at risk (Howell and Loeb 1969). Poor absorption or inadequate utilization of iron may also be responsible. Iron-deficiency anemia can also be caused by chronic diseases such as bronchitis, endocarditis, and various malignancies. In most instances, however, iron-deficiency anemia invariably means blood loss (Crosby 1977). This blood loss could be caused by gastrointestinal bleeding, urinary tract bleeding, or bleeding from varicose ulcers (Ehtisham and Cape 1977). Chronic blood loss may also result from hiatus hernia and diverticulum disease.

In the elderly, particularly those with rheumatoid arthritis and osteoarthritis, salicylate intake is likely high and prolonged, which can account for significant blood loss.

There is little valid evidence of a beneficial effect of iron administration in mild iron-deficiency anemia, which is most commonly said to be the cause of fatigue. It would seem, though, that anemia in the elderly may have more serious consequences, as it can impact on the circulatory system which might already be impaired by arteriosclerosis (Ehtisham and Cape 1977). A good response to iron therapy can be expected in elderly with low hemoglobin associated with chronic infections or arthritis, renal, or malignant diseases (Ehtisham and Cape 1977).

A definite duration of treatment should be set at the outset, which has been suggested at three or six months (Cook and Monsen 1976), sufficient to replenish iron stores if bleeding has stopped.

While there is disagreement on the effects of mild anemia, it is agreed that severe anemia causes a rapid circulation time, tachycardia, increased cardiac output, decreased vascular resistance, and reduced blood volume. These effects can be expected when the hemoglobin level is below seven or eight grams, and in patients with multiple pathology (Elwood and Hughes 1970). Treatment of anemia may lead to increased blood pressure, and high hemoglobin levels are a risk factor in cardiovascular disease (Birnbaum 1963; Dunn et al 1970). On the other hand, there is little evidence of any harmful effects of relatively low hemoglobin levels.

Generally, iron supplementation should not be used by any person without iron-deficiency anemia. Iron administration is contraindicated in patients receiving methyldopa, as they may be subject to autoimmune hemolysis. These patients may have elevated iron stores despite anemia, because of red cell breakdown. Additional iron may cause hemochromatosis (Cook and Monsen 1976). Iron is also contraindicated in patients receiving allopurinol. Increased hepatic iron concentrations may occur when iron salts and xanthine oxidase inhibitors are administered concurrently.

Drugs such as penicillin, probenecid, and the phenothiazines can cause hemolytic anemia from hypersensitivity reactions. In these cases iron administration is not advisable because it will further saturate iron stores (Cook and Monsen 1976). Finally, iron administration can interfere with testing for occult blood, unless the benzidine test is used.

Zinc Zinc deficiency can lead to anorexia, diarrhea, and dermatitis (Ulmer 1977). Zinc is needed for growth and development. It has been used in the treatment of idiopathic hypogeusia (Ulmer 1977; Henkins et al 1971). Zinc also may be beneficial for treatment of pressure sores, widespread among elderly institutionalized patients (Michocki and Lamy 1976). Wound healing seems to be delayed by zinc deficiency, but is restored to normal by zinc administration (Ulmer 1977). Dietary fiber decreases the availability and thus increases the need for zinc (Mertz 1978).

Potassium There is no RDA for potassium. However, dietary potassium deficiency in the elderly exists. In one study, almost half of the participants had insufficient potassium intake, which cannot readily be measured by serum potassium (Judge and Cowan 1971; Dall et al 1971). An elderly person in good health requires about 60 mEq/day, and insufficient intake may cause muscle weakness, apathy, depression, and fecal impaction.

Disturbances of the potassium balance in heart disease are complex (Flear 1972a). Clinically, potassium depletion impairs the functions of neuromuscular tissue, leading to cramps, paralytic ileus, and a fall in cardiac output. Enzyme activity may be reduced, leading to disturbances in cell and tissue metabolism. The structure of cells and tissues, particularly those of the kidney, heart, and skeletal muscle, may be irreversibly damaged if depletion is severe and prolonged.

Potassium depletion is, of course, frequently encountered in patients with congestive heart failure (CHF) receiving diuretics and digitalis. However, it is not simply a complication of therapy, it is also due to a progression of the disease (Flear 1972a). Circulation cannot meet the metabolic requirements of the tissues and cells cannot accumulate sufficient potassium. Patients with CHF receiving 20 mEq to 60 mEq may still lose 20 mEq to 180 mEq in the urine (Flear 1972a).

Some time ago, it was suggested that potassium be supplied solely through the use of potassium-rich foods, such as orange juice, bananas, or apricots. It has come to be recognized that this is not economically feasible in many instances, particularly in the elderly poor, and that the required quantity of such foods would be too large.

Potassium intoxication can occur. It should be noted that the so-called salt substitutes contain an appreciable amount of potassium, ranging anywhere from approximately nine milliequivalents to 13 mEq/mg (Oexmann-Wannamaker 1976). Sharp or persistent abdominal discomfort demands discontinuation of potassium supplements for a while, as do complaints of stiff fingers or a metallic taste in the mouth. Paresthesia in hands and feet accompanies a rapid rise in potassium serum level (Flear 1972b).

Vitamins

So much nonsense is written about vitamins that there has been misunderstanding, misrepresentation, and misuse. Three-quarters of the adult population believe that extra vitamins provide extra energy and well-being, and at least 20% attribute arthritis and cancer to vitamin and mineral deficiencies. Excessive intake of vitamins is probably the rule and not the exception. Patients and providers often do not distinguish between supplemental vitamins and therapeutic vitamins, which can lead to unnecessary economic expenditures or even adverse effects.

Vitamins are indispensable dietary components. They act as catalysts for biochemical reactions. Essentially, they function as coenzymes (Herbert 1977a). Vitamins A, B-1, B-2, B-6, B-12, C, D, E, niacin, and pantothenic acid are essential for human functions. Vitamin requirements remain substantially the same throughout adult life.

Complete dependency on vitamin supplementation in old age is undesirable (Howell and Loeb 1969). There must be a well-balanced diet of core foods, including citrus fruits and other fresh, frozen, or canned fruits and vegetables.

The elderly are probably at high risk to vitamin deficiency because of a lack of regular vitamin intake from natural sources. However, vitamin deficiencies could result from different factors:

- a) Inadequate intake, which in the elderly population could be caused by a switch to a higher carbohydrate intake and an increased intake of empty calories.
- b) Absorption disturbance can occur with advancing age. Vitamins B-6 and B-12, as well as folic acid, seem to

be absorbed with greater difficulty. Achlorhydria and diminished intestinal mucus secretion may also lead to decreased intestinal synthesis of vitamins (Howell and Loeb 1969).

c) Increased requirements may occur anytime, but occur particularly in the elderly population. Stress and disease states often demand increased vitamin intake in order to prevent deficiencies.

Vague symptoms may result from vitamin deficiency, including fatigue and weakness, all too easily ascribed to old age. In evaluating patients for vitamin sufficiency, it must be borne in mind that the elderly rarely suffer from a single vitamin deficiency and that it may take a prolonged time for a deficiency to manifest. Sometimes, symptoms will appear after a year of onset of deficiency, depending on the particular vitamin.

Much discussion has centered around automatic vitamin supplementation for the elderly. As a matter of fact, a variety of studies report that one-third to more than one-half of the elderly use vitamin supplements, with or without additional calcium and iron.

The usefulness of preventive vitamin therapy in the elderly has not yet been sufficiently documented (Libow 1973), but, on the other hand, as the toxicity of vitamin B complex components and vitamin C is extremely low, administration is advisable (Lehman and Ban 1974). Yet geriatric vitamins containing iron can mask iron-deficiency anemia in the elderly (Pauling 1974). A regimen of vitamin doses at least 10 times the recommended dietary allowance is referred to as megavitamin therapy (Herbert, 1977b). The frequent suggestion for megadoses of single vitamins or megavitamin therapy may reflect the unending search for the elusive "fountain of youth." Megadoses of vitamins cannot act as vitamins; once the basic human requirement is met, they can act only as chemicals with possible adverse effects (Herbert 1977a). For example, megadoses of vitamin C may raise uric acid levels and may, therefore, precipitate gout in those predisposed to this disease. False negative urine sugar tests with Testape and false positive tests with Clinitest may result as a consequence of intake of high doses of vitamin C. False negative occult test results may lead to misdiagnosis of intestinal disorders (Herbert 1977a).

The effectiveness of megavitamins in the treatment of schizophrenia has been suggested (Pauling 1974) and disputed (Task Force on Vitamin Therapy in Psychiatry 1974). Megadoses of niacin had no effect on prevention of heart attacks (Coronary Drug Project Research Group 1975).

The evidence for vitamin deficiency in the elderly is equivocal. In one study, almost 40% were found to be deficient in vitamin A and

16% were deficient in vitamin C (Schaefer and Ogden 1969). Others have reported that more than 10% of the elderly have several important vitamin deficiencies (Libow 1973). The evidence is difficult to evaluate; self-selected vitamin supplementation among the elderly seems high, one study reporting almost 50% of those in their sixth or seventh decade self-administering vitamins (Rose et al 1976).

Vitamin A This vitamin consists of retinol and 3-dehydroretinol. It plays an important role in the function of the retina. It is apparently needed for maintenance of the integrity of the epithelial cells and is probably involved in the formation of progesterone, androstenedione, and corticosterone. Vitamin A is fat-soluble and is, therefore, stored mainly in the liver.

Chronic diseases such as cancer, tuberculosis, pneumonia, nephritis, urinary tract infections, and prostatic diseases may be responsible for vitamin A deficiency, probably more so than dietary deficiency.

Mild vitamin A deficiency is easily overlooked. Serum levels usually remain normal until liver reserves have been substantially depleted. The first symptoms of vitamin A deficiency present as night blindness and xerosis of the conjuctiva. Epithelial drying at other body sites, nerve lesions, and increased pressure in the cerebrospinal fluid may also occur.

Ingestion of large doses may lead to toxicity, manifested by fatigue, malaise, and lethargy, among other signs.

Kidney, milk products, and eggs are particularly good sources of vitamin A. However, skim milk is not, and should not be used unless fortified with this vitamin.

Vitamin B-1 Thiamine is essential in carbohydrate metabolism. Thiamine requirements are related to a person's metabolic rate. It tends to be depleted under stress and thiamine deficiency should be considered in the differential diagnosis of high-output cardiac failure. Consumption of foods high in tannins can cause thiamine deficiency (Rungruangsak et al 1977), as tannic acid and thiamine react to form a modified thiamine derivative (Kositowattanakul et al 1977). Its deficiency has been cited as a possible cause of pseudosenility (Libow 1973).

Vitamin B-2 Riboflavin plays a vital role in the metabolism of respiratory proteins. Riboflavin requirements are related to energy expenditures. Deficiency states are manifested by a variety of symptoms, including ocular symptoms. Lack of riboflavin has also been cited as a possible cause of pseudosenility (Libow 1973).

Vitamin B-6 Pyridoxine is needed in the metabolism of amino acids. Age-related decreases in plasma pyridoxal phosphate (PLP) levels have been reported (Rose et al 1976) and, generally, B-6 levels in women are lower than in men. Its absence, too, might play a role in pseudosenility (Libow 1973). In patients with liver disease, not necessarily related to alcoholism, the biologically active form of pyridoxine (PLP) is degraded at an increased rate, leading to a vitamin B-6 deficiency (Labadarios et al 1977).

Vitamin B-12 Low serum levels of cyanocobalamin are common in the elderly (Shulman 1967) as a consequence of atrophic gastritis, achlorhydria, and lack of intrinsic factor. Vitamin B-12 is used to treat macrocytic anemia, in which CNS symptoms occur in 40% of patients (Libow 1973). Vitamin B-12 deficiency can lead to neurologic complications (Brain and Walton 1969) and dementia (Gordon 1977). Of 432 psychiatric patients tested, more than 14% had low B-12 levels (Carney and Sheffield 1970). Vitamin B-12 deficiency may not have any hematologic indices, and the B-12 level has to be determined (Gordon 1977). B-12 deficiency should be considered in the differential diagnosis of peripheral neuropathies, myopathies, and obscure neurologic disturbances, whether or not anemia is present. Anemic or postgastrectomy patients are candidates for B-12 deficiency, which should also be suspected in unexplained fatigue, confusional states, or dementia of unknown origin.

It has been suggested that the addition of ascorbic acid could be deleterious to vitamin B-12 in meals (Herbert and Jacob 1974), but this has not been substantiated (Newark et al 1976).

Vitamin C Extensive literature has accumulated about the use and misuse of ascorbic acid. Severe deficiency states, of course, result in scurvy, which is not seen among either the general population or the elderly. Ascorbic acid plays a role in amino acid and carbohydrate metabolism, and is thought to be involved also in the synthesis of adrenocorticosteroids. It is essential to collagen maintenance. Smoking appears to increase the vitamin C requirement. In one study, intake of ascorbic acid was less than 10 mg per day in approximately 5% of elderly participants (McLeod et al 1974a). Vitamin C is rapidly depleted with stress and poor nutrition (Libow 1973). It has been widely accepted that much ill health among the elderly is caused or aggravated by undiagnosed vitamin C deficiency. This has not been substantiated (Burr et al 1974), but is supported by pooled data of several studies involving more than 850 people (Bermond 1976). These data support evidence that low plasma ascorbic acid (PAA) levels are associated with higher morbidity and age. Similarly, it has been suggested that age-related changes in the tissue concentrations of vitamin C, as well as other vitamins, are likely to alter various metabolic processes that may account for the causes of aging (Patnaik 1971).

Vitamin D Vitamin D is essential for normal calcium and phosphate metabolism. It increases the intestinal absorption of calicum and the movement of calcium leads to increased phosphate absorption. In some cases, administration of vitamin D will not correct hypocalcemia (Medalle et al 1976). Magnesium depletion is associated with vitamin D resistance and can be overcome by the administration of magnesium (Medalle et al 1976). Bile is essential for adequate intestinal absorption of vitamin D, which may not be adequate in the elderly. Intake of vitamin D is low in a large percentage of older men and even lower in a higher percentage (33%) of women over the age of 65 years (McLeod et al 1974b).

Vitamin E Little is known about the consequences of vitamin E deficiency in humans. Its self-selected intake has increased sharply in the population at large; it is thought to act as an antioxidant, based on the free radical theory of aging. In growing animals, vitamin E is required for the maintenance of the structural and functional integrity of endocrine tissue, skeletal, cardiac, and smooth muscle, and the peripheral vascular system (Horwitt 1961). Despite the fact that there are few demonstrated cases of vitamin E deficiency and almost no valid indications for it, many proponents of vitamin E prescribe it essentially as a drug, to cure a variety of nondeficiency diseases. This includes diseases of the circulatory, reproductive, and nervous systems. Frequently, vitamin E is used in the belief that aging may be retarded by optimal intake of antioxidants, particularly vitamin E (Tappel et al 1973; Kohn 1971; Harman 1971). Vitamin E may protect the integrity of tissue (Horwitt 1976). There are some indications, though, that this vitamin may protect against the effects of air pollution (Institute of Food Technology 1977). While no adverse effects to vitamin E treatment have thus far been reported, adverse effects are possible (Farrell and Bieri 1975). In persons with vitamin E deficiency, erythrocytes are destroyed at a rate 8% to 10% faster than in controls (Horwitt 1963). Long-term treatment with vitamin E appears to be useful in intermittent claudication (Haeger 1974), and it may prolong plasma clotting time (Korsan-Bensten et al 1972). Therefore, if a patient is receiving vitamin E and warfarin concurrently, it may be advisable to adjust the level of warfarin.

In 1968, the Food and Nutrition Board allowed 30 IU of vitamin E per day for adult humans, which was lowered to 15 IU in 1974, with the provision that more would be needed by people who consume large amounts of polyunsaturated fatty acids. Canadian studies concluded that the adult requirement for vitamin E is less than 15 IU per day and that the vitamin E/PUFA ratio is not a useful indication of the adequacy of foods and diets (Thompson et al 1973).

Folic acid Pteroylglutamic acid is reduced in the body to its active form, tetrahydrofolic acid. It is necessary, as a coenzyme, in purine synthesis, pyrimidine nucleotide synthesis, and several amino acid conversions. There is an interrelation of folate and vitamin B-12 metabolism and vitamin B-6 metabolism. Folate deficiency is associated with megaloblastic anemia. Low serum folate levels are frequently found in the elderly (Girdwood 1969) and reports of subnormal folacin levels in the elderly range from 5% to 40% of populations surveyed (Liebman 1977). Thirty-three percent of 411 psychiatric patients suffered from folic acid deficiency (Kariks and Perry 1970), as did 16% of 113 patients admitted to a geriatric unit (Sneath et al 1973). In another group of 432 psychiatric patients, 22.5% had low folate levels (Carney and Sheffield 1970), and in England, it has been estimated that 80% of the elderly will have demonstrable folate deficiencies (J. Runcie, personal communication, March, 1977).

Folic acid deficiency can occur from insufficient intake. As a matter of fact, the elderly have been cited as one of three groups at particularly high risk to folate deficiency, generally caused by dietary insufficiency. Insufficiency may also be due to the fact that food folate is labile and is destroyed by heat and light. Many drugs (some used on a chronic basis) interfere with the absorption, metabolism, or utilization of folic acid. Among these are alcohol, barbiturates, cycloserine, diuretics, nitrofurantoin, phenothiazines, phenylbutazone, phenytoin, primidone, and salicylates (Girdwood 1969; Liebman 1977; Waxman et al 1970). Folacin status is also known to be altered by a number of disease states. CHF, chronic alcoholism, infections, skin diseases, certain hematologic disorders, liver malfunction, malabsorption, neoplasia, rheumatoid arthritis, and organic brain syndrome have all been associated with folate deficiency.

Folate deficiency predisposes a patient to overt nutritional megaloblastic anemia in case of a severe infection. Folate deficiency should be considered in the diagnosis of dementia, peripheral neuropathy, myelopathy, and macrocytic anemia. It can cause a spectrum of neurologic disorders, ranging from irritability to gross paranoid psychosis. There is a correlation between the restless-legs syndrome and folate deficiency in pregnancy (Botez 1976; Botez and Lambert 1977). A significant increase of organic brain syndrome and pyramidal tract damage was found in folate-deficient patients (Reynolds 1973), and patients with dementia had significantly lower red blood cell-folate levels than controls (National Center for Health Statistics 1974). The cause and effect of severe neurologic disturbances and folate deficiency are not clear. It is possible that dementia leads to poor dietary intake and to folate deficiency. On the other hand, folate deficiency may lead to impaired mental function. Some dementias are amenable to treatment; among those folic acid deficiency should be considered (Strachan and Henderson 1967). Neurologic involvement has been resolved with folic acid therapy (Pincus et al 1972), and folate-treated patients with organic psychoses, endogenous depression, and schizophrenia were in better clinical state at discharge (Carney and Sheffield 1970).

Many studies have shown that age-related vitamin deficiencies can easily be corrected by simple supplementation. Deficiencies can be reversed by administration of the specific vitamin.

OTHER DIETARY COMPONENTS

Fiber has been defined as the remnants of plant cells resistant to the alimentary enzymes of man (Trowell 1977). Dietary fiber may play an important role in lipid metabolism (Kritchevsky 1977), and it has been postulated that fiber acts as a protector against certain metabolic diseases, such as ischemic heart disease, diabetes mellitus, and obesity (Fuchs et al 1976; Walker 1974, 1976; Drasar and Jenkins 1976; Trowell 1976; Burkitt 1973).

The addition of fiber to the diet is associated with several objective alterations in colonic function, such as decreased stool transit time and increased stool bulk. It is not yet known which components of dietary fiber influence functions like fecal bulking, retention of water in the stool, or binding of bile salts (Walker 1974; Southgate 1977). Vegetable fiber is a physical complex that acts principally in the colon. It's water-holding, cation exchange, and adsorptive activities vary with the type of fruit or vegetable from which it is derived. Dietary fiber is desirable, although it will probably not be regarded as an essential nutrient. An intake of 30 to 60 gm/day has been suggested as both feasible and "protective" (Mendeloff 1977).

Adequate fluid intake is also important. Ordinarily, thirst will determine intake. However, in the elderly, thirst may be diminished. Incontinent patients may restrict their fluid intake, and ingrained habits may deemphasize fluid intake. In addition, the elderly may eat fewer times during the day, and thus drink less. It is important that enough fluids are consumed to yield a 24-hour urinary volume of 1000 ml to 1500 ml, which would require an intake of six to seven glasses of water per day.

CLINICAL SIGNS OF NUTRIENT DEFICIENCY

Subclinical malnutrition, the condition probably most often encountered among the elderly, can lead to poor health, apathy, and loss of interest. More importantly, during illness, subclinical malnutrition may change to a deficiency state. Thus, it is important to recognize early clinical signs of nutrient deficiency.

Early signs may be associated with low or extremely high blood and urinary levels of certain nutrients (normal values are listed in Table 12-4). Less efficient performance may occur. If undernutrition continues for prolonged periods of time, physical changes of the skin, hair, eyes, mouth, and tongue may appear. Only severe malnutrition will cause signs of frank deficiency. Some early signs of undernutrition are well known, such as magenta coloring of the tongue in riboflavin deficiency, or the beefy red tongue coloring caused by thiamine or niacin deficiency. Lack of vitamin C may lead to capillary bleeding in the skin or gum mucosa. (Other clinical signs of nutrient deficiency are listed in Table 12-5).

Table 12-4
Normal Values of Nutrition-Related Blood Tests

Blood		Serum	
Hematocrit		Total protein	6-8 gm/dl
Men	40-54%	Albumin	4.0-5.5 gm/dl
Women	37-47%	Vitamin A	40-120 IU/dl
		Vitamin C	0.4-1.0 mg/dl
Hemoglobin		Folic acid	7-16 ng/ml
Men	14-17 gm/dl	Vitamin B_1	3.4 μg/dl
Women	12-15 gm/dl	Vitamin B_2	20 μ/dl
		Vitamin B_{12}	350-750 μg/dl
Cell differential		Tocopherol	1.0-1.2 mg/dl
Lymphocytes	25-33%	Prothrombin time	10-15 sec
Monocytes	3-7%		
Neutrophils	54-62%	Calcium	4.5-5.5 mEq/liter
Eosinophils	1-3%	Chlorides	100-106 mEq/liter
Basophils	0-0.75%	Copper	130-230 μg/dl
		Protein-bound	
Transferrin	170-250 mg/dl	iodine	4-8 μg/dl
		Iron	80-180 μg/dl
Total iron-binding		Magnesium	1.6-2.4 mEq/liter
capacity	250-410 μg/dl	Phosphate	1.6-2.7 mEq/liter
		Phosphorus	3.0-4.5 mg/dl
Urea nitrogen	10-20 mg/dl	Potassium	4.0-5.0 mEq/liter
		Sodium	136-145 mEq/liter
Mean corpuscular			
volume	80-94 cu μ		

Reprinted with permission from Alfin-Slater, R., Anderson, J.J.B., Bozian, R.C. et al. Helping patients learn to eat right. *Patient Care* 12(5):120, 1978.

Nutritional Status of the Elderly

The relationship between health and nutrition in the elderly has assumed increasing importance with the great increase of the elderly population. It seems that poverty and health influence nutritional status more so than age per se. Nutritional deficiencies increase with decreased income, and malnutrition in the elderly is often secondary to disease and disability (Watkins 1975). Old people are vulnerable to malnutrition because of social isolation, depression, mental impairment, and lack of support from family or community (Exton-Smith 1968). Institutionalized elderly persons, in general, appear to be in poorer nutritional health than those living at home.

Table 12-5
Clinical Signs of Various Nutrient Deficiencies

Nutrient deficiency	High risk	Moderate risk	Low risk
Protein		Hepatomegaly Potbelly	
Riboflavin	Angular lesions of lips Angular scars of lips Magenta tongue	Cheilosis Nasolabial seborrhea	Conjunctival injection, eyes
Niacin	Filiform papillary atrophy of tongue Scarlet beefy tongue	Fungiform papillary hypertrophy of tongue Fissures of tongue	Serrations or swelling of tongue
Thiamine		Absent knee jerks Absent ankle jerks	
Vitamin D*		Bowed legs Knock knees	
Vitamin A		Follicular hyperkeratosis, arm	Follicular hyperkeratosis, upper back Dry, scaling skin (xerosis)
Vitamin C		Bleeding and swollen gums	Diffuse marginal inflammation Swollen red papillae of gingivae
Iodine	Thyroid enlargement, Group II	Thyroid enlargement, Group I	
Calcium		Positive Chvostek sign	

*The clinical signs listed here would indicate a moderate risk of having had the deficiency.
Preliminary Findings of the First Health and Nutrition Examination Survey, U.S., 1971–72. Anthropometric and clinical findings. DHEW Publ. No. (HRA) 75-1229. Rockville, Md.: National Center for Health Statistics, 1974.

The most recent estimate of the nutritional status of Americans was conducted under the name of the First Health and Nutrition Examination Survey (HANES), the preliminary findings of which were published (National Center for Health Statistics 1974; National Center for Health Statistics, 1975). The survey included noninstitutionalized persons aged one year to 74 years. It was the first program to collect measures of nutritional status for a scientifically designed sample, representative of the United States civilian population.

In general, preliminary data show a fairly low prevalence of high and moderate risk signs for most nutritional deficiencies. For all age groups, men had a lower prevalence of obesity than women, but in the older age groups, regardless of income, white men tend to be more obese than black men. In general, men had a higher prevalence of signs of protein, vitamin C, and vitamin D deficiencies. Women, on the other hand, showed symptoms of possible vitamin A, niacin, and calcium deficiencies (Table 12-6).

In older age groups, signs of protein deficiencies were observed more frequently in blacks of lower income groups than in whites with comparable income. Whites over age 60 tended toward riboflavin deficiency (2.4%), mostly prevalent in lower income groups. Thiamine deficiency was seen most frequently in blacks more than 60 years old (approximately 7.7%). In contrast, the rate of niacin deficiency was higher in all groups over age 45 with income above the poverty level. The report included specific findings on caloric intake. Among those with incomes above the poverty level, 16% of the white population and 18% of the black population consumed less than 1000 cal/day. Figures cited for those with incomes below the poverty level were 21% and 36%. Intake of protein and calories was related to income in both races.

Calcium intake was 37% below recommended standards for all participants over age 60. All groups had intakes of vitamin A 52% to 62% below the recommended standards. Vitamin C intake was below recommended standards in 39% to 59% of the participants. In blacks over the age of 60 years, 29.6% showed indications of low hemoglobin levels and 41.7% had low hematocrits.

Overall, the report concluded that there is no consistent evidence of poor nutritional status or marked deficiency of nutritional intake. However, significant numbers of study participants consumed less than the recommended amounts of protein, calcium, ascorbic acid, and vitamin A.

Other studies have found that caloric intake is less than optimal for the elderly. The elderly also consume, in general, less bulk than is necessary, although the quality of food seems acceptable. Calcium is frequently consumed in minimal quantities, as is vitamin A, vitamin C, iron, and folic acid. This may lead to "latent" deficiency disease states,

Table 12-6
Clinical Findings on Nutritional Status for Two Age Groups

Nutrient deficiency and clinical signs by risk category	Persons aged 45–59 years Total*	Persons aged 45–59 years White	Persons aged 45–59 years Black	Persons Aged 60 years and over Total*	Persons Aged 60 years and over White	Persons Aged 60 years and over Black
n	1143	871	263	1938	1486	435
N	34,232	30,796	3228	20,560	18,719	1791
Protein						
Hepatomegaly (M)	3.3	3.3	4.4	4.0	4.2	2.3
Potbelly (M)	—	—	—	—	—	—
Riboflavin						
Magenta tongue (H)	1.0	0.0	1.6	—	—	—
Angular lesions of lips (H)	1.0	1.0	—	1.2	1.3	—
Angular scars of lips (H)	0.0	0.0	0.0	0.0	0.0	0.0
Cheilosis (M)	0.0	0.0	0.0	0.0	0.0	0.0
Nasolabial seborrhea (M)	1.6	1.4	1.0	1.0	1.0	0.0
Conjunctival infection (L)	1.0	1.0	0.0			
Niacin						
Filiform papillary atrophy of tongue (H)	3.2	3.2	3.1	4.9	4.8	6.1
Scarlet beefy tongue (H)	0.0	0.0	—	1.0	1.0	0.0
Fungiform papillary hypertrophy of tongue (M)	2.1	1.9	4.0	1.7	1.6	2.8
Fissures of tongue (M)	8.6	9.0	5.0	13.2	13.1	14.6
Serrations or swelling of tongue (L)	8.9	8.8	8.9	6.1	6.4	3.3
Thiamine						
Absent knee jerks (M)	1.3	1.1	2.8	2.3	1.9	5.8
Absent ankle jerks (M)	3.0	2.6	6.5	7.1	6.5	13.6

Table 12-6 *(continued)*

Nutrient deficiency and clinical signs by risk category	Persons aged 45–59 years Total*	Persons aged 45–59 years White	Persons aged 45–59 years Black	Persons Aged 60 years and over Total*	Persons Aged 60 years and over White	Persons Aged 60 years and over Black
Vitamin D						
Bowed legs (M)	4.6	4.3	7.2	5.4	5.5	4.3
Knock knees (M)	1.0	1.0	3.5	1.0	1.0	2.5
Vitamin A and/or essential fatty acids						
Follicular hyperkeratosis of arms (M)	1.1	1.1	2.0	2.2	1.9	5.6
Follicular hyperkeratosis of upper back (L)	0.0	0.0	0.0	0.0	0.0	0.0
Dry or scaling skin (L)	3.5	3.4	3.9	9.2	9.4	7.4
Vitamin C						
Bleeding and swollen gums (M)	3.8	2.6	14.7	4.0	3.7	6.7
Swollen red papillae (L)	9.2	7.2	25.9	7.3	5.6	23.6
Diffuse marginal inflammation (L)	27.0	23.6	53.9	26.6	23.7	52.7
Iodine						
Thyroid enlargement						
Group I (M)	2.6	2.7	1.1	2.6	2.6	2.6
Group II (H)	1.4	1.0	5.0	1.1	1.0	3.2
Calcium						
Positive Chvostek's sign	2.9	2.3	8.4	1.3	1.2	2.8

*Total includes all races.

Notes: n = examined persons; N = estimated population in thousands; (H) = high risk indicator of possible deficiency; (M) = moderate risk indicator; (L) = low risk indicator.

Preliminary Findings of the First Health and Nutrition Examination Survey, U.S., 1971–72. Anthropometric and Clinical Findings. DHEW Publ. No. (HRA) 75-1229. Rockville, Md.: National Center for Health Statistics, 1975.

but does not necessarily limit health (Waxman et al 1970; Botez 1976; Botez and Lambert 1977; Reynolds et al 1973; Strachan and Henderson 1967; Pincus et al 1972; Walker 1974; Southgate 1977; Mendeloff 1977; Watkins 1975; Guthrie et al 1972; Balacki and Dobbins 1974; Rawson et al 1978). With increasing age, there is a significant decrease in the intake of fat and saturated fatty acids (Garcia et al 1977) and the nutritive value of diets decreases by about 85 kcal and 4 gm of protein for every increase of 10 years of age (Swanson et al 1959). Over 14 years, diets of women between 50 to 59 years decreased by 182 calories, between 60 to 69 years by 459 calories, and over 70 years by 320 calories (Steinkamp et al 1965). At other times, the average intake for men aged 55 years and over had been judged adequate, but thiamine intake of women was 13% deficient, riboflavin intake was 16% deficient, and calcium intake was 36% deficient, as measured against RDAs (United States Department of Agriculture 1968). A later study found that persons over the age of 60 years consumed far less food than is needed to meet nutritional standards set for their age, sex, and weight (Center for Disease Control 1972b).

Earlier studies identified deficient hematocrit values and thiamine and vitamin C deficiencies in both men and women (Brin et al 1965), and an evaluation of studies conducted during a 10-year period showed no marked inadequate intake, but did report less than recommended levels of protein, riboflavin, niacin, thiamine, iron, and particularly calcium, vitamin A, and vitamin C (Kelsay 1969). In South Wales, among 533 elderly persons, low levels of folate and vitamin B-12 were not associated with health impairment (Elwood et al 1971). Possibly, this finding relates to a report finding a decrement of vitamin B-12 levels of approximately 35% between the ages of 25 to 70 years (Gaffney et al 1957).

Several studies estimated protein and iron deficiency, in particular, their possible associations with anemia and low serum albumin, low hemoglobin, and low hematocrit levels. In England, 3% of an elderly population study were diagnosed as having protein-calorie malnutrition (PCM), often caused by an underlying medical condition (Department of Health and Social Security 1972). It is difficult to estimate protein deficiency, as levels of serum protein are relatively insensitive to marginal protein deficiencies. In a Medicare population of central Maine, men were more likely than women to have an inadequate intake (two-thirds of RDA). Thirty-six percent of those with protein intakes below RDA had low total serum proteins and low albumin, and were also judged to be anemic (Jordan 1976). An additional 16% had borderline protein deficiency. These subjects had adequate intake but were anemic. Among those, one-third had low serum protein values. Low or deficient levels of total serum protein and albumin were observed in 20% of 70 elderly women (Jansen and Harrill 1977). Two recent studies measured total protein and serum albumin as assessment of protein status (National Center for Health Statistics 1974; Center for Disease Control 1972a). HANES suggests that disease effect on blood protein could be related to low serum protein and albumin with age, while the ten-state survey (Center for Disease Control 1972a) is inconclusive regarding lowered albumin levels. Lowered levels could be caused by modification of protein utilization or could be directly age-related. In the study of 70 elderly women (Jansen and Harrill 1977), protein deficiency occurred more often than iron deficiency. Iron deficiency was found to be more prevalent in people over 60 years of age (Center for Disease Control 1972a) and HANES found a relatively high percentage of low hemoglobin values and a low incidence of low serum iron (National Center for Health Statistics 1974). The protein needs of the elderly may not differ from those of younger persons, but disease may increase the need. Serum protein and albumin deficiencies most often correlate with an intake of 0.8 gm/kg of body weight; thus, an intake of 1 gm protein/kg of body weight has been suggested (Young and Scrimshaw 1975).

A different picture emerges when one looks at elderly institutionalized patients, although the number of studies is quite low. It is not clear whether poor nutritional status has led to hospitalization, or whether certain disease states contribute directly to poor nutritional status. Probably both factors are responsible. In seriously ill patients, subnormal levels of certain nutrients exist frequently. Again, this may be a direct effect of disease (loss of protein in decubitus ulcer, for example), or it may be a drug effect (drugs used in rheumatoid arthritis).

Hospitalized patients, in general, have deficiencies in serum albumin, protein, vitamin A, vitamin C, hemoglobin, hematocrit, and body weight (Bollet and Owen 1973). In this study, protein deficiency was seen in hyperthyroid patients, and chronic obstructive pulmonary disease led to lowest mean body weight and highest hemoglobin and hematocrit values. Chronic congestive heart disease led to low serum albumin, and in these patients, low vitamin A and vitamin C levels were also observed. Low serum albumin was found in patients with rheumatoid arthritis, who also lacked vitamin C and showed low protein and hemoglobin values. Many individuals in American hospitals suffer from protein-calorie malnutrition (PCM), which is caused by stress and protein and caloric restrictions due to their disease states. Usually, skeletal muscle is the major site of net nitrogen loss (Bistrian 1977).

Severe vitamin C deficiency is found among the institutionalized elderly, mainly men (Exton-Smith 1968). Vitamin A deficiency is prevalent in about 10% of those admitted to institutions (Brewer et al

1956) and there is a high degree of thiamine, pyridoxine, and riboflavin deficiency (Hoorn et al 1975). Approximately one-half of the patients in one study had one or more deficiencies (Hoorn et al 1975), most likely caused by an interaction of diet, disease, and drugs. More than 70% of elderly hospitalized patients had inadequate diets and showed borderline or low levels of folic acid and B-12 (Whanger and Wang 1974). Low or deficient hemoglobin values were reported for 40% of elderly women in private nursing homes (Justic et al 1974).

As it may take up to one year to reverse deficiency problems, and disease may convert borderline deficiency states into states of frank deficiency, it is advisable to give daily vitamin supplements to institutionalized elderly patients.

NUTRITION AND DISEASE

Diets that do not provide sufficient vitamin C, vitamin D, calcium, iron, and protein in earlier life can lead to deterioration in later life (Exton-Smith and Stanton 1965). While this seems to be a reasonable dictum based on reasonable evidence, it is interesting to note that observations recur in the literature suggesting that dietary patterns during early life, although they may have been deficient in terms of current standards, may well be responsible for longevity. Evidence rests mainly on animal studies. Rats receiving essential nutrients, but lacking sufficient calories to promote growth and maturation, survived considerably longer than control rats (McCay 1952). Normal growth was achieved with adequate caloric intake. Restriction of dietary intake either throughout life, or from 12 weeks after weaning, prolonged the life span of rats (Nolen 1972).

The literature also presents presumptive evidence that the development of disease can be controlled to some degree by diet. If disease occurs as part of the aging process, dietary restriction should delay onset of specific diseases. Indeed, a 46% dietary reduction in rats increased life span by 25%, and delayed onset of chronic glomerulonephritis, muscular dystrophy, and carcinogenesis (Berg and Simms 1960). Restricted carbohydrate and caloric intake in rats also led to sharp reduction in the incidence of progressive glomerulonephrosis (Bras and Ross 1965), and low intakes of proteins, carbohydrates, and calories in rats reduced the incidence or number of tumors and delayed the age of appearance of tumors (Ross and Bras 1965).

Dietary intervention has also been shown to have a profound effect on the development of autoimmune disease of mice (Fernandes et al 1972). Thus, it would appear that in some animals certain forms of nutritional intervention in early life may modify life expectancy and disease risk (Ross and Lustbader 1976). Some correlation exists for the relationship between animal protein intake and cancer of the breast and colon (Drasar and Irving 1973), which is similar to the correlation between the intake of animal fats and cancer of the colon and rectum (Wynder et al 1969).

Disease-Nutrition

Many chronically ill patients fail to eat properly and, as a consequence, become malnourished. Still, it is not yet clear whether malnutrition is the primary cause of disease or secondary to other diseases (Butterworth 1974). Decrease in serum albumin levels, resulting from protein deficiency, has been cited as a possible cause of edema. This decrease can also lead to altered drug response of protein-bound drugs, which interferes with therapeutic management of disease states (Butterworth 1974).

While most studies fail to show a significant relationship between nutritional deficiencies and physiologic impairments, the evidence is stronger in certain cases than in others. In the case of osteoporosis, much has been written about the possible link with calcium intake. Incidence of osteoporosis is high among the elderly. Fifty percent of trabecular bone and 5% of cortical bone is lost between early and later life. The overall bone loss averages 15%, and the rate of loss is highest among postmenopausal women (Wynder et al 1969; Keys 1970). Statistics show 50% of women between 65 and 70 years of age have osteoporosis, which increases to 90% in those over 90 years of age. In comparison, only 15% of males between the ages of 65 and 70 years are so diagnosed, and that figure increases to 30% in those over 90 years of age. Reduced calcium intake, altered calcium-phosphorus ratio, decreased protein intake, and a change in the acid-base balance, could all contribute to bone loss (Garn 1970). Osteoporosis of old age may also be caused by impaired calcium absorption caused by vitamin D deficiency.

Emotional stress, observed frequently in the elderly, can lead to a negative nitrogen balance (Scrimshaw 1964) and a negative calcium balance (Todhunter 1965), and serum cholesterol levels can change with variations in emotional tension (King 1964). Patients with advanced breast cancer have significantly lowered plasma pyridoxal phosphate levels; bladder and breast cancer and Hodgkin disease cause elevated excretion of tryptophan metabolites, and an impaired immune response can be produced by vitamin B-6 deficiency (Potera et al 1977).

There is a direct relationship between infection and malnutrition. Malnutrition changes host resistance to infection, and infection exaggerates malnutrition, particularly protein nutrition. Infections can also precipitate avitaminoses in persons with latent vitamin deficiencies (Scrimshaw 1975).

It is clear that there are infection-induced alterations in amino acid and protein metabolism. During acute infections, there is an excess loss of 0.6 gm to 1.2 gm/kg of body weight per day of protein; thus, protein intake should be increased by 200% of minimal normal requirements during convalescence (Beisel 1977). Others have suggested a calorie intake increase of 125% during a convalescence period, and that the convalescence last three times as long as the illness.

However, there is still uncertainty about individual nutritional requirements in infectious disease states. While it is clear that there are alterations, it is not clear how disease might change nutritional requirements (Scrimshaw 1977). Individuals with infectious diseases usually have a negative protein and energy balance, and plasma, iron, and zinc levels may be lowered. Lipid metabolism (mainly of free fatty acids) is affected during infection (Blackburn 1977).

Chronic disease in the elderly can interfere with nutritional status either directly, by disruption of the nutrient chain leading to target tissues, or indirectly by a self-limited choice of foods. Depressive and involutional states may lead to anorexia and even refusal of food (Howell and Loeb 1969). Low-grade fevers of long duration may produce excess utilization of calories, incorrect dietary management may lead to hyperglycemia or hypoglycemia, and in hypertension there may be a significant protein loss in the urine (Howell and Loeb 1969). A relationship of nutrient intake to atherosclerosis has been documented and is disputed (Mann 1977); some relationship between nutrient intake and rheumatoid arthritis has been suggested. The preponderance of evidence seems to suggest that poor nutritional states can lead to certain diseases, and it is clear that disease, imposed on a poor nutritional state, may further deplete nutritional reserves.

Nutrition-Disease

A variety of nutritional deficiency states can result in conditions that simulate those frequently encountered in the elderly; but, it has not yet been determined that diet can protect the elderly from disease (Watkins 1958). However, considerable evidence shows a direct relationship between obesity and hypertension, and weight decrease can be related to a fall in blood pressure (Mann 1974; Tyroler et al 1975; Reisin et al 1978). Certainly, the first line of treatment of diabetes is dietary management leading to a reduction of total caloric intake and total body mass (Briant 1977).

Certain dietary components lead to nutritional deficiency states. For example, wheat bran decreases the availability and intestinal absorption of iron (by 72%) and of zinc (by 82.5%). Wholemeal bread acts in a similar manner (Ismail-Beigi et al 1977). Foods high in calcium, phosphorus, and proteins, such as milk and cheese, inhibit zinc absorption (Pecound et al 1975), and coffee reduces serum zinc levels. Recurrent stone formation in varied disorders has been controlled frequently with diet adjustment and adequate fluid intake, which should be sufficient to produce urinary output of at least 2500 ml per 24 hours (Smith et al 1978). Foods rich in oxalate, such as rhubarb, spinach, tea, cola drinks, and citrus fruits and juices may augment stone formation. Foods high in purine content tend to acidify the urine and thus increase urinary excretion of uric acid, a situation favorable for precipitation of uric acid crystals. Sucrose has been suggested as a major cause of atheroscleroisis, but the evidence is not convincing (Yudkin 1971). Subclinical deficiencies may cause loss of appetite, fatigue, irritability, anxiety, loss of recent memory, insomnia, and mild delusional states, which can be managed by specific dietary therapies (Keys et al 1950).

The possible influence of nutrition on psychologic functions of aging is only beginning to be realized. An early suggestion of such a relationship was made in 1958 (Bill 1958). Ten years later, it was suggested that psychologic symptoms may be the only apparent symptoms of dietary deficiencies, even long-standing deficiencies (Scrimshaw and Gordon 1968). The nervous system does not adapt to deficiency states but remains highly sensitive.

Research reports on a possible correlation between nutritional deficiency states and depression have appeared with some regularity. In the early 1940s, severe depression and mental confusion was related to deficiency in several B vitamins (Speis et al 1943). Situational depression in the elderly could be more severe or of longer duration in the presence of subclinical vitamin B deficiency. Experimental neurosis was produced by drastic, short-term starvation (Brozek and Keys 1945), and experimentally induced vitamin B deficiency produced confusion in a relatively short time (O'Shea et al 1942). It has been noted that mentally deteriorated elderly patients tend to have lower levels of vitamin C than normal persons, and as previously pointed out, stress can cause decreased vitamin C blood levels (Berkenau 1940). Slow mental performance has been related to iodine deficit and there also seems to be some relation between impairment of psychological performance and protein deficiency, as the response of nerve cells to stimuli becomes defective (Eichenwald and Fry 1969). Deficiencies of thiamine, niacin, folic acid, and ascorbic acid have long been suggested as causes of difficulty in orderly thinking, depression, apprehension, increased irritability, insomnia, memory loss, excitement, dementia, loss of well-being, lack of energy, and emotional instability (Bill 1958). It was reported that two vitamin deficiencies, pellagra and pernicious anemia, have a definite correlation with paranoid symptoms (Whanger 1976). This same observation was made almost 40 years ago (Speis et al 1943).

NUTRITIONAL STATUS, NUTRIENTS, AND DRUG ACTION

Various nutritional factors alter the absorption, distribution, metabolism, and excretion of drugs. Macronutrients, such as carbohydrates, proteins, and fats, as well as trace substances like vitamins and minerals, are often responsible. However, there are individual differences among patients. Nutrient components can change gastrointestinal motility, secretions involved in the digestive processes, blood flow rates, enzyme activity responsible for drug metabolism, and other factors (Gilette and Pang 1977; Prescott 1975). Much has been written on drug-dietary incompatibilities (Powell and Lamy 1977a; Powell and Lamy 1977b). The role of nutritional status and the possible action of nutrients on drug metabolism must be separated from a dietary role. Diets may include a variety of nonnutrient components, which can also affect drug action. While there is still no clear delineation of nutrient-drug interactions, evidence is strong that nutrition can be a major determinant of drug action (Campbell and Hayes 1974).

Altered absorption Acetaminophen absorption proceeds five times more rapidly in fasting subjects than in subjects consuming a high-carbohydrate meal (McGilveray and Mattock 1972). Carbohydrate nutrients, particularly those containing large amounts of pectin, delay acetaminophen absorption significantly, while proteins or lipids do not (Jaffe et al 1971). Lipids, on the other hand, double the absorption of griseofulvin in contrast to proteins, probably as griseofulvin is solubilized by bile secreted in response to lipid intake (Crounse 1970). Fasting causes a sevenfold increase in tetracycline absorption. In patients with delayed gastric emptying function, L-dopa may be ineffective (Heading et al 1973; Levine 1970; Prescott 1974).

Altered metabolism Nutritional factors are important in regulation of drug metabolism in humans. Weight, per se, does not seem to affect metabolism, as the half-lives of antipyrine and tolbutamide, drugs metabolized by the microsomal oxidation pathways, do not differ in healthy, normal or obese persons. The same results were obtained for drugs metabolized by acetylation (sulfisoxazole and isoniazid) and by the pseudocholinesterase hydrolysis pathway (procaine) (Reidenberg 1977). Others found that fasting enhances hepatic enzyme induction, but a long-term low-protein diet has the opposite effect (Cooksley and Powell 1971). Dietary protein deficiency can decrease cytochrome P-450 activity and increase the duration of barbiturate action by decreasing rates of metabolism and tissue clearance (Campbell 1977). High-protein, low-carbohydrate diets reduce the average plasma half-life of antipyrine by 41% and of theophylline by 36%, an effect counteracted by a low-protein, high-carbohydrate diet (Conney et al 1977). Diets that include animal fat and protein shorten antipyrine half-life by 50%, compared to the half-life observed in vegetarians (Fraser et al 1977).

Altered distribution No significant effect on drug distribution has yet been fully demonstrated. At one time, it had been suggested that dietary pyridoxine could inhibit the effect of levodopa as an antiparkinsonism drug, but it was later shown that not enough dietary vitamin B-6 could be consumed to bring about this effect (Mena and Cotzias 1975). Recently, though, an interesting concept was advanced (Markovitz and Fernstrom 1977). Large neutral amino acids share a common transport system located at the blood-brain barrier with methyldopa, a drug often used in the elderly. The drug and the natural neutral amino acid compete for brain uptake. Nutrients can affect serum amino acid patterns and can, thus, significantly influence the availability of amino acid drugs to the brain.

Enhancement of natural substances Choline and tryptophan are precursors of acetylcholine and serotonin, which are CNS neurotransmitters. Acetylcholine and serotonin are both involved in tardive dyskinesia. Administration of choline may be useful in stimulating acetylcholine to counteract tardive dyskinesia. Choline is normally present in foods like soybeans, liver, eggs, and products containing lecithin (Wurtman and Growdon 1978).

Altered excretion Diets deficient in glutathione can lead to reduced bromsulphthalein (BSP) excretion, as glutathione conjugation of BSP is essential for transport of BSP from liver to the bile (Combes 1962). In addition, the excretion of drugs sensitive to changes in urinary pH can be affected by changes in dietary patterns and, thus, urinary pH. Foods that can potentially acidify or alkalinize urine are listed in Table 12-7. Balanced protein diets will produce an acid urinary pH (pH 5.9), while low-protein diets usually result in an alkaline urinary pH (pH 7.5) (Weslay-Hadzija 1971). It should be noted that citrus fruit juices are responsible for an alkaline, and not an acid, urinary pH, probably because of their relatively high concentration of potassium (Harper 1971).

DRUG EFFECT ON NUTRITIONAL STATUS

Many different drug classes are capable of altering a patient's nutritional status. Among them are antacids, anorexiants, anticonvulsants, antidepressants, antimicrobials, autonomic agents, cathartics, corticosteroids, cytotoxic agents, diuretics, and hypocholes-

Table 12-7
Foods Potentially Causing Changes in Urinary pH

Foods potentially contributing to the acidification of urine	Foods potentially contributing to the alkalinization of urine

Meats
  Meat, fish, fowl, shellfish
  Eggs
  Cheese
  Peanut butter
	Milk products
	  Milk, cream, buttermilk
	
	Fats
	  Almonds, chestnuts, coconut

Vegetables
  Corn and lentils
	Vegetables
	  All types

Fat
  Bacon
  Nuts: Brazil, filberts, peanuts, walnuts
	Fruit
	  Citrus fruits

Fruit
  Cranberries
  Plums
  Prunes	

Breads
  Breads (all types), crackers
  Macaroni, spaghetti, noodles	

Dessert Cakes, cookies	

teremic agents (Lamy 1979). Many of these drugs are used in the treatment of chronic diseases frequently encountered among the elderly. Long-term use of these drugs could, therefore, enhance the drug's capacity to alter a patient's nutritional status. These interactions may be responsible for many diverse results, including malabsorption syndromes. Effectiveness of nutrients depends on many factors, and drugs can interfere with the nutrient chain (Table 12-8). Drugs can cause appetite depression, irritation of the stomach, nausea, and decreased nutrient absorption. They can alter electrolyte balance, carbohydrate and fat metabolism, and may interfere with normal serum protein functions (Christakis and Miridjanian 1968). Griseofulvin, clofibrate, and lincomycin, among others, can cause altered taste sensations (Fagan 1971) and thus depress appetite, while phenothiazines, and the tricyclic antidepressants, because of a positive effect on a patient's mental status, can cause increased food intake and weight gain (Pierpaoli 1972). Patients on chronic antacid therapy may be subject to thiamine deficiency (Levy and Hewitt 1971), and cathartics, frequently used in skilled nursing facilities and long-term care facilities, tend to diminish nutrient absorption by reducing exposure of gastrointestinal contents to absorption sites (Krondl 1970). Drugs can alter the pancreatic or intestinal phase of digestion (see Table 12-9) (Gray 1973).

Table 12-8
Mechanisms for the Effects of Drugs on Nutritional Status

1. Appetite Suppression or Stimulation
2. Altered Nutrient Absorption
   a. Altered Gastrointestinal pH
   b. Interference with Bile Acid Activity
   c. Impaired or Enhanced Gastrointestinal Motility
   d. Inactivation of Absorptive Enzyme Systems
   e. Competitive Inhibition of Nutrient Absorption
   f. Damage to Absorptive Mucosal Cells
   g. Complexation of Nutrients by Drugs
3. Impaired Nutrient Metabolism and Utilization
4. Altered Nutrient Excretion

Although Parkinson disease can affect the metabolism and absorption of phenylalanine (Bianchine et al 1971), absorption of this amino acid and tyrosine may be further impaired by L-dopa used in the treatment of parkinsonism (Granerus et al 1971). This condition can be exacerbated if a patient is maintained on a low-protein diet. A number of drugs, including colchicine, can damage the intestinal mucosa leading to impaired absorption of nutrients like fats, vitamin B-12, and folic acid (Waxman et al 1970; Race et al 1970).

Glucocorticoids can lower serum calcium by reducing absorption, and osteomalacia results from chronic intake of anticonvulsants. Prednisone, phenobarbital, phenytoins, primidone, and others have all been shown to cause calcium malabsorption by different mechanisms (Roe 1974). Aspirin, used frequently to treat rheumatoid arthritis, has been associated with folate deficiency, as have been many other drugs, including cycloserine and phenobarbital. Hypokalemia may develop in patients with Parkinson disease treated with L-dopa, as a result of increased urinary excretion of potassium (Granerus et al 1977).

Some of the drug effects on nutritional status have been summarized in Table 12-10 (Hethcox and Stanaszek 1974). The elderly are particularly at risk to these effects for several reasons. Usually, they receive several prescribed drugs concurrently, which are added to self-prescribed, nonprescription drugs. The elderly are often on marginal diets and their nutritional status may also be impaired by chronic diseases (Roe 1974). Thus, nutritional deficiencies may result from

Table 12-9
Drugs and Carbohydrate Absorption

Drug	Principal biological action	Effect on carbohydrate digestion-absorption	Probable mechanism of action
Saccharides	Dietary carbohydrates	↑ Disaccharidases	Stabilization of sucrase
Neomycin	Antibiotic	↓ Lactase, 75%	Intestinal mucosal damage
Colchicine	Block of cell mitosis	↓ All disaccharidases, especially lactase up to 85%	Failure of intestinal cells to acquire disaccharidases
Atropine	Anticholinergic	↑ Monosaccharide absorption	Increased contact-time between carbohydrates and mucosa
Epinephrine, norepinephrine	Adrenergic agents	↑ Glucose absorption, 60%	? Mediated by cyclic AMP
Digitoxin	Cardiac glycoside	↓ Glucose absorption, 50%	Competition for glucose transport
Cortisone	Adrenal steroid	↑ Sucrase in neonate	Precocious development of intestinal surface
Phenformin	Biguanide type anti-diabetic agent	↓ Glucose absorption	Related to log of dose ? competition for energy sources
Ethacrynic acid	Diuretic agent	↓ Glucose absorption	? Interference with formation of glucose-Na^+-carrier complex

G.M. Gray. Drugs, malnutrition, and carbohydrate absorption. *Am J Clin Nutr.* 26:121, 1973. Reprinted with permission.

Table 12-10
Reported Drug Interferences with Nutrients

Drug	Interference
Analgesics	
Colchicine	damage to intestinal wall → nonspecific ↓ in absorption
	↓ absorption of vitamin B_{12}, carotene, fat, lactose, d-xylose, electrolytes
Anorexiants	appetite suppression → growth retardation
Antacids	alkaline destruction of thiamine → thiamine deficiency
Anticonvulsants	
Barbiturates	inhibition of absorptive enzymes or ↑ metabolism and turnover → deficiency in body folate and vitamin D
	↓ vitamin B_{12} and d-xylose absorption
Hydantoins	inhibition of absorptive enzymes or ↑ metabolism and turnover → deficiency in body folate, vitamin D
Antidepressants	
Tricyclic antidepressants	stimulation of appetite → weight gain
Antimetabolites	
Methotrexate	damage to intestinal wall → nonspecific ↓ in absorption
	inhibition of enzyme system
	↓ in vitamin B_{12} and d-xylose absorption
Antimicrobials	appetite suppression and diarrhea → ↓ nutrient absorption
Chloramphenicol	↓ protein synthesis
Isoniazid	complexation of vitamin B_6 → ↑ excretion of vitamin B_6
Para-aminosalicyclic acid	inhibition of absorptive enzymes → ↓ vitamin B_{12} absorption
Penicillin	aftertaste with food → suppression of appetite
	inhibition of glutathione
Sulfonamides	↓ synthesis of folic acid, B vitamins, vitamin K
Tetracyclines	binding of bone calcium
Autonomics	
Ganglionic blockers	↓ peristalsis → ↓ nutrient absorption
Anticholinergics	↓ peristalsis → ↓ nutrient absorption

J.M. Hethcox, and W.F. Stanaszek. Interactions of drugs and diet. *Hosp Pharm.* 9:373, 1974. Reprinted with permission.

chronic diseases or the treatment of these diseases. Dose, duration of treatment, and multiple drug regimens should be monitored carefully in the elderly.

DIET-DRUG INTERACTIONS

Food can delay the speed with which drugs reach the general circulation and, thus, delay the onset of action of certain drugs. There may be a decrease in the onset of action, but often the rate of absorption is affected by food. This has been confirmed with many drugs, most recently for digoxin (White et al 1971; Sanchez et al 1973; Greenblatt et al 1974). This is not clinically important if a patient is receiving drugs chronically (*Br Med J.* 1977).

A series of articles (Bates et al 1974; Levy et al 1975; Melander et al 1977a; Melander et al 1977b; Melander et al 1977c) report on the enhancement of the rate and extent of absorption of carbamazepine, hydralazine, nitrofurantoin, propranolol, and spironolactone by concurrent food administration. The effect is not negligible because two to three times as much hydralazine enters the general circulation when the drug is taken with food than when it is taken on an empty stomach.

The elderly exhibit individual variations to drug administration more so than any other age group; and anything that might decrease that variation and increase predictability of drug response should be carefully investigated.

RECOMMENDATIONS

Many elderly probably follow a nutritional intake acquired by habit throughout life which has not changed with physiology and decreased activity. Furthermore, it is difficult to change this ingrained habit. In the elderly, an imbalanced nutritional status or subclinical malnutrition can be produced by undernutrition, chronic disease, or treatment. Undernutrition may be the result of excessive intake of empty calories, or caused by a lack of a nutrient.

Ideally, caloric intake should be reduced with age. There should be a decreased intake of fats, and a sufficient intake of proteins, but certain proteins do not supply all of the needed amino acids. Fluid and dietary fiber intake should not be neglected. In England, it has been suggested that men between the ages of 65 and 75 years consume 2350 calories daily, and those over 75 should not consume more than 2100 calories per day. For women, comparable intake should be 2050 calories and 1900 calories, respectively (Department of Health and Social Security 1969). In the United States, the following daily standards have been suggested for those 60 years and older (Table 12-11) (National Center for Health Statistics 1974).

Table 12-11
Suggested Daily Standards

	Calories/kg	Protein gm/kg	Ca mg	Iron mg	A IU	C mg
M	34	1.0	400	10	3500	60
F	29	1.0	600	10	3500	55

In developing an individualized nutritional regimen, consideration must be given to individual preferences as well as social, religious, racial, and psychologic factors. The lifestyle of the patient must be considered, as well as the patient's ability to prepare foods. Older people probably do not seek variety and novelty in foods, but prefer familiar foods. It may prove difficult to introduce the desired beneficial nutrients into the patient's dietary regimen, thus, educational methods must be chosen carefully.

At one time, it was thought that desire for longevity, retention of youthful appearance and energy, and good health could not necessarily be used to gain compliance with a selected nutrition program (Riley and Foner 1968). However, in those patients with diabetes, arthritis, and hypertension, a desire to stay healthy has been used successfully as a basis for patient acceptance of nutritional regimens. Counseling increases awareness of nutrition and improvement of knowledge of nutrition and food selection. However, the elderly are probably not interested in why certain foods should or should not be included; rather, they want to know what to buy and eat (Marshall 1971; Rae and Burke 1978). An excellent cookbook will help elderly people plan nourishing meals (Davies 1972).

REFERENCES

Aaron, J.E., Gallagher, J.C., Anderson, J. et al. Frequency of osteomalacia and osteoporosis in fracture of the proximal femur. *Lancet* 1:229, 1974.

Ahrens, E.H., Jr. The management of hyperlipidemias: whether, rather than how. *Ann Intern Med.* 85:87, 1976.

Albanese, A.A. Osteoporosis. *J Am Pharm Assoc.* NS17:252, 1977.

Alfin-Slater, R., Anderson, J.J.B., Bozian, R.C. et al. Helping patients learn to eat right. *Patient Care* 12(5):120, 1978a.

Alfin-Slater, R., Anderson, J.J.B., Bozian, R.C. et al. Dietary answers to common problems. *Patient Care* 12(7):42, 1978b.

Alfin-Slater, R., Anderson, J.J.B., Bozian, R.C. et al. Nutrition in everyday practice. *Patient Care* 12(4):76, 1978c.

Anderson, E.L. Eating patterns before and after dentures. *J Am Diet Assoc.* 58:421, 1971.

Balacki, J.A., and Dobbins, W.O. Maldigestion and malabsorption: making up for lost nutrients. *Geriatrics* 29:157, 1974.

Bates, T.R., Sequeira, J.A., and Tembo, A.V. Effect of food on nitrofurantoin absorption. *Clin Pharmacol Ther.* 16:63, 1974.

Beal, R.W. Haematinics. I. Patho-physiological and clinical aspects. *Drugs* 2:190, 1971.

Beisel, W.R. Impact of infection on nutritional status: concluding comments and summary. *Am J Clin Nutr.* 30:1564, 1977.

Berg, B.N., and Simms, H.S. Nutrition and longevity in rats. II. Longevity and onset of disease with different levels of food intake. *J Nutr.* 71:255, 1960.

Berkenau, P. Vitamin C in senile psychoses. *J Ment Sci.* 86:675, 1940.

Bermond, P. Clinical symptoms of malnutrition and plasma ascorbic acid levels. *Am J Clin Nutr.* 29:493, 1976.

Bianchine, J.R., Calimlim, L.R., Morgan, J.P. et al. Metabolism and absorption of L-3, 3-dihydroxy-phenylalanine in patients with Parkinson's disease. *Ann NY Acad Sci.* 179:126, 1971.

Bill, E.C. Nutritional deficiencies and emotional disturbances. *J Psychol.* 45:47, 1958.

Birnbaum, N. Normal hemoglobin level and coronary heart disease. *Am Heart.* 65:136, 1963.

Bistrian, B.R. Interaction of nutrition and infection in the hospital setting. *Am J Clin Nutr.* 30:1228, 1977.

Blackburn, G.L. Lipid metabolism in infection. *Am J Clin Nutr.* 30:1321, 1977.

Blackburn, H. How nutrition influences mass hyperlipidemia and atherosclerosis. *Geriatrics* 33(2):42, 1978.

Bollet, A.J., and Owen, S. Evaluation of nutritional status of selected hospitalized patients. *Am J Clin Nutr.* 26:931, 1973.

Botez, M.I. Folate deficiency and neurological disorders in adults. *Med Hypothesis.* 2:135, 1976.

Botez, M.I., and Lambert, B. Folate deficiency and restless-legs syndrome in pregnancy. *N Engl J Med.* 297:670, 1977.

Boykin, L.S. Iron deficiency anemia in postmenopausal women. *J Am Geriatr Soc.* 24:558, 1976.

Brain, L., and Walton, J.M. *Brain's Diseases of the Nervous System.* London: Oxford University Press, 1969.

Bras, G., and Ross, M.H. Kidney disease and nutrition in the rat. *Toxicol Appl Pharmacol.* 6:247, 1965.

Brewer, W.D., Furnivall, M.E., Wagoner, A. et al. Nutritional status of the aged in Michigan. *J Am Diet Assoc.* 32:810, 1956.

Briant, R.H. Drug treatment in the elderly: problems and prescribing rules. *Drugs* 13:225, 1977.

Brin, M., Dibble, M.V., Peel, A. et al. Some preliminary findings on the nutritional status of the aged in Onondaga County, New York. *Am J Clin Nutr.* 17:240, 1965.

British Medical Journal. Editorial. Food and the handling of drugs. 1:1304, 1977.

Brock, J.F. Protein deficiency in adults. *Prog Food Nutr Sci.* 1(6):359, 1975.

Brozek, J., and Keys, A. Interdisciplinary research in human biology with special reference to behavior studies. *Am Sci.* 33:103, 1945.

Burkitt, D.P. Some diseases characteristic of modern Western civilization. *Br Med J.* 1:274, 1973.

Burr, M.L., Elwood, P.C., Hole, D.J. et al. Plasma and leukocyte ascorbic acid levels in the elderly. *Am J Clin Nutr.* 27:144, 1974.

Butterworth, E.E. Iatrogenic malnutrition: the skeleton in the hospital closet. *Nutr Today.* 9:4, 1974.

Campbell, T.C. Nutrition and drug-metabolizing enzymes. *Clin Pharmacol Ther.* 22:699, 1977.

Campbell, T.C., and Hayes, J.R. Role of nutrition in the drug-metabolizing enzyme system. *Pharmacol Rev.* 26:171, 1974.

Carney, M.W.P., and Sheffield, B.F. Associations of subnormal folate and vitamin B-12 values and effects of replacement therapy. *J Nerv Ment Dis.* 150:404, 1970.

Center for Disease Control. *Ten-State Nutrition Survey, 1968–1970, IV. Biochemical.* DHEW Publ. No. (HMS) 72-8132. Atlanta, Ga., 1972a.

Center for Disease Control. *Ten-State Nutrition Survey, 1968–1970.* DHEW Publ. No. (HMS) 72-8134, Health Services and Mental Health Administration. Washington, D.C., 1972b.

Central Maryland Health Systems Agency. *Health Systems Plan and Annual Implementation Plan.* Baltimore, Md., 1978.

Chinn, A.B. Working With Older People. Vol. IV. *Clinical Aspects of Aging.* PHS Publ. No. 1459. Washington, D.C.: U.S. Government Printing Office, 1971.

Christakis, G., and Miridjanian, A. Diets, drugs, and their interrelationships. *J Am Diet Assoc.* 52:21, 1968.

Civin, W.H., Ejarque, P.M., Hines, C. et al. Diet vs drugs in hyperlipidemia. *Patient Care* 10(14):20, 1976.

Combes, B. Importance of conjugation with glutathione on sulfobromophthalein transport blood to bile. *J Clin Invest.* 41:1351, 1962.

Conney, A.H., Pantuck, E.J., Kuntzman, R. et al. Nutrition and chemical biotransformation in man. *Clin Pharmacol Ther.* 22:707, 1977.

Cook, J.C., Monsen, E.R. Food iron absorption in human subjects. III. Comparison of the effect of animal protein on non-heme iron absorption. *Am J Clin Nutr.* 29:859, 1976.

Cooksley, W.G.E., and Powell, L.W. Drug metabolism and interaction with particular reference to the liver. *Drugs* 2:177, 1971.

Coronary Drug Project Research Group. Clofibrate and niacin in coronary disease. *JAMA.* 231:4, 1975.

Crosby, W.H. Current concepts: who needs iron? *N Engl J Med.* 297:543, 1977.

Crounse, R.R. Human pharmacology of griseofulvin: the effect of fat intake in a human subject. *J Pharm Sci.* 59:595, 1970.

Dall, J.L.C., Paulose, S., and Ferguson, F.A. Potassium intakes of elderly patients in hospital. *Gerontol Clin.* 13:114, 1971.

Davies, I.J.T. *The Clinical Significance of the Essential Biological Metals.* London: Charles C Thomas, 1972.

Davies, L. *Easy Cooking for One or Two.* New York: Penguin Books, 1972.

Department of Health and Social Security, Panel on Recommended Allowances of Nutrients. Recommended intakes of nutrients for the United Kingdom. London: HMSO, 1969.

Department of Health and Social Security. Nutrition of the elderly. London: HMSO, 1972.

Diamond, M.C. The aging brain: some enlightening and optimistic results. *Am Sci.* 66:66, 1978.

Drasar, B.S., and Irving, D. Environmental factors and cancer of the colon and breast. *Br J Cancer.* 27:167, 1973.

Drasar, B.S., and Jenkins, D.J.A. Bacteria, diet, and large bowel cancer. *Am J Clin Nutr.* 29:1410, 1976.

Dunn, J.P., Ipsen, J., Elson, K.O. et al. Risk factors in coronary artery disease, hypertension, and diabetes. *Am J Med Sci.* 259:309, 1970.

Ehtisham, M., and Cape, R.D.T. Protocol for diagnosing and treating anemia. *Geriatrics* 32(11):91, 1977.

Eichenwald, H.F., and Fry, P.C. Nutrition and learning. *Science* 190:163, 1969.

Elwood, P.C., and Hughes, D. Clinical trial of iron therapy on psychomotor function in anaemic women. *Br Med J.* 3:254, 1970.

Elwood, P.C., Shinton, N.K., Wilson, C.I.D. et al. Haemoglobin, vitamin B-12, and folate levels in the elderly. *J Haematol.* 12:557, 1971.

Exton-Smith, A.N. The problem of subclinical malnutrition in the elderly. Edited by A.N. Exton-Smith, and D.L. Scott. In *Vitamins in the Elderly.* Bristol: John Wright and Sons, Ltd., 1968.

Exton-Smith, A.N. Problems of diet in old age. *J R Coll Phys.* (London) 9(2):148, 1975.

Exton-Smith, A.N., and Stanton, B.R. Report of an investigation into the dietary habits of elderly women living alone. London: King Edward's Hospital Fund, 1965.

Fagan, L. Griseofulvin and dysgeusia: implications? *Ann Intern Med.* 74:795, 1971.

Farrell, P.M., and Bieri, J.G. Megavitamin E supplementation in man. *Am J Clin Nutr.* 28:1381, 1975.

Fernandes, G., Yunis, E.J., Smith, J. et al. Dietary influence on breeding behavior, hemolytic anemia, and longevity in NZB mice. *Proc Soc Exp Biol Med.* 139:1189, 1972.

Finch, C.A., and Monsen, E.R. Iron nutrition and the fortification of food with iron. *JAMA.* 219:1462, 1972.

Flear, C.T.G. Potassium problems in heart disease, Part I. *Adv Drug Reaction Bull.* 32:96, 1972a.

Flear, C.T.G. Potassium problems in heart disease, Part II. *Adv Drug Reaction Bull.* 33:100, 1972b.

Flynn, M.A. The cholesterol controversy. *Contemp Nutr.* 3(3), 1978.

Food and Nutrition Board, National Research Council. *Recommended Dietary Allowances,* 8th ed. Washington, D.C.: National Academy of Sciences, 1974.

Fraser, H.S., Mucklow, J.C., Bulpitt, C.J. et al. Environmental effects on antipyrine half-life in man. *Clin Pharmacol Ther.* 22:799, 1977.

Fry, P.C., Fox, H.M., and Linkswiler, J. Nutrient intakes of healthy older women. *J Am Diet Assoc.* 42:218, 1963.

Fuchs, H.M., Dorfman, S., and Floch, M.H. The effect of dietary fiber supplementation in man. II. Alteration in fecal physiology and bacterial flora. *Am J Clin Nutr.* 29:1443, 1976.

Gaffney, G.W., Horonick, A., Okuda, K. et al. Vitamin B-12 serum concentrations in 528 apparently healthy human subjects of ages 12–94. *J Gerontol.* 12:32, 1957.

Garbus, S.B., and Lamy, P.P. Managing the aging hypertensive. *Patient Care,* 1976.

Garcia, P.A., Battese, G.E., and Brewer, W.D. Longitudinal study of the age and cohort influences on dietary patterns. *J Gerontol.* 30:349, 1977.

Garn, S.M. *The Earlier Gain and the Later Loss of Cortical Bone in Nutritional Perspective.* Springfield, Ill.: Charles C Thomas, 1970.

Garn, S.M. Bone loss on aging. Edited by M. Rockstein. In *Physiology and Pathology of Human Aging.* New York: Academic Press, 1975.

Gilette, J.R., and Pang, K.S. Theoretic aspects of pharmacokinetic drug interactions. *Clin Pharmacol Ther.* 22:623, 1977.

Girdwood, R.H. Nutritional folate deficiency in the United Kingdom. *Scot Med J.* 14:296, 1969.

Goffman, E. *The Presentation of Self in Everyday Life.* New York: Doubleday & Co., Inc., 1959.

Goffman, E. The characteristics of total institutions. Edited by A. Etzioni. In *Complex Organizations.* New York: Atherton Press, 1961.

Goldstein, S. Changing income and consumption patterns of the aged. *Gerontologist* 8:17, 1968.

Gordon, B. Neurological aspects of dementia in the elderly. Presented at the Fifth Annual Symposium on Geriatric Medicine, Baltimore City Hospitals. Baltimore, 1977.

Granerus, A.K., Jagenburg, R., Rodgers, S. et al. Inhibition of L-phenylalanine absorption in patients treated with L-dopa for parkinsonism. *Proc Soc Exp Biol Med.* 137:942, 1971.

Granerus, A.K., Jagenburg, R., and Svanborg, A. Kaliuretic effect of L-dopa treatment in parkinsonian patients. *Acta Med Scand.* 201:291, 1977.

Gray, G.M. Drugs, malnutrition and carbohydrate absorption. *Am J Clin Nutr.* 26:121, 1973.

Greenblatt, D.J., Duhme, D.W., Koch-Weser, J. et al. Bioavailability of digoxin tablets and elixir in the fasting and postprandial state. *Clin Pharmacol Ther.* 16:444, 1974.

Guthrie, H.A., Black, K., and Madden, J.P. Nutritional practices of elderly citizens in rural Pennsylvania. *Gerontologist* 27:330, 1972.

Haeger, K. Long-term treatment of intermittent claudication with vitamin E. *Am J Clin Nutr.* 27:1179, 1974.

Harman, D. Free radical theory of aging: effect of the amount and degree of unsaturation of dietary fat on mortality rate. *J Gerontol.* 26:451, 1971.

Harper, H.A. *Review of Physiological Chemistry.* Los Angeles: Lange Medical Publications, 1971.

Harper, A.E. Recommended dietary allowances for the elderly. *Geriatrics* 33(5):73, 1978.

Heading, R.C., Nimmo, J., Prescott, L.F. et al. The dependence of paracetamol absorption on the rate of gastric emptying. *Br Med J.* 47:415, 1973.

Hearney, R.P., Recker, R.R., and Saville, P.D. Calcium balance and calcium requirements in middle-aged women. *Am J Clin Nutr.* 30:1603, 1977.

Henkins, R.I., Schechter, P.J., Hoye, R. et al. Idiopathic hypogeusia with dysgeusia, hyposmia and dysosmia. *JAMA.* 217:434, 1971.

Herbert, V., and Jacob, E. Destruction of vitamin B-12 by ascorbic acid. *JAMA.* 230:241, 1974.

Herbert, V.D. Megavitamin therapy. *Contemp Nutr.* 2(10), 1977a.

Herbert, V.D. Megavitamin therapy. *J Am Pharm Assoc.* NS17:764, 1977b.

Hethcox, J.M., and Stanaszek, W.F. Interactions of drugs and diets. *Hosp Pharm.* 9:373, 1974.

Hoorn, R.K.J., Flikwert, J.P., and Westerink, D. Vitamin B-1, B-2, and B-6 deficiencies in geriatric patients, measured by coenzyme stimulation of enzyme activities. *Clin Chem Acta.* 61:151, 1975.

Horwitt, M.K. Vitamin E in human nutrition–an interpretive review. *Rev Nutr Res.* 22:1, 1961.

Horwitt, M.K., Century, B., and Zeman, A.A. Erythrocyte survival time and reticulocyte levels after tocopherol depletion in man. *Am J Clin Nutr.* 12:99, 1963.

Horwitt, M.K. Vitamin E: a reexamination. *Am J Clin Nutr.* 29:569, 1976.

Howell, S.C., and Loeb, M.B. Nutrition, health and society: research review. *Gerontologist* 9(3):1–116, 1969.

Hughes, G. Changes in taste sensitivity with advancing age. *Gerontol Clin.* 11:225, 1969.

Institute of Food Technologists' Expert Panel on Food Safety and Nutrition and the Committee on Public Information. Vitamin E. *Contemp Nutr.* 2(11):1, 1977.

Inter-Society Commission on Heart Disease. Resources report: the primary prevention of atherosclerosis. *Circulation* 42:A-55, 1970.

Ismail-Beigi, F., Faraji, B., and Reinhold, J.G. Binding of zinc and iron to wheat bread, wheat bran, and their components. *Am J Clin Nutr.* 30:1721, 1977.

Jaffe, M.J., Colaizi, J.L., and Barry, H. Effects of dietary components on GI absorption of acetaminophen tablets in man. *J Pharm Sci.* 60:1646, 1971.

Jansen, C., and Harrill, I. Intakes and serum levels of protein and iron for 70 elderly women. *Am J Clin Nutr.* 30:1414, 1977.

Johnson, B., and Feniak, E. Food practices and nutrient intake of elderly home-bound individuals. *Can Nutr Notes.* 21:61, 1965.

Jordan, V.E. Protein status of the elderly as measured by dietary intake, hair tissue, and serum albumin. *Am J Clin Nutr.* 29:522, 1976.

Judge, T.G., and Cowan, N.R. Dietary potassium intake and grip strength in older people. *Gerontol Clin.* 13:221, 1971.

Justic, C.L., Howe, J.M., and Clark, H.C. Dietary intakes and nutritional status of elderly patients. *J Am Diet Assoc.* 65:639, 1974.

Kariks, J., and Perry, S.W. Folic acid deficiency in psychiatric patients. *Med J Aust.* p. 1192, June 13, 1970.

Kaunitz, H. Dietary lipids and arteriosclerosis. *J Am Chem Soc.* 58(8):293, 1975.

Kelly, J.T. Nutritional problems of the elderly. *Geriatrics* 33(2):41, 1978.

Kelsay, J.L. A compendium of nutritional status studies and dietary evaluation studies conducted in the United States 1957–1967. *J Nutr.* 99(suppl 1):119, 1969.

Keys, A., Brozek, J., Henschel, A. et al. *The Biology of Human Starvation*, Vol. II. Minneapolis: University of Minnesota Press, 1950.

Keys, A. (Ed.). Coronary heart disease in seven countries. *Circulation* 41(suppl 1): 1970.

King, S.H. Social psychological factors in illness. Edited by H.E. Freeman, S. Levin, and L.G. Reeder. In *Handbook of Medical Sociology*. Englewood Cliffs, N.J.: Prentice-Hall, Inc., 1964.

Kohn, R.R. Effect of antioxidants on life span of C57 BL mice. *J Gerontol.* 26:378, 1971.

Korsan-Bensten, K., Wilhelmsen, L., Elmfeldt, D. et al. Blood coagulation and fibrinolysis in man after myocardial infarction compared with a representative sample. *Atherosclerosis* 16:83, 1972.

Kositowattanakul, T., Tosukhowong, P., Vimokessant, S.L. et al. Chemical interactions between thiamin and tannic acid. II. Separation of products. *Am J Clin Nutr.* 30:1686, 1977.

Kritchevsky, D. Dietary (sic) fiber and other dietary factors in hypercholesteremia. *Am J Clin Nutr.* 30:979, 1977.

Krondl, A. Present understanding of interactions of drugs and foods during absorption. *Can Med Assoc J.* 103:360, 1970.

Labadarios, E., Rossouw, J.E., McConnell, J.B. et al. Vitamin B-6 deficiency in chronic liver disease–evidence for increased degradation of pyridoxal-5-phosphate. *Gut* 18:23, 1977.

Lamy, P.P. Aging: how human physiology responds. Edited by E.W. Busse. In *Theory and Therapeutics of Aging.* New York: MedCom, Inc., 1973.

Lamy, P.P. Drug-food interactions. Edited by M.C. Smith, and T.R. Brown. In *Handbook of Institutional Pharmacy Practice.* Baltimore: Williams and Wilkins, 1979.

Lamy, P.P., and Kitler, M.E. The geriatric patient: age-dependent physiologic and pathologic changes. *J Am Geriatr Soc.* 19:871, 1971.

LeBovit, C. The food of older people living at home. *J Am Diet Assoc.* 46:285, 1965.

Lehman, E., and Ban, T.A. Chemotherapy of aged psychiatric patients. *Can Psychiatr Assoc J.* 14:361, 1251, 1974.

Levine, R.R. The factors affecting gastrointestinal absorption of drugs. *Am J Dig Dis.* 15:171, 1970.

Levy, G., and Hewitt, R.R. Riboflavin and thiamine transport mechanisms. *Am J Clin Nutr.* 24:401, 1971.

Levy, R.H., Pitlick, W.H., Troupin, A.S. et al. Pharmacokinetics of carbamazepine in normal man. *Clin Pharmacol Ther.* 17:657, 1975.

Libow, L.S. Pseudo-senility: acute and reversible organic brain syndromes. *J Am Geriatr Soc.* 21:112, 1973.

Liebman, B.F. Determinants of folacin status in institutionalized elderly individuals. Thesis presented to the Graduate School, Cornell University, Ithaca, N.Y., 1977.

Maines, M.D., and Kappas, A. Regulation of cytochrome P-450-dependent microsomal drug metabolizing enzymes by nickel, cobalt, and iron. *Clin Pharmacol Ther.* 22:780, 1977.

Mann, G.V. The influence of obesity on health. *N Engl J Med.* 291:178, 1974.

Mann, G.V. Current concepts: diet-heart; end of an era. *N Engl J Med.* 297:644, 1977.

Markovitz, D.C., and Fernstrom, J.D. Diet and uptake of aldomet by the brain: competition with natural large neutral amino acids. *Science* 197:1014, 1977.

Marshall, W.H. Educational directions. *J Am Diet Assoc.* 58:509, 1971.

Mayer, J. Testimony before Select Committee on Nutrition. Nutrition needs of older Americans. Part 2. Washington, D.C.: U.S. Government Printing Office, 1972.

McCay, C.M. Chemical aspects of aging and the effect of diet upon aging. Edited by A.I. Lansing. In *Cowdry's Problems of Aging,* 3rd ed. Baltimore: Williams & Wilkins Co., 1952.

McGandy, R.B., Barrow, C.H., Spanias, A. et al. Nutrient intakes and energy expenditure in men of different ages. *J Gerontol.* 21:581, 1966.

McGilveray, I.J., and Mattock, G. Some factors affecting the absorption of paracetamol. *J Pharm Sci.* 24:615, 1972.

McLeod, C., Judge, T.G., and Caird, F.I. Nutrition of the elderly at home. I. Intakes of energy, protein, carbohydrate, and fat. *Age Ageing.* 3:158, 1974a.

McLeod, C., Judge, T.G., and Caird, F.I. Nutrition of the elderly at home. II. Intakes of vitamins. *Age Ageing.* 3:209, 1974b.

Medalle, R., Waterhouse, C., and Hahn, T.J. Vitamin D resistance in magnesium deficiency. *Am J Clin Nutr.* 29:854, 1976.

Medical Letter. Oral iron. 20(10):45, 1978.

Melander, A., Danielson, K., Scherten, B. et al. Enhancement by food of canrenone bioavailability from spironolactone. *Clin Pharmacol Ther.* 22:100, 1977a.

Melander A., Danielson, K., Hanson, A. et al. Enhancement of hydralazine bioavailability by food. *Clin Pharmacol Ther.* 22:104, 1977b.

Melander, A., Danielson, K., Shersten, B. et al. Enhancement of the bioavailability of propranolol and metropolol by food. *Clin Pharmacol Ther.* 22:108, 1977c.

Mena, I., and Cotzias, G.C. Protein intake and treatment of Parkinson's disease with levodopa. *N Engl J Med.* 292:181, 1975.

Mendeloff, A.I. Current concepts: dietary fiber and human health. *N Engl J Med.* 297:811, 1977.

Mertz, W. Trace elements. *Contemp Nutr.* 3(2), 1978.

Michocki, R.J., and Lamy, P.P. The care of decubitus ulcers (pressure sores). *J Am Geriatr Soc.* 24:217, 1976.

Morgan, R.H. Anemia in elderly housebound patients. *Br Med J.* 1:171, 1967.

Myrant, N.B. The influence of some dietary factors on cholesterol metabolism. *Proc Nutr Soc.* 34:271, 1975.

National Academy of Sciences, Food and Nutrition Board, National Research Council. Recommended dietary allowances, 8th ed. Washington, D.C.: National Academy of Sciences, 1974.

National Academy of Sciences. Committee on nutritional misinformation. *JAMA.* 233:898, 1975.

National Center for Health Statistics. Preliminary findings of the first health and nutrition examination survey, U.S., 1971-1972. Dietary intake and biochemical findings. DHEW Publ. No. (HRA) 74-1219-1. Hyattsville, Md.: National Center for Health Statistics, 1974.

National Center for Health Statistics. Preliminary findings of the first health and nutrition examination survey, U.S., 1971-1972. Anthropometric and clinical findings. DHEW Publ. No. (HRA) 75-1229. Hyattsville, Md.: National Center for Health Statistics, 1975.

National Heart and Lung Institute. *Task Force on Arteriosclerosis,* Vol. 2. Washington, D.C.: National Heart and Lung Institute, 1971.

Neugarten, B.L., Moore, J.W., and Lowe, J.C. Age norms, age constraints and adult socialization. Edited by B.L. Neugarten. In *Middle Age and Aging.* Chicago: University of Chicago Press, 1968.

Newark, H.L., Scheiner, J., Marcus, M. et al. Stability of vitamin B-12 in the presence of ascorbic acid. *Am J Clin Nutr.* 29:645, 1976.

Nolen, G.A. Effect of various restricted dietary regimens on the growth, health, and longevity of albino rats. *J Nutr* 102:1477, 1972.

Nordin, B.E.C., Barnett, E., MacGregor, J. et al. Lumbar spine densitometry. *Br Med J.* 1:1973, 1962.

Nutrition Canada: A report of nutrition Canada to the Department of National Health and Welfare, Ottawa, Canada, 1973.

Oexmann-Wannamaker, M.J. Salt substitutes. *Am J Clin Nutr.* 29:599, 1976.

Olson, R. Responses to dietary goals: eggs. *AIN Nutr Notes.* 13(3):1, 1977.

O'Shea, H.E., Elsom, K.O., and Higbe, R.V. Studies of the B vitamins in the human subject. IV. Mental changes in experimental deficiency. *Am J Med Sci.* 203:388, 1942.

Patnaik, B.K. Age-related studies on ascorbic acid metabolism. *Gerontologia* 17:122, 1971.

Pauling, L. On the orthomolecular environment of the mind: orthomolecular theory. *Am J Psychiatr.* 131:1251, 1974.

Pecound, A., Donzel, P., and Schelling, J.L. Effect of foodstuffs on the absorption of zinc sulfate. *Clin Pharmacol Ther.* 17:469, 1975.

Pierpaoli, P.G. Drug therapy and diet. *Drug Intell Clin Pharm.* 6:89, 1972.

Pincus, J.H., Reynolds, E.H., and Glaser, G.H. Subacute combined system degeneration with folate deficiency. *JAMA.* 221:496, 1972.

Potera, C., Rose, D.P., and Brown, R.R. Vitamin B-6 deficiency in cancer patients. *Am J Clin Nutr.* 30:1677, 1977.

Powell, M.F., and Lamy, P.P. Drug-dietary incompatibilities. I. Effects on nutritional status. *Hosp Formulary.* 12:774, 1977a.

Powell, M.F., and Lamy, P.P. Drug-dietary incompatibilities. II. Effects on drug therapy. *Hosp Formulary.* 12:870, 1977b.

Prasad, A.S. *Trace Elements in Human Health and Disease,* Vols. 1 and 2. New York: Academic Press, 1976.

Prescott, L.F. Gastrointestinal absorption of drugs. *Med Clin North Am.* 58:907, 1974.

Prescott, L.F. Pathological and physiological factors affecting drug absorption, distribution, elimination, and response in man. Edited by J.R. Gillette, and J.R. Mitchell. In *Concepts in Biochemical Pharmacology,* Part 3. New York: Springer Verlag, 1975.

Race, T.R., Paes, I.C., and Faloon, W.W. Intestinal malabsorption induced by oral colchicine. *Am J Med Sci.* 259:321, 1970.

Rae, J., and Burke, A.L. Counseling the elderly on nutrition in a community health care system. *J Am Geriatr Soc.* 26:130, 1978.

Rao, D.B. Problems of nutrition in the aged. *J Am Geriatr Soc.* 21:362, 1973.

Rawson, I.G., Weinberg, E.I., Herold, J.A. et al. Nutrition of rural elderly in southwestern Pennsylvania. *Gerontologist* 18:24, 1978.

Reidenberg, M.M. Obesity and fasting–effects on drug metabolism and drug action in man. *Clin Pharmacol Ther.* 22:729, 1977.

Reisin, E., Abel, R., Modan, M. et al. Effect of weight loss without salt restriction on the reduction of blood pressure in overweight hypertensive patients. *N Engl J Med.* 298:1, 1978.

Reynolds, E.H., Rothfield, P., and Pincus, J.H. Neurological disease associated with folate deficiency. *Br Med M.* 2:398, 1973.

Riley, M.W., and Foner, A. *Aging and Society. I. An Inventory of Research Findings.* New York: Russell Sage Foundation, 1968.

Roe, D.A. Effects of drugs on nutrition. *Life Sciences* 15:1219, 1974.

Rose, C.S., Gyorgy, P., Butler, M. et al. Age differences in vitamin B-6 status of 617 men. *Am J Clin Nutr.* 29:847, 1976.

Ross, M.H., Bras, G. Tumor incidence patterns and nutrition in the rat. *J Nutr.* 87:245, 1965.

Ross, M.H., and Lustbader, E. Dietary practices and growth responses as predicators of longevity. *Nature* 262:548, 1976.

Rungruangsak, K., Tosukhowong, P., Panijpan, B. et al. Chemical interactions between thiamin and tannic acid. I. Kinetics, oxygen dependence, and inhibition by ascorbic acid. *Am J Clin Nutr.* 30:1680, 1977.

Sanchez, N., Sheiner, L.B., Halkin, H. et al. Pharmacokinetics of digoxin: interpreting bioavailability. *Br Med J.* 4:132, 1973.

Savin, M.A. A practical approach to the treatment of iron deficiency. *Rational Drug Ther.* 11(9):1, 1977.

Schaefer, A.E., and Ogden, C.J. Are we well fed? The search for the answer. *Nutr Today.* 4:2, 1969.

Scrimshaw, N.S. Nutrition and stress. Edited by G.E.W. Wolstenholme, and M. O'Connor. In *Diet and Bodily Constitution.* Boston: Little, Brown and Co., 1964.

Scrimshaw, N.S. Nutrition and infection. *Prog Food Nutr Sci.* 1(6):393, 1975.

Scrimshaw, N.S. Effect of infection on nutrient requirements. *Am J Clin Nutr.* 30:1536, 1977.

Scrimshaw, N.S., and Gordon, J.E. *Malnutrition, Learning and Behavior.* Cambridge, Mass.: The MIT Press, 1968.

Sevringhaus, E.L. Nutritional problems after fifty. *Food Nutr News.* 43:5, 1972.

Shulman, R. Psychiatric aspects of pernicious anemia: a prospective controlled investigation. *Br Med J.* 3:226, 1967.

Smith, L.H., Van Den Berg, C.J., and Wilson, D.M. Nutrition and urolithiasis. *N Engl J Med.* 298:87, 1978.

Southgate, D.A.T. The definition and analysis of dietary fiber. *Nutr Rev.* 35(3):31, 1977.

Speis, T.D., Bradley, J., Rosenbaum, M. et al. Emotional disturbances in persons with pellagra, beriberi, and associated deficiency states. *Res Nerv Ment Dis.* 22:122, 1943.

Steinkamp, R.C., Cohen, N.L., and Walsh, H.E. Resurvey of an aging population fourteen-year follow-up. The San Mateo nutrition study. *J Am Diet Assoc.* 46:103, 1965.

Stenback, A. Object loss and depression. *Arch Gen Psychiatry.* 12:144, 1965.

Strachan, R.W., and Henderson, J.G. Dementia and folate deficiency. *Q J Med.* New Series. 36(142):189, 1967.

Swanson, P., Willis, E., Jebe, E. et al. *Food Intakes of 2189 Women in Five North Central States.* Iowa Agricultural and Home Economics Experiment Station Research Bulletin, 486. Ames, Iowa: Iowa State College, 1959.

Tappel, A., Fletcher, B., and Deamer, D. Effect of antioxidants and nutrients on lipid peroxidation fluorescent products and aging parameters in the mouse. *J Gerontol.* 28:415, 1973.

Task Force on Vitamin Therapy in Psychiatry. Megavitamin and orthomolecular therapy in psychiatry. Washington, D.C.: American Psychiatric Association, 1974.

Thomas, J.H. Anaemia in the elderly. *Br Med J.* 4:288, 1973.

Thompson, J.N., Beare-Rogers, J.L., Erodoedy, P. et al. Appraisal of human vitamin E requirements based on examination of individual meals and a composite Canadian diet. *Am J Clin Nutr.* 26:1349, 1973.

Todhunter, E.N. The evolution of nutrition concepts–perspectives and new horizons. *J Am Diet Assoc.* 46:123, 1965.

Trowell, H. Definition of dietary fiber and hypotheses that it is a protective factor in certain diseases. *Am J Clin Nutr.* 29:417, 1976.

Trowell, H. Food and dietary fibre. *Nutr Rev.* 35(3):6, 1977.

Tyroler, H.A., Heyden, S., and Hames, G.G. Weight and hypertension: Evans County study of blacks and whites. Edited by O. Paul. In *Epidemiology and Control of Hypertension.* New York: Stratton Intercontinental Medical Books, 1975.

Ulmer, D.D. Trace elements. *N Engl J Med.* 297:318, 1977.

Underwood, E.J. *Trace Elements in Human and Animal Nutrition,* 4th ed. New York: Academic Press, 1977.

U.S. Department of Agriculture, Consumer and Food Economics Research Division, Agricultural Research Service. *Food Consumption and Dietary Levels of Older Households in Rochester, New York.* Washington, D.C.: Home Economics Research Report No. 25, 1957.

U.S. Department of Agriculture. *Consumption of Households in the United States, Spring 1965.* Washington, D.C.: Household Food Consumption Survey 1965–66, Report No. 1, 1968.

U.S. Department of Agriculture. *Nutrition Programs for the Elderly: A Guide to Menu Planning, Buying and the Care of Food for Community Programs.* Washington, D.C., 1975.

U.S. Department of Labor, Bureau of Labor Statistics. *Prices Charged in Food Stores Located in Low and Higher Income Areas of Six Large Cities.* Washington, D.C., 1966.

U.S. Senate, Special Committee on Aging, Hearings. Usefulness of the model cities program to the elderly, Part 1. Washington, D.C., July 23, 1968.

Walker, A.R.P. Dietary fiber and the pattern of diseases. *Ann Intern Med.* 80:663, 1974.

Walker, A.R.P. Colon cancer and diet, with special reference to intakes of fat and fiber. *Am J Clin Nutr.* 29:1417, 1976.

Watkins, D.M. The assessment of protein nutrition in aged man. *Ann NY Acad Sci.* 60:902, 1958.

Watkins, D.M. The impact of nutrition on the biochemistry of aging in man. *World Rev Nutr Diet.* 6:124, 1966.

Watkins, D.M. Nutrition for the elderly of today and tomorrow. *Nutr News.* 38, 1975.

Waxman, S., Corcino, J.J., and Herbert, V. Drugs, toxins, and dietary amino acids affecting vitamin B-12 or folic acid absorption or utilization. *Am J Med.* 48:599, 1970.

Weit, D.R., and Houser, H.D. Problems in the evaluation of nutritional status in chronic illness. *Am J Clin Nutr.* 12:278, 1963.

Wesley-Hadzija, B. A note on the influence of diet in West Africa on urinary pH and excretion of amphetamine in man. *J Pharm Pharmacol.* 23:366, 1971.

Whanger, A.D. Paranoid syndromes of the senium. Edited by C. Eisdorfer, and W.E. Fann. In *Psychopharmacology and Aging.* New York: Plenum Press, 1976.

Whanger, A.D., and Wang, H.S. Vitamin B-12 deficiency in normal aged and elderly psychiatric patients. Edited by E. Palmore. In *Normal Aging,* Vol. 2. Durham, N.C.: Duke University Press, 1974.

Whedon, G.D. Effects of high calcium intakes on bones, blood, and soft tissues. Relationship of calcium intake to balance in osteoporosis. *Fed Proc.* 18:1112, 1959.

White, R.J., Chamberlain, D.A., Howard, M. et al. Plasma concentrations of digoxin after oral administration in the fasting and postprandial state. *Br Med J.* 1:380, 1971.

White House Conference on Aging, 1st Reader. *Recommendations on Nutrition.* DHEW Publ. No. (AOA) 147. Washington, D.C., 1971.

WHO Expert Committee. Trace metals in human nutrition. WHO Technical Report Series No. 532. Geneva, 1973.

Williams, E.I., and Nixon, J.V. Hemoglobin levels in a group of 75-year-old patients studied in general practice. *Gerontol Clin.* 16:210, 1974.

Winick, M. Nutrition and aging. *J Am Pharm Assoc.* NS17:585, 1977.

Wurtman, R.J., and Growdon, J.H. Dietary enchancement of CNS neurotransmitters. *Hosp Practice.* 13(3):71, 1978.

Wylie, C.M. Hospitalization for fractures and bone loss in adults. *Public Health Rep.* 92:33, 1977.

Wynder, E.L., Kajitani, T., Ishikawa, S. et al. Environmental factors of cancer of the colon and rectum. II. Japanese epidemiological data. *Cancer* 23:1210, 1969.

Young, V. Nutrient utilization and requirements of the aged. Presented at

Biomedical Aspects of Senile Dementia and Related Disorders. Symposium, South Central Regional Medical Educational Center, VA Hospital. St. Louis, 1978.

Young, V.R., and Scrimshaw, N.S. Protein needs of the elderly. *Nutr Notes*. 11:6, 1975.

Yudkin, J. Sugar. Edited by J. Yudkin, J. Edelman, and L. Hough. In *Chemical, Biological, and Nutritional Aspects of Sucrose*. London: Butterworth, 1971.

APPENDIX A

PRUDENT NUTRITION FOR THE OLDER PERSON*

Goals

1. To control calories and maintain a desirable weight.
2. To meet the daily requirements for protein, minerals, especially calcium, iron, and vitamins.
3. To increase the use of more complex sugars and starches and reduce the intake of refined sugar.
4. To use more polyunsaturated fat and less saturated fat.

Guidelines

To meet the goals, the older person can follow these guidelines. Include in your diet daily:

A. Four servings of fruits and vegetables (a serving is ½ cup). Choose one green or yellow vegetable daily.

Fruits and vegetables are low in fat content and are lower in calories than the meats and dairy products. Vitamin C (ascorbic acid) is a water-soluble vitamin, not readily stored in the body, so a good source of vitamin C should be used each day. Good sources are: oranges, grapefruit, tangerines, lemons, limes, tomatoes, strawberries, cantaloupe, papayas, broccoli, sprouts, and green pepper.

B. Four servings of cereals and bread (a serving is one slice of bread or ½ cup cereal). Choose wholegrain rye or enriched spaghetti, rice, noodles, breads, cereals (read the labels).

C. Two-ounce portions of meat, poultry, fish. Limit egg yolks to 3 per week. Limit use of shrimp, organ meats, and cheese. Two ounces may be substituted for 1 egg yolk. Use fish, chicken, turkey, and veal as often as possible. Limit beef, lamb, and pork to moderate size portions a day. Cut off visible fat. Meat should be broiled, roasted, stewed, baked. Avoid meat drippings and poultry skin. This will help in the control of saturated fat.

D. Dairy products—1 pint of milk daily. If the person has a problem of too much weight, skim or buttermilk should be used. Milk is a source of easily absorbed calcium so necessary for good bones and teeth.

---

*Reproduced with permission from the Maryland Office of Aging.

Tips on Cooking

Use vegetable oils and soft margarine that are rich in polyunsaturated fats in place of butter and other cooking fats that are solid or hydrogenated.

Nuts, with the exception of cashew and macadamia, may be used. Avoid coconut and chocolate. Peanut butter, however, is fine and a good substitute for meat.

If you must watch your weight, use skim milk and cheeses made with skim milk.

Use plain bread and rolls in place of pancakes, waffles, pastries, rich cakes, and pies. Choose desserts from the following: fruit, gelatins, skim milk puddings, sherbets, water ice, angel food cake.

Reduce your intake of salt. Try tasting your food before salting. It may not need extra salt. Use spices and herbs in cooking to spruce up that vegetable.

Avoid luncheon rolls or loaves. They are high in salt and saturated fats. Use them for an occasional treat.

Water is our most important nutrient. Drink 6 to 8 glasses daily. You can count coffee, tea, milk, juice, soup as part of your fluid intake. Water is necessary for the good function of your kidneys and elimination system.

Fiber   Cellulose is the framework of the cells making up plant fiber. It is found in fruit and vegetables and outside coverings of cereal grains. The human digestive tract is unable to reduce cellulose so that it can be absorbed.

Cellulose and other indigestible materials contained in plant fiber serve a useful purpose in enhancing the movement of the large intestine. If you eat your fruits, vegetables and cereals daily, you will not need to eat additional fiber as graham flakes, etc.

Eating is Fun

Try something new. There are all kinds of prepared mixes for breads, puddings, that add zest to a meal. Read the labels for instructions for 1 or 2 servings.

Invite a friend to share a meal. Organize a pot luck meal with each guest bringing their specialty. (Watch out for extra calories here.) Have a variety in what you eat. Consult your local library for cook books for one or two. READ THE LABELS OF THE FOODS YOU BUY. Spices and herbs can add zest to your food. They are calorie-free and salt-free.

Use Leftovers

Try to find new ways of using leftovers. Add strips of meat, chicken, to a salad. Mix cooked and fresh vegetables in a salad. Delicious with your favorite dressing. Use leftover meat and vegetables in an omelet, using two of your eggs. Add fruit or crisp vegetables to cottage cheese. Make soup with leftover meat, vegetables, and vegetable juices. Use your imagination in concocting casseroles with leftovers combined with rice, noodles, spaghetti, or other pasta.

Shopping Hints

Make a list of foods you need to prepare meals you have planned. Check newspaper ads, compare prices, buy at stores with majority of best prices. Take advantage of "cents off" coupons. Read labels, check prices, amounts of package. Most often the medium size is the best buy. Plan on second servings, using leftovers in another dish.

Cuts of meat high in bone, fat, or gristle are often more expensive than lean meat even if they are priced low.

How Many Meals Should An Older Person Eat?

Meals may be spaced according to the person's usual habits as long as the amount of food in the guide is used. If the individual has difficulty maintaining his weight or gaining weight, regular meal times should be established. The person with a finicky appetite may do better with more frequent meals and smaller amounts of food.

Exercise—Join the Active People Over 60!

Stimulate your appetite by exercising. This may be light exercise as walking.

13 Altered Pharmacokinetics in the Elderly

DRUG ACTION

Elderly patients often are more sensitive to drug actions than younger people (Trounce 1975), possibly because of age-related changes in one or both of the major factors that govern drug response in man:

1. Pharmacodynamics—govern the effect of a drug at the site of action or target organs
2. Pharmacokinetics—embrace the processes of drug absorption, distribution, metabolism, and excretion

The Effect of Aging on Pharmacodynamics

In general, there are still not sufficient data to support the concept of age-related changes in the pharmacodynamics of drug action; however, there have been suggestions of increased target sensitivity as age proceeds (Castleden et al 1977b), and there is some evidence that differences in tissue sensitivity to drugs become more pronounced with age (Bender 1974; Frolkis et al 1972). Changes in receptor activity may be responsible, as well as a decline in cellular viability and the homeostatic mechanism. Progressive physiologic changes that affect tissue reactivity, sensitivity, and tolerance to a drug are often cited (Triggs and Nation 1975; Brunaud 1975) as reasons for age-related pharmacodynamic changes. The well-known sensitivity of the elderly to the depressant action of morphine is one example of changing pharmacodynamics. It has been postulated that the aging brain becomes more sensitive to drugs which depress certain aspects of central nervous function.

The elderly are also more sensitive to nitrazepam (Castleden et al 1977a), diazepam, and chlordiazepoxide (Boston Collaborative Drug Surveillance Program 1973a), than are the young. Interestingly, diazepam clearance is not impaired in most elderly (Klotz et al 1975) but the metabolic clearance of chlordiazepoxide is impaired even in healthy, elderly persons (Shader et al 1977). The sensitivity of the central nervous system to the depressant effect of flurazepam may be greater in the elderly than in younger persons (Greenblatt et al 1977). At 15 mg per day, adverse effects occur in about 1.3% of the elderly, but at double that dose, 12.3% of elderly patients might be affected. This apparent increased sensitivity may not be limited to the central nervous system. The elderly also exhibit increased sensitivity to the action of warfarin, which does not appear to be related to such pharmacokinetic parameters as plasma kinetics or protein binding (Shepherd and Stevenson 1978). It has also been suggested that some receptor sites may decrease in sensitivity with age and that the ability of the older person to maintain homeostasis and thereby limit drug effects is also impaired.

Although there is altered sensitivity to some drugs in the elderly, the reasons for these changes are still not clear. It has been suggested that altered drug action is probably most often caused by altered drug kinetics (Rawlins 1974).

The Effect of Aging on Pharmacokinetics

The term pharmacokinetics was introduced in 1953 to describe the movement of a drug through the body. Biologic rate processes control the onset, intensity, and duration of action of any drug by determining the concentration of the drug, its active metabolites, or both at the receptor site (Azarnoff 1973).

Alterations in the pharmacokinetic processes may result in either increased or decreased drug response (Richey 1975). Age-related changes in drug action caused by pharmacokinetic changes have been documented for numerous drugs, such as digoxin, dihydrostreptomycin, indomethacin, kanamycin, phenytoin, and sulfamethizole. Others include (Table 13-1):

Table 13-1
Some Drugs Demonstrating Age-related Changes in Pharmacokinetics

Drug	Reference
Aminopyrine	Jori et al 1972
Antipyrine	O'Malley et al 1975
	Vestal et al 1975
Barbiturates	Irvine et al 1974
Benzodiazepines	Klotz et al 1975
Meperidine	Chan et al 1975
Morphine	Berkowitz et al 1975
Penicillin	Kampman et al 1972
Phenylbutazone	O'Malley et al 1971
Propranolol	Castleden et al 1975

Explicit guidelines to enhance the effectiveness or to decrease the toxicity of drugs are lacking, so the clinician must be familiar with both the pharmacodynamics and the pharmacokinetics of a drug. This is particularly true when selecting a specific therapeutic regimen for an elderly patient, as both factors may exhibit age-related changes.

BASIC PRINCIPLES OF PHARMACOKINETICS

There is a quantitative relationship between the pharmacokinetic processes and the blood level of an orally administered drug. In turn, there is generally a relationship between the steady state concentration of the drug at the receptor site or target organ and the drug's therapeutic effect. This is particularly true for drugs which bind reversibly, such as reserpine. Theoretically, if input factors (absorption) and disposition factors (distribution, metabolism, and excretion) can be predicted and controlled, it should be possible to predict and control a drug's therapeutic effect. However, the fate of an orally administered drug is complex. A two-compartment model theory has been developed to explain the pharmacokinetic rate processes (Figure 13-1).

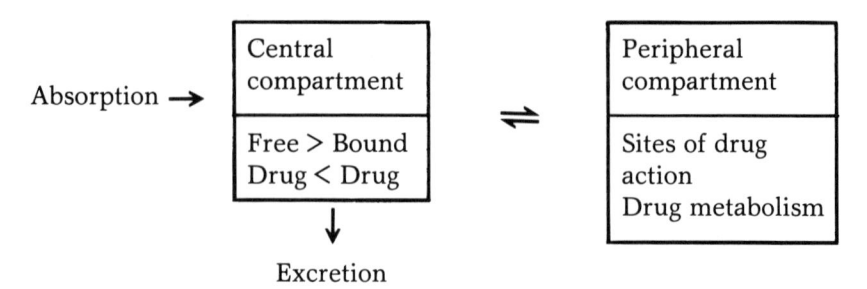

```
Absorption →  | Central          |  ⇌  | Peripheral        |
              | compartment      |     | compartment       |
              |                  |     |                   |
              | Free > Bound     |     | Sites of drug     |
              | Drug < Drug      |     | action            |
              |        ↓         |     | Drug metabolism   |
              
              Excretion
```

Figure 13-1 Two-compartment model of pharmacokinetic rate processes.

The drug is absorbed from the gastrointestinal tract into the blood stream, which distributes it rapidly throughout the blood and the rapidly perfused tissues, collectively represented by the small compartment (Figure 13-1). The free (unbound) drug is then distributed slowly to the larger, peripheral compartment, consisting of the less well perfused tissues. Part of this larger compartment is the liver, which plays the major role in drug metabolism. Drug metabolites are returned to the central compartment from which they are excreted by renal and nonrenal processes.

The steady state concentration, which is thought to determine the intensity and duration of drug action, depends on a number of factors:

$$\text{Steady state concentration} = \frac{\text{Amount of dose absorbed} \times \text{Elimination half-life}}{\text{Apparent volume of distribution} \times \text{Dosage interval}}$$

The formula shows that the steady state blood level of a drug is directly proportional to the amount of drug absorbed and to its elimination half-life. It is inversely proportional to the drug's apparent volume of distribution and the time interval between doses. The steady state level of drugs eliminated by first-order kinetics can be reached in approximately five half-lives if these drugs are given at a fixed dose and at intervals less than or equal to the half-life (Greenblatt and Koch-Weser 1975). The steady state concentration depicts the concentration of drug in plasma when input and disposition factors are in equilibrium. Although this correlates well with some drugs' pharmacologic action, the steady state is highly variable.

The half-life simply denotes the time required for drug levels to decrease by one-half. Most drugs are eliminated by first-order kinetics and the half-life remains the same regardless of the dosage. The half-life can change, however, with changing distribution, elimination characteristics, and disease states.

The apparent volume of distribution is determined by various physiologic factors, such as body size and composition and by certain properties of the drug, such as solubility. The volume of distribution indicates roughly the overall extent of distribution and binding of drug in the body. It includes total body fluid (TBF), extracellular fluid (ECF), and intracellular fluid (ICF), as well as the tissues in which the drug is distributed (Table 13-2):

Table 13-2
Major Fluid Compartments

Compartment	Volume (liters)	Body weight (%)
Intracellular	3-4	4
Extracellular	12	17-20
Total body water	41	58

Thus, a drug distributed exclusively throughout total body water would have an apparent volume of distribution of 41 liters. However, most drugs do not follow that pattern, but are concentrated in specific tissues, such as the brain, the liver, or fatty tissues. A drug with an exceedingly high volume of distribution is assumed to be selectively distributed to particular tissues. Nortriptyline, for example, has an apparent volume of distribution of 500 to 1000 liters in humans (Sjoeqvist et al 1971).

A highly lipid soluble drug, such as diazepam, which is also bound to tissue, would also have a large volume of distribution and low plasma levels. On the other hand, a drug which is distributed mostly into extracellular fluids would have a volume approximating 20% of body weight. If the amount of dose absorbed, the half-life of the drug, and the dose administration interval are kept constant, the steady state blood level is inversely proportional to the apparent volume of distribution.

SOME FACTORS CAUSING VARIATIONS IN PHARMACOKINETICS

Various factors can alter the pharmacokinetics of a drug, particularly in the elderly. Bed rest, cardiovascular function, dehydration, diet, diseases, drugs, enzyme induction or inhibition, fever, gastrointestinal function, hepatic blood flow, humidity, infection, malnutrition, stress, and temperature are among those factors. In the elderly, disease effects on drug action are particularly important because the elderly usually present with multiple pathology and problems, often involving altered states of cardiovascular, endocrine, hepatic, hormonal, and nervous systems. Bed rest, often prescribed for the elderly, can alter the pharmacokinetics of drugs (Levy 1967). Acetaminophen plasma concentrations are significantly higher in bedbound than in ambulatory patients (Prescott 1975). Patients recovering from myocardial infarction have impaired orthostatic tolerance after bed rest.

Diuretics, insulin, laxatives, and salicylates can induce hypokalemia and digitalis toxicity. Neomycin alters gastrointestinal flora and reduces the absorption of digoxin (Lindenbaum et al 1976). Fever reduces gentamicin concentrations by 40% after intramuscular injection of the drug (Pennington et al 1975), possibly because of increased renal blood flow in fever. In patients with achlorhydria, aspirin is absorbed faster and produces higher blood levels than in normal subjects (Prescott 1974) and slow gastric emptying may make L-dopa ineffective (Bianchine et al 1971). Folic acid absorption can be diminished in jejunal disease and impairment of the transport of bile acids may impair gastrointestinal absorption of the fat-soluble vitamins (Hepner et al 1968).

It is well known that thyroid status can sharply influence metabolic reactions of the liver mixed-function oxidases. Hyperthyroid patients need larger than normal digitalis doses, while hypothyroid patients should receive smaller than normal doses.

Decreased cardiac output in CHF leads to diminished renal and hepatic perfusion. Prolonged prothrombin times are typical in patients with CHF. Plasma drug clearance in CHF patients is approximately 70% that of control subjects and quinidine plasma concentrations are significantly higher in CHF patients (Ueda and Dzindzio 1978). The absorption rate of quinidine from the gastrointestinal tract is reduced in CHF because of reduction in the rate of splanchnic blood flow (Crouthamel 1974; Crouthamel 1975). Due, perhaps to factors such as decreased renal excretion or decreased metabolism, acute congestive heart failure (and its treatment) may impact on theophylline kinetics (Jenne et al 1977), and maintenance dose reduction is necessary in such patients. Lidocaine half-life is significantly prolonged in patients with cardiac failure. The extended half-life is most likely caused by reduced hepatic blood flow (Prescott et al 1976).

In uremia, there is reduced binding of amobarbital (Ehrnebo and Odar-Cederlof 1975), clofibrate (Reidenberg 1974), diazoxide (O'Malley et al 1975), digitoxin (Shoeman and Azarnoff 1972), furosemide (Prandota and Pruitt 1975), pentobarbital (Ehrnebo and Odar-Cederlof 1975), phenylbutazone (Mussche et al 1975), phenytoin and salicylate (Andreason 1973), sulfonamides (Anton and Corey 1971), thyroxine (Arango et al 1968), and triamterene (Buettner et al 1969). Drugs with unchanged elimination rate in uremia include phenobarbital, propranolol, quinidine, and tolbutamide (Reidenberg 1974).

Renal excretion data often deal only with the aging but undiseased kidney. Even if the elderly have apparently normal serum creatinine levels, it is possible that reduced renal function may alter the normal biotransformation pathways of the drug, which could lead to abnormal tissue sensitivity or toxicity (Kronenberg and Drage 1973). In addition, the elderly are likely to suffer from renal impairment caused by CHF, dehydration, diabetes, or urinary retention. In nephritis, hypoproteinemia and hypoalbuminemia are present. In such cases, it is likely that the free fraction of the drug will be elevated, leading possibly to intensified drug effects and increased adverse drug reactions. Renal impairment may also lead to varying degrees of water loading, which may lead to modification of drug concentrations in the fluid compartments of the body, including the plasma. Drugs, which are transformed to active metabolites, should be administered with extreme caution to patients with renal disease. Elimination of metabolites may be extremely slow in severely uremic patients, and the metabolites may accumulate even if the dosage has been adapted to the functional renal capacity of the patient. On the other hand, the effect of severe renal failure on drug pharmacokinetics cannot be predicted with certainty. The half-life of furosemide may be normal or substantially prolonged in patients with advanced renal failure (Beerman et al 1977).

Liver disease can alter the disposition of many drugs (Shand 1977) and in liver disease, theophylline plasma half-life is greatly increased while plasma clearance is decreased. Liver disease may lead to subnormal serum albumin levels and a decreased prothrombin time ratio. In such patients, lidocaine is eliminated at only 16% the normal rate (Forrest et al 1977). Hepatic damage may lead to reduced liver blood flow and altered parenchymal, synthetic, and metabolic function, as well as biliary excretion. When there is decreased hepatic perfusion, as is the case in CHF, drugs with a high metabolic clearance would be affected. Aldosterone, isoproterenol, lidocaine, meperidine, morphine, nortriptyline, organic nitrates, pentazocine, propranolol, and propoxyphene would, therefore, be affected. Altered enzyme activity affects mainly drugs with low metabolic clearance whose half-life could be considerably lengthened. Acetaminophen, antipyrine, carbenicillin, chloramphenicol, diazepam, isoniazid, meprobamate, phenobarbital, phenylbutazone, prednisolone, rifampin, and theophylline would be affected by altered enzyme activity.

Thus, many factors which affect the elderly also affect the pharmacokinetics of drugs often prescribed for the elderly.

PHARMACOKINETICS IN THE ELDERLY

Input Factors

Absorption Most drugs are absorbed according to simple, first-order kinetics, but a number of drugs follow zero-order kinetics and are absorbed at a constant rate. Among those are alcohol, erythromycin, griseofulvin, hydroflumethiazide, and sulfisoxazole.

Gastrointestinal absorption involves several processes, which occur both simultaneously and sequentially, involving dissolution of the drug, absorption from different sites, and gastric emptying. Little attention has been given to possible changes in the absorptive processes with age but, as most drugs are absorbed by passive diffusion, it is unlikely that aging would affect their absorption (Trounce 1974). It might be reasoned that drugs absorbed by active transport may well be affected, as enzyme systems involved might be affected by age changes. Absorption efficiency is described in terms of both the amount of drug that reaches the general circulation and the rate of this process (Wagner 1974). There is usually a minimum effective concentration of drug in the blood that must be reached to obtain the desired therapeutic effect. Interference with either or both factors may affect the clinical efficacy of a drug. For drugs administered repeatedly at a fixed dose, the rate of absorption is less important than the fraction absorbed, as accumulation will occur as long as there is a sufficiently short administration interval. There is little direct evidence that any change occurs in the absorption of drugs from the gastrointestinal tract of elderly patients (Gorrod 1974). In the absence of frank gastrointestinal pathology, the rate and extent of drug absorption does not seem to be markedly affected by the aging process (Lamy and Kitler 1971; Lamy 1973). This has been shown to be true in the case of acetaminophen, aspirin, and sulfamethizole (Castleden et al 1977b) as well as phenylbutazone (Triggs 1975). Even highly lipid-soluble drugs do not seem to be affected (Triggs et al 1975). On the other hand, a slower rate of absorption of chlordiazepoxide in the elderly has been suggested (Shader et al 1977). An age-related decrease in absorption of some sugars, calcium, iron, and thiamine occurs (Bender 1974) and based on this, a similar decrease has been suggested for drugs. As nutrients are absorbed by active transport and most drugs by passive diffusion, there is probably no correlation between the two. However, there has been much speculation that decreased absorption could occur because of several age-related changes in the gastrointestinal tract, such as decreased total gastric acidity, a reduction in peristaltic activity, a change in gastric emptying, or a change in arterial sufficiency (Salzman et al 1970).

In the elderly, there is a decrease in fluid volume of the gastrointestinal tract. Poorly soluble drugs like ampicillin, digoxin, griseofulvin, and tolbutamide may, therefore, be absorbed more slowly. It has also been suggested that, as a corollary, their prolonged presence may lead to adverse local effects.

Passive diffusion of a drug depends on its solubility, which depends on its degree of ionization. Ionization, in turn, depends on the acidity of the gastric milieu and the pK of the drug molecule. In elderly persons, there is an age-related decrease in the acidity of the gastric fluids. Achlorhydria or hypochlorhydria occurs ten times as frequently in older as in younger persons. Thus, weakly acidic drugs, such as barbiturates, might not be well absorbed in the elderly. (This could not be shown for acetaminophen, aspirin, or some sulfonamides.)

The absorption of weakly basic drugs, such as amitriptyline, diazepam, L-dopa, or pentazocine, takes place from the less acidic intestine. The stomach emptying rate can then become a critical factor if food intake varies. Furthermore, gastric emptying is under the control of the CNS, which may lose efficiency with advancing age. Emotional stress also can inhibit gastric emptying, thus decreasing the absorption of weakly basic drugs (Johnson et al 1971).

A reduction in the absorbing surface size may also lead to lessened absorption, but one aspect that has not as yet been investigated is the possibility that the intestinal mucosa might become less of a barrier to drugs with age.

It is not unreasonable to assume that intestinal blood supply may be reduced in the elderly. Intestinal blood flow may be reduced by as much as 50% by age 65. Emotional stress can decrease intestinal blood flow, causing drug absorption to become slow and erratic (Johnson et al 1971). In CHF, there is diminished intestinal blood flow and slower and erratic drug absorption. Low blood pressure may exert a similar effect, and decreased absorption of drugs should also be expected because of diminished perfusion from shock or hypothermia. In contrast, hyperthermia and excitement may cause increased blood flow and, consequently, increased absorption.

Drug administration can influence absorption of concurrently administered drugs. The elderly frequently are given antacids containing magnesium or calcium, which can reduce drug dissolution or bind drugs in the gastrointestinal tract, inhibiting absorption of such drugs as chlordiazepoxide, chlorpromazine, digoxin, or tetracycline (Hurwitz 1977). Of particular interest for the elderly, who may already be affected by subclinical vitamin deficiency, is the fact that absorption of vitamins or trace elements like vitamin A, calcium, iron salts, and phosphorus can be adversely affected by antacid therapy (Hurwitz 1977). On the other hand, antacids containing magnesium-aluminum hydroxide can enhance levodopa absorption in man (Rivera-Calimlim et al 1971). Therefore, while there is no clear evidence that absorption is affected by the aging process, diseases and drugs in the elderly may decrease absorption of drugs, which may result in lower drug plasma levels and failure to achieve a desired therapeutic effect.

Drug Disposition Factors

Drug disposition involves events that take place after the drug reaches the fluids of distribution. Involved are the processes of distribution, metabolism, and excretion. Disposition factors may be affected by such physiologic factors as body weight, body position, urinary pH, and urinary flow rate. Nutritional and disease states also may impact on disposition factors (Wagner 1974). For many drugs, there is a greater individual variation in the delivery to and removal from target organs or tissues than there is with regard to the sensitivities of the receptor sites. There may be plasma alterations and possibly tissue binding, as reduced concentrations of plasma albumin may lead to a reduction in the binding capacity for certain drugs. The apparent volume distribution may change, as may metabolism and excretion (Triggs and Nation 1975).

Distribution Only if an adequate amount of drug reaches and penetrates the target organ or tissue is a desired therapeutic effect achieved. Thus, impaired distribution can seriously affect the outcome of a specific regimen. In the elderly, there is decreased cardiac output, increased circulation time and, often, cardiovascular pathology. These factors can cause impaired drug distribution (Salzman et al 1970). The result may be delayed onset of action or a prolonged effect, as removal to the site of metabolism could also be delayed.

Changes in body weight and composition have been associated with changes in drug distribution and, thus, drug action. Loss in weight might influence drug concentrations in body fluids either directly or indirectly. Increase in weight because of an increase in fatty tissue or fluid retention would tend to change the apparent volume of distribution. Total body fluid (TBF) decreases significantly with age. Between the ages of 30 and 80 years, TBF decreases by 18.3% in males and 13.4% in females. The volume of distribution decreases proportionally with decreasing total body fluid. A change in this volume, coupled with a change in the elimination rate constant of a drug, can affect drug clearance and result in a prolonged drug half-life (Triggs et al 1975). Significant changes in the apparent volume of distribution with age have been documented for propicillin (Simon et al 1972) and the active metabolite of lidocaine (Nation et al 1977). Higher peak levels of ethanol have also been related to the smaller volume of water in the elderly (Vestal et al 1977). Thus, it may be advantageous at times to determine the volume of distribution. A simple and rapid method for doing this has been developed, which can be used for the rapid individualization of dosage regimens (Chiou et al 1978).

In the elderly, active metabolic tissue is replaced by fatty tissue, even if there is no weight change. This is ascribed to the fact that adipose tissue increases and lean tissue decreases with age (Novak 1972). Between the ages of 18 and 55 years, body fat in men increases from 18% to 36%, and in women from 33% to 48%. As fatty tissue increases and lean body weight decreases, the volume of distribution of lipid-soluble drugs will increase. Such drugs as chlorpromazine, diazepam, and phenobarbital may be stored in fatty tissue to a larger extent in the elderly, and if these drugs are prescribed on the basis of body weight, the elderly may exhibit increased sensitivity to these drugs (Hayes et al 1975b; Trounce 1975). Concurrently, the volume of distribution for water-soluble drugs would decrease.

A drug's effect on the target organ may also be altered if there are changes in protein binding or if subnormal albumin levels are present. The fate of many drugs in the body is influenced greatly by their binding to serum albumin. The extent of plasma protein binding of several drugs is listed in Tables 13-3–13-7 (Bennett et al 1977). Adsorption of drugs on the surface of plasma proteins is called protein binding. Plasma proteins facilitate the transfer of drugs from the intestine to the blood. At any time, a certain percent of a drug in serum is bound to protein. The bound drug is in reversible equilibrium with the unbound (free) drug. Some of the drug-protein complex continuously dissociates as free drug diffuses out of the blood through capillary membranes. Only the free drug in the central compartment, which is in equilibrium with body tissues, is active. Binding, therefore, influences drug activity by determining the proportion of the dose absorbed which is available to the sites of action in the tissues. For example, the bound drug is unable to cross the blood brain barrier. Furthermore, binding makes the drug unavailable for metabolism and elimination. Thus, it is clear that reduced binding can affect the clinical effect of a drug. Changed binding in the elderly can occur as plasma protein concentrations change with age. There is generally a fall in albumin levels and a rise in gamma globulin (Woodford-Williams et al 1964) with advancing age. The clinical effect of changes in protein binding is variable and depends on several factors. Large changes in protein binding of drugs, such as gentamicin, which are only bound to a limited degree, also would not have any apparent clinical consequences, while a change of only 1% of a highly bound drug may lead to serious clinical effects. A more intense clinical effect can be produced by reduced protein binding. With warfarin (97% bound), reduced protein binding leads to greater diffusion of free drug into the tissues, resulting in a more intense effect (Hayes et al 1975a), although the extent of protein binding is not the sole determinant of anticoagulant response of patients to a given concentration of warfarin and the cause of reduced binding is not clear (Yacobi et al 1976). On the other hand, reduced binding of phenytoin (90% bound) leads to faster clearance and possibly to a less intense and shorter duration of action (Hayes et al 1975a).

Table 13-3
Plasma Protein Binding of Some Antimicrobial Drugs

Drug	Percent bound
Antifungals	
Amphotericin B	90
5-Fluorocytocine	10
Antituberculars	
Aminosalicylic acid	60–70
Ethambutol	10
Isoniazid	10
Rifampin	60–90
Aminoglycosides	
Amikacin	0
Gentamicin	0–20
Kanamycin	0–20
Streptomycin	35
Cephalosporins	
Cefamandole	75
Cefazolin	75–85
Cephalexin	15
Cephalothin	65
Cephapirin	45
Cephradine	10
Others	
Chloramphenicol	60
Chloroquine	55
Clindamycin	60
Colistimethate	75
Erythromycin	70
Lincomycin	70
Metronidazole	20
Nalidixic acid	93
Quinine	70
Vancomycin	10
Penicillins	
Amoxicillin	15–25
Ampicillin	16–20
Carbenicillin	50
Cloxacillin	94
Dicloxacillin	96
Methicillin	37
Nafcillin	90
Oxacillin	92
Penicillin G	20–60
Ticarcillin	45
Sulfas	
Sulfamethoxazole-trimethoprim	40–70
Sulfisoxazole	85
Tetracyclines	
Tetracycline	55–65
Doxycycline	80–93
Minocycline	75

Table 13-4
Plasma Protein Binding of Some Cardiovascular Drugs

Drug	Percent bound
Antiarrhythmics	
Lidocaine	66
Procainamide	14-23
Propranolol	90-96
Quinidine	82
Antihypertensives	
Guanethidine	0
Hydralazine	87
Methyldopa	0
Minoxidil	0
Prazosin	97
Reserpine	40
Cardiac Glycosides	
Digitoxin	94
Digoxin	20-30
Diuretics	
Acetazolamide	70-90
Chlorthalidone	85-95
Ethacrynic acid	High
Furosemide	95
Metolazone	90
Spironolactone	98
Thiazides	60
Triamterene	40-70

Table 13-5
Plasma Protein Binding of Some Sedatives, Hypnotics, and Tranquilizers

Drugs	Percent bound
Barbiturates	
Pentobarbital	61
Phenobarbital	20-40
Secobarbital	44
Benzodiazepines	
Chlordiazepoxide	86-93
Diazepam	97-98
Others	
Ethchlorvynol	35-50
Glutethimide	45
Lithium	0
Meprobamate	30
Methaqualone	80
Phenothiazines	
Chlorpromazine	90

Table 13-5 (continued)

Drugs	Percent bound
Tricyclics	
Amitryptiline	96
Desmethylimipramine	90–92
Imipramine	96
Nortriptyline	94

Table 13-6
Plasma Protein Binding of Some Antiarthritic and Antigout Drugs

Drug	Percent bound
Allopurinol	0
Colchicine	10–20
Gold sodium thiomalate	95
Indomethacin	99
Phenylbutazone	90
Probenecid	80

Table 13-7
Plasma Protein Binding of Some Analgesic Drugs

Drug	Percent bound
Acetaminophen	25–50
Acetylsalicylic acid	87
Meperidine	40–60
Morphine	35
Pentazocine	50–75
Propoxyphene	10 (?)

Age-related changes in protein binding seem to be related to changing albumin concentrations. Decreased protein binding of phenytoin and warfarin occurred only when patients had lowered albumin concentrations (Hayes et al 1975a; Hayes et al 1975b).

Adverse reactions to phenytoin were recorded in more than 11% of patients with a serum albumin concentration of less than 3 gm/100 ml, but in only 3.8% of patients with normal albumin levels (Boston Collaborative Drug Surveillance Program 1973b), and serum albumin concentrations have been correlated with the clearance of antipyrine, diazepam, and propranolol (Levi et al 1968; Mawer et al 1972).

While drug binding is most likely under genetic control, a variety of diseases can also influence protein binding (Wallace et al 1976).

Changes in protein binding in nephrotic patients have been identified (Gugler et al 1975) and in both nephrotic and uremic patients a twofold increase in the fraction of free drug in plasma has been observed (Gibaldi and McNamara 1977). Reduced plasma binding in nephrotic patients was ascribed to hypoalbuminemia, whereas changes in the molecular structure of albumin were thought to be responsible for reduced binding in uremic patients.

Similarly, decreased albumin binding capacity and alteration in albumin composition have been suggested as reasons for decreased binding in renal disease (Boobis 1977).

Multiple drug use, which is more often than not the rule in the medical management of the elderly, seems to affect protein binding. Concurrent drug administration may affect protein binding. For example, it has been proposed that heparin causes release of free fatty acids which displace digitoxin and digoxin from their albumin binding sites (Storstein and Janssen 1976). Free levels of phenylbutazone, salicylate, and sulfadiazine were significantly higher in the elderly on multiple drug therapy, while in patients receiving only one drug, only phenylbutazone binding decreased with age (Wallace et al 1976).

Finally, it has been shown that binding to red blood cells can change with age (Chan et al 1975). Meperidine binds to red blood cells much more in younger than in older persons, leading to higher plasma concentrations of the drug in the elderly. Acetazolamide and chlorthalidone are bound to red blood cells, most likely to the carbonic anhydrase fraction; acetazolamide displaces chlorthalidone from this binding site (Beerman et al 1975).

Thus, from the data available, there is no question that drug distribution is affected by changes in age, which in general lead to higher blood levels and more intense drug effects or more adverse drug reactions.

Metabolism A number of metabolic processes can take place in plasma and other body fluids and in the intestinal mucosa, but the liver is the main organ of metabolism.

Drugs under polymorphic control, ie, such drugs as hydralazine, isoniazid, procainamide, and many sulfonamides undergo hepatic acetylation, using a nonmicrosomal enzyme pathway. People are either fast or slow acetylators (Zacest and Koch-Weser 1972; Farah et al 1977). Most drugs, however, and particularly such drugs frequently used by the elderly as psychotropics, oral anticoagulants, and oral hypoglycemic agents, are under polygenic control and are metabolized by microsomal oxidation in the liver. There are pharmacokinetic reasons for reducing the dosage of the drugs in the elderly for those that are metabolized by oxidation, but not for those metabolized by acetylation (Farah et al 1977).

The chief site for liver metabolism of drugs is in the lipid membranes surrounding the liver microsomes. Thus, liver metabolism is an enzyme-mediated, probably saturable process. Metabolism in the liver serves to change fat-soluble to water-soluble drugs so that they may be excreted. If lipid-soluble drugs are excreted into the glomerular filtrate, primary bile, or the gastrointestinal contents, they will be readily reabsorbed through the lipoidal membranes, prolonging their action. Thus, to be excreted, drugs must be sufficiently water-soluble.

Most drugs undergo metabolic conversions, which occur most often in two phases. The purpose of phase I metabolism is to introduce an anion into the drug molecule which can then react with a conjugating agent in phase II of metabolism. Phase I commonly occurs as an oxidation, reduction, or hydrolytic reaction. Aromatic and aliphatic hydroxylation, S-oxidation, O-dealkylation, N-dealkylation, deamination, S-dealkylation, N-oxidation, and N-hydroxylation occur most commonly. These reactions happen mostly in the endoplasmic reticulum of the cell. A common oxidizing system involving cytochrome P-450 has been proposed for most but not all xenobiotics (Gwilt et al 1963b).

Reduction reactions are catalyzed by cytochrome reductase. In some cases, reactions in phase I are enough to make the drug sufficiently water-soluble for excretion either by the renal or biliary route. Most often, though, the transformation step is followed by a synthesis step. The drug (or other foreign agent) is conjugated with an endogenous substance, such as glucuronic or sulfuric acid (Hanninen 1975). The product of this step may be a glycoside, an acyl amino acid, sulfate, or some other compound, depending on the endogenous substance which reacts with the drug. The second phase usually abolishes the action of the drug undergoing metabolism.

Liver metabolism has variable effects on drug action. If the activity resides in the original drug molecule, the metabolic processes will eliminate activity of that drug. However, if metabolism results in the formation of one or more active metabolites, as in the case of the tricyclics, then the effect will depend on the activity of the metabolite, which can increase both the intensity and duration of pharmacologic action (Dencker et al 1976).

Drugs absorbed from the stomach or intestine are delivered via the hepatic portal vein to the liver before reaching the general circulation (enterohepatic circulation). As metabolism is an enzyme-mediated process, it is probably a saturable process. Thus, if a drug enters the liver quickly, the system may only be partially saturated, permitting more of the unmetabolized drug to reach the general circulation. If, on the other hand, a drug enters slowly, more of the drug will be metabolized.

The amount of liver metabolism which takes place following absorption (first-pass effect) can significantly influence the fraction of a dose that reaches the general circulation (Wilkinson and Shand 1975). Hepatic clearance is the product of liver blood flow and liver extraction ratio. Normal liver blood flow is approximately 1.5 liters/min. Thus, a drug with an extraction ratio of 0.5 (50% of the drug is removed during the first pass through the liver) would have a clearance of 0.75 liters/min. Hepatic clearance has been used to categorize drugs (Kauffman and Habersang 1977).

The first of these includes drugs with an extraction ratio greater than 0.7. The hepatic clearance of these drugs is primarily determined by hepatic blood flow. Decreased clearance of these drugs would be expected in diseases which decrease hepatic blood flow, such as CHF. Lidocaine, meperidine, morphine, propranolol, and propoxyphene fall into this category.

The clearance of drugs with a low extraction ratio (0.2) depends primarily on hepatocellular function and is not significantly affected by hepatic blood flow. This holds true for acetaminophen, antipyrine, chloramphenicol, and theophylline. Finally, there are drugs, such as clindamycin, diazepam, phenytoin, and warfarin, which have a low extraction ratio but which are highly bound to serum proteins. Their clearance will not be affected by changes in hepatic blood flow, but will be influenced by changes in hepatocellular function and/or protein binding.

Biliary excretion can also significantly affect the amount of drug that reaches the general circulation (Wilkinson and Shand 1975). Excretion in bile is a relatively minor route of elimination of unmetabolized drugs, but is the major route of elimination of drug metabolites, particularly of the conjugates.

Very few studies have been conducted to elicit the possible effect of aging on human drug metabolism. Most studies have been performed in animals, and many aspects of drug metabolism and changes which might occur with age are still poorly understood. This, probably, is caused at least partly by the fact that there is no direct measure of metabolic activity and, therefore, only indirect measures such as half-life and elimination rate can be used to study metabolism. In addition, none of the conventional liver function tests, such as SGOT, SGPT, LDH, alkaline phosphatase, bilirubin, and BSP clearance, correlate well with alterations in hepatic drug metabolism and disposition.

During adult years, drug metabolism decreases with age. Factors like alcohol, drugs, and atmospheric pollutants can induce the microsomal enzyme system. It is very difficult to separate the possible effects of prior exposure to drugs, which occurs frequently in the elderly, and prior exposure to air pollutants, which may exert a particularly significant effect in the elderly urban poor, from simple age-related effects. The elderly may also be faced more often than younger persons with diseases of the metabolic organ which can be caused by drug administration (Rosenstein and Lamy 1970; Hyams 1973) (Table 13-8).

While certain drugs can decrease liver enzyme activity (isoniazid, chloramphenicol, and phenytoin), others can stimulate increased liver

Table 13-8
Hepatic Effects of Some Drugs Frequently Prescribed for the Elderly

Effect	Drug
Hepatic necrosis	Acetaminophen (overdose) Cytotoxic drugs Iron (overdose) Heavy metals Tetracycline (IV)
Fatty liver	Alcohol
Hepatitis-like reaction	Anticonvulsants Antidepressants Antirheumatics Antituberculars Halothane
Intrahepatic cholestasis due to hypersensitivity	Antidepressants Antithyroid drugs Benzodiazepines Chlorpromazine Hypoglycemic agents (oral) Phenylbutazone Sulfonamides Thiazides
Intrahepatic cholestasis without hypersensitivity	Anabolic agents (oral) Methyltestosterone
Mixed	Antituberculars Erythromycin estolate Hypoglycemic agents (oral) Methyldopa Sulfonamides

enzyme activity (barbiturates), which can lead to a decreased intensity and duration of effect. Chronic use of some drugs, too, can lead to self-stimulated increase of liver enzyme systems, leading to "tolerance" to the drug and the need for higher doses in order to achieve a desired therapeutic effect. Atmospheric pollutants often stimulate enzyme activity.

The elderly have been shown to suffer often from subclinical malnutrition. Vitamin C deficiency, which occurs commonly in the elderly, is known to impair drug metabolism in humans. Similarly, folate deficiency may limit microsomal metabolism of phenytoin. It has also been suggested that vitamin A deficiency can impair oxidative hepatic metabolism. Patients with low levels of vitamin C, folic acid, vitamin A, and vitamin B-12, either singly or in combination, had significantly longer antipyrine half-lives, which was related to declining microsomal enzyme activity caused by poor nutrition (Smithard and Langman 1977). In protein-calorie malnutrition (PCM), the plasma half-life and metabolic clearance rate of antipyrine are decreased significantly (Narang et al 1977). In PCM the liver is enlarged and there is fatty infiltration of the liver. There is also slower conjugation of chloramphenicol in PCM (Mehta et al 1975), but nutritional rehabilitation restores normal enzyme activity. A sufficient protein intake is needed for the synthesis of the enzymes and, thus, reduced intake can lead to reduced enzyme activity. Although the metabolic clearance of drugs can be reduced in the elderly even when they are apparently healthy (Ochs et al 1977), disease states such as anemia and those causing changed cardiac output are also implicated in changed metabolic rates in the elderly (Fraser et al 1976). Reduction of hepatic blood flow in the elderly may hinder metabolic transformation of some drugs.

Changes in liver metabolism with age have been suggested for such drugs as phenylbutazone (Crooks et al 1976), warfarin (Hewick et al 1975), amobarbital (Irvine et al 1974), and propranolol (Castleden et al 1975) which, incidentally, functions to reduce hepatic blood flow itself. Liver impairment seems to play a role in a prolonged half-life of the active metabolite of lidocaine (Nation et al 1977). The metabolism rate of some barbiturates is influenced by age (Nies et al 1977). There is an age-related metabolic clearance of chlordiazepoxide (Shader et al 1977) and drugs, such as warfarin and dicumarol, which are eliminated from the body by oxidative biotransformation, show pronounced variation in their elimination kinetics (Yacobi et al 1976). Antipyrine is often studied to elucidate the function of the mixed oxidative enzyme system and it is metabolized slower in the elderly (O'Malley et al 1971). The pharmacokinetics of the benzodiazepines are also influenced by age, probably due to a gradual decrease in specific activities of drug metabolizing enzymes in the liver (Klotz et al 1975). This effect might also be due to the fact that liver mass changes in relation to body size with age. Finally, it has also been documented that the biliary excretion of indomethacin might be increased in the elderly, leading to a significantly lower proportion of unchanged free drug in the elderly (Traeger et al 1973).

Thus, it seems clear that the metabolic processes change with age, either due to physiological processes, disease states, prior drug exposure, or exposure to atmospheric pollutants. A knowledge of these factors and their effects in the elderly can help to eliminate variability in drug response and to prevent or anticipate drug interactions (Logie et al 1976).

Excretion Renal elimination of drugs from the body occurs only if drugs reach the kidney as polar, water-soluble substances. Several processes govern renal excretion. The first is glomerular filtration. Bowman's capsule filters out molecules of molecular weight of 66,000 and higher. The concentration of drug in the glomerular filtrate usually equals the concentration of free drug in the serum. A protein-bound drug is protected from glomerular filtration and the rate of glomerular filtration of a drug is inversely proportional to the extent of drug-protein binding. By means of renal tubular diffusion, lipid molecules in the glomerular filtrate are reabsorbed into the blood stream until equilibrium is reached between plasma and urinary drug concentrations. Reabsorption of weak electrolytes is highly pH-dependent. Acidic drugs are extensively reabsorbed when urine is acidic; if urine is alkaline, basic drugs such as quinidine will be reabsorbed. Finally, weakly acidic drugs such as penicillin, the thiazides (Beerman et al 1976), and glucuronide metabolites of many drugs are excreted by this mechanism, which principally involves the proximal tubule. Basic drugs in their ionized form are also excreted by this mechanism. Drug-albumin interactions do not generally limit the tubular excretion of drugs.

Age-related changes can have important effects on drug elimination. By age 65, there is a 40% to 50% reduction of blood flow to the kidney (Davies and Shock 1950) with a concomitant decrease in glomerular filtration rate and urea clearance. Some drugs, which elderly patients receive, may further decrease the glomerular filtration rate (GFR). Tubular excretory capacity and creatinine clearance are also reduced in the elderly (Baylis et al 1972; Leikola and Vartia 1957).

The renal blood flow rate begins to decrease about age 40. If the rate is 600 ml per minute at age 40, it reduces by half, to about 300 ml per minute, at age 85. The glomerular filtration rate is also reduced as a function of "normal" aging, from 100 to 120 ml per minute in a person at age 40, to 60 to 70 ml per minute at age 85. There is also thought to be a reduction in the number of functioning tubules. These changes mean that the maximum rate of urine flow diminishes in aging patients, as well as the diluting ability of the kidney. Decreased renal clearance may affect the elimination of metabolites and further contribute to tissue aging.

Most aging individuals also suffer from pyelonephritis and benign nephrosclerosis, yet there are no specific diseases of the aging kidney. The kidney is chief among the body organs to lose functioning cells with aging, and age-sequential changes of the kidney often relate to the clinical status of a geriatric patient. Many elderly patients can have sharply reduced renal function even in the absence of symptomatology.

Renal impairment is most likely caused by the effects of age-induced changes, arteriosclerosis, and infections. The kidney is also severely affected by hypertension. The more pronounced the blood pressure elevation, the more severe the damage. In assessing a patient prior to therapy, a physician must consider the possible effects of renal senescence and frequency of kidney infections, as well as possible impaired vascular and humoral responses. Consideration of possible or probable reduced renal blood flow is important for several reasons. Reduction of blood supply to any organ reduces its capacity to respond to stress produced by the administration of drugs. Thus, reduction of the reserve capacity of the kidney can have serious consquences if the kidney is overloaded with drugs. The effect of poor renal function is clinically important for many water-soluble drugs, such as digoxin (Ewy et al 1969), the aminoglycoside antibiotics, the long-acting sulfonamides, the penicillins and tetracyclines, phenobarbital, procainamide, and most hypotensive agents. Whether or not reduced renal excretion will be clinically significant depends entirely on the toxicity that may result due to reduced clearance and concurrent accumulation. Accumulation of drugs can be very pronounced in anuric patients (Table 13-9) (Dettli et al 1971).

The clinical effect of poor renal function regarding lipid-soluble drugs is not easily predictable. When metabolism of such drugs leads to the formation of inactive metabolites which cause no side effects, no adverse effect can be expected. Chloramphenicol is an example of a drug which forms an inactive metabolite and would, thus, not be affected by poor renal function. On the other hand, oral sulfonylureas form active

Table 13-9
Increases in Elimination Rate Constants in Anuric Patients

Drug	Increase
Ampicillin	5 ×
Cephalexin	23 ×
Cephaloridine	13 ×
Cephalothin	23 ×
Chloramphenicol	1.5×
Chlortetracycline	1.5×
Colistin	4 ×
Digitoxin	1.3×
Digoxin	2 ×
Erythromycin	4 ×
Gentamicin	15 ×
Kanamycin	25 ×
Lincomycin	3 ×
Methicillin	8 ×
Oxacillin	4 ×
Penicillin G	47 ×
Polymyxin B	8 ×
Streptomycin	27 ×
Tetracycline	10 ×

metabolites, and accumulation in patients with reduced renal function may be very hazardous (Brater 1976; Reidenberg 1976). In order to avoid toxic accumulation of drugs, many different methods have been described to determine renal function. Determination of blood urea nitrogen (BUN) is one, but it is affected by protein intake, which has been shown to be low in many elderly patients, and the general nutritional state of patients, which often is not optimal in elderly patients. Serum creatinine and creatinine clearance are useful indicators of renal function. A nomogram (Rowe et al 1976) can aid the physician to determine creatinine clearance changes with age (Figure 13-2). However, it must be realized that the impaired capacity of the kidneys to excrete

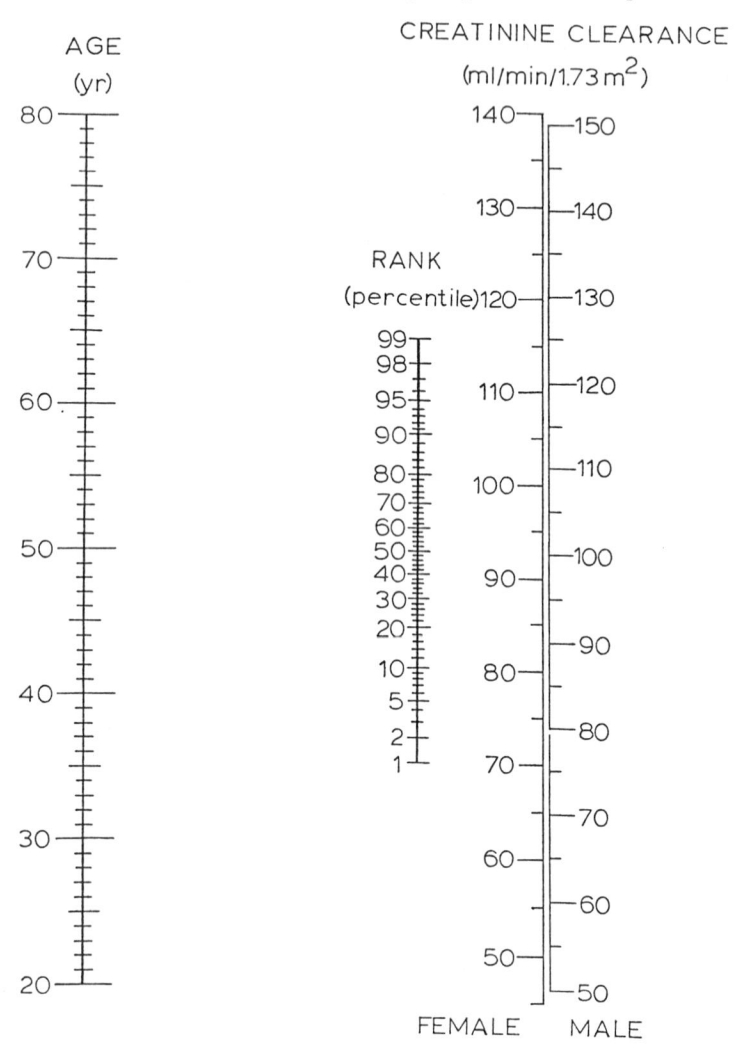

Figure 13-2 Nomogram to determine age-related creatinine clearance. J.W. Row, R. Andres, J.D. Tobin et al. *Ann Intern Med.* 84:567, 1967. Reprinted with permission.

drugs may not be detectable by the determination of serum creatinine, as these levels are not affected until creatinine clearance has been reduced by about 50% (Siersback-Nielsen et al 1971).

There has been some dispute as to whether or not creatinine determination delineates total kidney impairment. The Intact Nephron Hypothesis states that the diseased kidney simply represents an organ in which the remaining nephrons are normal or intact. If this concept is accepted, it follows that tubular function and glomerular function in a particular patient deviate to the same degree from the normal state. Thus, any test of glomerular function characterizes both glomerular filtration and tubular secretion.

Therefore, one can set the renal elimination constant proportional to the endogenous creatinine clearance, whether or not the drug undergoes glomerular filtration or additional tubular secretion and reabsorption. Caution, though, should be exercised, as this hypothesis may not hold true for all patients with kidney disease.

There has also been some dispute regarding drug effect on the GFR. High doses of oral salicylates may depress the GFR (Kimberly and Plotz 1977), but this has been disputed (Bennett and Porter 1977) and others have found no change in GFR as a result of salicylate administration (Leonard 1977). The GFR has been correlated with lack of clinical effectiveness of some drugs (Table 13-10) (Bennett et al 1977).

Recently, it has also been suggested that, contrary to general belief, there is compensatory renal hypertrophy in the elderly, and that GFR and tubular secretion, both of which depend essentially on renal blood flow, increase with renal compensatory hypertrophy (Ekelund and Goethlin 1976). A drug classification based on creatinine clearance

Table 13-10
Glomerular Filtration Rate (GFR) and Clinical Effect

Drug	GFR (ml/min)
	Ineffective in urinary infection when GFR:
Cephalothin	< 20
Cephapirin	< 10
Chloramphenicol	< 40
Carbenicillin	< 20
Tetracyclines	< 20
	Hyperkalemia common when GFR:
Spironolactone	< 25
Triamterene	< 25
	Ineffective when GFR:
Thiazides	< 25

may be helpful in predicting possible effects of renal impairment. Three types of drugs have been described (Kunin and Finland 1959). Type A drugs are agents which normally are eliminated almost entirely by the kidneys. The half-life of a type A drug will increase slightly with decreasing values of creatinine clearance, until a critical clearance value has been reached. Beyond that critical value (clearance of 10 to 20 ml/min) the half-life will increase dramatically with further decreases in clearance values. Type A drugs would include polar, water-soluble drugs. Type B drugs are those which are almost exclusively eliminated by extrarenal mechanisms. Their half-lives would remain practically unchanged with decreasing clearance values. Finally, type C drugs are those which are partially eliminated by the kidneys and partially by extrarenal mechanisms. These would be most difficult to assess, because clear understanding of their action and the action of their metabolites would be necessary.

As mentioned, tubular reabsorption of some drugs follows pH-dependent kinetics. Weakly acidic drugs would show increased excretion in the presence of alkaline urine. Conversely, weakly basic drugs would show increased excretion in the presence of acidic urine.

However, in the elderly, nutritional factors may affect urinary pH to a larger extent than in younger patients. High protein diets usually produce an acidic urinary pH. As many elderly switch to low protein diets with advancing age (because of economic and other considerations), an alkaline urinary pH may occur and, thus, tubular reabsorption may be affected and altered. It is not unreasonable to assume that renal disease can cause hypoalbuminemia, which can lead to increased adverse drug reaction as more free drug would be present in the plasma.

Any change in drug elimination must be carefully evaluated. Many drugs are excreted through a combined effect of extrarenal and renal elimination. When extrarenal elimination predominates, blood flow and metabolic capacity should be evaluated (Triggs et al 1975). If renal clearance predominates, drugs eliminated primarily by the kidney should be used with caution, particularly drugs having a low margin of therapeutic safety.

Several methods and concepts have evolved in order to achieve maximum drug effect with minimum toxicity in renal impairment. In principle, a dosage regimen can be adjusted either by lowering the maintenance dose or by prolonging the dosage interval. The theoretical goal would be to retain an effective plasma concentration at the beginning of every dose interval. This is impossible, as the descending part of the elimination curve is always steeper in normal than in uremic patients.

However, some guidelines for selecting either of the two methods are available. When significant toxicity occurs at peak plasma concentrations following a daily dose, there is clinical reason for divided doses. In the case of bacteriocidal agents, it is important to provide the maximum concentration necessary for drug effectiveness. For bacteriostatic agents, the minimum inhibitory concentration must still be maintained at the end of the dosage schedule (Krueger-Thiemer 1960).

It is often necessary to reach and maintain a maximum or minimum therapeutic concentration of drug in the body which, once established, is maintained by multiple dosing. During the course of treatment, the drug concentration will fluctuate between a maximum and minimum level. Selection of a particular method of administration should proceed according to particular characteristics of the drug.

To avoid toxic effects, which would occur at unnecessarily high plasma levels, drugs that follow the minimum inhibitory concentration (MIC) should be administered by reducing the dosage and maintaining normal dosing intervals. A minimum effective concentration (MEC) must be reached and maintained; higher levels do not increase the drug's effectiveness. Such drugs, therefore, should be administered by reducing their dose and maintaining normal dosing intervals (Ritschel 1976). If the dose were maintained at normal levels and the administration interval were lengthened, toxic levels might be reached. The dosage reduction method has also been recommended for drugs for which a relatively constant blood level is desired, such as the anticoagulants, the antidiabetics, and the corticosteroids. However, by reducing the dose, one also lengthens the time needed to reach an effective level, thus, a loading dose of the drug is recommended.

For many analgesics, cardiovascular agents, and antibacterial agents, the interval extension method is recommended. While this permits the attainment of necessary maximum levels, it also may lead to greater fluctuations in drug concentrations.

In selecting a method, the peak-trough differences and possible toxicities at peak levels must be considered, in addition to the half-life of the drug. Tables 13-11–13-18 list drugs and their dosage adjustments (Bennett et al 1977). There are dosage guides for gentamicin administration (Lamy and Vestal 1976), but there may be difficulty in establishing a drug regimen for patients based on measures of renal function, and these dose adjustment methods may not be reliable (Chan et al 1972; Mawer et al 1974; Sawchuk et al 1977). It has been suggested that dosing intervals and infusion rates for gentamicin be calculated based on the patient's kinetic parameters and desired steady state peaks and nadirs (Sawchuk et al 1977). A different formula has been developed for kanamycin to be administered to patients with stabilized renal disease (Cabana and Dittert 1975):

$$\text{Dosing interval} = 9 \times \text{serum creatinine (mg\%)}$$

Table 13-11
Antimicrobials Administered by Dosage Reduction in Renal Failure

Drug	Major Excretion Route
Antituberculars	
Rifampin	Hepatic
Aminoglycosides	
Gentamicin	Renal
Kanamycin	Renal
Cephalosporins	
Cefamandole	Renal
Cefazolin	Renal
Cephradine	Renal
Others	
Chloramphenicol	Hepatic (renal)
Chloroquine	Nonrenal
Clindamycin	Hepatic (renal)
Colistimethate	Renal
Erythromycin	Hepatic
Methenamine mandelate	Renal
Nalidixic acid	Renal
Pyrimethamine	Nonrenal
Penicillins	
Carbenicillin	Renal (hepatic)
Penicillin G	Renal (hepatic)
Ticarcillin	Renal
Tetracyclines	
Doxycycline	Renal (hepatic)

Table 13-12
Analgesics Administered by Dosage Reduction in Renal Failure

Drug	Major Excretion Route
Codeine	Hepatic (renal)
Meperidine	Hepatic (renal)
Morphine	Hepatic (renal, GI)
Naloxone	Hepatic
Pentazocine	Hepatic (renal)
Propoxyphene	Hepatic (renal)

**Table 13-13
Central Nervous System Drugs Administered
by Dosage Reduction in Renal Failure**

Drug	Major Excretion Route
Barbiturates	
Pentobarbital	Hepatic
Secobarbital	Hepatic
Benzodiazepines	
Chlordiazepoxide	Hepatic
Diazepam	Hepatic (renal)
Flurazepam	GI (renal)
Others	
Ethchlorvynol	Hepatic (renal)
Glutethimide	Hepatic
Haloperidol	Hepatic (renal, GI)
Lithium carbonate	Renal
Methaqualone	Hepatic
Phenothiazines	
Chlorpromazine	Hepatic
Tricyclics	
Amitriptyline	Hepatic (renal)
Desmethylimipramine	Hepatic (renal)
Imipramine	Hepatic (renal)
Nortriptyline	Hepatic (renal)

**Table 13-14
Cardiovascular Drugs Administered
by Dosage Reduction in Renal Failure**

Drug	Major Excretion Route
Antiarrythmics	
Lidocaine	Hepatic (renal)
Propranolol	Hepatic
Antihypertensives	
Clonidine	Nonrenal
Diazoxide	Renal (nonrenal)
Minoxidil	Nonrenal
Prazosin	Hepatic
Reserpine	Nonrenal
Cardiac glycosides	
Digitoxin	Hepatic (renal)
Digoxin	Renal (nonrenal)
Diuretics	
Furosemide	Renal
Metolazone	Renal
Thiazides	Renal

**Table 13-15
Analgesics Administered by Interval Extension in Renal Failure**

Drug	Major Excretion Route
Acetaminophen	Hepatic
Acetylsalicylic acid	Renal (hepatic)
Methadone	Hepatic (renal)
Phenazopyridine	Renal

**Table 13-16
Central Nervous System Drugs Administered by Interval Extension in Renal Failure**

Drug	Major Excretion Route
Meprobamate	Hepatic (renal)
Phenobarbital	Hepatic (renal)

**Table 13-17
Cardiovascular Drugs Administered by Interval Extension in Renal Failure**

Drug	Major Excretion Route
Antiarrhythmics	
Procainamide	Renal (hepatic)
Quinidine	Nonrenal (renal)
Antihypertensives	
Guanethidine	Renal (nonrenal)
Hydralazine	Hepatic (renal)
Methyldopa	Renal (hepatic)
Diuretics	
Acetazolamide	Renal
Chlorthalidone	Renal (nonrenal)
Ethacrynic acid	Hepatic
Mercurials	Renal
Spironolactone	Hepatic
Triamterene	Hepatic (renal)

Table 13-18
Antimicrobials Administered by Interval Extension in Renal Failure

Drug	Major Excretion Route
Antifungals	
Amphotericin B	Nonrenal
5-Fluorocytocine	Renal
Antituberculars	
Aminosalicylic acid	Renal (hepatic)
Ethambutol	Renal
Isoniazid	Hepatic (renal)
Aminoglycosides	
Amikacin	Renal
Gentamicin	Renal
Kanamycin	Renal
Neomycin	Renal
Streptomycin	Renal
Cephalosporins	
Cefamandole	Renal
Cefazolin	Renal
Cephalexin	Renal
Cephalothin	Renal (hepatic)
Cephapirin	Renal (hepatic)
Others	
Lincomycin	Hepatic (renal)
Metronidazole	Renal (hepatic)
Quinine	Nonrenal
Vancomycin	Renal
Penicillins	
Amoxicillin	Renal
Ampicillin	Renal (hepatic)
Carbenicillin	Renal (hepatic)
Cloxacillin	Hepatic (renal)
Dicloxacillin	Renal (hepatic)
Methicillin	Renal (hepatic)
Nafcillin	Hepatic
Oxacillin	Renal (hepatic)
Penicillin G	Renal (hepatic)
Ticarcillin	Renal
Sulfas	
Sulfamethoxazole-trimethoprim	Renal
Sulfisoxazole	Renal
Tetracyclines	
Minocycline	Hepatic
Tetracycline	Renal (hepatic)

A simple method has also been suggested to estimate individual dosage regimens of drugs in patients with renal disease from the endogenous creatinine clearance or from serum creatinine concentrations (Dettli 1974), although wide variations seem possible with this instrument. The necessary dosage of other drugs has also been correlated with creatinine clearance (Ohnhaus and Spring 1975), but whatever method is chosen, clinical observation of the patient prior to and following therapy remains mandatory, and one must be ready to adjust the dose based on patient response.

USE OF PHARMACOKINETICS IN THERAPY

With the advance in clinical, analytic chemistry and the realization of the possible marked variations in drug disposition kinetics, individualization of dosing regimens for potent drugs based on pharmacokinetic principles and blood or plasma level monitoring has been recommended (Gibaldi and Levy 1976a; Gibaldi and Levy 1976b). There exists for every drug a level at which it exerts its full therapeutic action. Lower levels would lead to reduced effects, while higher levels may produce harmful effects. Caution must be exercised in using drug level data, as they can serve only as a guide in adjusting drug dosage. Additionally, the plasma is not always the site of action and, thus, plasma levels may not correlate well with therapeutic action (Sakalis et al 1972). Therefore, it would probably be of greater interest to measure drug concentration at the receptor site, but this is very difficult or, in some cases, impossible to achieve. In most instances, though, it is believed that drug concentration at the receptor site is proportional to drug plasma levels. It must also be realized that plasma levels of a particular drug may not be an indicator; as the drug's metabolite may exert a greater or more prolonged drug action, and its concentration would be important to know.

Plasma levels are not needed if a drug produces an immediate clinical response. They are, however, most useful when toxic effects precede therapeutic effects (as is the case with the tricyclics) or if therapeutic effects are delayed. Plasma levels are also useful when wide individual fluctuations in response to fixed doses are expected. A clear relationship between plasma levels and clinical response has been established only for a limited number of drugs (Table 13-19). With some drugs, it is probably best to measure both the free and bound drug concentration, while in others (like propranolol), it is better to relate the free drug alone to clinical effect (McDevitt et al 1976). Caution must be used in interpreting these data, as not all clinicians agree on particular levels and broad, individual differences exist.

Table 13-19
Suggested Therapeutic Plasma Levels

Drug	Therapeutic Range (mcg/ml)	Reference
Acetaminophen	10-20	Gwilt et al 1963a
Amitriptyline	0.3-0.9	Wallace and Dahl 1967
Carbamazepine	4-8	Kutt and Penry 1974
		Cereghino et al 1974
Carisoprodol	10-40	Maes et al 1969
Chlordiazepoxide	1-2	deSilvia and D'Acronte 1969
Chlorpromazine	0.5-0.7	Curry 1968
Clonazepam	0.012-0.072	Dreifuss et al 1975
		Medical Letter 18(6):25, 1976
Clorazepate	0.075	Solow et al 1974
Diazepam	0.05-0.2	Solow et al 1974
Digitoxin	0.014-0.30	Koch-Weser 1972
Digoxin	0.0009-0.002	Koch-Weser 1972
Ethosuximide	40-80	Kolmodin et al 1969
		Solow and Green 1971
Flurazepam	0.05	deSilvia et al 1974
Glutethimide	0.02-0.4	Goldbaum and Williams 1960
Lidocaine	1.5-4.0	Koch-Weser 1972
Lithium	0.5-1.3 (mEq/liter)	Koch-Weser 1972
Phenytoin	10-20	Koch-Weser 1972
Procainamide	4-8	Koch-Weser and Klein 1971
Propranolol	0.02-0.05	Koch-Weser 1972
	0.035-0.20	Shand et al 1970
Quinidine	2-5	Koch-Weser 1972
Salicylate	150-300	Koch-Weser 1972
Analgesic	50-100	Williams et al 1959
Antiarthritic	350-400	Williams et al 1959
Thioridazine	0.04-0.3	Mellinger and Keeler 1964
Tolbutamide	50-95	Forist et al 1957

Caution—Other Levels Differ

Much work has been done to correlate drug levels with the therapeutic effect of the tricyclics. The concept of the "therapeutic window" states that below a certain minimum level, there will be no therapeutic response, while above a certain maximum level, there will be no further therapeutic response. For example, for nortriptyline, used in endogenous depression, there will be a therapeutic response only when plasma levels are above 50 ng/ml and below 150 to 180 ng/ml. Above that level, patients respond poorly (Gram 1977; Montgomery et al 1978). As only 50% to 70% of depressed patients usually benefit from treatment with tricyclics, response failure may be associated with levels outside the therapeutic window, and blood level measurements could lead to increased therapeutic response. Nortriptyline plasma level data is given in Table 13-20.

Table 13-20
Nortriptyline Plasma Levels and Therapeutic Response*

Plasma Levels (ng/ml)		
Good responders	*Poor or no responders*	References
50–140	< 50 and > 140	Asberg et al 1971
50–175	> 175	Kragh-Sørenson et al 1976
< 140	> 140	Ziegler et al 1976

*In endogenous depression

It has been suggested that only two-thirds of those receiving nortriptyline are treated adequately. Furthermore, female and older patients tend to have a slower plasma nortriptyline clearance and a longer half-life. Depressed patients also tend to have longer half-lives than do healthy persons. However, the steady state plasma level achieved in individual patients is quite reproducible (Braithwaite et al 1978). On the other hand, several investigators have not been able to correlate nortriptyline plasma levels with therapeutic response (Burrows et al 1972; Burrows et al 1974). In amitriptyline-treated patients, nortriptyline plasma levels showed no age relationship. No explanation has been offered, but it has been suggested that clinical treatment of depressed, older patients with nortriptyline might therefore be less complicated than with other tricyclics (Nies et al 1977). In contrast, there was a significant correlation between imipramine, amitriptyline, and desipramine steady state levels and age.

For imipramine, there was no indication of an upper limit; plasma levels of 1000 ng/ml were recorded. Nevertheless, it has been suggested that the best response is obtained when plasma levels range between 150 to 240 ng/ml. Below 150 ng/ml, response rate is similar to that of spontaneous remission in endogenous depression (Table 13-21).

Patient variability was also seen with amitriptyline levels. Although there was some overlap in the plasma levels of responders and nonresponders, it has been suggested that the best response can be obtained when the combined plasma level of parent compound and metabolite is between 80 to 120 ng/ml (Table 13-22).

A 3600% variation in plasma steady state desipramine levels has been reported in patients receiving equal amounts of the drug based on body weight (Hammer et al 1967).

There may be a critical upper plasma concentration level for protriptyline, as patients with levels above 270 ng/ml did not respond as well as those with lower levels (Whyte et al 1976; Moody et al 1977). Response to doxepin is poor when combined plasma levels of doxepin and desmethyldoxepin were below 50 ng/ml and adequate when levels

Table 13-21
Imipramine Plasma Levels and Therapeutic Response*

Plasma Levels (ng/ml)				
Good responders		Poor or no responders		References
Imipramine (a)	Desipramine (b)	(a)	(b)	
High	Not given	Low	Not given	Walter 1971
a + b	~ 200	—	—	Olivier-Martin et al 1975
> 45	> 75	< 45	< 75	Gram et al 1976
a + b > 180		a + b < 180		Glassman et al 1977
a + b > 240		a + b < 240		Gram 1977

*In endogenous depression

Table 13-22
Amitriptyline Plasma Levels and Therapeutic Response*

Plasma Levels (ng/ml)		
Good responders	Poor or no responders	References
Amitriptyline (a) Nortriptyline (b)	—	
a + b > 90	a + b < 70	Braithwaite et al 1972
—	a + b < 120	Montgomery and Braithwaite 1975
a + b > 100	a + b < 100	Ziegler et al 1978

*In endogenous depression

were above 100 ng/ml, although individual patient variation was again observed (Friedel and Raskind 1975).

Antianxiety effects of diazepam correlate well with blood levels. A level of 400 ng/ml is the minimum, effective steady state level that must be achieved (Dasberg et al 1974).

Clinical correlates of plasma chlorpromazine in psychiatric patients have not yet been established (Rivera-Calimlim 1976). There are sharp, individual differences in plasma levels in patients treated with the same dose (Curry et al 1970). One reason may be that there is no relation between the free and bound drug, as the drug must penetrate the blood brain barrier and only the free drug can do that (Curry 1970a; Curry 1970b; Curry et al 1971) and concentration in the human brain is estimated at five times that in plasma (Sakalis et al 1972). Chlorpromazine blood levels peak relatively early and then decline, possibly because chlorpromazine causes enzyme induction and thus accelerates its own metabolism. Patients' metabolic pathways differ, some produce active metabolites and others inactive ones, which leads to a greater variability of response (Sakalis et al 1972). Patients with higher chlorpromazine plasma levels experience more side effects (Lader 1976; Loga et al 1975), and patients with cirrhosis exhibit greater CNS toxicity due to chlorpromazine (Maxwell et al 1972).

Current knowledge on chlorpromazine has been summarized as follows:

1. There is no clinical improvement if plasma levels are not greater than 50 ng/ml.
2. If plasma levels are greater than 50 ng/ml there will be variable improvement.
3. There is a reasonable correlation between plasma levels and improvement in thought disorders and paranoid delusions, but poor correlation with improvement in depression and withdrawal retardation symptoms.
4. Plasma levels above 500 ng/ml will result in toxicity in the form of parkinsonism, akathisia, and seizures.

Furthermore, there is no way to predict chlorpromazine plasma levels from the dose administered (Rivera-Calimlim 1976). Some information is available on the correlation of the toxicity of some drugs and their plasma levels. Clinically significant elevations in serum creatinine and blood urea nitrogen (BUN) have been reported with peak gentamicin levels exceeding 12 mcg/ml and trough concentrations greater than 2 to 4 mcg/ml (Hewitt 1974). Toxicity with kanamycin has been reported when blood levels exceed 30 mcg/ml. Toxicities of aminoglycosides are dose-related and can be avoided if blood levels are controlled by maintaining minimum inhibitory concentrations. There is also a clear relationship between the ototoxicity of aminoglycosides and high concentrations attained in the inner ear fluids. In renal disease, serum concentrations tend to rise leading to elevated levels in the labyrinthine fluids (Neu and Bendush 1976; Federspii et al 1976). Ototoxicity of vancomycin should be expected when levels reach 80 to 100 mcg/ml (Bennett et al 1977).

There seems to be a good correlation between digoxin toxicity and serum levels. Toxicity should be expected when serum levels reach 1.6 ng/ml (Waldorff and Buch 1978), although other levels have also been reported.

Diazepam blood levels of 100 ng/ml are associated with significant electroencephalogram (EEG) effects (Fink et al 1976), and T-wave malformation occurs when plasma concentrations of the thioridazine ring sulfoxide, an inactive metabolite, reaches 0.9 mcg/ml—but not in all patients (Rosenquist et al 1971; Gottschalk et al 1978).

The incidence of EEG abnormalities caused by the tricyclics seems to be dose-related while the severity seems to be related to chronologic age (Thornton and Wendkis 1971).

Apparently, for most drugs, there are no established correlations of plasma levels and clinical response or toxicity. The guidelines that are available can be useful to the clinician, but clinical observation cannot be replaced.

DIGOXIN—A PHARMACOKINETIC PROFILE

Digoxin is often used in the elderly and its toxicity has been the subject of many publications.

According to the two-compartment model, digoxin distributes into an initial volume of distribution and a final, larger volume of 7 liters/kg. Myocardial response is to the drug distributed into the larger compartment. The volume of distribution is affected by thyroid function (Croxson and Ibbertson 1975), which changes by approximately 30% both in hyperthyroidism and hypothyroidism. Digoxin is eliminated by both liver metabolism and renal excretion. If cardiac output is reasonable, clearance is about 0.82 liter per kg per day, but in CHF, this is reduced by about one-half. Hepatic clearance becomes important as renal function declines (Koup et al 1975), and digoxin half-life in patients with renal failure is five to seven days, as opposed to two days in patients with normal renal function (Lawrence et al 1977). The fraction of the dose absorbed depends on the dosage form administered. If tablets are used, 0.65 of the dose will be absorbed, the elixir will yield an absorption of 0.80, and the drug will be 100% absorbed if given intravenously (Johnson and Bye 1975). Plasma digoxin levels do not appear to correlate well with the degree of renal impairment if measured by creatinine clearance (Baylis et al 1972), and the serum levels associated with a satisfactory therapeutic response without causing undue toxicity are generally accepted as between 0.5 to 2.0 ng/ml (Smith and Haber 1970; Smith 1975). Frequently, patients require levels above those suggested and exhibit toxicity (Brater and Morrelli 1977).

In general, the effects of aging on pharmacokinetics prolong drug elimination half-lives, reduce total drug clearance, cause inconsistent changes in volume of distribution, and no changes in albumin binding, although free drug concentration in the elderly may be higher because of lower serum albumin concentrations. Application of pharmacokinetic principles to prescribing for the elderly, if applied cautiously and correctly (Fell and Stevens 1975), should yield the following information:

Is drug readily absorbed?
Is drug excreted unchanged?
Does metabolism result in formation of one or more active metabolites?
What is the major route of elimination?
Are metabolites active or toxic, and what are their excretion characteristics?
What is the onset and duration of pharmacologic action?

If, in establishing a dosage schedule, a therapeutic plasma range is used, caution must be exercised because of the broad variations in response. The effect of a calculated dose will be determined by many interrelated factors. Pharmacokinetic principles must be combined with careful observation of and reaction to the clinical response of the patient in establishing a dosage regimen for an elderly patient.

REFERENCES

Andreason, F. Protein binding of drugs in plasma from patients with acute renal failure. *Acta Pharmacol Toxicol.* 32:417, 1973.

Anton, A.H., and Corey, W.T. Interindividual differences in the protein binding of sulfonamides: the effect of disease and drugs. *Acta Pharmacol Toxicol.* 29(suppl 3):134, 1971.

Arango, G., Mayberry, W.E., Hochert, T.J. et al. Total and free human serum thyroxine in normal and abnormal thyroid states. *Mayo Clin Proc.* 43:503, 1968.

Asberg, M., Cronholm, B., Sjoeqvist, F. et al. Relation between plasma level and therapeutic effect of nortriptyline. *Br Med J.* 33:331, 1971.

Azarnoff, D.L., Use of pharmacokinetic principles in therapy. Editorial *N Engl J Med.* 289:635, 1973.

Baylis, E.M., Hall, M.S., Lewis, G. et al. Effects of renal function on plasma digoxin levels in elderly ambulant patients in domiciliary practice. *Br Med J.* 1:338, 1972.

Beerman, B., Hellstroem, K., Lindstroem, B. et al. Binding-site interaction of chlorthalidone and acetazolamide, two drugs transported by red blood cells. *Clin Pharmacol Ther.* 17:424, 1975.

Beerman, B., Groschinsky-Grind, M., and Rosen, A. Absorption, metabolism, and excretion of hydrochlorothiazide. *Clin Pharmacol Ther.* 19:531, 1976.

Beerman, B., Dalen, E., and Lindstroem, B. Elimination of furosemide in healthy subjects and in those with renal failure. *Clin Pharmacol Ther.* 22:70, 1977.

Bender, A.D. Pharmacodynamic principles of drug therapy in the aged. *J Am Geriatr Soc.* 22:296, 1974.

Bennett, W.M., and Porter, G.A. Aspirin and renal function. Letter to the Editor. *N Engl J Med.* 296:1168, 1977.

Bennett, W. M., Singer, I., Golper, T. et al. Guidelines for drug therapy in renal failure. *Ann Intern Med.* 86:754, 1977.

Berkowitz, B.A., Ngai, S.H., Yang, J.C. et al. The disposition of morphine in surgical patients. *Clin Pharmacol Ther.* 17:629, 1975.

Bianchine, J.R., Calimlim, L.R., Morgan, J.P. et al. Metabolism and absorption of L-3,4 dihydroxyphenylalanine in patients with Parkinson's disease. *Ann NY Acad Sci.* 179:126, 1971.

Boobis, S.W. Alteration of plasma albumin in relation to decreased drug binding in uremia. *Clin Pharmacol Ther.* 22:147, 1977.

Boston Collaborative Drug Surveillance Program. Clinical depression of the central nervous system due to diazepam and chlordiazepoxide in relation to cigarette smoking and age. *N Engl J Med.* 288:277, 1973a.

Boston Collaborative Drug Surveillance Program. Diphenylhydantoin side effects and serum albumin levels. *Clin Pharmacol Ther.* 14:529, 1973b.

Braithwaite, R.A., Goulding, R., Theano, G. et al. Plasma concentration of amitriptyline and clinical response. *Lancet* 1:1297, 1972.

Braithwaite, R.A., Montgomery, S., and Dawling, S. Nortriptyline in depressed patients with high plasma levels. II. *Clin Pharmacol Ther.* 23:303,1978.

Brater, D.C. Renal insufficiency. *Drug Ther.* 6(10):191, 1976.

Brater, D.C., and Morrelli, H.F. Digoxin toxicity in patients with normokalemic potassium depletion. *Clin Pharmacol Ther.* 22:21, 1977.

Brunaud, M. Toxicite et pharmacodynamie des medicaments chez les animaux ages. *Therapie* 30(3):321, 1975.

Buettner, H.F., Protuick, E.M., and Staudt, N. Zur pharmakokineticks von sulfonamiden unter pathologischen bedingungen. *Klin Wochenschr.* 42:103, 1969.

Burrows, G.D., Davies, B., and Scoggins, B.A. Plasma concentration of nortriptyline and clinical response in depressive illness. *Lancet* 2:619, 1972.

Burrows, G.D., Davies, B., Scoggins, B.A. et al. Plasma nortriptyline and clinical response. *Clin Pharmacol Ther.* 16:639, 1974.

Cabana, B.E., and Dittert, L.W. Drug absorption and disposition as monitors of safety and efficacy. *J Pharmacokinet Biopharm.* 3:143, 1975.

Castleden, C.M., Kaye, C.M., and Parson, R.L. The effect of age on plasma levels of propranolol and practolol in man. *Br J Clin Pharmacol.* 2:303, 1975.

Castleden, C.M., George, C.F., Marcer, D. et al. Increased sensitivity to nitrazepam in old age. *Br Med J.* 1:10, 1977a.

Castleden, C.M., Volans, C.N., and Raymond, K. The effect of aging on drug absorption from the gut. *Age Ageing.* 6:138, 1977b.

Cereghino, J.J., Brock, J.T., Van Meter, J.C. et al. Carbamazepine for epilepsy. *Neurology* 24:401, 1974.

Chan, K., Kendell, M.J., Mitchard, M. et al. The effect of aging on plasma pethidine concentration. *Br J Clin Pharmacol.* 2:297, 1975.

Chan, R.A., Benner, E.J., and Hoeprich, P.D. Gentamicin therapy in renal failure: a nomogram for dosage. *Ann Intern Med.* 76:773, 1972.

Chiou, W.L., Peng, G.W., and Nation, R.L. Rapid estimation of volume of distribution after a short intravenous infusion and its application to dosing adjustments. *J Clin Pharmacol.* 18:266, 1978.

Crooks, J., O'Malley, K., and Stevenson, I.H. Pharmacokinetics in the elderly. *Clin Pharmacokinet.* 1:280, 1976.

Crouthamel, W.G. Elimination of quinidine in congestive heart failure. Letter to the Editor. *N Engl J Med.* 290:1379, 1974.

Crouthamel, W.G. The effect of congestive heart failure on quinidine pharmacokinetics. *Am Heart J.* 90:335, 1975.

Croxson, M.S., and Ibbertson, H.K. Serum digoxin in patients with thyroid disease. *Br Med J.* 3:566, 1975.

Curry, S.H. Determination of nanogram quantities of chlorpromazine and some of its metabolites in plasma using gas-liquid chromatography with an electron capture detector. *Anal Chem.* 40:1251, 1968.

Curry, S.H. Plasma-protein binding of chlorpromazine. *J Pharm Pharmacol.* 22:193, 1970a.

Curry, S.H. Theoretical changes in drug distribution resulting from changes in binding to plasma proteins and to tissues. *J Pharm Pharmacol.* 22:753, 1970b.

Curry, S.H., Marshall, J.H.L., Davies, J.M. et al. Factors affecting chlorpromazine plasma levels in psychiatric patients. *Arch Gen Psychiatry.* 22:209, 1970.

Curry, S.H., D'Mello, A., and Mould, G.P. Destruction of chlorpromazine during absorption in the rat in vivo and in vitro. *Br J Pharmacol.* 42:403, 1971.

Dasberg, H.H., van der Kleign, E., Guelen, P.J.R. et al. Plasma concentrations of diazepam and of its metabolite N-desmethyldiazepam in relation to angiolytic effect. *Clin Pharmacol Ther.* 15:473, 1974.

Davies, D.N., and Shock, N.W. Age changes in glomerular filtration rate, effective renal plasma flow, and tubular excretory capacity in adult males. *J Clin Invest.* 29:496, 1950.

Dencker, H., Dencker, S.J., Green, A. et al. Intestinal absorption, demethylation, and enterohepatic circulation of imipramine. *Clin Pharmacol Ther.* 19:584, 1976.

deSilvia, J.A., and D'Acronte, L. The use of spectrophotofluorometry in the analysis of drugs in biological materials. *J Forensic Sci.* 14:184, 1969.

deSilvia, J.A., Puglisi, C.V., Brooks, M.A. et al. Determination of flurazepam (Dalmane) and its major metabolite in blood by electron-capture gas-liquid chromatography and in urine by differential pulse polarography. *J Chromatogr.* 99:461, 1974.

Dettli, L. Individualization of drug dosage in patients with renal disease. *Med Clin North Am.* 58(5):977, 1974.

Dettli, L., Spring, P., and Ryter, S. Multiple dose kinetics and drug dosage in patients with kidney disease. *Acta Pharmacol Toxicol Scand.* 29(suppl 3): 211, 1971.

Dreifuss, F.E., Penry, J.K., Rose, S.W. et al. Serum clonazepam concentrations in children with absence seizures. *Neurology* 25:255, 1975.

Ehrnebo, M., and Odar-Cederlof, I. Binding of amobarbital, pentobarbital and diphenylhydantoin to blood cells and plasma proteins in healthy volunteers and uraemic patients. *Eur J Clin Pharmacol.* 8:445, 1975.

Ekelund, L., and Goethlin, J. Compensatory renal enlargement in older patients. *Am J Roentgenol.* 127:713, 1976.

Ewy, G.A., Kapadia, G.G., Yao, L. et al. Digoxin metabolism in the elderly. *Circulation* 39:449, 1969.

Farah, F., Taylor, W., Rawlins, M.D. et al. Hepatic drug acetylation and oxidation: effects of aging in man. *Br Med J.* 2:155, 1977.

Federspii, P., Schaetzle, W., and Tiesler, E. Pharmacokinetics and ototoxicity of gentamicin, tobramycin, and amikacin. *J Infect Dis.* 134:S200, 1976.

Fell, P.J., and Stevens, M.T. Pharmacokinetics—uses and abuses. *Eur J Clin Pharmacol.* 8:241, 1975.

Fink, M., Irwin, P., Weinfeld, R.E. et al. Blood levels and electroencephalographic effects of diazepam and bromazepam. *Clin Pharmacol Ther.* 20:184, 1976.

Forist, A.A., Miller, W.L., Krake, J. et al. Determination of levels of tolbutamide (1-Butul-3-p-tolylsulfonyl-urea, Orinase) (23425). *Proc Soc Exp Biol Med.* 96:180, 1957.

Forrest, J.A.H., Finlayson, N.D.C., Adjepon-Yamoah, K.K. et al. Antipyrine, paracetamol, and lignocaine elimination in chronic liver disease. *Br Med J.* 1:1384, 1977.

Fraser, H.S., Bulpitt, C.J., Kahn, C. et al. Factors affecting antipyrine metabolism in West African villagers. *Clin Pharmacol Ther.* 20:369, 1976.

Friedel, R.O., and Raskind, M.A. Relationship of blood levels of Sinequan to clinical effects in the treatment of depression in aged patients. Edited by L. Mendels. In *Sinequan—A Monograph of Recent Clinical Studies.* Amsterdam: Excerpta Medica, 1975.

Frolkis, V.V., Berzrukov, V.V., Kuplenko, Y.K. et al. The hypothalamus in aging. *Exp Gerontol.* 7:169, 1972.

Gibaldi, M., and Levy, G. Pharmacokinetics in clinical practice. I. Concepts. *JAMA.* 235:1864, 1976a.

Gibaldi, M., and Levy, G. Pharmacokinetics in clinical practice. II. Applications. *JAMA.* 235:1987, 1976b.

Gibaldi, M., and McNamara, P.J. Tissue binding of drugs. Letter to the Editor. *J Pharm Sci.* 66:1211, 1977.

Glassman, A.H., Perel, J.M., Shostak, M. et al. Clinical implications of imipramine plasma levels for depressive illness. *Arch Gen Psychiatry.* 34:197, 1977.

Goldbaum, L.R., and Williams, M.A. Determination of glutethimide in biological fluids. *Anal Chem.* 32:81, 1960.

Gorrod, J.W. Absorption, metabolism, and excretion of drugs in geriatric subjects. *Gerontol Clin.* 16:30, 1974.

Gottschalk, L.A., Dinovo, E., Biener, R. et al. Plasma concentrations of thioridazine metabolites and ECG abnormalities. *J Pharm Sci.* 67:155, 1978.

Gram, L.F. Plasma level monitoring of tricyclic antidepressant therapy. *Clin Pharmacokinet.* 2:237, 1977.

Gram, L.F., Reisby, N., Iben, I. et al. Plasma levels and antidepressive effect of imipramine. *Clin Pharmacol Ther.* 19:318, 1976.

Greenblatt, D.J., and Koch-Weser, J. Clinical pharmacokinetics, Part II. *N Engl J Med.* 293:964, 1975.

Greenblatt, D.J., Allen, M.D., and Shader, R.I. Toxicity of high-dose flurazepam in the elderly. *Clin Pharmacol Ther.* 21:355, 1977.

Gugler, R., Shoeman, D.W., Huffman, D.H. et al. Pharmacokinetics of drugs in patients with the nephrotic syndrome. *J Clin Invest.* 55:1182, 1975.

Gwilt, J.R., Robertson, A., and McChesney, E.W. Determination of blood and other tissue concentration of paracetamol in dog and man. *J Pharm Pharmacol.* 15:440, 1963a.

Gwilt, J.R., Robertson, A., Goldman, L. et al. The absorption characteristics of paracetamol tablets in man. *J Pharm Pharmacol.* 15:445, 1963b.

Hammer, W., Idelstroem, C.M., and Sjoeqvist, F. Chemical control of antidepressant drug therapy. Edited by S. Garattini, and M.N.G. Dukes. In *Proceedings First International Symposium on Antidepressant Drugs.* Amsterdam: Excerpta Medica, 1967.

Hanninen, O. Age and exposure factors in drug metabolism. *Acta Pharmacologia.* 36(suppl 2):3, 1975.

Hayes, M.J., Langman, M.J.S., and Short, A.H. Changes in drug metabolism with increasing age. I. Warfarin binding and plasma proteins. *Br J Clin Pharmacol.* 2:73, 1975a.

Hayes, M.J., Langman, M.J.S., and Short, A.H. Changes in drug metabolism with increasing age. II. Phenytoin clearance and protein binding. *Br J Clin Pharmacol.* 2:69, 1975b.

Hepner, G.W., Booth, C.C., Cowan, J. et al. Absorption of crystalline folic acid in man. *Lancet* 2:302, 1968.

Hewick, D.S., Moreland, T.A., Shepherd, A.M.M. et al. The effect of age on sensitivity to warfarin sodium. *Br J Clin Pharmacol.* 2:189P, 1975.

Hewitt, W.L. Gentamicin: toxicity in perspective. *Postgrad Med J.* 50(suppl 7):55, 1974.

Hurwitz, A. Antacid therapy and drug kinetics. *Clin Pharmacokinet.* 2:269, 1977.

Hyams, D.E. The liver and biliary system. Edited by J.C. Brocklehurst. In *Textbook of Geriatric Medicine and Gerontology.* London: Churchill Livingstone, 1973.

Irvine, R.E., Grove, J., Toseland, P.A. et al. The effect of age on the hydroxylation of amylobarbitone sodium in man. *Br J Clin Pharmacol.* 1:41, 1974.

Jenne, J.W., Chick, T.W., Miller, B.A. et al. Apparent theophylline half-life fluctuations during treatment of acute left ventricular failure. *Am J Hosp Pharm.* 34:408, 1977.

Johnson, B.F., and Bye, C. Maximal intestinal absorption of digoxin and its relation to steady-state plasma concentration. *Br Heart J.* 37:203, 1975.

Johnson, G., Sjogren, J., and Solvell, L. Beta-blocking effect of alprenolol in man after administration of ordinary and sustained-release tablets. *Eur J Clin Pharmacol.* 3:74, 1971.

Jori, A., DiSalle, E., and Quadri, A. Rate of aminopyrine disappearance from plasma in young and aged humans. *Pharmacology* 8:273, 1972.

Kampman, J., Hansen, J.M., Siersback-Nielsen, K. et al. Effect of some drugs on penicillin half-life in blood. *Clin Pharmacol Ther.* 13:516, 1972.

Kauffman, R.E., and Habersang, R. A pediatric perspective. Presented at the Symposium on Clinical Pharmacology and Therapeutics. Minneapolis, 1977.

Kimberly, R.P., and Plotz, P.H. Aspirin-induced depression of renal function. *N Engl J Med.* 296:418, 1977.

Klotz, U., Avant, G.R., Hoyumpa, A. et al. Effects of age and liver disease on disposition and elimination of diazepam in adult man. *J Clin Invest.* 55:347, 1975.

Koch-Weser, J. Serum drug concentrations as therapeutic guides. *N Engl J Med.* 287:227, 1972.

Koch-Weser, J., and Klein, S.W. Procainamide dosage schedules, plasma concentrations and clinical effects. *JAMA.* 215:1454, 1971.

Kolmodin, B., Azarnoff, D.L., and Sjoeqvist, F. Effect of environmental factors on drug metabolism-decreased plasma half-life of antipyrine in workers exposed to chlorinated hydrocarbon insecticides. *Clin Pharmacol Ther.* 10:638, 1969.

Koup, J.R., Juski, W.J., Elmwood, C.M. et al. Digoxin pharmacokinetics–role of renal failure in dosage regimen design. *Clin Pharmacol Ther.* 18:9, 1975.

Kragh-Sørenson, P., Hansen, C.E., Basstrup, P.C. et al. Self-inhibiting action of nortriptyline's antidepressive effect at high plasma levels-randomized double-blind study controlled by plasma concentrations in patients with endogenous depression. *Psychopharmacologia* 45:305, 1976.

Kronenberg, R.S., and Drage, C.W. Attenuation of ventilatory and heart rate responses to hypoxia and hypercapnia with aging in normal men. *J Clin Invest.* 52:1812, 1973.

Krueger-Thiemer, E. Dosage schedule and pharmacokinetics in chemotherapy. *J Am Pharm Assoc.* 49:311, 1960.

Kunin, C.M., and Finland, M. Persistence of antibiotics in blood of patients with acute renal failure. III. Penicillin, streptomycin, erythromycin and kanamycin. *J Clin Invest.* 38:1509, 1959.

Kutt, H., and Penry, J.K. Usefulness of blood levels of antiepileptic drugs. *Arch Neurol.* 31:283, 1974.

Lader, M. Monitoring plasma concentrations of neuroleptics. *Pharmacopsychology* 9:170, 1976.

Lamy, P.P. Aging: how human physiology responds. Edited by E.W. Busse. In *Theory and Therapeutics of Aging.* New York: MedCom, Inc., 1973.

Lamy, P.P., and Kitler, M.E. The geriatric patient: age-dependent physiologic and pathologic changes. *J Am Geriatr Soc.* 19:871, 1971.

Lamy, P.P., and Vestal, R.E. Drug prescribing for the elderly. *Hosp Practice.* 11(1):111, 1976.

Lawrence, J.R., Sumner, D.J., Kalk, W.J. et al. Digoxin kinetics in patients with thyroid dysfunction. *Clin Pharmacol Ther.* 22:7, 1977.

Leikola, E., and Vartia, K.O. On oral penicillin levels in young and geriatric patients. *J Gerontol.* 12:48, 1957.

Leonard, A. Aspirin and renal function. *N Engl J Med.* 296:1168, 1977.

Levi, A.J., Sherlock, S., and Walker, D. Phenylbutazone and isoniazid metabolism in patients with liver disease in relation to previous drug therapy. *Lancet* 1:1275, 1968.

Levy, G. Effect of bed rest on distribution and elimination of drugs. Letter to the Editor. *J Pharm Sci.* 56:928, 1967.

Lindenbaum, J., Maulitz, R.M., and Butler, V.P. Inhibition of digoxin absorption by neomycin. *Gastroenterology* 71:399, 1976.

Loga, S., Curry, S., and Lader, M. Interactions of orphenadrine and phenobarbitone with chlorpromazine: plasma concentrations and effects in man. *Br J Clin Pharmacol.* 2:197, 1975.

Logie, A.W., Galloway, D.B., and Petrie, J.C. Drug interactions and long-term antidiabetic therapy. *Br J Clin Pharmacol.* 3:1027, 1976.

Maes, R., Hodnett, N., Landesman, H.H. et al. The gas chromatographic determination of selected sedatives (ethchlorvynol, paraldehyde, meprobamate, and carisoprodol) in biological material. *J Forensic Sci.* 14:235, 1969.

Mawer, G.E., Miller, N.E., and Turnberg, L.A. Metabolism of amylobarbitone in patients with chronic liver disease. *Br J Pharmacol.* 44:549, 1972.

Mawer, G.E., Ahmad, R., Dobbs, S.M. et al. Prescribing aids for gentamicin. *Br J Clin Pharmacol.* 1:45, 1974.

Maxwell, J.M., Carrella, J.D., Parkes, R. et al. Plasma disappearance and cerebral effects of chlorpromazine in cirrhosis. *Clin Sci.* 43:143, 1972.

McDevitt, D.G., Frisk-Holmberg, M., Hollifield, J.W. et al. Plasma binding and the affinity of propranolol for a beta receptor in man. *Clin Pharmacol Ther.* 20:152, 1976.

Medical Letter. Drugs for epilepsy. 18(6):25, 1976.

Mehta, S., Kalsi, H.K., Jayaraman, S. et al. Chloramphenicol metabolism in children with protein-calorie malnutrition. *Am J Clin Nutr.* 28:977, 1975.

Mellinger, T.J., and Keeler, C.E. Factors influencing spectrofluorometry of phenothiazine drugs. *Anal Chem.* 36:1840, 1964.

Montgomery, S., and Braithwaite, R. The relationship between plasma concentration of amitriptyline and therapeutic response. Presented at the British Association of Psychopharmacologists Meeting. London, July 1975.

Montgomery, S., Braithwaite, R., Dawling, S. et al. High plasma nortriptyline levels in the treatment of depression. *Clin Pharmacol Ther.* 23:309, 1978.

Moody, J.P., Whyte, S.F., Macdonald, A.J. et al. Pharmacokinetic aspects of protriptyline plasma levels. *Eur J Clin Pharmacol.* 11:51, 1977.

Mussche, M.M., Belpaire, F.M., and Bogaert, M.G. Plasma-protein binding of phenylbutazone during recovery from acute renal failure. *Eur J Clin Pharmacol.* 9:69, 1975.

Narang, R.K., Mehta, S., and Mathur, V.S. Pharmacokinetic study in malnourished children. *Am J Clin Nutr.* 30:1979, 1977.

Nation, R.L., Triggs, E.J., and Selig, M. Lignocaine kinetics in cardiac patients and aged subjects. *Br J Clin Pharmacol.* 4:439, 1977.

Neu, H.C., and Bendush, C.L. Ototoxicity of tobramycin: a clinical overview. *J Infect Dis.* 134:S206, 1976.

Nies, A., Robinson, D.S., Friedman, M.J. et al. Relationship between age and tricyclic antidepressant plasma levels. *Am J Psychiatry.* 134(7):790, 1977.

Novak, L.P. Aging, total body potassium, fat-free mass, and cell mass in males and females between ages 18 and 85 years. *J Gerontol.* 27:438, 1972.

Ochs, H.R., Greenblatt, D.J., Woo, E. et al. Reduced clearance of quinidine in elderly humans. *Clin Res.* 25:513A, 1977.

Ohnhaus, E.E., and Spring, P. Elimination kinetics of sulfadiazine in patients with normal and impaired renal function. *J Pharmacokinet Biopharm.* 3:171, 1975.

Olivier-Martin, R., Marzin, D., Buschenschutz, E. et al. Concentrations plasmatiques de l'imipramine et de la desmethylimipramine et effet antidepresseur au cours dun traitement controle (Plasma levels of imipramine and desmethylimipramine and antidepressant effect during controlled therapy). *Psychopharmacologia* 41:187, 1975.

O'Malley, K., Crooks, J., Duke, E. et al. Effect of age and sex on human drug metabolism. *Br Med J.* 3:607, 1971.

O'Malley, K., Velasco, M., Pruitt, A.W. et al. Decreased plasma-protein binding of diazoxide in uremia. *Clin Pharmacol Ther.* 18:53, 1975.

Pennington, J.E., Dale, D.C., Reynolds, H.Y. et al. Gentamicin sulfate pharmacokinetics: lower levels of gentamicin in blood during fever. *J Infect Dis.* 132:270, 1975.

Prandota, J., and Pruitt, A.W. Furosemide binding to human albumin and plasma of nephrotic children. *Clin Pharmacol Ther.* 17:159, 1975.

Prescott, L.F. Gastrointestinal absorption of drugs. *Med Clin North Am.* 58(5):907, 1974.

Prescott, L.F. Pathological and physiological factors affecting drug absorption, distribution, elimination and response in man. Edited by J.R. Gillette, and J.R. Mitchell. In *Concepts in Biochemical Pharmacology*, Part 3. New York: Springer Verlag, 1975.

Prescott, L.F., Adjepon-Yamoah, K.K., and Talbot, R.C. Impaired lignocaine metabolism in patients with myocardial infarction and cardiac failure. *Br Med J.* 1:939, 1976.

Rawlins, M.D. Variability in response to drugs. *Br Med J.* 4:91, 1974.

Reidenberg, M.M. Kidney disease and drug metabolism. *Med Clin North Am.* 58(5):1059, 1974.

Reidenberg, M.M. Drug metabolism and distribution in patients with poor renal function. *Drug Ther.* 6(11):190, 1976.

Richey, D.P. Effects of human aging on drug absorption and metabolism. Edited by R. Goldman, M. Rockstein, and M.L. Sussman. In *The Physiology and Pathology of Human Aging.* New York: Academic Press, 1975.

Ritschel, W.A. Pharmacokinetic approach to drug dosing in the aged. *J Am*

Geriatr Soc. 24:344, 1976.

Rivera-Calimlim, L. Chlorpromazine-trihexyphenidyl interaction. *Drug Ther.* 6(11):196, 1976.

Rivera-Calimlim, L., Dujuvne, C.A., Morgan, J.P. et al. Absorption and metabolism of L-dopa by the human stomach. *Eur J Clin Invest.* 1:313, 1971.

Rosenquist, R.J., Brauer, W.W., and Mark, J.N. Recurrent major ventricular arrhythmias associated with thioridazine therapy. *Minn Med.* 54:877, 1971.

Rosenstein, S., and Lamy, P.P. Drug-induced diseases. I. The liver. *Hosp Form Mangmt.* 5(6):11, 1970.

Rowe, J.W., Andres, R., Tobin, J.D. et al. Age-adjusted standards for creatinine clearance. *Ann Intern Med.* 84:567, 1976.

Sakalis, G., Curry, S.H., Mould, G.P. et al. Physiologic and clinical effects of chlorpromazine and their relationship to plasma level. *Clin Pharmacol Ther.* 13:931, 1972.

Salzman, C., Shader, R.I., Pearlman, M. Psychopharmacology and the elderly. Edited by R.I. Shader, and A. DiMascio. In *Psychotropic Drug Side Effects: Clinical and Theoretical Perspectives.* Baltimore: Williams and Wilkins Co., 1970.

Sawchuck, R.J., Zaske, D.E., Cipolle, R.J. et al. Kinetic model for gentamicin dosing with use of individual patient parameters. *Clin Pharmacol Ther.* 21:362, 1977.

Shader, R.I., Greenblatt, D.J., Harmatz, J.S. et al. Absorption and disposition of chlordiazepoxide in young and elderly male volunteers. *J Clin Pharmacol.* 17: 709, 1977.

Shand, D.G. Drug disposition in liver disease. Editorial. *N Engl J Med.* 296:1527, 1977.

Shand, D.G., Nuckolls, E.M., and Oates, J.A. Plasma propranolol levels in adults. *Clin Pharmacol Ther.* 11:112, 1970.

Shepherd, A.M.M., and Stevenson, I.H. Warfarin protein-binding in young and elderly subjects. *Clin Pharmacol Ther.* 23:129, 1978.

Shoeman, D.W., and Azarnoff, D.L. The alteration of plasma proteins in uremia as reflected in their ability to bind digitoxin and diphenylhydantoin. *Pharmacology* 7:169, 1972.

Siersback-Nielsen, K., Møholm-Hansen, J.M., Kampmann, J. et al. Rapid evaluation of creatinine clearance. Letter to the Editor. *Lancet* 1:1133, 1971.

Simon, C., Malerczyk, V., Mueller, U. et al. Pharmacokinetics of procillin in elderly and young adults. *Dtsche Med Wochenschr.* 97:1999, 1972.

Sjoeqvist, F., Alexanderson, B., Asberg, M. et al. Pharmacokinetics and biological effects of nortriptyline in man. *Acta Pharmacol Toxicol.* 29(suppl 3):255, 1971.

Smith, T.W. Digitalis toxicity: epidemiology and clinical use of serum concentration measurements. *Am J Med.* 58:470, 1975.

Smith, T.W., and Haber, E. Digoxin intoxication: the relationship of clinical presentation to serum digoxin concentration. *J Clin Invest.* 49:2377, 1970.

Smithard, D.J., and Langman, M.J.S. Drug metabolism in the elderly. *Br Med J.* 2:520, 1977.

Solow, E., and Green, J.B. The determination of ethosuximide in serum by gas chromatography, preliminary results of clinical application. *Clin Chim Acta.* 33:87, 1971.

Solow, E., Freeman, R., and Metaxas, J. Gas-chromatographic method for serum levels of diazepam and metabolites using micro blood samples. *Clin Chem.* 20:861, 1974.

Storstein, L., and Janssen, J. Studies on digitalis. VI. The effect of heparin on serum protein binding of digitoxin and digoxin. *Clin Pharmacol Ther.* 20:15, 1976.

Thornton, C., and Wendkis, M.H. EKG-T wave distortions among thioridazine-treated psychiatric patients (some correlates of the incidence and severity). *Dis Nerv Syst.* 32:320, 1971.

Traeger, A., Kunze, M., Stein, G. et al. Zur pharmakokinetik von indomethazin bei alten menschen. *Z Alternsforsch.* 27:151, 1973.

Triggs, E.J., and Nation, R.L. Pharmacokinetics in the aged: a review. *J Pharmacokinet Biopharm.* 3:387, 1975.

Triggs, E.J., Nation, R.L., and Ashley, J.J. Pharmacokinetics in the elderly. *Eur J Clin Pharmacol.* 8:55, 1975.

Trounce, J.R. Drug metabolism in the elderly. *Mod Geriatr.* 4:330, 1974.

Trounce, J.R. Drug metabolism in the elderly. *Br J Clin Pharmacol.* 2:289, 1975.

Ueda, C.T., and Dzindzio, B.S. Quinidine kinetics in congestive heart failure. *Clin Pharmacol Ther.* 23:158, 1978.

Vestal, R.E., Norris, A.H., Tobin, J.D. et al. Antipyrine metabolism in man: influence of age, alcohol, caffeine, and smoking. *Clin Pharmacol Ther.* 18:425, 1975.

Vestal, R.E., McGuire, E.A., Tobin, J.D. et al. Aging and ethanol metabolism. *Clin Pharmacol Ther.* 21:343, 1977.

Wagner, J.G. An overview of determinants of drug activity. Edited by F.G. McMahon. In *Pharmacokinetics, Drug Metabolism, and Drug Interactions, Principles and Techniques of Human Research and Therapeutics,* Vol. 3. New York: Futura Publishing Co., 1974.

Waldorff, S., and Buch, J. Serum digoxin and empirical methods in identification of digitoxicity. *Clin Pharmacol Ther.* 23:19, 1978.

Wallace, J.E., and Dahl, E.V. The determination of amitriptyline by ultraviolet spectrophotometry. *J Forensic Sci.* 12:484, 1967.

Wallace, S., Whiting, B., and Runcie, J. Factors affecting drug binding in plasma of elderly patients. *Br J Clin Pharmacol.* 3:327, 1976.

Walter, C.J.S. Drug plasma levels and clinical effect. *Proc R Soc Med.* 64:282, 1971.

Whyte, S.F., MacDonald, A.J., Naylor, G.J. et al. Plasma concentrations of protriptyline and clinical effects in depressed women. *Br J Psychiatry.* 128:384, 1976.

Wilkinson, G.R., and Shand, D.G. A physiological approach to hepatic drug clearance. *Clin Pharmacol Ther.* 18:377, 1975.

Williams, L.A., Linn, R.A., and Zak, B. Differential ultraviolet spectrophotometric determination of serum salicylates. *J Lab Clin Med.* 53:156, 1959.

Woodford-Williams, E., Alvares, A.S., Webster, D. et al. Serum protein patterns in "normal" and pathological aging. *Gerontologia* 9-10:86, 1964.

Yacobi, A., Udall, J.A., and Levy, G. Serum protein binding as a determinant of warfarin body clearance and anticoagulant effect. *Clin Pharmacol Ther.* 19:552, 1976.

Zacest, R., and Koch-Weser, J. Relation of hydralazine plasma concentration to dosage and hypotensive action. *Clin Pharmacol Ther.* 13:420, 1972.

Ziegler, V.E., Co, B.T., Taylor, J.R. et al. Amitriptyline plasma levels and therapeutic response. *Clin Pharmacol Ther.* 19:795, 1976.

Ziegler, V.E., Clayton, P.J., Taylor, J.R. et al. Nortriptyline plasma levels and therapeutic response. *Clin Pharmacol Ther.* 20:458, 1978.

14 Adverse Effects of Drugs in the Elderly

"All of us have at some time been distressed by the adverse and often paradoxic reactions and interactions that occur...(in) older people....We don't know nearly enough about the age-related and disease-related effects (of drugs)"

R.N. Butler

Health care for older people involves dealing with the effects of aging as well as with the effects of particular diseases. Advancing age increases vulnerability to diseases and variability in response to drug therapy, and inhibits capability to recover from disease. The relationship between somatic, psychologic, and interpersonal alterations brought about by aging must be recognized, as well as the interactions between somatic therapy and the altered biologic, cognitive, and emotional functions in advanced age (Salzman et al 1976). There may be considerable decrease in the aged patient's reserve functional capacities, energy metabolism, and enzymatic processes (Lamy and Kitler 1971).

In the elderly, sedatives can cause stupor, confusion, and sometimes overexcitement. Rashes are common, as is intestinal bleeding caused by administration of drugs like aspirin or phenylbutazone. Steroid therapy may precipitate peptic ulcers, fungal infections, or osteoporosis.

Cholinergic blocking agents, used in ophthalmology, should be given in lower doses because of a more intense action in the aged. The heart of the elderly patient is less responsive to cardiac stimulation and the brain is more sensitive to depressants, but less sensitive to stimulants. Narcotic analgesics, particularly in older patients, can cause significant respiratory depression even in very small doses, probably because of decreased responsiveness of the brain stem to carbon dioxide increases. Therapeutic doses of salicylates can be as potent as some sulfonylureas in lowering blood sugar levels, probably caused by increased utilization of glucose by peripheral tissues and decreased carbohydrate metabolism.

The usual maintenance dose of digoxin for patients with congestive heart failure may be toxic for those with impaired renal function or hypokalemia. Increased cardiac sensitivity to digoxin is also associated with hypokalemia.

For the elderly, this may be the age of safe surgery and dangerous medicine (Lamy 1972). No drug should be considered completely harmless, even if used correctly. The finesse and skill with which a drug is used will largely determine drug response. Most likely, elderly patients will not respond in the same manner as younger people to a therapeutic dose of a given drug. Many factors influence an elderly person's response to a drug, changing the normal dose to a subtherapeutic or toxic dose, which can result in adverse drug reactions (ADRs).

ADVERSE DRUG REACTIONS

Definition

It is extremely difficult to find consensus regarding adverse drug reactions. There is not even agreement about a definition. The World Health Organization defines an adverse reaction as "any response to a drug which is noxious and unintended and which occurs at doses used in man for prophylaxis, diagnosis, or therapy." Objections have been raised, particularly to the word "unintended." Dry mouth, resulting from administration of anticholinergics, may be unintended, but it would be expected. Thus, adverse reactions are "harmful responses to medications that occur unintentionally during routine, appropriate use of a drug" (Karch 1977). They have also been called "unexpected pharmacologic effects, uncommon drug effects, and drug effects which are influenced by disease states or patient characteristics which cannot be anticipated or predicted in many instances and, in new drugs, cannot be fully evaluated prior to general use of the drug" (Jick 1976). The difficulty in assessing ADRs, exacerbated as failure to achieve an intended therapeutic benefit, may be caused by an interaction (Karch and Lasagna 1977).

There is still no generally accepted definition of an adverse drug reaction (Karch 1977). ADRs are difficult to assess accurately (Karch et al 1976; Koch-Weser and Greenblatt 1976) and the most important aspect of adverse drug reactions, ie, the incidence rate, is still to be determined (Karch and Lasagna 1975; Ingelfinger 1976).

Incidence

Many statistics on ADRs are being questioned (Wiener 1973). While there is thought to be overreporting, it is more likely that drug reactions which result in increased or new toxicities attract most attention. Those that decrease a specific therapeutic effect or negate an expected therapeutic outcome may seldom be reported, thus, the incidence of ADRs may be seriously underreported.

ADRs in hospitalized medical patients can range from 6% to 15%, in surgical patients from 2% to 3%, and in psychiatric patients from 2% to 6% (Karch and Lasagna 1974). It is said that about 5% of all hospital admissions are necessitated by adverse drug reactions (Melmon 1971). This figure is based on several epidemiologic assessments conducted in the 1960s. Two recent investigations have again confirmed that ADRs constitute a major cause of hospital admissions (Caranasos et al 1974; Miller 1974).

The ambiguity in definition and the parameters used for reporting are reflected in the published incidence rates (Table 14-1):

Table 14-1
Incidence of Adverse Drug Reactions

Approximate rate (%)	Reference
10	Hurwitz and Wade 1969
36	Meleny and Fraser 1969
16	Learoyd 1972
3	Caranasos et al 1974
4	Miller 1974
2.6	Jansen et al 1975
20	Vakil et al 1975
27	Irey 1976
12	May et al 1977

Six percent to 7% of all adverse drug reactions contribute directly or indirectly to death (Seidl et al 1966; Caranasos et al 1974). Most of the fatal drug reactions seem to be caused by older, standard drugs (Karch and Lasagna 1974). In one study, the ten most frequently cited drugs had all been available for at least 15 years (Irey 1976). The majority of reported ADRs, though, are minor functional gastrointestinal disturbances. These, together with rashes, itching, drowsiness, insomnia, weakness, headache, tremulousness, muscle twitches, and fever account for up to 71% of reported ADRs (Karch and Lasagna 1974). While these may be categorized as "minor," they could be important to the vulnerable, elderly patient.

The Patient at Risk

Adverse reactions are more common in whites than in blacks (Seidl et al 1966; Cluff et al 1964; Caranasos et al 1974), and more common in women than in men (Cluff et al 1964; Stewart and Cluff 1971; Caranasos et al 1974; Mulroy 1973; Vakil et al 1975). The risk to adverse reactions can be depicted as:

$$\text{white women} \gg \text{black women} > \text{white men} > \text{black men}$$

The clinical significance of this is not quite clear, as white women seem to suffer most often from gastrointestinal effects. It is also possible that the greater incidence of ADRs in elderly women compared to elderly men may be related to differences in drug metabolism.

Age as a Risk Factor

Aging alters drug effects and drug effects alter senescent functions, making the elderly more susceptible to adverse drug effects (Freeman 1974). The elderly are more sensitive to some drugs than younger people (Trounce 1975) and decreased renal drug clearance may be the single most important reason for the increased incidence of ADRs in the elderly. The elderly are also particularly at risk to iatrogenic drug reactions as they often have complicated drug regimens and may administer drugs incorrectly. Drug toxicities may manifest as confusional states which could further increase the risk of ADRs (Shaw and Opit 1976). One major reason for an increased incidence of ADRs in the elderly may be a lack of a desired therapeutic endpoint, therapeutic regimens may be continued indefinitely, and toxicity then may become a direct extension of the desired pharmacologic effect (Melmon 1971).

Others agree that the incidence of ADRs increases with increasing age, calling the increased incidence variously slight, common, or sharp (Hurwitz and Wade 1969; Wade 1972; Hall 1973; Azarnoff 1974). In one study, those over 70 years of age had significantly more admissions to a hospital because of ADRs (Caranasos et al 1974) and another (Seidl et al 1966) showed the following age-related incidence of ADRs (Table 14-2):

Table 14-2
Adverse Drug Reactions

Age in years	Incidence (%)
All ages	13.6
51–60	14.3
61–70	15.7
71–80	18.3
81+	24.0

There seems to be considerable evidence that the incidence of ADRs increases with increasing age, for a variety of reasons. On the other hand, in one study involving 338 patients, there was no age difference (Vakil et al 1975), another could not demonstrate a difference among those over 65 years of age compared with younger people (Davies 1977), and a third study, involving 6200 ambulatory patients, showed that incidence of reactions in those over 60 years of age was no higher than in other adult groups (Mulroy 1973).

Perhaps these differences can be reconciled by noting that, often, differences are shown among hospitalized patients or after admission to an institution, and it is reasonable to assume that the disease forcing institutionalization may make the elderly more vulnerable to ADRs.

Drugs Most Often Involved

Arthritis, congestive heart failure, diabetes, hypertension, prostatic hypertrophy, psychiatric illness, pyelonephritis, upper respiratory tract infections, and urethritis all are treated with drugs likely to cause ADRs. However, with the possible exception of diabetic acidosis, no disease seems to predispose a patient significantly to drug reactions (Seidl et al 1966).

There seems to be agreement that a limited number of classes of drugs (Table 14-3) is most often involved, but it is not clear whether their involvement stems from inherent drug toxicity or frequency of use (Barr 1955; Schimmel 1964; MacDonald and MacKay 1964; Seidl et al 1966; Ogilvie and Ruedy 1967; Meleny and Fraser 1969; Hurwitz and Wade 1969; Stewart and Cluff 1971; Agaard 1972; Mulroy 1973; Caranasos et al 1974; Kaiser 1975; Irey 1976; May et al 1977).

Table 14-3
Drugs Most Often Responsible for Adverse Drug Reactions

Analgesics (aspirin)	Antihypertensives
Antacids	Cardiac glycosides
Antiarthritics	CNS drugs
Antimicrobials	Diuretics
Anticoagulants	Steroids

It is interesting to note that digitalis accounts for 21% of all drug reactions in hospitals (Melmon 1971) and that such reactions were lethal in 30% of cases in one study (Ogilvie and Ruedy 1967). Antibiotics were responsible for nearly 22% of all ADRs in another study (Mulroy 1973).

Almost 15 years ago, the psychotherapeutic agents and the cardiovascular drugs were thought to present the greatest danger (MacGregor 1965). In a similar vein, outpatients receiving anticoagulants and/or antihypertensives were considered at greatest risk, needing particular care during additional drug therapy or when they used nonprescription drugs (Starr and Petrie 1972). Recently, patients receiving anticoagulants or antihypertensives were found to be at greatest risk to ADRs (May et al 1977).

Nonprescription Drugs and ADRs

Data on nonprescription drugs are not easily available. It seems clear, however, that the over-the-counter (OTC) drugs contribute importantly to the incidence of ADRs. In one study, aspirin was responsible for more than 15% of all adverse reactions (Stewart and Cluff 1971). Fatal adverse reactions to phenolphthalein, in the form of a laxative or cold tablet, have been reported. The patients developed erythema multiforme (Seidl et al 1966). In another study, 18% of all identified ADRs were caused by OTC drugs; aspirin was most often involved, but antacids and phenolphthalein were being implicated (Caranasos et al 1974). In patients receiving warfarin, salicylates were responsible for 9% of adverse reactions because of the combination of the two drugs (Starr and Petrie 1972).

Among outpatients receiving prescription drugs, more than 98% also used OTC drugs, and increased age led to increased OTC drug use (Stewart and Cluff 1971) (Table 14-4).

Table 14-4
Prescription and Nonprescription Drug Use

Age in years	Number of prescription drugs		Number of OTC drugs	
	Male	*Female*	*Male*	*Female*
All ages	2.2	3.8	2.6	3.1
50–64	2.4	4.2	3.0	3.1
65+	4.1	5.7	3.7	3.2

It is important to question elderly patients about OTC drug use. In one study, 35% of men and 43% of women used OTC drugs in addition to prescribed drugs, and there was no record of this use (Starr and Petrie 1972). Thirty-four percent of diabetic patients participating in a survey were taking one to four self-prescribed medications (Logie et al 1976), many of which could interfere with the hypoglycemic treatment.

Dose Relationship

Patients aged 65 years and older frequently deteriorated with increased drug dosage (Learoyd 1972). In one study, 78% of all recorded ADRs were dose-related (Seidl et al 1966). Only 2% of patients over 70 years of age experienced adverse reactions to flurazepam when they received 15 mg per day, but when the daily dose was doubled, the incidence of ADRs increased to 31% (Greenblatt et al 1977). The increased frequency of ADRs with an increased daily dose is related to the ability of the liver to metabolize a variety of drugs which decreases in the elderly (Boston Collaborative Drug Surveillance Program 1973), reinforcing the dictum that the elderly should receive as few drugs as possible in the lowest dosage possible.

Multiple Drug Therapy

Many reports call attention to the fact that as the number of drugs administered to a patient increases, the probability of adverse reactions also increases. This is not a simple increase but an exponential one. Multiple drug therapy decreases the benefit/risk ratio for each drug used in a total regimen. Yet, multiple pathology in the elderly often mandates multiple drug use, and it is of prime importance to keep the number of drugs used in a particular regimen to the absolute minimum. Still, multiple drug use among the elderly is frequent; often there are no defined therapeutic endpoints and drugs should be continued only if specific objectives have been established. Furthermore, drugs should be added to an existing regimen under the same criterion (Melmon 1971). Two of three persons over the age of 60 had repeat prescriptions and in 62% of all cases, it was the original physician who had started and continued repeat regimens for long-term use (Balint 1970). Drugs that probably tend to be used continuously without careful patient reevaluation include the antihypertensives, diuretics, cardiac glycosides, oral hypoglycemics, and steroids used to treat arthritic conditions.

Of more than 150 patients 75 years and older, 87% were on a specific treatment regimen, 34% taking three or four different drugs each day (Law and Chalmers 1976). Among diabetic patients questioned on drug use, 63% were taking between one and nine drugs, in addition to the prescribed hypoglycemic agent, as well as OTC drugs (Logie et al 1976). Digitalis toxicity was found in 10% of patients, but the incidence increased to about 26% when diuretics were added to that regimen (Melmon 1971). Twelve percent of patients exhibited untoward drug effects when they received between one and three drugs; the percentage increased to nearly 23% when more than three drugs were used (Vakil et al 1975). Multiple drug therapy is a major determinant of adverse drug reactions. Table 14-5 shows the effects of multiple drug therapy in one study (Cluff et al 1964).

Table 14-5
Multiple Drug Therapy: Effect on Incidence of Adverse Drug Reactions

Number of drugs	Approximate rate (%)
Up to 5	4
6–10	7
11–15	24
16–20	40
21+	45

Influence of Disease

Primary aging, ie, the decrease in level of function of several physiologic systems, may cause increased and variable response to drugs in the elderly, leading to unanticipated adverse reactions. Furthermore, the elderly may suffer from diseases that make multiple drug therapy almost mandatory, such as diabetes, hypertension, and psychiatric illness, which would predispose the elderly to a greater incidence of adverse reactions. Finally, certain diseases affect systems involved in the pharmacokinetics of drugs, ie, drug absorption, distribution, metabolism, and excretion.

Endocrine disorders, neurologic disorders, or mental confusion predispose the elderly to hypothermia, especially those who may be immobilized by physical or mental disorders or who are socially isolated. Drugs such as the phenothiazines could intensify this effect.

In patients with experimentally-induced fever, antipyrine metabolic clearance rate was reduced by 16%, which could be considerably greater in patients with cardiovascular, hepatic, renal, or thyroid disease (Elin et al 1975). The plasma antipyrine half-life is also significantly increased in liver diseases (Andreasen and Vessell 1974). The liver furthermore, is the sole source of plasma albumins to which drugs are bound to various degrees. In liver disease, therefore, serum albumin concentration can decrease. Hypoalbuminemia can be accompanied by a substantial decrease in the bound fraction of a drug, leading to a higher concentration of the active part of the drug, which can lead to a more intense drug reaction, but the effect of hepatic disease on drug metabolism varies with the nature and severity of the disease.

Reduced renal function, either from disease or the normal aging process, may be one of the most important reasons for the increased incidence of adverse reactions with advancing age. For example, a patient with normal renal function loses approximately 25% of the normal digoxin dose per day. However, anuric patients may lose only 14%, leading to cumulation and toxicity.

The aminoglycosides cause a high incidence of adverse reactions in patients with renal disease, as the kidney provides the only route of elimination for these drugs. Thus, one would expect both auditory and vestibular effects to occur more readily in the elderly, and those with renal failure should be treated carefully with aminoglycosides (Dorff 1978). Wide variations in plasma steady state levels and drug half-lives have been documented for a wide variety of drugs (Conney et al 1974). The pharmacokinetics of the drug should be taken into consideration when prescribing. For example, doxycycline is often used in renal insufficiency because it is mainly eliminated by the liver. However, as it is eliminated by the liver, it is subject to the effects of enzyme induction by concurrently administered drugs, eg, phenytoin and carbamazepine can reduce its half-life by approximately 50%.

The effects of drugs on certain diseases frequently encountered in the elderly are shown in Table 14-6 (Davison 1972).

Table 14-6
Some Drug Effects in Frequently Encountered Diseases of the Elderly

Disease state	Drug	Effect
Uremia	Antibiotics Barbiturates	Are likely to cause neurologic symptoms
Chronic renal failure	Tetracyclines	Marked reduction of renal function
Asymptomatic organic brain disease	Atropine Digoxin Trihexyphenidyl	Can precipitate confusion
Organic dementia	Amantadine Barbiturates L-dopa Opiates Trihexyphenidyl	Mental confusion, nightmares, auditory-visual hallucinations
Ischemic heart disease	Glyceryl trinitrate	Postural hypotension
Ischemic brain disease	Chlorpromazine	Postural hypotension
Cerebrovascular insufficiency	Antidepressants Diuretics Sedatives Tranquilizers Vasodilators	Syncope
Cerebrovascular disease	Any drug that lessens cerebral control; increases bladder irritability	Precipitate incontinence

Influence of Genetics

Genetic factors can play a role in drug reactions. This conclusion is based on a wide number of studies. One showed that concordance rates were generally higher in monozygotic than dizygotic twins (Lader et al 1974). For example, rapid metabolizers of propranolol are apparently more sensitive to this drug's action than slow metabolizers (Zacest and Koch-Weser 1972), but slow acetylators develop sensitivity to phenytoin when isoniazid is added to that regimen (Kutt et al 1970).

TYPE OF ADVERSE DRUG REACTION

ADRs have been classified in various ways. ADRs can be due to side reactions (in 47% of patients), toxic reactions (in 31% of patients), allergic reactions (in 14% of patients), superinfections (in more than

1% of patients), and caused by a primary irritant action of a drug (in less than 1% of patients); the others are unclassified (Seidl et al 1966). Simple drug intoxication would produce reactions like lethargy, confusion, and disorientation; secondary drug effects would lead to hypotensive syncope, respiratory depression associated with chest infection, urinary retention, or gastrointestinal ileus (Learoyd 1972). A drug-induced disease could occur from an overdose, a drug interaction, idiosyncracy, or hypersensitivity (Maudlin 1973). Hypersensitivity is related to a subject's immunologic response to a standard dose of a drug, while an idiosyncracy is described as an inordinate response to the usual or less than usual dose of a drug (Melmon 1971). These two factors, as well as drug tolerance to which an individual may be genetically predisposed, are not predictable. However, in combination they account for only 20% to 30% of all ADRs. Of all ADRs 70% to 80% are predictable and should, therefore, be preventable (Melmon 1971).

Tissue sensitivity to drugs may become more apparent with age-related changes in receptor activity or with the decline of cellular viability and the homeostatic mechanism observed with aging (Rawlins 1974). These, then, may not be predictable, but it would not be unreasonable to expect these reactions. Furthermore, it would not be unreasonable to suspect that unanticipated reactions may have occurred from an overdose based on inappropriate drug ingestion and poor drug compliance (Crooks et al 1975).

Individuals who are allergic to food are generally sensitive to drugs (North American Contact Dermatitis Group 1973), but it is probably unreasonable to hope that blood levels could routinely be used to prevent ADRs. They cannot help differentiate those patients with an intrinsic clinical response to a drug which is different from the response expected in a normal population (Perrier and Gibaldi 1974), and plasma levels among patients receiving the same dose of a drug can vary widely (Breckenridge and Orme 1973).

When all possible causes of an ADR are considered, it is clear that the two major factors involved seem to be either pharmacodynamic or pharmacokinetic; most of which are predictable and, therefore, preventable.

ALTERED TISSUE SENSITIVITY

For some drugs, changes in tissue reactivity can be important. As yet, however, the nature of differences in tissue responsiveness is still unclear, as is the number of drugs which may be involved.

It has been suggested that certain tissues of the elderly are hypersensitive to drug action (Harman 1971; Chouinard 1975), and increased sensitivity of brain tissue to depressant drugs like nitrazepam

(Castleden et al 1977) is often cited. On the other hand, there are studies that proclaim decreased tissue sensitivity in the elderly (Hall 1975). For example, clinically, elderly patients seem to develop tolerance to side effects of neuroleptics such as sedation and postural hypotension. This tolerance is thought to be a tissue tolerance (Curry et al 1970). Finally, the great variation in response to warfarin is explained on the basis of broad individual differences in tissue sensitivity (Breckenridge and Orme 1973).

It seems that various tissues in the elderly may exhibit altered tissue sensitivity, either increased or decreased, to a variety of drugs, and that this altered tissue sensitivity can lead to either an increase or decrease in adverse drug reactions.

DRUG INTERACTIONS

The first major conference on drug interactions was held at the Royal Society of Medicine in London in 1965. Since then, there have been many reviews and discussions on drug interactions (Lamy 1970; Kosman 1974; Lamy 1975a, 1975b), but the information is often conflicting, incomplete, and sometimes misleading (Lamy 1972). Fortunately, several books are available, which provide adequate information on drug interactions (Hansten 1975; American Pharmaceutical Association 1976). Only a few articles have addressed themselves to interactions and the elderly (Cohon 1974; MacLennan 1974a; Block 1977).

The term "drug interaction" not only refers to drug-drug reactions, but also to interactions with nutrients and sociologic, psychologic, and disease factors. Also, an understanding of the mechanisms involved in these interactions is mandatory for their prevention.

When two (or more) drugs are administered concurrently, the result may be indifference, synergism, potentiation, or antagonism. Synergism is rare, and the term should be applied to the result of an interaction only when the combined action of two mildly acting drugs exceeds summation (homergic drugs). Synergism also denotes the result of an interaction of an inactive drug with an active drug (heterergic drugs), the clinical effect being greater than the effect of the active drug alone. Potentiation denotes the fact that two active drugs produce a more marked effect than could be predicted on the basis of their dose-response curve. Antagonism is a widely criticized term which denotes that the clinical effect of one drug is reduced or negated by a concurrently administered drug.

Pharmaceutical interactions can lead to physical or chemical incompatibilities, pharmacokinetic interactions can lead to decreased bioavailability, and pharmacodynamic interactions can lead to a reduced response (Ariens 1969). In short, different drugs can interact at different body sites, involving various mechanisms and leading to various outcomes (Bleehen and Edwards 1973).

Mechanisms of Drug Interactions

There are a number of valuable discussions on the mechanisms of drug interactions (Anders 1971; Hurwitz and Sheehan 1971; Stockley 1971; Wang and Ober 1971; Kabins 1972; Rosenoer and Gill 1972; Prescott 1973; Matilla 1974; MacLennan 1974b; Sjoeqvist 1975). The different mechanisms are listed in Table 14-7.

Table 14-7
Some Mechanisms of Drug Interactions

Alterations of absorption
  Chelation or adsorption of drug
  Changes in gastrointestinal motility
  Changes in gastric emptying
  Changes in gastrointestinal pH
  Toxic effect on gastrointestinal tract
  Unknown mechanism

Drug binding interactions
  Displacement from plasma protein
  Displacement from tissue protein

Interaction at the end-organ receptor site
  Displacement from receptor site
  Blockade at receptor site
  Competition for specific uptake mechanisms

Modification of liver metabolism
  Enzyme induction
  Enzyme inhibition

Modification of excretion
  Competition for tubular transport mechanism
  Change in urinary pH

Disturbance of electrolyte or fluid balance

Alteration of absorption Chelation or adsorption of drugs in the gastrointestinal tract may cause a drastic depression in both the rate and the extent of drug absorption. This mechanism is responsible for most clinically important absorption interactions. Many drugs, such as the anticoagulants, antibiotics, and aspirin may be affected.

The best-known interaction is probably the one involving the heavy metal ions (aluminum, calcium, magnesium) found in antacids and iron supplements with the tetracyclines. Poorly soluble precipitates or large complexes are formed that cannot be absorbed from the gastrointestinal tract.

Decreased gut motility may be induced by a wide range of drugs used by the elderly, such as the anticholinergics, phenothiazines, and tricyclics. Reduced motility prevents efficient mixing, which, in turn, may reduce the rate of absorption and increase the possibility of enzymatic inactivation of such drugs as erythromycin. Increased gastrointestinal motility caused by strongly acting laxatives shortens the transit time of many drugs, reducing the opportunity for absorption. This may be of particular importance with extended release medications.

For drugs absorbed from the intestine, gastric emptying assumes a rate-limiting function in the absorptive processes. Antacids containing the aluminum ion inhibit gastric emptying and can markedly slow the drug absorption rate.

The unionized moiety of a drug is absorbed through the lipoprotein membrane of the gastrointestinal tract. Antacids alter this drug characteristic and increase the ionization of acidic drugs and decrease it for basic drugs. The effect is a lesser absorption of acidic drugs and increased absorption of basic drugs.

Some drugs, such as the antigout drug colchicine, exert a toxic effect on the gastrointestinal tract on long-term use, causing malabsorption syndromes. Best known in this category would be the folic acid depletion in patients chronically treated with colchicine.

Phenobarbital interferes with the absorption of griseofulvin, heptabarbital reduces warfarin absorption, and aspirin is thought to reduce indomethacin absorption. The mechanisms for these interactions have not yet been elucidated.

Drug binding interactions Displacement of a bound drug from its plasma binding site by another drug will not be clinically significant when the first drug is bound less than 80% to 85%. However, displacement of a highly bound drug (eg, one that is bound 99%) can be highly clinically significant, even if only 1% of the bound drug is displaced, as this would double the amount of the free, circulating drug.

Displacement can occur when two acidic drugs, both having a volume of distribution of less than 0.5 liters/kg reach the plasma. During displacement, it is possible that there is a decreased concentration of the displaced drug in plasma because of an increased volume distribution. It is more likely, however, that there will be an increased concentration of unbound drug in plasma and tissues, which leads to an increased pharmacologic or toxic effect.

Displacement interactions are not clinically important when a drug binds extensively to tissue proteins. Such drugs have a large volume of distribution (above 1 liter/kg) and less than 4% of the drug will be found in the plasma.

Phenylbutazone, salicylates, and sulfonamides can displace tolbutamide from its binding site, leading to hypoglycemia. Concurrent administration of clofibrate and warfarin demands a reduction of the warfarin dose from one-third to one-half because of the displacement of warfarin from its plasma protein binding sites. Phenylbutazone has a small volume of distributions and is highly bound. The same is true for oral anticoagulants, thus, this type of interaction should be anticipated and prevented.

Interaction at the end-organ receptor site Several mechanisms are responsible for interactions at the receptor site. Displacement interactions lead to a diminished response of the displaced drug. On the other hand, drugs sharing an anticholinergic effect, such as the antihistamines and antidepressants, can exhibit toxic effects, such as paralysis of the intestine or bladder.

Access to the receptor may be denied one drug by another. Propranolol, a beta blocker, reverses the effect of sympathomimetics in this fashion. Finally, drugs may compete for specific uptake mechanisms. For example, guanethidine is taken up into the sympathetic neuron by the so-called membrane pump, catalyzed by an active, enzymatic process. The principal mechanism of action of the tricyclics is to inhibit that pump. Thus, concurrent administration of the antihypertensive drug and an antidepressant tricyclic will completely block the action of guanethidine.

Modification of liver metabolism Many drugs stimulate microsomal liver metabolism of other drugs; some even stimulate their own metabolism on chronic administration. Conversely, other drugs are responsible for inhibition of liver metabolism.

Phenobarbital stimulates enzyme induction and increases the metabolism of the oral anticoagulants and decreases the magnitude and duration of their action. While this interaction can be anticipated and prevented, serious clinical consequences occur when phenobarbital is withdrawn from the regimen. Anticoagulant metabolism will then decrease and the action of the anticoagulant will increase causing toxic effects, unless the anticoagulant dose is reduced.

It should be noted that enzyme induction does not necessarily lead to reduced drug action. If metabolism leads to the formation of a metabolite that is more active than the parent drug, then enzyme induction can lead to an increased drug effect, cumulation, and toxicity.

Chloramphenicol inhibits the metabolism of anticoagulants by decreasing their rate of removal from the body and consequently increasing the magnitude and duration of their action. Thus, inhibition of liver metabolism can lead to prolonged drug action. To prevent serious hemorrhage, anticoagulant dosage must be reduced as long as both drugs are administered simultaneously. By means of the same mechanism, the oral anticoagulants and isoniazid inhibit enzyme metabolism of phenytoin, increasing that drug's activity.

It has been suggested that metabolic interactions are the most frequent pharmacokinetic drug interactions.

Modification of excretion Two types of interactions can modify drug excretion. The excretion of drugs that are actively secreted or reabsorbed by the tubular cells can be influenced by drugs which compete for the same transport mechanism. In general, there will be prolonged drug action, which increases the possibility of cumulation and toxicity. In this manner, salicylates inhibit the action of uricosuric drugs. The best example of this type interaction is a desired interaction. Penicillin is mainly excreted by active tubular secretion. Addition of probenecid to a penicillin regimen will block penicillin excretion, prolonging its action.

Drug excretion can also be changed by changes in urinary pH. The renal clearance of basic drugs is increased in acid urine and decreased in alkaline urine (Figure 14-1). In contrast, the excretion of acidic drugs

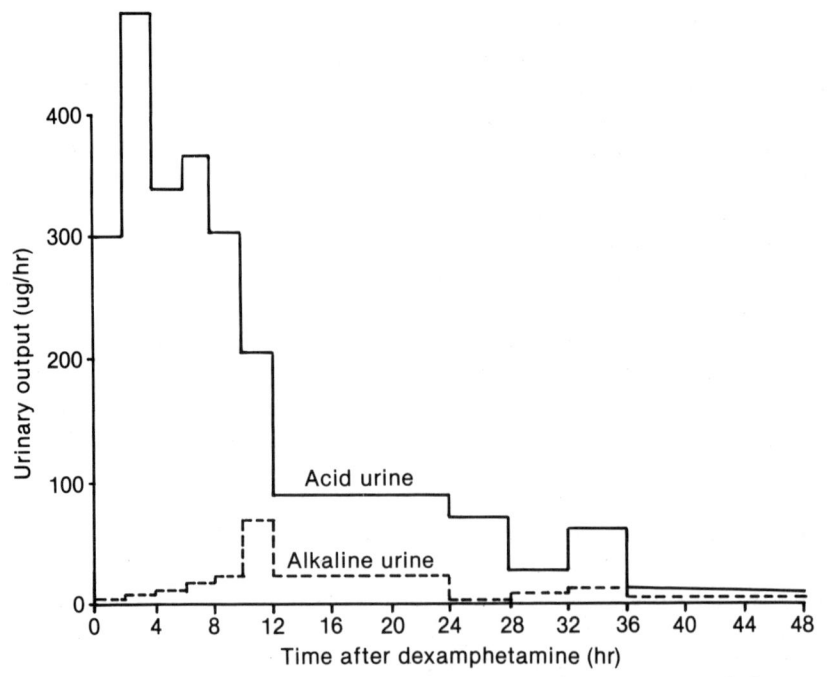

Figure 14-1 The influence of urinary pH on the excretion of dexamphetamine. A.M. Asatoor, B.R. Galman, J.R. Johnson, and M.D. Milne. *Br J Pharmacol.* 24:293, 1965. Reproduced with permission.

is enhanced in alkaline urine and decreased in acid urine. Changes in urinary pH can occur because of prolonged administration of antacids and changes in dietary intake.

Disturbance of electrolyte or fluid balance   The elderly are particularly sensitive to changes in electrolyte or fluid balance. These changes could result either in increased or decreased drug action. Chronic administration of the thiazide diuretics may induce hypokalemia, which would then potentiate the effects of digitalis, frequently leading to digitalis toxicity.

There is no question that elderly patients are more at risk to adverse drug effects than younger patients. Elderly patients frequently deteriorate with an increased number of drugs and increasing dosage of drugs administered, although in the elderly even the "usual" dose may cause unanticipated and unwanted drug effects.

Inappropriate drug ingestion, multiple drug therapy, and poor drug compliance contribute to the heightened incidence of adverse drug effects in the elderly. In general, though, adverse reactions that are caused by intolerance, idiosyncracies, or hypersensitivities, ie, unpredictable reactions, account for only 20% to 30% of all adverse reactions. In other words, 70% to 80% of all adverse reactions can be predicted and therefore prevented or their effects can at least be ameliorated. Foremost among those are the reactions caused by the altered drug handling capability of the elderly, their impaired homeostatic mechanisms and their intercurrent diseases which can contribute to altered drug response. Among the predictable but often unanticipated adverse reactions are the drug-drug interactions and drug interactions with nutrients. These should be suspected, particularly when chronic care drugs are used.

REFERENCES

Agaard, G.N. Drug therapy in the aged. *Postgrad Med.* 52(8):115, 1972.

American Pharmaceutical Association. *Evaluations of Drug Interactions.* Washington, D.C., 1976.

Anders, M.W. Enhancement and inhibition of drug metabolism. *Ann Rev Pharmacol.* 11:37, 1971.

Andreasen, P.B., and Vessell, E.S. Comparison of plasma levels of antipyrine, tolbutamide, and warfarin after oral and intravenous administration. *Clin Pharmacol Ther.* 16:1059, 1974.

Ariens, E.J. Reduction of drug action by drug combination. *J Mond Pharm.* 3:263, 1969.

Azarnoff, D.L. Drug interactions. *Isr J Med Sci.* 10:346, 1974.

Balint, M. Repeat-prescription patients, are they an indefinable group? Edited by M. Balint. In *Treatment or Diagnosis.* Philadelphia: J.B. Lippincott Co., 1970.

Barr, D.P. Hazards of modern diagnosis and therapy–the price we pay. *JAMA*. 159:1452, 1955.

Bleehen, S.S., Edwards, I.R. Drug interaction I. *Br J Dermatol*. 88:625, 1973.

Block, L.H. Drug interactions and the elderly. *US Pharmacist* 2(10):46, 1977.

Boston Collaborative Drug Surveillance Program. Clinical depression of the central nervous system due to diazepam and chlordiazepoxide in relation to cigarette smoking and age. *N Engl J Med*. 288:277, 1973.

Breckenridge, A., and Orme, M.L.E. Measurement of plasma warfarin concentrations in clinical practice. Edited by D.S. Davies, and B.N.C. Prichard. In *Biological Effects of Drugs in Relation to their Plasma Concentrations*. London: MacMillan and Co., 1973.

Caranasos, G.J., Stewart, R.B., and Cluff, L.E. Drug-induced illness leading to hospitalization. *JAMA*. 288:713, 1974.

Castleden, C.M., George, C.F., Marcer, D. et al. Increased sensitivity to nitrazepam in old age. *Br Med J*. 1:10, 1977.

Chouinard G. Psychopharmacology. Editorial *Mod Geriatr*. 5(8):2, 1975.

Cluff, L.E., Thornton, C.F., and Seidl, L.G. Studies of the epidemiology of adverse drug reactions. *JAMA*. 188:976, 1964.

Cohon, M.S. Drug interactions unique to the geriatric patient. *Wisc Pharm Ext Bull*. 17(12):1, 1974.

Conney, A.H., Kuntzman, R., Carver, B. et al. Drug metabolism in normal and disease states. Edited by T. Teorell, R.L. Diedrick, and P.G. Condliffe. In *Pharmacology and Pharmacokinetics*. New York: Plenum Publishing Co., 1974.

Crooks, J., Shepherd, A.M.M., and Stevenson, I.H. Drugs and the elderly: the nature of the problem. *Health Bull*. (Edinburgh) 33(5):222, 1975.

Curry, S.H., Marshall, J.H.L., Davis, J.M. et al. Factors affecting chlorpromazine plasma levels in psychiatric patients. *Arch Gen Psychiatry*. 22:209, 1970.

Davies, D.M. History and epidemiology. Edited by D.M. Davies. In *Textbook of Adverse Drug Rections*. Oxford: Oxford University Press, 1977.

Davison, W. Unwanted drug effects in the elderly. Edited by L. Meyler, and H.M. Peck. In *Drug-Induced Diseases*. Amsterdam: Excerpta Medica, 1972.

Dorff, G.J. Avoiding aminoglycoside toxicity. *Drug Ther*. 8(8):153, 1978.

Elin, R.J., Vessell, E.S., and Wolff, S.M. Effects of etiocholanolone-induced fever on plasma antipyrine half-lives and metabolic clearance. *Clin Pharmacol Ther*. 17:447, 1975.

Freeman, J.T. Some principles of medication in geriatrics. *J Am Geriatr Soc*. 22:289, 1974.

Greenblatt, D.J., Allen, M.D., and Shader, R.I. Toxicity of high-dose flurazepam in the elderly. *Clin Pharmacol Ther*. 21:355, 1977.

Hall, M.R.P. Drug therapy in the elderly. *Br Med J*. 3:582, 1973.

Hall, M.R.P. Use of drugs in elderly patients. *NY State J Med*. 75:67, 1975.

Hansten, P.D. *Drug Interactions*. Philadelphia: Lea and Febiger, 1975.

Harman, J.B. Prescribing for the elderly. *Prescriber's J*. 11:142, 1971.

Hurwitz, A., and Sheehan, M.B. The effects of antacids on the absorption of orally administered pentobarbital in the rat. *J Pharmacol Exp Ther*. 179:124, 1971.

Hurwitz, N., and Wade, O.L. Intensive hospital monitoring of adverse reactions to drugs. *Br Med J*. 1:531, 1969.

Ingelfinger, F.J. Counting adverse drug reactions that count. Editorial *N Engl J Med*. 294:1003, 1976.

Irey, N.S. Adverse drug reactions and death, a review of 827 cases. *JAMA*.

236:575, 1976.

Jansen, H.H., Hopker, W.W., Doernberger, V. et al. Unerwuenschte medikamentoese nebenwirkungen im alter aus pathologischer-anatomischer sicht. *Z Gerontol.* 8:339, 1975.

Jick, H. Introduction. Edited by R.R. Miller, and D.J. Greenblatt. In *Drug Effects in Hospitalized Patients.* New York: John Wiley and Sons, 1976.

Kabins, S.A. Interactions among antibiotics and other drugs. *JAMA.* 219:206, 1972.

Kaiser, H. Klinisch-pharmacologische problems in der geriatrie. *Aktuel Gerontol.* 5:83, 1975.

Karch, F.E. What is an adverse drug reaction. *Drug Ther.* 7(9):24, 1977.

Karch, F.E. and Lasagna, L. *Adverse Drug Reactions in the United States–An Analysis of the Scope of the Problem and Recommendations for Future Approaches.* Washington, D.C.: Medicine Public Interest, 1974.

Karch, F.E., and Lasagna, L. Adverse drug reactions. *JAMA.* 234:1236, 1975.

Karch, F.E., and Lasagna, L. Adverse drug reactions–a matter of opinion. *Clin Pharmacol Ther.* 21:247, 1977.

Karch, F.E., Smith, C.L., Kerzner, B. et al. Toward the operational identification of adverse drug reactions. *Clin Pharmacol Ther.* 19:489, 1976.

Koch-Weser, J., and Greenblatt, D.J. The ambiguity of adverse drug reactions. *Clin Pharmacol Ther.* 19:110, 1976.

Kosman, M.E. Pharmacokinetic drug interactions: sedative, hypnotic, and antianxiety agents. *JAMA.* 229:1485, 1974.

Kutt, H., Brennan, R., Dehejia, H. et al. Diphenylhydantoin intoxication a complication of isoniazid therapy. *Am Rev Respir Dis.* 101:377, 1970.

Lader, M., Kendell, R., and Kasriel, J. The genetic contribution to unwanted drug effects. *Clin Pharmacol Ther.* 16:343, 1974.

Lamy, P.P. Therapeutic incompatibilities. Edited by J.B. Sprowls. In *Prescription Pharmacy.* Philadelphia: J.B. Lippincott Co., 1970.

Lamy, P.P. Classification of drug interactions. *Drug Inform J.* 6(1):99, 1972.

Lamy, P.P. Drug interactions: a growing problem, Part I. *Hosp Form Management.* 10(2):60, 1975a.

Lamy, P.P. Drug interactions: a growing problem, Part II. *Hosp Form Management.* 10(4):161, 1975b.

Lamy, P.P. and Kitler, M.E. Drugs and the geriatric patient. *J Am Geriatr Soc.* 19:23, 1971.

Law, R., and Chalmers, C. Medicines and elderly people: a general practice survey. *Br Med J.* 1:565, 1976.

Learoyd, B.M. Psychotropic drugs and the elderly patient. *Med J Aust.* 1:1131, 1972.

Logie, A.W., Galloway, D.B., and Petrie, J.C. Drug interactions and long-term antidiabetic therapy. *Br J Clin Pharmacol.* 3:1027, 1976.

MacDonald, M.G., and MacKay, B.R. Adverse drug reactions: experience of Mary Fletcher Hospital during 1962. *JAMA.* 190:1071, 1964.

MacGregor, A.G. Review of points at which drugs can interact. *Proc R Soc Med.* 58:943, 1965.

MacLennan, W.J. The identification of drug interactions in old age. *Mod Geriatr.* 4(8):334, 1974a.

MacLennan, W.J. Drug interactions. *Gerontol Clin.* 16:18, 1974b.

Matilla, J. Effect of sodium sulfate and castor oil on drug absorption from the human intestine. *Ann Clin Res.* 6:19, 1974.

Maudlin, R.K. Drug-induced diseases. *J Am Pharm Assoc.* NS13:316, 1973.

May, F.E., Stewart, R.B., and Cluff, L.E. Drug interactions and multiple drug administration. *Clin Pharmacol Ther.* 22:323, 1977.

Meleny, H.E., and Fraser, M.L. A retrospective study of drug usage and adverse drug reactions in hospital outpatients: final report. *Drug Inform Bull.* 3:124, 1969.

Melmon, K.L. Preventable drug reactions–causes and cures. *N Engl J Med.* 284:1361, 1971.

Miller, R. Hospital admissions due to adverse drug reactions. A report from the Boston Collaborative Drug Surveillance Program. *Arch Intern Med.* 134:219, 1974.

Mulroy, R. Iatrogenic disease in general practice: its incidence and effects. *Br Med J.* 2:407, 1973.

North American Contact Dermatitis Group. Epidemiology of contact dermatitis in North America: 1972. *Arch Dermatol.* 108:537, 1973.

Ogilvie, R.I., and Ruedy, J. Adverse drug reactions during hospitalization. *Can Med Assoc J.* 97:1450, 1967.

Perrier, D., and Gibaldi, M. Drug concentrations in the plasma as an index of pharmacologic effect. *J Clin Pharmacol.* 14:415, 1974.

Prescott, L.F. Clinically important drug interactions. *Drugs* 5:161, 1973.

Rawlins, M.D. Variability in response to drugs. *Br Med J.* 4:91, 1974.

Rosenoer, V.M., and Gill, G.M. Drug interactions in clinical medicine. *Med Clin North Am.* 56:585, 1972.

Salzman, C., Shader, R.I., and Van Der Kolk, B.A. Clinical psychopharmacology and the elderly patient. *NY State J Med.* 76:71, 1976.

Schimmel, E.M. The hazards of hospitalization. *Ann Intern Med.* 60:100, 1964.

Seidl, L.G., Thornton, G.F., Smith, J.W. et al. Studies on the epidemiology of adverse drug reactions. III. Reaction in patients on a general medical service. *Bull Johns Hopkins Hosp.* 119:299, 1966.

Shaw, S.M., and Opit, L.J. Need for supervision in the elderly receiving long-term prescribed medications. *Br Med J.* 1:505, 1976.

Sjoeqvist, F. Drug interactions. *Triangle* 14(3):143, 1975.

Starr, K.J., and Petrie, J.C. Drug interactions in patients on long-term oral anticoagulant and antihypertensive adrenergic neuron-blocking drugs. *Br Med J.* 4:133, 1972.

Stewart, R.B., and Cluff, L.E. Studies on the epidemiology of adverse drug reactions. VI. Utilization and interactions of prescription and nonprescription drugs in outpatients. *Johns Hopkins Med J.* 129:319, 1971.

Stockley, I.H. Some mechanisms of drug interaction. *Pharm J.* 206:277, 1971.

Trounce, J.R. Drugs in the elderly. Editorial *Br J Clin Pharmacol.* 2:289, 1975.

Vakil, B.J., Kulkarni, R.D., Chabria, N.L. et al. Intense surveillance of adverse drug reactions. *J Clin Pharmacol.* 15:435, 1975.

Wade, O.L. Drug therapy in the elderly. *Age Ageing.* 1:65, 1972.

Wang, R.I.H., and Ober, K.F. A survey of drug reactions for the practicing physician. *Drug Ther.* 1(10):48, 1971.

Wiener, H. Approval of new drugs. Letter to the Editor. *Science* 181:110, 1973.

Zacest, R., and Koch-Weser, J. Relation of propranolol level to B-blockade during oral therapy. *Pharmacology* 7:178, 1972.

15 Nonprescription Drugs

Nonprescription drugs, also called over-the-counter (OTC) drugs, can contribute to the well-being of patients, if used intelligently and according to specific label directions.

Unfortunately, many of these agents are viewed as nondrug drugs by patients and physicians. Alcohol, aspirin, Tums, vitamins, and other, sometimes potent drugs are not viewed as such by the public and, in some instances, by the physician.

Self-medication is based on self-diagnosis, and the elderly patient cannot always make a correct diagnosis. Self-selection of a particular OTC drug may be erroneous, and self-treatment may lead to unfortunate clinical consequences. For example, persistent use of cough remedies could delay diagnosis of serious respiratory illness. Patients not following label instructions could self-administer an amount equal to that found in a prescription drug. Many OTC drugs contain active ingredients which, at higher doses, would only be available on prescription (Lamy and Kitler 1971a; Lamy and Kitler 1971b; Lamy 1975a;

Lamy 1975b). Correct judgment by patients cannot be assumed as shown by the fact that even unused portions of antibiotics are used for self-treatment, most often incorrectly (Chretien et al 1976). Self-treatment, instead of medical care or as a supplement to medical care, is common (Jeffreys et al 1960). The physician should not take for granted that the patient is using only those drugs which have been prescribed (Lamy 1977), but should question the patient closely about the possible use of OTC drugs (Lamy et al 1975).

USE OF NONPRESCRIPTION DRUGS BY THE ELDERLY

Few studies have addressed the issue of nonprescription drug use by the elderly. In general, there is agreement that 25% to 60% of the population in any Western country use prescription drugs and approximately 25% to 40% in addition use nonprescription drugs. Physicians have thus far exerted little influence on OTC drug use, ceding to the elderly patient the role of diagnostician, prescriber, and consumer. In France, about 15 years ago, it was estimated that elderly persons used approximately 7.2 OTC drugs yearly, or 80% more than persons between the ages of 30 and 49 years. About five years ago, in the United States, it was estimated that expenditures for nonprescription drugs increase with age and that persons over 65 years of age spend one-third the dollar volume on OTC drugs per year as on prescription drugs.

A Canadian study (Chaiton et al 1976) found no relationship between self-medication and medical consultation. Fifty-eight percent of the study population used at least one OTC drug within 48 hours of being surveyed. Of those, 25% used two, and 20% used three OTC drugs simultaneously. Vitamins, analgesics, cold remedies, and laxatives were most frequently used (Table 15-1). The use of OTC drugs seemed to be influenced by sex and age of the persons surveyed (Table 15-2).

Table 15-1
Medication Use by a Community Population

	Percent Population Using	
	Prescribed drugs	*Nonprescribed drugs*
Vitamins and tonics	8.9	14.4
Aspirin and other analgesics	5.4	14.3
Cold remedies	3.1	6.2
Laxatives and stomach medicines	4.1	4.3

Table 15-2
Influence of Age and Sex on OTC Drug Use

	Percent Population Using	
Years of age	*Male*	*Female*
40–49	54.3	71.4
50–59	55.6	73.0
Over 59	54.8	80.8

Another study found almost 50% of elderly persons self-administered vitamins (Rose et al 1970). In Washington, DC, more than two-thirds of elderly ambulant patients in a study used OTC drugs. More than one-half of the OTC drugs used were internal analgesics, with cough and cold preparations accounting for about 13%. Only 8% of those surveyed felt that they needed OTC drugs for performance of regular daily activities, while 40% needed prescription drugs to meet daily requirements. Of interest is the fact that only 12% of the study population consulted a physician about OTC drug use (Guttman 1977). In another study, 28 day treatment center participants followed for eight weeks, were found to use more than 200 OTC drugs. Patients used an average of 7.25 OTC drugs as opposed to 3.8 prescription drugs. Internal analgesics and gastrointestinal drugs were used most often (Boykin et al 1978).

Thus, it appears that the elderly use nonprescription drugs (analgesics, antacids, cough and cold preparations, laxatives, and vitamins) frequently, and that most often they do not consult their physician about their use.

INTERNAL ANALGESICS

Many different kinds of pains plague the elderly patient. Prolonged use of phenacetin-containing analgesics carries the risk of papillary necrosis (Shelley 1967). The combination of aspirin, phenacetin, and caffeine has not been found to be superior to aspirin, in providing analgesia, and should not be recommended to elderly patients (AMA Drug Evaluations 1973; Beaver 1966). The most frequently used OTC analgesics are aspirin and acetaminophen. It is important that their use by the elderly be monitored closely, as analgesic abuse may lead to analgesic nephropathy (females are afflicted three times as often as males) (Goldberger and Talner 1975; Murray and Goldbery 1975; Wilson 1972). Hypertension may accompany analgesic nephropathy (Prescott 1972). The patients most at risk are those with long-standing backaches, headaches, or arthritis.

Both aspirin and acetaminophen are equally effective in providing analgesia for mild to moderate pain, including musculoskeletal pain of nonrheumatic origin. Neither is effective in intense pain such as biliary pain or the pain associated with intestinal or ureteral colic.

Aspirin

Aspirin is the most frequently used OTC drug. Over 200 aspirin-containing products, both prescription and nonprescription, are listed (Leist and Banwell 1974), many with names that do not clearly indicate the aspirin content. Aspirin acts peripherally. It has been proposed that it prevents prostaglandin release in inflammation, thereby preventing sensitization of pain receptors to stimulation (Lim et al 1964). It is used prophylactically in rheumatoid arthritis to prevent symptoms of arthritic pain. There is no tolerance to its effect and it therefore lends itself to chronic administration. In treating inflammatory conditions, blood levels must be maintained at optimal levels. If a patient ceases to take the medication when experiencing pain relief, salicylate blood levels will be reduced below optimal levels, and inflammation and pain will recur (Kantor 1976).

Aspirin provides ascending analgesia that is dose-related. It is probably the best OTC analgesic for mixed acute and chronic pain. Its site of action is the pain site. Aspirin can elicit many unanticipated or adverse reactions (Lamy and Kitler 1971b). The most serious ones include hypersensitivity reactions, gastrointestinal blood loss, and interactions with oral anticoagulants and uricosuric agents. Symptoms of salicylate toxicity appear at lower doses in the elderly, manifesting themselves as confusion, irritability, and deafness. Salicylates induce dyspepsia in 6% of randomly chosen patients and in 10% of patients with rheumatoid arthritis (Davies and Gold 1977). Salicylates can also cause a 50% decrease in sodium and chloride excretion which, in turn, can lead to expansion of intracellular water. This might be of concern in patients on low sodium diets or those with congestive heart failure (Lamy 1975b). Chronic use of moderate doses of salicylates may cause sufficient blood loss to cause iron deficiency anemia in patients with low iron reserves and inadequate dietary iron. As iron-deficient anemia is not uncommon among the elderly (Morgan 1967), the need for aspirin use among this population should be carefully evaluated.

Patients with a history of anemia should avoid aspirin if possible (Leonards et al 1973). Ingestion of a single dose of 0.3 to 1.2 gm of aspirin can prolong bleeding time by several minutes (Weiss 1974). A single aspirin tablet can cause focal lesions, predominantly in the glandular (fundic) and antral mucosa; the nonglandular parts of the stomach are much less susceptible to aspirin injury. There is an association between the amount of aspirin ingested and the frequency of gastrointestinal bleeding, but there is a much clearer association between aspirin ingestion and chronic ulceration as opposed to acute ulceration. (Douglas and Johnson 1961; Gillies and Skyring 1968; Levy 1974). Use of 3 gm per day will likely cause an occult or overt blood loss of 3 to 6 ml daily, and 15% of patients may lose as much as 10 ml. Thus, the elderly suffering from rheumatoid arthritis or osteoarthritis are particularly at risk.

These problems can be exacerbated when incontinent elderly patients attempt to limit their fluid intake and use insufficient fluids when taking aspirin (at least one full glass of water is recommended), which could lead to increased gastrointestinal insult. Furthermore, concurrent use of salicylates with alcohol, which is present in many OTC cough preparations, can cause increased gastrointestinal bleeding.

Anything that modifies the body's ability to regulate temperature can contribute to the development of hypothermia or hyperthermia. The normal physiologic mechanisms that compensate for temperature variations are least efficient in the elderly (Butler 1977). One manifestation of salicylate intoxication is hyperthermia. Excessive heat, as well as the use of diuretics, makes the elderly prone to hyperthermia, especially in a high humidity environment (Hall 1972), so the combination of these three factors should be carefully avoided. In contrast, hypothermia can easily develop in the elderly. A possible association with chronic aspirin use has been suggested (Fox et al 1973). Shivering and feeling cold is sometimes the only complaint of elderly chronic rheumatic patients who may develop subnormal temperatures spontaneously. In those cases, an electric blanket controlled by the patient can be very helpful (Meerloo 1973).

It is important to note that salicylates can interfere with a number of laboratory test values (Table 15-3). Salicylate consumption of 4 gm per day for 10 days may invalidate the creatinine clearance test as an index of renal function; this dose causes more than a one-third increase in plasma creatinine and a one-fourth decrease in creatinine clearance (Burry and Dieppe 1976). Possible interactions of salicylates with prescription drugs are listed in Table 15-4.

Table 15-3
Influence of Salicylates on Some Laboratory Test Values

Laboratory Test	Effect of salicylates on laboratory test values
Benedict's test	Elevated or false positive
Phenyl ketone in urine	Possible false positive or negative
Cholesterol in serum	Decreased or false negative

Table 15-3 *(continued)*

Laboratory Test	Effect of salicylates on laboratory test values
CO_2 content in serum	Elevated or false positive
	Decreased or false negative
Diacetic acid in urine	Elevated or false positive
Fasting glucose	Decreased or false negative
PBI	Decreased or false negative
Potassium in serum	Decreased or false negative
Proteins in spinal fluid (Follin-Ciocalteu method)	Elevated or false positive
Proteins in urine	Elevated or false positive
Prothrombin time	Elevated or false positive
Thrombocytes	Decreased or false negative
Triiodothyronine uptake	Elevated or false positive when given in high doses
Uric acid in serum	Elevated or false positive
Uric acid in urine	Elevated or false positive

Table 15-4
Interactions of Salicylates with Other Drugs

Drug	Result of Interaction
Urinary alkalinizers	Decreased effect of salicylates because of increased excretion rate
Aminosalicylic acid (PAS)	Increased danger of salicylate toxicity
Anticoagulants	May enhance anticoagulant effect especially in doses exceeding one gram per day
Corticosteroids	Increased danger of gastrointestinal ulceration
Methotrexate	Drug may be displaced from albumin binding sites resulting in increased toxicity
Phenobarbital	Decreased effect of salicylates caused by enzyme induction
Phenylbutazone	Increased danger of gastrointestinal ulceration
Phenytoin	Large doses may enhance drug effect
Probenecid	Uricosuric activity of drug is antagonized
Sulfinpyrazone	Uricosuric activity of drug is antagonized
Sulfonylureas	Hypoglycemic response may be enhanced

Acetaminophen

Acetaminophen has been used for more than 75 years. It is marketed under approximately 50 brand names and in almost 200 proprietary combinations. Its advantages and disadvantages have been extensively discussed (Beaver 1965; Koch-Weser 1976; Ameer and Greenblatt 1977). Acetaminophen has analgesic and antipyretic properties similar to those of aspirin. Both drugs are equally effective in lowering body temperature of febrile patients. Thus, acetaminophen is a suitable substitute for aspirin when it is used as an analgesic or antipyretic. Acetaminophen in the recommended dosage will not produce gastric irritation, erosion, or occult blood loss. Furthermore, it does not interfere with platelet function and does not appreciably potentiate the action of oral anticoagulants (Mielke and Britten 1970; Koch-Weser and Sellers 1971). Because it also does not affect uric acid excretion, it is preferred over aspirin for patients receiving oral anticoagulants and for those with hyperuricemia, gouty arthritis, asthma, or peptic ulcer.

However, aspirin is superior to acetaminophen for treatment of rheumatoid arthritis. Aspirin has an antiinflammatory action that acetaminophen lacks (Hajnal et al 1959; DiCyan and Hessman 1972).

Acetaminophen effects can be enhanced with dosage increase to 500 to 600 mg. Further increase will not lead to increased effectiveness. The drug is not effective for any severe pain, and aspirin remains the drug of choice when antiinflammatory action is required for relief of a painful condition. Acetaminophen overdoses can lead to very serious hepatotoxicity (Proudfoot and Wright 1970), but the major disadvantage of acetaminophen as compared to aspirin is its high cost.

Buffered aspirin seems to be no more efficient or effective than regular aspirin, and the use of enteric-coated aspirin may lead to erratic absorption, without providing an additional safety factor. Aspirin in effervescent form is less irritating to the gastric mucosa than regular aspirin. However, this dosage form should not be used for high dosage or chronic administration, as patients would ingest too much sodium and potassium. Acetaminophen should be used in patients with anemia, asthma, or ulcers, and in those taking oral anticoagulants, probenecid, or methotrexate. Some interactions are summarized in Table 15-5.

Table 15-5
OTC Drug Interactions of Clinical Significance

R Drug	OTC Drug	Possible Effect
Alcohol[3]	Salicylates	Gastrointestinal bleeding
Anticoagulants[1] (coumarin-type)	Salicylates	Increased anticoagulant effect
Digitalis[1]	Laxatives (prolonged use)	Increased digitalis toxicity
Hypoglycemic agents[2]	Salicylates	Increased hypoglycemia
MAO inhibitors[1]	Sympathomimetic amines	Hypertensive crisis
Methotrexate[2]	Salicylates	Increased effect and toxicity of methotrexate
Probenecid[1]	Salicylates	Decreased uricosuric effect
Sulfinpyrazone[2]	Salicylates	Decreased uricosuric effect
Tricyclic antidepressants[1]	Sympathomimetic amines	Hypertensive crisis

[1]*The Medical Letter.* 12(23):93, 1970.
[2]*The Medical Letter.* 15(19):77, 1973.
[3]*The Medical Letter.* 16(22):92, 1974.

ANTACIDS

About 15% to 20% of Americans suffer from symptoms of excessive gastric acidity and call it "acid indigestion," "upset stomach," and "heartburn." They, as well as the 10% of the population afflicted with peptic ulcers, usually treat themselves with antacids (*Federal Register 1973*). The rationale of antacid therapy rests with the assumption that neutralization of gastric acidity will relieve pain, discomfort, and promote healing.

In considering the choice of antacids, several factors have to be taken into account, such as potency, palatability, calcium carbonate content, sodium content, and known side effects.

Potency In general, the onset of action of antacids may be as short as one to two minutes. They reduce gastric acidity for about 20 to 40 minutes; if administered one hour after meals, their duration of action is prolonged. Although the desirable pH achieved by antacid therapy is still being disputed, there seems to be general agreement that in peptic ulcers, an antacid should produce a gastric milieu of at least pH 5.5.

The labeled content of antacids does not reveal functional neutralization capacity. Antacids differ widely in their neutralizing efficiency, and even preparations of the same substance may vary considerably. Maalox, Kolantyl, Gelusil, and Dicarbosil had the best antacid capacity in one study, while Aludrox, Amphojel, and Mylanta failed to increase gastric pH to 5.5 (Ritschel and Erni 1978). These results are at variance with other published results (Table 15-6) (Fordtran et al 1973; Sklar et al 1977).

Table 15-6
Neutralizing Capacity of Some Antacids

Antacid	Ingredients	Dose (ml) containing 80 mEq	mEq HCl/ ml antacid
Delcid	a,b	10	8.46
Ducon	a,b,c	11	7.04
Mylanta II	a,b, and simethicone	19	4.14
Titralac	c and glycine	21	3.87
Camalox	a,b,c	22	3.59
Basaljel	aluminum carbonate	24	3.29
Maalox	a,b	31	2.58
Di-Gel	a,b, and simethicone	33	2.45
Mylanta	a,b, and simethicone	34	2.38
Riopan	a,b	36	2.21
Amphojel	a	42	1.93
Kolantyl	a,b, dicyclomine HCl	46	1.69
Gelusil*	a, alginates, magnesium trisilicate	60	1.33

Key: a = aluminum hydroxide
b = magnesium hydroxide
c = calcium carbonate
*Gelusil has been reformulated. The dose containing 80 mEq is now approximately 33 ml, and for Gelusil II is approximately 17 ml.

A 15 ml dose of Maalox given one hour after breakfast, brought gastrointestinal pH above 3.5 for 36 minutes, while Ducon kept pH above 3.5 for 67 minutes (Littman and Pine 1975).

Appreciation of the varying potencies of antacids is particularly important for elderly patients, as achlorhydria and hypochlorhydria occur ten times as frequently in older than in younger patients, and different dosages may be indicated. On the other hand, in peptic ulcer therapy, large quantities of antacids are often needed, sometimes as much as 200 ml. In those instances, the palatability of antacids is important.

Palatability It may well be the taste of an antacid preparation that determines compliance with an antacid regimen. In old age, the number of taste buds is reduced (Chinn 1971; Hughes 1959) and this, coupled with an appreciable loss of salivary secretion, may change the taste sensation considerably. Little has been done to test the acceptance of antacids, based on palatability. It has been suggested that

Marblen (peach/apricot flavor), Titralac (spearmint flavor), Kudrox, Mylanta II, and Camalox (vanilla-mint flavor) are the best-tasting antacids. One study ranked antacids according to taste acceptability, but this may not be applicable to elderly patients, as the subjects ranged in age from 25 to 43 years. Ranking did not show a statistically significant difference (Table 15-7).

Table 15-7
Taste Comparison of Some Common Antacids

Antacid	Rank
Mylanta	1
Mylanta II	2
Titralac and Maalox	3
Maalox Lemon or Maalox Plus	4
Kolantyl	5
Di-Gel and Riopan	6
Delcid	7
Basaljel	8
Camalox	9
Gelusil	10
Ducon	11
Amphojel	12

Calcium carbonate content Calcium carbonate can cause gastric hypersecretion, or "acid rebound" (Barreras 1973; Case 1973). While it is an excellent antacid (Harvey 1970), it also has constipating properties which argue against its chronic use, particularly in the elderly who frequently complain about constipation. Magnesium trisilicate, which is less effective as an antacid but does not cause acid rebound, may be preferred. Other commonly used antacid ingredients do not cause acid rebound.

Aluminum and magnesium content Aluminum hydroxide has a constipating effect that is counteracted in many preparations by the inclusion of magnesium salts, which have a diarrheal effect. Intestinal obstruction in elderly patients, particularly those with decreased bowel motility or those on fluid restriction, is possible if aluminum-containing antacids are used, but not if a preparation contains both aluminum and magnesium (Morrissey and Barreras, 1974). Dementia can result when elderly uremic patients are placed on long-term antacid therapy with preparations containing aluminum hydroxide (Ambre and Fischer 1973).

Sodium content Sodium retention has clinical consequences when sodium-containing antacids are used in large doses or in individuals with decreased renal function. Hyponatremia and fluid retention has been reported in patients with congestive heart failure using antacids for gastrointestinal distress (Rimer and Frankland 1968), and it has been suggested that even healthy elderly persons should not consume more than 100 mEq (2300 mg) of sodium derived from antacids per day. OTC antacids containing more than 5 mEq of sodium per maximum dose must carry an appropriate cautionary label (*Federal Register* 1973). Fortunately, most antacids contain only small amounts of sodium (Table 15-8). Effervescent preparations and those containing sodium bicarbonate are the major exceptions.

Table 15-8
Some Antacids Containing Relatively High Amounts of Sodium Per Dose

Product	Dose	Milligrams of sodium per dose
Alka-Seltzer (blue)	tablet	521
Alka-Seltzer (gold)	tablet	276
Bell-Ans	tablet	147
Bisodol	powder	157
Brioschi	powder	710
Bromo-Seltzer	powder	758
Carbamine	powder	499
Citrocarbonate	powder	701
Eno	powder	780
Fizrin	powder	674
Gelusil Lac	powder	112
Kolantyl	tablet	20
Rolaids	tablet	53
Soda Mint	tablet	89
Willard's	tablet	230

Side Effects and Interactions

Several clinically important drug interactions with antacids may occur (Hurwitz 1977). Antacids may increase the absorption of acidic drugs and decrease the absorption of basic drugs by changing intestinal pH. Drugs may be adsorbed by antacids and (in the case of levodopa) antacids can accelerate the passage of the drug from the gut, thus decreasing its inactivation by the gastric mucosa. By delaying gastric emptying, antacids can also delay absorption of drugs that are primarily absorbed from the intestine. The elderly may be particularly vulnerable to these effects as they are likely being maintained on multiple drug therapy. It is difficult to arrive at general conclusions, however; some drugs may be affected by aluminum-containing antacids, others by magnesium-containing antacids, and still others by carbonates. Frequently, the specific antacid involved in an interaction is not mentioned.

It is thought that antacids may cause decreased absorption of the following drugs:

> Anticoagulants
> Barbiturates
> Chlordiazepoxide
> Chlorpromazine
> Digoxin
> Isoniazid
> Lithium carbonate
> Nitrofurantoin
> Penicillin G
> Phenytoin
> Salicylates
> Tetracyclines
> Vitamins

Conversely, they may increase the absorption of:

> Dicoumarol (only
>   magnesium hydroxide)
> Levodopa
> Nalidixic acid
> Sulfonamides

As many of these are drugs frequently prescribed for the elderly, failure to react to drug therapy as anticipated should be evaluated in terms of possible concurrent antacid use by the patient.

The elimination processes of some drugs can also be influenced by agents that affect urinary pH. An increase in urinary pH, which can be caused by antacid therapy, can lead to increased excretion of acidic drugs and decreased excretion of basic drugs, which changes blood levels and the intensity and duration of drug effects. Antacids have been shown to affect urinary pH to varying degrees (Table 15-9) (Gibaldi et al 1974).

Urinary pH also has a pronounced effect on the efficacy of several drugs used to treat urinary tract infection. Methenamine and the tetracyclines are most active when urinary pH is 5.5 or less and antacids could, therefore, negate their effect. The effectiveness of

Table 15-9
Effect of Some Antacids on Urinary pH

Preparation	Increase in urinary pH (units)
Robalate	None
Titralac	0.41
Phillip's Milk of Magnesia	0.48
Maalox	0.86

erythromycin against gram-negative bacterial infection can be maximized if the urine is alkalinized and the dose of gentamicin and kanamycin can be decreased, thus decreasing their toxicity, to which the elderly are especially sensitive, when the urine is alkaline (Hussar 1971).

Use of antacids and their specific ingredients has been shown to affect the elderly patient's status and concurrent drug therapy. Thus, it is important to ascertain whether or not elderly patients use these products.

COUGH AND COLD PREPARATIONS

The common cold is a self-limiting respiratory infection caused by one or more viruses. Its course may extend for 7 to 14 days, and while it is rarely serious in the younger adult, its effects may be much more serious in elderly persons who suffer already from multiple diseases, a compromised respiratory system, and subclinical malnutrition. The elderly are also more susceptible to secondary bacterial infections, as their cellular and humoral defense mechanisms may fail to resist pathogenic microorganisms.

The common cold occurs most often in autumn, major incidence peaks also are observed during late winter and early spring. The incidence of the common cold decreases with advancing age because of increasing immunity. The first symptoms of the common cold are usually a dry throat and nose, followed by accumulation of secretions in the air passages, nose, throat, and bronchial tubes.

Diseases associated with common colds are pharyngitis, sinusitis, laryngitis, bronchiolitis, bronchitis, pneumonia, and influenza.

OTC cough and cold products afford some relief, usually temporary, from the symptoms of the common cold (Adams 1967; Lamy and Rotkovitz 1972; Lamy 1973).

In general, OTC antitussives are designed to diminish coughs associated with acute, self-limiting conditions that irritate the respiratory tract. They should not be used for persistent or chronic cough that occurs with asthma or emphysema. Expectorants facilitate the evacuation of secretions from the bronchial airways. They are useful in treatment of an irritating, nonproductive cough. These products, too, should not be used in chronic conditions.

Elderly patients may be more susceptible to the action of the ingredients, singly or combined, of the cough and cold preparations.

Alcohol Many of the liquid cough and cold preparations contain a minimal amount of alcohol, and clinically significant drug interactions probably would not occur. However, some products contain as much as 40% alcohol (Table 15-10). Elderly patients self administering those products and also receiving phenothiazines or sedatives are exposed to a possible potentiated effect of the prescription drug.

Table 15-10
The Alcohol Content of Some OTC Cough and Cold Preparations*

Product	Alcohol concentration (%)
Actol Expectorant	12.5
Anatuss Syrup	12.0
Breacol	10.0
Broncho-Tussin	40.0
Coldene Adult Cough Formula	15.0
Consotus Antitussive	10.0
Dristan Liquid	12.0
Formula 44-D	10.0
GG-Cen Syrup	10.0
Halls Cough Syrup	22.0
Novahistine DMX Liquid	10.0
Nyquil	25.0
Quiet-Nite Syrup	25.0
Romilar III Syrup	10.0
Terpin Hydrate Elixir	43.0
Trind Syrup	15.0
Trind DM Syrup	15.0
Tussend Expectorant	15.0

*Listing includes only those products containing at least 10% alcohol.

Antihistamines Antihistamines, in small doses, are included in many of these products to suppress symptoms caused by histamine release, such as sniffles, watery eyes, and itching. The antihistamines differ in their adverse effects and patients' responses also vary markedly (*Medical Letter* 1977a). The most frequently encountered adverse effect is sedation, to which the elderly are probably more susceptible than are younger adults. As the antihistamines may cause drowsiness, concurrent alcohol intake is not advised. Elderly patients with asthma, glaucoma, and men with prostate gland enlargement should be advised against using products containing antihistamines.

Anticholinergics Belladonna alkaloids, such as atropine, are often included in cold preparations to inhibit excessive nasal and lacrimal secretions. The elderly may be particularly at risk to the side effects of these agents, because of diseases (eg, glaucoma), or they may already be receiving drugs with anticholinergic properties, such as the phenothiazines or the antiparkinsonism drugs. Elderly patients should discontinue these OTC drugs when constipation, excessive dryness of mouth, insomnia, excitement, confusion, rapid pulse, or blurred vision occur. Such side effects may be difficult to ascertain, as the elderly patient may already suffer from insomnia. Other drugs may be responsible for confusional states. Digoxin may cause blurred vision, and the phenothiazines may cause mouth dryness.

In any case, these products should not be taken by elderly patients with asthma, glaucoma, or an enlarged prostate gland. Nine percent of the elderly may suffer from glaucoma, and patients with angle closure glaucoma are particularly susceptible to increasing intraocular pressure caused by anticholinergic agents (Lund 1972).

Finally, excessive use of atropine slows ciliary beat and will eventually cause complete loss of ciliary movement (Burn 1954), depriving the body of an essential defense mechanism, which may already be compromised in the elderly.

Bronchodilators and decongestants These are mainly sympathomimetic amines. Bronchodilators are used for the symptomatic relief of wheezing and shortness of breath associated with asthma. They are less useful in relieving the shortness of breath of chronic bronchitis and emphysema. Nasal decongestants, which can be used topically as nose drops or orally as tablets, reduce nasal obstruction in patients with acute or chronic rhinitis. Nearly all cold preparations contain a sympathomimetic amine (Table 15-11).

Some of these products, particularly the oral dosage forms, may cause nervousness, dizziness, or insomnia (McLaurin et al 1961). The sympathomimetic amines also facilitate glycogen breakdown, causing increased blood sugar levels, therefore directly opposing the action of insulin. This has to be considered in determining the insulin dosage for a diabetic patient.

The elderly (who probably read cautionary labels as infrequently as others), should be told that products with these ingredients are contraindicated in patients with high blood pressure, those who take antidepressants, as well as diabetic and thyroid patients.

Table 15-11
Some OTC Cough and Cold Products Containing Antihistamines and/or Sympathomimetic Amines

Inhalation products	Tablets and capsules
Adrenalin Chloride	4 Way Cold Tablets
AsthmaNefrin	Allerest
Breatheasy	Bronitin
Bronkaid Mist	Bromo-Quinine
Epinephrine Solution	Bronkaid
Medihaler-Epi	Cheracol Cold Capsules
Primatene Mist	Chexit
	Citrisum
Liquids	Colchek
Coldene	Contac
Novahistine	Coricidin
Orthoxicol	Coricidin-D
Robitussin	Coryban-D
Romilar CF	Dondril
Sudafed	Dristan
Super Anahist Cough Syrup	Fedrazil
Triaminic	Thephorin
Triaminicol	Thephorin-AC
Trind	Theracin
Nasal sprays and nose drops	Triaminicin
Alconefrine	Tri-Span
Contac	Tussagesic
Drilitol	Ursinus Inlay-Tabs
Neo-Synephrine	Zantrate
NTZ	
Privine	
Sinex	
St. Joseph's Nose Drops for Children	
Super Anahist	
Vasoxyl	

Sugar Some of the liquid cough and cold preparations contain high amounts of sugar, and may be contraindicated in diabetic patients who are hard to control. Some of these products are listed in Table 15-12.

OTC cough and cold preparations are useful in treating symptoms of the common cold. However, they do contain ingredients to which the elderly in particular may react adversely. Furthermore, some of the ingredients are contraindicated in diseases and conditions frequently encountered among the elderly. Therefore, these products should be used only episodically with advice, and preferably under the supervision of a primary care provider.

Table 15-12
The Approximate Sucrose Content of Some OTC
Cough and Cold Preparations

Product	Sucrose gm/5 ml*
Chlortrimeton	3.0
Coricidin	3.5
Dristan	3.0
Robitussin	2.8
St. Joseph's	3.9
Triaminic	3.6
Trind	2.5

*Expressed in the usual dose. Most likely, a patient will consume this dose three to four times daily.

LAXATIVES

The Past Revisited*

The public has two common misconceptions regarding the use of laxatives. The first is that a daily bowel movement is absolutely essential to health and the second is that the use of laxatives is harmless and without danger. The facts are...that with the average adult a daily bowel movement is not a necessity for a state of health and, further, cathartics are habit-producing drugs which should be used only in cases of temporary disturbance and only occasionally by the normal person and never habitually. Some years ago, a British physician urged that advertisements of laxatives should be attacked by the medical profession as inimical to the public health.

What the public does not realize is that laxative drugs are probably among the most frequent causes of constipation, for such drugs produce evacuation from over-stimulation of the intestinal tract. As Fantus has well put it: 'Even the mildest and blandest laxatives as well as enemas must be charged with a tendency to get the bowel into sluggish habits, for the very ease with which soft or liquid contents pass along the large bowel diminishes the necessity for muscular effort and leads to atony and ultimate atrophy.'

*From: A.J. Cramp. *Nostrums and Quackery and Pseudo-Medicine*. Chicago, Ill.: American Medical Association, 1936.

Laxatives are the single most frequently used class of drugs in nursing homes and extended care facilities. Almost 60% of all patients receive at least one laxative daily (US Department of Health, Education and Welfare 1976). As Table 15-13 shows, there is considerable qualitative and quantitative difference in the use of laxatives between long-term care institutions and short-term hospitals, as well as among long-term care institutions. Overall, the majority of laxatives used in nursing homes are saline laxatives; a greater variety is used in short-term hospitals.

In long-term care institutions, milk of magnesia is used twice as often as stool softeners; the difference is not as great in short-term hospitals. The most commonly used laxatives and their site of action are listed in Table 15-14.

Table 15-13
Institutional Use of Cathartics

	Percentages		
Type	LTC*	SNF	STH
Saline	37.5	17.8	29.8
Stimulant	27.0	20.5	10.3
Stool softeners	21.5	19.5	39.7
Total	86.0	58.0	59.6

*LTC = Long-Term Care (US Department of Health, Education and Welfare 1976)
SNF = Skilled Nursing Facility (Lamy and Krug 1978)
STH = Short-Term Hospital (Miller 1976)

Table 15-14
Commonly Used Laxatives

Name	Site of Action
Bulk Laxatives	
Methylcellulose	Small and large intestine
Psyllium	Small and large intestine
Saline laxatives	
Magnesium citrate	Small and large intestine
Magnesium sulfate	Small and large intestine
Sodium phosphate	Small and large intestine
Stimulant laxatives	
Aloe	Colon
Bisacodyl	Colon
Cascara sagrada	Colon
Castor oil	Colon
Danthron	Colon
Phenolphthalein	Colon
Senna	Colon
Stool softeners	
Calcium and Dioctyl sodium sulfosuccinate	Colon

Among elderly ambulant patients, laxative use is also high. It has been estimated that between 30% and 50% of the elderly use laxatives (Cummings 1974; Hyams 1974). Those over 70 years of age are thought to use laxatives twice as often as people between 40 and 50 years of age.

Constipation

Constipation is a decrease in frequency of bowel movements, accompanied by a prolonged and difficult passage of stool, followed by a sensation of incomplete evacuation (Derezin 1975). Alternatively, constipation has been defined as an infrequent and difficult evacuation of feces. In constipation, mean colonic transit time is significantly slowed, but gastric emptying time and small intestinal transit time do not change (Walter 1975).

Preoccupation with bowel function is common in old age. Many older people believe themselves to be constipated, and many are. Statistics (National Center for Health Statistics 1973) show that there is an increasing incidence of constipation with age and that low-income, female patients most often complain about constipation (Table 15-15).

Table 15-15
Prevalence of Constipation per 1000 Population

Characteristics	All ages	65 years and over
Total	23.8	96.3
Male	13.7	62.5
Female	33.1	121.9
White	23.8	96.5
All other	23.7	94.7
Northeast residence	18.1	73.6
North central	19.6	79.4
South	34.5	137.8
West	19.1	85.9
Low income	46.5	115.9
Medium	18.2	67.5
High	12.3	58.1

It is not at all clear whether or not complaints about constipation do coincide with actual constipation. Often, patient complaints revolve around misconceptions of normal bowel function and the belief that serious consequences could result if the bowel is not evacuated daily. In fact, there is no consistent alteration of bowel frequency with advancing age. A healthy, male population averaged an interval between bowel evacuations of almost 28 hours, ranging between 9 and 57 hours (Rendtorf and Kashgarian 1967). No relationship of decreased bowel frequency and age has been demonstrated (Connell et al 1965).

Possible causes of constipation Poor dentition is often cited as a contributing factor; it can lead to poor nutrition, both qualitative and quantitative. Poor dietary intake may also be related to anorexia caused by an impaired sense of smell and taste, bland food, or various organic disease states. The elderly ambulant patient may lack the ability or facility to cook, or other socioeconomic reasons may be responsible for poor nutrition. Lack of adequate fluid intake, particularly by incontinent patients, contributes to the problem. Lack of exercise is also a factor, most certainly with bedbound patients.

Slow transit time, incomplete emptying, and diminished awareness of a loaded or overloaded rectum may also be causative factors (Hyams 1974). Elderly prone to constipation should avoid milk, as ingestion of cow's milk is a common cause of constipation, obstipation, and fecal impaction in the elderly (Fingl 1975). Small, hard, infrequent stools are often caused by diets low in fruit or vegetable fiber and insufficient fluid intake.

A multitude of mechanical, physiologic, and psychologic factors can cause constipation (Table 15-16).

Diverticular disease, neurologic disease, fissures, or hemorrhoids may be involved, in addition to hypokalemia or hypothyroidism, depression, or stress (Almy 1954). Drugs are frequently involved. Ganglionic blocking agents are frequently cited (Davies and Gold 1977). The tricyclic antidepressants, frequently prescribed for the

Table 15-16
Some Causes of Constipation

Disease
  Cancer
  Diverticulosis
  Fissures
  Hemorrhoids
  Hypokalemia
  Hypothyroidism

Nutritional Status
  Inadequate bulk intake
  Inadequate fluid intake
  Obesity

Other Patient Characteristics
  Depression
  Diminished physical activity
  Emotional stress

elderly, are constipating because of their direct, atropine-like effect on colonic smooth muscle (Ayd 1961). The antihistamines, antiparkinsonism drugs, glutethimide, meperidine, and phenothiazines are all anticholinergic drugs. Among the elderly, use of more than one anticholinergic occurs often, and additive anticholinergic effects are produced at the receptor sites, which leads to constipation (Hootnick 1956). Other drugs, such as aluminum or calcium carbonate-containing antacids, iron salts, sedatives, and opiates can also be responsible for constipation in the elderly (Pietrusko 1977).

Diagnosis Before laxative use is initiated, a definite diagnosis is necessary. The elderly suffer from three forms of constipation: hypertonic, hypotonic, and dyschezial; hypotonic constipation is most common (Palmer 1976). This is characterized by a partially full colon and soft, putty-like stool so that stool softeners are of little benefit. In many elderly institutionalized patients, presbycolon, in which constipation is combined with colon gas and impaction, is common (Palmer 1976). Among elderly ambulant patients, the dyschezial constipation should be suspected. It is based on habitual laxative use. In an effort to maintain daily bowel movements, increased doses of a laxative are used by the patient, or the patient switches to a stronger laxative. Laxatives can provoke a "cathartic colon," or the irritable bowel syndrome (Cummings 1974). Diagnosis of laxative abuse and its resultant disorders is often difficult as patients may deny this habit or would not volunteer information (LaRusso and McGill 1975; Gossain and Wrk 1972). Watery diarrhea, weight loss, and weakness may be signs of chronic intake of large doses of laxatives (Wittoesch et al 1958). Over 90% of patients suffering chronic ill health from laxative abuse are women (Cummings 1974). Morbid anatomic changes in cathartic colon, which can only be diagnosed by biopsy, include damage and loss of the intrinsic innervation, atrophy of the smooth muscle coat, and melanosis coli (Smith 1973). This pigment indicates chronic use of the anthraquinone cathartics, such as aloe, cascara, rhubarb, or senna.

Appropriate Use

Valid indications for laxative use are limited (Fingl 1975). The need for their use is clear in patients who must avoid straining, those with coronary artery disease, aortic aneurysm, or cerebrovascular accident. Otherwise, laxative use should be carefully evaluated in view of the fact that constipation can lead to fecal incontinence, intestinal obstruction, mental disturbances, retention of urine, or rectal bleeding (Hyams 1974). Appropriate laxatives must be used in patients 1) whose abdominal and perineal muscles have become atrophied, 2) with diminished food intake, 3) who have lost partial or complete rectal reflex, 4) with altered bowel motility caused by drug therapy (*AMA Drug Evaluations* 1977).

The Food and Drug Administration (*Federal Register* 1975) suggests laxative use when there is need to increase bowel frequency, to soften stool, or to increase bulk. It has been suggested that for elderly patients with weak muscles, a bulk-forming agent combined with small doses of a stimulant is effective (*AMA Drug Evaluations* 1977). Often, suggested management of constipation in the elderly revolves around the use of naturally laxative foods, such as fruits and vegetables, oatmeal, cracked wheat bread, or bran, as well as exercise and maintenance of regular bowel habits. However, it may be difficult, if not impossible, to retrain a chronically abused, malfunctioning, dyskinetic colon (Palmer 1976). In such cases, the least harmful laxative should be chosen and administered in a dose sufficient to produce the desired action.

Bulk laxatives If a constipating, low-residue diet cannot be corrected, bulk laxatives are indicated (Fingl 1975). Bulk laxatives, rather than enemas or stronger laxatives, are also indicated in the treatment of constipation caused by uncomplicated diverticular disease. However, when colon strictures are present, bulk laxatives are contraindicated. Some bulk laxatives are also marketed in an effervescent form that usually contains a large amount of sodium.

Stool softeners Stool softeners are commonly used by the elderly. They promote defecation merely by a modest softening of the stool and do not promote peristalsis, either directly or indirectly. Surface-active properties permit water to penetrate the fecal mass, thus softening the stool. Their clinical usefulness is limited (Fingl 1975), but they appear to be most useful in relieving constipation caused by hard, dry stools in persons with normal intestinal tone. They are recommended for prevention of constipation induced by the use of tricyclic antidepressants (Stimmel 1975). Much of their advantage in chronic constipation appears to be lost by combining them with cathartic drugs (Aviado 1972).

Saline laxatives Saline laxatives attract water to the intestinal lumen, where the water is retained, creating intestinal motility. They are widely used, although strong-acting cathartics are not recommended for the elderly (Hyams 1974); they can cause dehydration and considerable damage to gut physiology. Sodium phosphate, a saline laxative, should be avoided in patients with hypocalcemia. Milk of magnesia is probably the safest and most widely used saline laxative.

Stimulant laxatives The stimulant laxatives are viewed favorably for use by the elderly. They increase peristaltic activity by acting on intestinal nerves and muscles, but prolonged and chronic use can lead to laxative dependency. There are two types of stimulant laxatives. Those containing anthraquinone are cascara, danthron, and senna. Bisacodyl and phenolphthalein are diphenylmethane derivatives.

Dietary fiber The incidence of noninfectious diseases in East Africa and in Western industrialized nations was studied and compared to dietary intake. Among those were colonic diseases, including constipation and diverticular disease. It was concluded that there may be a correlation between these diseases and dietary fiber intake (Trowell 1960; Burkitt 1973; Walker 1974; Burkitt and Trowell 1975). However, it is still not known which components of dietary fiber influence fecal bulking or water retention in the stool. The association of dietary fiber with objective alterations in colonic functions, such as decreased stool transit and increased stool bulk has so far rested exclusively on epidemiologic evidence, but there are now data available based on a controlled, clinical trial that shows improvement of bowel habits in one-half of the study patients because of high fiber diet (Mannin et al 1977). The Food and Drug Administration (*Federal Register* 1975) views dietary bran as a bulk-forming laxative. Bran is safe and effective in doses of 6 gm to 16 gm daily when there is adequate (one to two full glasses) water intake (Payler 1973; Cummings, 1973; *Medical Letter* 1973).

Bran-rich breakfast cereals and whole wheat bread are convenient sources. One hundred grams of bran flakes contain between 2.7 and 6.5 gm of crude fiber, and one slice of whole wheat bread contains between 1 and 2 gm. Bran should not be given to patients with partial digestive tract obstruction; it may lead to complete obstruction. Unprocessed bran should be used with caution because of its high phytic acid content, which may impair calcium absorption in patients with a vitamin D deficiency (Hyams 1974).

Adverse Effects of Laxatives

Castor oil, mineral oil, or phenolphthalein should not be used by the elderly. All of the other laxatives may also cause adverse effects, to which the elderly are especially sensitive (Miller 1976) (Table 15-17).

Table 15-17
Failure Rates and Adverse Effects of Laxatives in Hospital Patients

Name	Failure rate (%)	Adverse reactions of recipients (%)
Bisacodyl	10	3.2
Cascara	10	2.6
Dioctyl sodium sulfosuccinate	8	2.5
Magnesium citrate	9	2.5
Milk of magnesia	9	1.8
Psyllium	15	1.8
Sodium phosphate	12	1.0

Bulk laxatives The bulk laxatives, ie, the hydrophilic agents and mucilaginous substances, should be administered with large volumes of water to avoid the hazard of intestinal obstruction. They can be especially dangerous if there is a narrowing of the gut or if the patient is dehydrated. Some bulk laxatives may contain as much as 50% dextrose. Plant gums can also cause allergies. Bulk laxatives, though, are probably least likely to cause laxative abuse (*AMA Drug Evaluations* 1977). Apparently, they do not interfere with intestinal absorption of essential nutrients. As they only act when fully hydrated, their full effect may not manifest for 72 hours.

Stool softeners The toxicity of stool softeners, whether potential or real, has been discussed frequently. Animal studies indicate that dioctyl sodium sulfosuccinate is toxic to hepatic cells and may contribute to the hepatotoxicity of other drugs (*Medical Letter* 1977b), but evidence is inconclusive and the incidence of this toxicity may be negligible (Bond 1977). Other adverse effects of this laxative manifest as rash, fever, and incontinence, which are more likely to occur in elderly than in younger patients (Miller 1976).

Saline laxatives The major hazard of saline laxatives is their ability to cause electrolyte disturbances. The elderly exhibit a diminished capacity to return a disturbed fluid and electrolyte balance to a normal level; in fact, the electrolyte balance may already be disturbed by the use of diuretics. Older persons also lose some ability to concentrate urine, which can lead to dehydration if fluid intake is inadequate. This can exacerbate fluid loss caused by saline laxative use. Excessive use may also lead to gastrointestinal loss of potassium and, thus, to hypokalemia. Dehydration can lead to fever, flushing, tachycardia, and personality changes.

Disturbance of the water and electrolyte balance is particularly undesirable in older patients with concurrent cardiac difficulties. In uremic patients, there is an increased risk of magnesium toxicity (Jameson 1972), and preparations containing large amounts of sodium may be hazardous to patients with edema or congestive heart failure. Interactions, of course, can also occur. For example, sodium sulfate decreases the absorption and urinary excretion of INH (Matilla 1974).

Stimulant laxatives Excessive use of stimulant laxatives can lead to electrolyte disturbances, particularly to hypokalemia, to changes in the colonic rectal mucosa, and to a "cathartic colon" (Houghton and Pears 1958; Aitchison 1958). Some cause cramps, diarrhea, and dehydration. Senna is unlikely to disturb the fluid and electrolyte balance and its use is recommended, particularly for institutionalized elderly patients (Hyams 1974).

Some interactions of laxatives involve mineral oil, which should not be used in the elderly (Table 15-18).

The elderly use laxatives frequently, probably more than the general population. Although there is no valid reason for frequent use,

Table 15-18
Interactions of Laxatives with Some Other Drugs

Laxative	Other Drug	Result of Interaction
Dioctyl sodium sulfosuccinate	Mineral oil	Absorption of mineral oil may be increased. Should not be given concurrently for prolonged period of time.
Bisacodyl (enteric coated)	Antacids	Increased pH may cause disintegration of the coating and release the drug in stomach. May result in vomiting and nausea.
Mineral oil	Oral anticoagulants	Variable alterations of the anticoagulant effect have occurred.
	Poloxalkol	Absorption of mineral oil may be increased. Should not be given concurrently over prolonged period of time.
	Vitamins	Prolonged administration of mineral oil may reduce the absorption of oil-soluble vitamins (A,D,E,K).

occasional use is probably safe and effective. Chronic use can lead to electrolyte and water balance disturbances and, in some instances, to pathologic tissue changes. Correct dietary and fluid intake and exercise may help, if the colon is not chronically abused, malfunctioning, and dyskinetic.

VITAMINS

While the evidence for vitamin deficiency in the elderly is equivocal, use of vitamin supplementation appears high. It has been suggested that excessive intake is probably the rule, not the exception.

Although vitamins are not prescription drugs, excessive intake can lead to unanticipated clinical consequences, especially in the elderly. There is extensive literature on the toxicities of megadoses of vitamins A and D (DiPalma and Ritchie 1977). There is also some evidence that excess thiamine intake affects the cardiovascular and nervous systems. Niacin, if taken in excess, is responsible for abnormal liver function and high blood levels of uric acid and glucose. Excessive intake of riboflavin is associated with convulsive disorders but, on the other hand, large doses of pyridoxine interfere with normal utilization of riboflavin. Excessive folic acid intake may lead to toxicities involving the CNS and renal system. Megadoses of vitamin C may cause precipitation of cystine and oxalate stones in the urinary tract, may block utilization of vitamin B-12, and may shorten prothrombin time when heparin or warfarin is used (Rosenthal 1971).

Vitamins can also interfere with many laboratory test results. Some possible interactions are listed in Table 15-19:

Table 15-19
Effect of Some Vitamins on Some Laboratory Test Values

Laboratory test	Vitamin	Effect of vitamin on laboratory test values
Alkaline phosphatase	Vitamin D	Decreased or false negative
Bilirubin and icteric index	Vitamin K and K$_2$ (large doses in newborn)	Elevated or false positive
Calcium in serum	Vitamin D	Elevated or false positive
Calcium in urine	Vitamin D	Elevated or false positive
Cholesterol	Vitamin A	Elevated or false positive
Erythrocyte count and/or hemoglobin	Vitamin A (excess dose and use)	Decreased or false negative
Glucose (Benedict's)	Ascorbic acid	Elevated or false positive
Glucose (oxidase)	Ascorbic acid	Decreased or false negative
Leukocytes	Vitamin A (prolonged use)	Decreased or false negative
NPN	Vitamin D	Elevated or false positive
Occult blood in stool	Ascorbic acid (high doses)	Decreased or false negative
Occult blood in urine (Guaiac test)	Ascorbic acid (high doses)	Decreased or false negative
PBI	Vitamin A and D (Cod liver oil preparation)	Elevated or false positive
Phosphate (inorganic) in serum	Vitamin D	Elevated or false positive
Protein in urine	Vitamin D	Decreased or false negative
Prothrombin time	Vitamin A, Vitamin K	Elevated or false positive
Sedimentation rate	Vitamin A	Elevated or false positive
Uric acid in serum	Ascorbic acid	Elevated or false positive

The primary provider caring for the elderly receiving chronic drug treatment must also be aware that many drugs used in chronic care can induce vitamin deficiency states (Tables 15-20 and 15-21).

There are many complex nutrient interrelationships and the balance between vitamins, minerals, and sources of energy, ie, proteins, fats, and carbohydrates, is very important. Many studies have shown that the elderly may suffer from subclinical vitamin deficiencies, that may be excacerbated by chronic use of drugs, certain diseases and stress. Vitamin deficiencies, which may manifest a year after the beginning of the deficiency, can be corrected by simple supplementation, but complete dependency on vitamin supplementation in old age is undesirable. There must be a well-balanced diet of core foods and vitamins. Excessive use of vitamins leads to adverse effects.

Table 15-20
Drugs That May Induce Deficiency of Fat-Soluble Vitamins

Drug	Vitamin
Antacids Cholestyramine Colchicine Mineral oil	A
Barbiturates (anticonvulsants) Cholestyramine Mineral oil Phenytoin Primidone	D
Alcohol Chloramphenicol Cholestyramine Coumarins Kanamycin Mineral oil Neomycin Polymyxin Sulfonamides Tetracyclines	K

Table 15-21
Drugs That May Induce Deficiency of Water-Soluble Vitamins

Drug	Vitamin
Alcohol Antacids	B-1 (thiamine)
Hydralazine Isoniazid Penicillamine	B-6 (pyridoxine)
Cholestyramine Colchicine Kanamycin Neomycin Para-aminosalicylic acid Trifluperazine	B-12 (cyanocobalamin)
Aspirin Alcohol	C (ascorbic acid)
Aspirin Barbiturates (anticonvulsants) Cycloserine Methotrexate Nitrofurantoin Para-aminosalicylic acid Phenytoin Primidone Pyrimethamine Sulfasalazine Trimethoprim	Folic acid

OTC PRODUCTS AND ANTICOAGULANTS

As elderly patients are frequently receiving anticoagulants, Table 15-22 summarizes the possible interactions of OTC products and anticoagulants (Bernstein 1974).

Table 15-22
Interactions of Some OTC Products
With Coumarin-type Anticoagulants

Product	Possible effect
Acetaminophen (8 tablets per day)	Potentiation
Antipyrine	Inhibition
Ascorbic acid	Potentiation
Aspirin (more than 1 gm/day)	Potentiation
Laxatives (oxyphenisatin, phenolphthalein)	Potentiation
Mineral oil	Potentiation
Psyllium hydrophilic mucilloid	Inhibition
Vitamin A (excessive intake)	Inhibition

REFERENCES

Adams, J.M. *Viruses and Cold, The Modern Plague.* New York: Elsevier North Holland, Inc., 1967.

Aitchison, J.D. Hypokalaemia following chronic diarrhoea from overuse of cascara and a deficient diet. *Lancet* 2:75, 1958.

Almy, T.P. Physiological and psychological factors in the production of constipation. *Ann NY Acad Sci.* 58:398, 1954.

American Medical Association. *Drug Evaluations,* 2nd ed. Acton, Mass.: Publishing Sciences Group, 1973.

American Medical Association. *Drug Evaluations,* 3rd ed. Littleton, Mass.: PSG Publishing Company, Inc., 1977.

Ambre, J.J., and Fischer, L.J. Effect of coadministration of aluminum and magnesium hydroxides on absorption of anticoagulants in man. *Clin Pharmacol Ther.* 14:231, 1973.

Ameer, B., and Greenblatt, D.J. Acetaminophen. *Ann Intern Med.* 87:202, 1977.

Aviado, D.M. (Ed.). *Krantz and Carr's Pharmacologic Principles of Medical Practice.* Baltimore, Md.: Williams and Wilkins Co., 1972.

Ayd, D.F. Antidepressants: a critique. *Dis Nerv Syst.* 22(suppl):32, 1961.

Barreras, R.F. Calcium and gastric secretion. *Gastroenterology.* 64:1168, 1973.

Beaver, W.T. Mild analgesics: a review of their clinical pharmacology. *Am J Med Sci.* 250:577, 1965.

Beaver, W.T. Mild analgesics: a review of their clinical pharmacology, Part II. *Am J Med Sci.* 251:576, 1966.

Bernstein, D. Drugs known to react with coumarin-type anticoagulants, revised. *Drug Intell Clin Pharm.* 8:172, 1974.

Bond, W.S. Safety of stool softeners. *J Am Pharm Assoc.* 17:588, 1977.

Boykin, S.P., Burkhart, V.P., and Lamy, P.P. Drug use in a day treatment center. *Am J Hosp Pharm.* 35:155, 1978.

Burkitt, D.P. Some diseases characteristic of modern Western civilization. *Br Med J.* 1:274, 1973.

Burkitt, D.P., and Trowell, H.C. (Eds.). *Refined Carbohydrate Foods and Disease, Some Implications of Dietary Fibre.* London: Academic Press, 1975.

Burn, J.H. Acetylcholine as a local hormone for ciliary movement and the heart. *Pharmacol Rev.* 6:107, 1954.

Burry, H.C., and Dieppe, P.A. Apparent reduction of endogenous creatinine clearance by salicylate treatment. *Br Med J.* 2:16, 1976.

Butler, R.N. *Energy and Aging.* Washington, D.C.: National Institute of Aging, 1977.

Case, R.M. Calcium and gastrointestinal secretion. *Digestion* 8:269, 1973.

Chaiton, A., Spitzer, W.O., Roberts, R.S. et al. Patterns of medical drug use–a community focus. *Can Med Assoc J.* 114:33, 1976.

Chinn, A.B. Clinical aspects of aging. In *Working With Older People,* Vol. 4. PHS Publ. No. 1459. Washington, D.C.: U.S. Government Printing Office, 1971.

Chretien, J.H., Esswein, J.G., McGarvey, M.A. et al. Self-treatment with antibiotics. *Hosp Form.* 11(5):260, 1976.

Connell, A.M., Hilton, C., Irvinennard-Jones, G. et al. Variation of bowel habit in two population samples. *Br Med J.* 2:1095, 1965.

Cummings, J.H. Progress report. Dietary fibre. *Gut* 14:69, 1973.

Cummings, J.H. Progress report. Laxative abuse. *Gut* 15:758, 1974.

Davies, D.M., and Gold, R.G. Cardiac disorders. Edited by D.M. Davies. In *Textbook of Adverse Drug Reactions.* Oxford: Oxford University Press, 1977.

Derezin, M. Laxatives and fecal modifiers. *Am Fam Physician.* 10:126, 1975.

DiCyan, E., Hessman, L. *Without Prescription.* New York: Simon and Schuster, 1972.

DiPalma, J.R., and Ritchie, D.M. Vitamin toxicity. *Ann Rev Pharmacol Toxicol.* 17:133, 1977.

Douglas, R.A., and Johnson, E.D. Aspirin and chronic gastric ulcer. *Med J Aust.* 11:893, 1961.

Federal Register. 38(65):8710, 5 April 1973.

Federal Register. 40(56):12904-12908, 21 March 1975.

Fingl, E. Laxatives and cathartics. Edited by L.S. Goodman, and A. Gilman. In *The Pharmacological Basis of Therapeutics.* New York: MacMillan Publishing Company, Inc., 1975.

Fordtran, J.S., Morawski, S.G., and Richardson, C.T. In vivo and in vitro evaluation of liquid antacids. *N Engl J Med.* 288:923, 1973.

Fox, R.H., MacGibbon, R., Davies, L. et al. Problem of the old and the cold. *Br Med J.* 1:21, 1973.

Gibaldi, M., Gurndhofer, B., and Levy, G. Effect of antacids on pH of urine. *Clin Pharmacol Ther.* 16:520, 1974.

Gillies, M., and Skyring, A. Gastric ulcer, duodenal ulcer and gastric carcinoma: a case-control study of certain social and environmental factors. *Med J Aust.* 2:1132, 1968.

Goldberger, L.E., and Talner, L.B. Analgesic abuse syndrome: a frequently overlooked cause of reversible renal failure. *Urology* 5:728, 1975.

Gossain, V.V., and Wrk, E.E. Surreptitious laxation and hypokalemia. Letter to the Editor *Ann Intern Med.* 76:671, 1972.

Guttman, D. *A Survey of Drug-Taking Behavior of the Elderly.* Washington, D.C.: Catholic University, 1977.

Hajnal, J., Sharp, J., and Popert, A.J. A method for testing analgesics in rheumatoid arthritis using a sequential procedure. *Ann Rheum Dis.* 18:189, 1959.

Hall, M.R.P. Drugs and the elderly. *Adv Drug Reactions Bull.* 35:108, 1972.

Harvey, S.C. Gastric antacids and digestants. Edited by L.S. Goodman, and A. Gilman. In *The Pharmacological Basis of Therapeutics.* New York: MacMillan Publishing Company, Inc., 1970.

Hootnick, H.L. Constipation in elderly patients due to drug therapy. *J Am Geriatr Soc.* 4:1021, 1956.

Houghton, B.J., and Pears, M.A. Chronic potassium depletion due to purgation with cascara. *Br Med J.* 1:1328, 1958.

Hughes, G. Changes in taste sensitivity with advancing age. *Gerontol Clin.* 11:225, 1959.

Hurwitz, A. Antacid therapy and drug kinetics. *Clin Pharmacokinet.* 2:269, 1977.

Hussar, D.A. Factors predisposing a patient to drug interactions. *Am J Pharm.* 143:177, 1971.

Hyams, D.E. Gastrointestinal problems in the old. *Br Med J.* 1:107, 1974.

Jameson, S. Magnesium-containing antacids to patients with uremia–an intoxication risk. *Scand J Urol Nephrol.* 6:260, 1972.

Jeffreys, M., Brotherston, J.H.F., and Cartwright, A. Consumption of medicines in a working-class housing estate. *Br J Prevent Soc Med.* 14:64, 1960.

Kantor, T.G. When analgesics are interchangeable and when they are not. *Drug Ther.* 6(4):169, 1976.

Koch-Weser, J. Acetaminophen. *N Engl J Med.* 295:1297, 1976.

Koch-Weser, J., and Sellers, E.M. Drug interactions with coumarin anticoagulants, Part 1. *N Engl J Med.* 285:487, 1971.

Lamy, P.P. Cold medicines. Edited by G.B. Griffenhagen, and L.L. Hawkins. In *Handbook of Non-Prescription Drugs.* Washington, D.C.: American Pharmaceutical Association, 1973.

Lamy, P.P. OTC drugs and the ambulant patient, Part I. *Hosp Form.* 10(9):451, 1975a.

Lamy, P.P. OTC drugs and the ambulant patient, Part II. *Hosp Form.* 10(10):499, 1975b.

Lamy, P.P. What the physician should keep in mind when prescribing drugs for an elderly patient. *Geriatrics* 32(5):37, 1977.

Lamy, P.P., and Kitler, M.E. Untoward effects of drugs, Part I. (Including non-prescription drugs). *Dis Nerv Syst.* 32: 18, 1971a.

Lamy, P.P., and Kitler, M.E. Untoward effects of drugs, Part II. (Including non-prescription drugs). *Dis Nerv Syst.* 32:105, 1971b.

Lamy, P.P., and Krug, B.H. Review of laxative utilization in a skilled nursing facility. *J Am Geriatr Soc.* 26:544, 1978.

Lamy, P.P., and Rotkovitz, I.I. The common cold and its management. *J Am Pharm Assoc.* NS12:582, 1972.

Lamy, P.P., Reichel, W., and Weg, R. Make age a factor in the drug equation. *Patient Care* 9(14):136, 1975.

LaRusso, N.F., and McGill, D.S. Surreptitious laxative ingestion. Delayed recognition of a serious condition: a case report. *Mayo Clin Proc.* 50:706, 1975.

Leist, E.R., and Banwell, J.G. Products containing aspirin. *N Engl J Med.* 291:710, 1974.

Leonards, J.R., Levy, G., and Niemezura, R. Gastrointestinal blood loss during prolonged aspirin administration. *N Engl J Med.* 289:1020, 1973.

Levy, G. Aspirin use in patients with major upper gastrointestinal bleeding and peptic ulcer disease. *N Engl J Med.* 290:1158, 1974.

Lim, R.K.S., Guzman, R., Rodgers, D.W. et al. Site of action of narcotic and non-narcotic analgesics determined by blocking bradykinin-evoked visceral pain. *Arch Int Pharmacodyn Ther.* 152:25, 1964.

Littman, A., and Pine, B.H. Antacids and anticholinergic drugs. *Ann Intern Med.* 82:544, 1975.

Lund, O.E. Second roundtable: medical therapy of glaucoma. *Doc Ophthalmol.* 33(1):245, 1972.

Mannin, A.P., Heaton, K.W., Harvey, R.F. et al. Wheat fibre and irritable bowel syndrome. *Lancet* 2:417, 1977.

Matilla, J. Effect of sodium sulfate and castor oil on drug absorption from the human intestine. *Ann Clin Res.* 6:19, 1974.

McLaurin, J.W., Shipman, W.F., and Rosedale, R. Oral decongestants. *Laryngoscope* 71:54, 1961.

Medical Letter. Laxatives and dietary fiber. 15:98, 1973.

Medical Letter. Prazosin (Minipress) for hypertension. 19:1, 1977a.

Medical Letter. Safety of stool softeners. 19:45, 1977b.

Meerloo, J.A.M. The concept of cybernosis. *Sandorama.* 5:4, 1973.

Mielke, C.H., and Britten, A.F.H. Use of aspirin or acetaminophen in hemophilia. Letter to the Editor *N Engl J Med.* 282:1270, 1970.

Miller, R.R. Cathartics. Edited by R.R. Miller, and D.J. Greenblatt. In *Drug Effects in Hospitalized Patients.* New York: John Wiley and Sons, 1976.

Morgan, R.H. Anemia in elderly house-bound patients. *Br Med J.* 4:171, 1967.

Morrissey, J.F., and Barreras, R.F. Antacid therapy. *N Engl J Med.* 290:550, 1974.

Murray, T., and Goldbery, M. Chronic interstitial nephritis: etiologic factors. *Ann Intern Med.* 82:453, 1975.

National Center for Health Statistics. Prevalence of selected chronic digestive conditions, United States, July–December 1968. DHEW Publ. No. (HRA) 74-1510. Rockville, Md., 1973.

Palmer, E.D. Presbycolon problems in the nursing home. *JAMA.* 235:1150, 1976.

Payler, D.K. Food fibre and bowel behavior. Letter to the Editor *Lancet* 1:1394, 1973.

Pietrusko, R.G. Use and abuse of laxatives. *Am J Hosp Pharm.* 34:291, 1977.

Prescott, L.F. Antipyretic analgesics and drugs used in rheumatic diseases and gout. Edited by L. Meyler, and A. Herxheimer. In *Side Effects of Drugs.* Amsterdam: Excerpta Medica, 1972.

Proudfoot, A.T., and Wright, N. Acute paracetamol poisoning. *Br Med J.* 3:557, 1970.

Rendtorff, R.C., and Kashgarian, M. Stool patterns of healthy adult males. *Dis Colon Rect.* 10:222, 1967.

Rimer, D.G., and Frankland, M. Sodium content of antacids. *JAMA.* 173:995, 1968.

Ritschel, W.A., and Erni, W. Evaluation of antacids in man using the Heidelberg capsule. *Drug Dev Ind Pharm.* 4:305, 1978.

Rose, C.S., Gyorgy, P., Butler, M. et al. Age differences in vitamin B-6 status of 617 men. *Am J Clin Nutr.* 29:847, 1970.

Rosenthal, G. Interaction of ascorbic acid and warfarin. *JAMA.* 215:1671, 1971.

Shelley, J.H. Phenacetin, through looking glass. *Clin Pharmacol Ther.* 8:427, 1967.

Sklar, D., Liang, M.H., and Porta, J. Antacids: cost, taste and buffering. *N Engl J Med.* 296:1007, 1977.

Smith, B. Pathologic changes in the colon produced by anthraquinone purgatives. *Dis Colon Rect.* 16:455, 1973.

Stimmel, G.I. Depression. Edited by L.Y. Young, and M. Kimble. In *Applied Therapeutics for Clinical Pharmacists.* San Francisco, Calif.: Applied Therapeutics, 1975.

Trowell, H.C. *Non-Infective Diseases in Africa.* London: Edward Arnold, 1960.

United States Department of Health, Education and Welfare. Long-term care facility improvement campaign. Monograph No. 2. Physicians' drug prescribing patterns in skilled nursing facilities. DHEW Publ. No. (OS)76-50050. Washington, D.C.: U.S. Government Printing Office, 1976.

Walker, A.R.P. Dietary fibre and the pattern of diseases. *Ann Intern Med.* 80:663, 1974.

Walter, S. Differential measurement of small and large bowel transit times in constipation and diarrhoea: a new approach. *Gut* 16:372, 1975.

Weiss, H.J. Aspirin–a dangerous drug? *JAMA.* 229:1221, 1974.

Wilson, D.R., II. Analgesic nephropathy in Canada: a retrospective study of 351 cases. *Can Med Assoc J.* 107:752, 1972.

Wittoesch, J., Jackman, R., and McDonald, J. Melanosis coli: general review and study of 887 cases. *Dis Colon Rect.* 1:172, 1958.

16 Analgesic and Antiinflammatory Drugs

ANALGESICS

Pain, which may be the first sign of a disease, is one of the major reasons that patients seek medical help and advice. The elderly though, often accept pain stoically as an inevitable byproduct of aging. Furthermore, the elderly commonly have difficulty giving an accurate description of the character and locus of pain; pain perception is altered. Pain at the site of origin is rarer than in younger people, but referred pain occurs more often. Pain originating from internal organs can be referred to locomotor regions and referred pain in the superficial tissues is not uncommon (Hunt 1976). Myocardial pain might be referred to the arm or jaw, diaphragmatic pain to the shoulders, and hip pain to the knee. Diffuse pain in the lower extremities may be caused by diabetes or uremia, and diffuse back and pelvic pain in elderly women by osteoporosis. Cervical osteoarthritis or depression, on the other hand, frequently present as muscle-tension headaches in the elderly, to be treated with drugs, moist heat, massage, and other modalities.

Migraine headache occurs less frequently with advancing age. However, vascular headache associated with giant cell arteritis is more prevalent, and could be caused by congestive heart failure, transient ischemia, and metabolic disorders. Any suddenly appearing headache in an elderly patient should trigger a serious investigation, as it may be caused by giant cell arteritis or lesions. Conversely, a sudden onset of a behavioral disorder may be the only sign of a painful state.

General Management of Pain

In the elderly, it may be difficult to differentiate between pain and depression, particularly as chronic pain in the elderly often leads to depression. The patient may also claim to have pain in an effort to explain or cover up a functional impairment, using a "painful condition" as a form of self-protection (Fordyce 1978). For patients with chronic pain, this can lead to a feeling of loss of control of one's life (Sternbach 1978).

Pain seems to be influenced by attention, anxiety, prior conditioning, and other psychologic variables. Some pain may be exacerbated by treatment. Often, pharmacologic, sensory, and psychologic methods must be combined in order to achieve pain relief for the patient (Melzack and Taenzer 1977).

Chronic pain Pain lasting longer than six months is considered chronic pain and can lead to feelings of suspicion, anger, and depression in affected patients. There seems to be a direct relationship between intensity of chronic pain and depression. The effects of this type pain have been called the chronic intractable benign pain syndrome (CIBPS). The range of treatment modalities, fashionable or not, attests to the difficulties one encounters in treating chronic pain. Among them are acupuncture, transcutaneous electrical stimulation, hypnosis, biofeedback training, and others (Pinsky 1978).

Pharmacologic management of pain* There is some dispute regarding the most effective method of pain control using drugs. Control is difficult to achieve. It has been argued that it is impossible to abolish pain by regular analgesic use and that the analgesic can only remove the most severe impact of pain. There is agreement, though, that for institutionalized patients, the delivery of pain medication may be influenced by the nursing staff, who tend to withhold stronger

---

*Only systemic analgesics will be presented. A discussion of external analgesic preparations (most often nonprescription drugs) is beyond the scope of this chapter. However, many people, particularly the elderly, use external preparations extensively for the "aches and pains of rheumatism and arthritis." Such preparations as Yager's Liniment (Yager Drug Co., Baltimore, Md.), based on the traditional ammonia liniment formula, are very popular and their ingredients have been found safe and effective by the recent FDA OTC Review Panel.

medications from the elderly or tend to ask for analgesics to be prescribed "as needed." This is a highly undesirable type of administration, as drugs will then be given on a pain-contingent basis, which may reinforce a patient's pain behavior. Thus, there seems to be no disagreement that pain, particularly chronic pain, should be treated on a time-contingent or fixed-time schedule and not a pain-contingent schedule.

Analgesic usage always follows a set schedule, even in severe pain. Most often, analgesics are administered three or four times per day. However, this usual fixed-time schedule is insufficient. Patients are probably overdosed in the first hour, reasonably well dosed for the next two hours, and underdosed during the last hour. Therefore, analgesics must be given more frequently in order to abolish pain. It has been suggested that administration intervals should be sufficiently close to avoid swings in pain levels. A schedule, once established, should be strictly followed.

It has also been proposed that analgesics should be administered according to an individual schedule. The patient should be observed for pain response. Once this has been established, an analgesic should be administered before the effect of the prior dose has disappeared, even before the patient deems the dose necessary. This would erase both pain and fear of pain.

Whatever administration schedule is chosen, pain should be treated first with the weakest analgesic available, and drug administration should be titrated against the patient's pain. The dose should be increased gradually, or a stronger analgesic should be selected and administered. This process is continued until the patient is pain-free.

Aspirin and Other Salicylates

Aspirin, which is discussed in detail elsewhere, is still the backbone of analgesic therapy. If taken with food, significant gastrointestinal disturbance occurs only rarely. Bleeding can be intensified when gastric contents are acid, but it also occurs in patients with achlorhydria (St. John and McDermott 1970). Aspirin-induced gastric damage appears to be age-related (Rainsford 1975; Abrishami and Thomas 1977). The degree of gastric hemorrhage caused by aspirin is of particular concern in the elderly, as they probably have a reduced blood volume and a reduced hematocrit. Stress is also implicated in hemorrhage caused by aspirin. Tinnitus serves as an important warning symptom of aspirin toxicity (Mongan et al 1973). The metabolite of aspirin, salicylic acid, is pharmacologically active. The metabolic conversion of salicylate becomes less efficient as the dose of aspirin increases. The half-life of aspirin ranges from two to four hours with doses of less than 0.5 gm, to approximately 20 hours when doses greater than 10 gm are administered. When it is important to ascertain if a patient is taking any aspirin-containing drug, it must be remembered that many drugs are marketed with names that do not indicate the presence of aspirin or some other salicylate.

Some literature claims that choline magnesium trisalicylate compares favorably with aspirin. It may be given in a twice daily dosage and is said to cause less gastrointestinal bleeding than aspirin. Furthermore, it does not appear to inhibit platelet aggregation or serotonin release, two effects of aspirin therapy (Cohen and Garber 1978; Cohen 1978; Cohen et al 1978).

Combinations

Many analgesic combinations are available. There has been some dispute as to the effectiveness of analgesic combinations. Apparently, combinations of mild analgesics do not offer greater pain relief than an increased dose of a single effective agent. For example, acetaminophen, in high doses, is significantly more effective in reducing pain intensity and in providing pain relief than a combination of propoxyphen and acetaminophen (Hopkinson et al 1976). Similar data have been presented for a propoxyphen-APC combination versus high doses of acetaminophen (Smith et al 1975).

Narcotic (Schedule II) Analgesics

Narcotic analgesics are poorly tolerated by the elderly. They may precipitate hypotensive periods, particularly in patients with a decreased blood volume. There appears to be a lack of awareness that chronic use of these drugs can lead to major cognitive deficits in elderly patients. Narcotic analgesics can also interfere with sphincter action, particularly the sphincter of Oddi, which is seen in patients with pancreatitis.

Morphine use should be restricted. It has a strong depressant action and should probably not be used at all in patients over 70 years of age (Sale 1952). If its use is unavoidable, the initial dose should be two-thirds the usual adult dose. At times, the use of meperidine has been advocated instead of morphine, but there is no proof that meperidine causes less respiratory depression than morphine (*Medical Letter* 1973). The metabolism of meperidine increases with age (Chan et al 1975).

Codeine should be avoided as it has constipating action and, if not given in therapeutically adjusted doses, may cause dizziness and drowsiness (Davison 1968). Other authorities view codeine as a helpful analgesic in gaining sleep, arguing that adjustment of the diet for a mild laxative effect can counteract its constipating action.

Antidepressants and tranquilizers have been suggested as good adjuncts in the treatment of pain of malignant disease (Davison 1972). Older people tend to respond to placebos with greater frequency of pain relief than younger ones (Lasagna 1971).

Within the past five years, there has been a surge in the use of Brompton's Mixture for the treatment of pain in terminally ill patients (LeShan 1964; Saunders 1967; Forrest et al 1973; Marks and Sachar 1973; Twycross 1973; Twycross 1974a; Twycross 1974b, 1975; Twycross et al 1974; Craven et al 1975; Lipman 1975; Mount 1976; Mount et al 1976; Melzack et al 1976; Weintraub 1977; Maljovec et al 1977).

Brompton's Mixture, also known as Brompton's Elixir or Cocktail, bears the name of the Brompton Chest Hospital in England. Suggested for use in terminally ill patients when nonnarcotic and milder narcotic preparations are found to be ineffective, it was officially recognized by being placed in the British Pharmaceutical Codex in 1973. The original formula contained:

Diamorphine HCl (heroin)	0.0025 (or more)
Cocaine HCl	0.010
Ethyl Alcohol	2.5
Syrup	5.0
Chloroform Water qs ad	20.0

In the United States, chloroform water is not used and morphine is substituted for heroin. It is assumed that 15 mg morphine are equivalent to 10 mg heroin orally.

Morphine is thought to be as effective as heroin as an analgesic. It is less efficiently absorbed when given orally instead of parenterally, but has a prolonged action when given orally. Therefore, it is thought to be efficacious when given orally in the management of chronic pain. The morphine dose can be adjusted up to 120 mg, although most patients will probably respond positively to a dose of 2.5 to 20 mg. One advantage of the liquid oral dosage form, of course, rests with the opportunity to increase the strength of morphine per dose without creating patient awareness of the increase. Some hospitals use methadone instead of morphine, as it is more effective and has a longer half-life. Other hospitals have added amphetamines to the formula in an effort to achieve potentiation of morphine. Amphetamines also serve to antagonize the sedating effect of the narcotic analgesic. The reason for inclusion of cocaine in the formula is controversial. It is thought to act as a mood elevator, but it does not seem to increase patient alertness significantly. However, subjective "highs" in many patients can be greater after intranasal administration (Van Dyke et al

1978). There is no question that some of it is absorbed orally (Inaba et al 1978); plasma levels appear about 30 minutes after oral administration. Cocaine is also thought to counteract the sedation and the possible respiratory depression caused by the narcotic analgesic as well.

The alcohol concentration is relatively high (23 proof) and some patients complain about the high alcohol content. Instead of alcohol, gin, brandy, and vermouth have all been tried in various formulas. Alcohol is added to increase the palatability of the preparation and to act as a mood elevator. Another means used to increase palatability is the use of honey or aromatic elixir instead of simple syrup.

The Cocktail is sometimes administered concurrently with phenothiazines to prevent nausea and vomiting. Prochlorperazine, 5 mg/5 ml, is usually effective as an antiemetic or antinausea agent. In case of restlessness or agitation, chlorpromazine, 10 to 25 mg/5 ml, may be used. Initially, the Cocktail and the phenothiazine liquid should be dispensed separately. Once the patient has been stabilized and the analgesic dose has been established, the two liquids can be combined into one preparation.

Based on the half-life of morphine, the Cocktail should be administered in 20 ml doses every four hours around the clock. Night-time doses should be omitted only if the patient remains pain-free, although some patients experience excessive CNS stimulation and, therefore, this preparation should not be given at bedtime. Once pain control has been achieved, the dose may be individualized and reduced.

If administration is scheduled in this manner, the patient will not experience apprehension and fear of pain, which serves to decrease pain intensity. For most effective use, it has been suggested that patients should swish the liquid around the inside of the mouth to increase absorption of cocaine from mucous membranes.

Side effects of this mixture are those that are usually encountered with narcotic analgesics. Sedation, nausea, and vomiting are common, with sedation decreasing after a few days of treatment. Constipation may be a problem but can be handled in the usual manner. Tolerance and dependence develop slowly but are not of clinical significance in treating terminally ill patients.

ANALGESIC AND ANTIINFLAMMATORY AGENTS

Rheumatism has been called the hallmark of aging. By retirement age, 80% of the population has some rheumatic complaints. Treatment is required by 40% of the elderly. Arthritis in the elderly comprises many different diseases:

Chondrocalcinosis
Gout
Osteoarthritis
Osteoporosis
Polyarthritis nodosa
Polymyalgia rheumatica
Polymyositis and dermatomyositis
Progressive systemic sclerosis
Rheumatoid arthritis
Systemic lupus erythematosus

Rheumatic diseases are one of the major causes of disability in the elderly. They are common among the elderly (Table 16-1), and the incidence is much higher than in younger patients. However, more than one-third of patients complaining of arthritis may not have arthritis at all, as many diseases resemble arthritis (Blau 1976). Pain originating in bones, joints, and tendons induces muscle spasms and pain in supportive skeletal muscles. Pain most often starts with "tight" regional musculature rather than from direct action on a sensory nerve. Muscle spasms and resulting injury are actually part of an involuntary defense mechanism, an attempt to immobilize a painful joint by increasing the tone of the muscles serving the skeletal area. This leads to chronic complaints which gradually erode the patient's health.

Twenty million Americans are afflicted with arthritis. Of these, 3.6 million have rheumatoid arthritis, at least half are 50 years of age and older. Arthritis ranks second only to heart disease as a cause of prolonged disability among those suffering from chronic disorders. The

Table 16-1
Musculoskeletal Conditions*

Condition	All ages A	65 years and over B	B/A
Arthritis (unspecified)	92.9	380.3	4.1
Rheumatism (unspecified)	6.1	23.2	3.8
Gout	4.8	12.7	2.6
Synovitis, bursitis, etc	16.5	27.7	1.7

*Rate per 1000 persons
Source: Prevalence of Chronic Skin and Musculoskeletal Conditions, U.S. 1969. DHEW Publ. No. (HRA) 75-1519, Rockville, Md.: National Center for Health Statistics, 1974.

economic costs of arthritis are staggering. In 1975, approximately 34.4 million physician visits cost arthritis patients $859 million. Prescription drugs cost these patients $690 million, while the patients spent an additional $575 million on nonprescription drugs.

The incidence of rheumatoid arthritis increases with age (Table 16-2). Rheumatoid arthritis is the most crippling of the various types of arthritis. The cause is unknown (National Commission on Arthritis 1976), but there is sufficient evidence to suggest that immunologic events play a major role in causing or continuing the inflammation in synovial fluid. In the elderly, the course of the disorder differs, possibly because of diminished immunocompetence. The disease primarily affects the connective tissues but damages mostly the joints. The disease can be accompanied by increased fatigue, malaise, low grade fever, and complications like anemia. Arthritic joints may develop misalignment as the disease progresses, which produces particular sensitivity to changes in the weather. Blood vessels, the heart, and the lungs may also be affected. Three times as many women as men are affected. Rheumatoid arthritis usually begins between the ages of 35 and 50 years. If pain on motion or tenderness in at least one joint, swelling in one or more joints, symmetrical joint swelling, and morning stiffness occur for more than six weeks, the condition is classified as rheumatoid arthritis (Kolodny and Klipper 1976).

Table 16-2
Prevalence of Rheumatoid Arthritis*

Age (years)	Both sexes	Men	Women
All ages	3.2	1.7	4.6
55–64	6.3	4.2	8.3
65–74	9.2	3.1	14.1
75–79	18.8	14.1	23.5

*Rate per 100 adults
Source: National Center for Health Statistics, 1963.

In about 20% of patients with rheumatoid arthritis, the disorder will terminate without deformity after about two years. Another 70% of patients will experience an intermittent course of the condition. There will be spontaneous and unpredictable remissions and exacerbations. The remaining 10% of patients will suffer from an unremitting course of the diseases, which will ultimately lead to progressive polyarthritis and severe deformities.

Immobilization will result in muscle atrophy and joint contractures. Therefore, the therapeutic goal of treatment is to suppress joint pain and inflammation, promote activity and prevent immobilization.

Treatment remains empirical. The basic management plan consists of drugs, rest, exercise, good nutrition, and, where indicated, orthopedic measures.

Treatment of Rheumatoid Arthritis

No currently marketed drug will cure rheumatoid arthritis. The present treatment is largely palliative, directed at decreasing inflammation and preserving or restoring function. The commonly used antiinflammatory agents do not alter the course of the disease but are used mainly to control inflammation and pain and to minimize immobility (Fye and Talal 1975). The placebo response is said to be very high.

The nonsteroidal antiinflammatory agents (Table 16-3) are not capable of completely abrogating inflammation in rheumatoid

Table 16-3
Nonsteroidal Antiinflammatory Agents

Name	Indications
Aspirin	Rheumatoid arthritis
	Osteoarthritis
Choline salicylate	Rheumatoid arthritis
	Osteoarthritis
Choline magnesium trisalicylate	Rheumatoid arthritis
	Osteoarthritis
Magnesium salicylate	Rheumatoid arthritis
	Osteoarthritis
	Bursitis
Salsalate	Rheumatoid arthritis
	Osteoarthritis
Fenoprofen	Rheumatoid arthritis
	Osteoarthritis
Ibuprofen	Rheumatoid arthritis
	Osteoarthritis
Indomethacin	Rheumatoid arthritis
	Ankylosing spondylitis
	Osteoarthritis of hip
	Gout
Naproxen	Rheumatoid arthritis
Oxyphenbutazone	Rheumatoid arthritis
	Gout
	Psoriatic arthritis
Phenylbutazone	Osteoarthritis
	Ankylosing spondylitis
Tolmetin	Rheumatoid arthritis

arthritis. They merely ameliorate the inflammation, acting primarily by blocking the production of local mediators of inflammation, including the kinins and prostaglandins. They do not inhibit histamine effects active in the early phases of inflammation, nor the serotonin-induced blood vessel changes. They also do not inhibit the lysosomal enzymes and complement, which are significant mediators of tissue injury in inflammation.

In any case, both provider and patient must understand that drugs must be used regularly and continuously over a long period of time. In addition, the patient must expect to take a large number of drugs daily. Analgesics, antiinflammatory nonsteroidal agents, corticosteroids, gold therapy, psychotropic drugs, antibiotics, vitamins, and minerals may all be used at some stage of the disease. The multitude of drugs used can only be understood when it is realized that rheumatoid arthritis demands management of pain and inflammation, as well as emotional and environmental factors. Additional management procedures include the use of heat, exercise, rest, and gait training.

Aspirin Aspirin is still the first choice of treatment for rheumatoid arthritis (Fritz et al 1978). It is the most widely used and most effective drug currently available for the management of rheumatoid arthritis. Like other nonsteroidal antiinflammatory drugs, it has an immediate effect. Patients with mild and moderate arthritis usually respond reasonably well to aspirin, supported by the necessary adjunctive measures. Its most effective action is inhibition of prostaglandin synthetase, thereby blocking the synthesis of prostaglandins, which are responsible for many aspects of inflammation, especially pain.

Aspirin has been judged clinically useful in the treatment of rheumatoid arthritis in a dosage of 3.6 gm/day (Multz et al 1974), but a starting dose as high as 5 to 6 gm per day has been suggested (Blechman 1976) and it must be given at times in doses as high as 8 gm per day, if the patient can tolerate such high doses (Fye and Talal 1975). The dose should be increased by two tablets every three to four days.

It is important that the patient understand the need to continue taking the drug even if pain has receded. Thus, if aspirin does not show effectiveness, one of the first steps should be a determination whether or not the patient has, indeed, taken the drug as prescribed. The desired blood level is usually listed as 20 to 30 mg/100 ml, but toxic levels in the elderly may be as low as 20 mg/100 ml. Therefore, blood levels should be checked periodically. In elderly on multi-drug therapy, higher than expected blood levels can occur (Wallace et al 1976). As tinnitus is an early warning of aspirin toxicity, it is important to establish, through a careful patient history, whether the patient already suffers from ringing in the ears. In addition, the elderly may experience tinnitus at blood levels below effective antiinflammatory levels (Bayles 1968). The first adverse effects a patient may experience might include abdominal pain, heartburn, and nausea. This could be followed by tinnitus, hyperventilation, tremors, confusion, loss of memory, and fluid retention, which is of special concern in the elderly patient with congestive heart failure (Greer 1965; Elliott 1964). Aspirin also has a certain diaphoretic effect that can be a deterrent in very warm climates. When control has been established, an attempt should be made to reduce drug dosage, but this should be done in slow steps.

Periodically, a patient may complain that the drug is not effective. This may be the result of the beneficial effect of the drug which permits the patient to have increased activity. The symptoms produced by increased activity may equal those of the restricted state, leading the patient to believe that the drug is not effective.

In general, though, aspirin is, dose for dose, the most effective and least expensive antiinflammatory drug. If aspirin does not produce sufficient pain relief in doses of 5 to 6 gm, codeine, dextropropoxyphen, or pentazocine may be added to the regimen (Bienenstock and Fernando 1976). Sodium salicylate and calcium salicylate, while they produce less gastrointestinal toxicity, usually are not as effective. While the same has been said for choline salicylate, a small number of studies seem to indicate that it has significant antiinflammatory and analgesic effects. One advantage (which may be important for the elderly) is that it is marketed as a mint-flavored liquid, while there are no stable aspirin liquids available.

Other antiinflammatory agents There are alternatives to aspirin therapy and, given "with enthusiasm, they may provide relief" (Blechman et al 1976). Their analgesic properties make them clear choices for treatment of the symptoms of rheumatoid arthritis. Their antiinflammatory properties are comparable to those of aspirin and all seem to have a lower incidence of gastrointestinal side effects than aspirin. However, all do have the potential for causing gastrointestinal distress; ulceration and bleeding are the most toxic manifestations (Blechman et al 1978). The propionic derivatives (fenoprofen, ibuprofen, naproxen) seem to be somewhat less toxic than the others, but withdrawal may be a problem with drugs of the propionic acid group. There are currently about 20 other antiinflammatory agents under investigation, but it would appear that one cannot expect that they will substantially differ from those already being marketed.

Fenoprofen is a phenylpropionic acid derivative which also has an antipyretic effect. It is rapidly absorbed, reaches peak serum levels in 90 minutes and has a plasma half-life of 160 minutes. It may possibly cause asthmatic and gastrointestinal side effects (DiPalma 1977).

Ibuprofen is rapidly absorbed from the small intestine, the rate of absorption being decreased by food. It is primarily metabolized in the liver and its plasma half-life is two hours. Serum blood levels of ibuprofen are reduced by aspirin.

Naproxen is a phenylpropionic acid derivative. It is rapidly absorbed and reaches peak serum levels in one to two hours. Its half-life of about 13 hours permits twice daily administration. It has a very low hepatic extraction ratio, but is highly bound to plasma proteins.

Tolmetin is an indomethacin derivative. It reaches peak plasma levels in 30 to 60 minutes and has a mean half-life of one hour. It is extensively bound to plasma proteins and probably has a high hepatic extraction ratio. It is contraindicated in patients allergic to aspirin, has the potential to cause hyperthermia (Brown and Weir 1978) and at least one case has been reported in which tolmetin, given to a 52-year-old woman with rheumatoid arthritis (400 mg three times daily for five weeks) caused shock, overwhelming sepsis, and death (Sakai and Joseph 1978).

No substantial studies have been published comparing the effectiveness of these drugs. However, if a patient does not respond to any one of these, it is not unreasonable to try another. All but fenoprofen should be given with food or milk. If significant inflammation remains after treatment with aspirin or the newer, nonsteroidal antiinflammatory agents, antimalarial drugs are sometimes tried. Hydroxychloroquine could be added to the basic regimen in a dose of 200 mg at bedtime. After one or two months, the patient should be seen by an ophthalmologist to check for drug deposits in the eye. If they appear, the drug must be withdrawn (Kolodny and Klipper 1976).

Gold therapy is an alternative to the antimalarials. Gold salts may require several months or a year before any effectiveness is demonstrated. They can cause dermatologic, hematologic, and renal complications. A new gold compound, auranofin, appears to be more potent and less toxic than other antiarthritic gold medications. Moreover, the new compound can be administered orally and need not be given parenterally. In a preliminary note from the Memorial Hospital Medical Center at Long Beach, California, it has been reported that a limited number of patients have benefitted from a twice daily administration for 16 weeks, without experiencing any serious side effects.

Cyclophosphamide can provide dramatic relief of symptoms and disability of rheumatoid arthritis, but can cause serious adverse reactions. It should, therefore, be reserved for severe, active progression, unresponsive to optimum conventional therapy.

The pyrazolone derivatives, oxyphenbutazone and phenylbutazone, are not primary drugs in the treatment of rheumatoid arthritis, but may occasionally be used in acute flare-ups for a short time. Similarly, the indole derivative, indomethacin, is only used in the treatment of acute rheumatoid arthritis unresponsive to conventional therapy, and may also be used in acute flare-ups. It probably causes the most gastrointestinal irritation of all drugs, and diarrhea is common in elderly patients treated with indomethacin. Rectal hemorrhage, severe headache, dizziness, and confusion have also been observed (Blechman et al 1978). Indomethacin should not be given concurrently with aspirin, as the two drugs compete with the same receptor sites. Recently, it has been suggested that a combination of indomethacin and diazepam should be considered the treatment of choice in the control of night pain and morning stiffness in rheumatoid arthritis.

The adrenocorticosteroids should only be used after all other treatment modalities have been tried and exhausted. Although they provide dramatic and effective relief, they also fail to alter the course of the disease. It is sometimes necessary to use steroids in patients over the age of 70 years with acute rheumatoid arthritis, mainly to prevent immobilization until such time as conventional therapy becomes effective. Thus, steroids, if used at all in the elderly, should be used only as adjuncts to nonsteroidal therapy. Their dose should be kept at the lowest level possible, and they should be discontinued as soon as possible. Their use and the need for continued therapy should be reviewed periodically, but in many patients, no review takes place (Eastwood 1974).

Corticosteroids, given on a chronic basis, increase bone resorption and decrease bone formation. They also increase urinary calcium excretion (Ditunno and Ehrlich 1970; Gifford 1973). As the elderly may suffer from osteoporosis, corticosteroids would increase the risk of fractures. Corticosteroids may also depress serum albumin levels, which may already be diminished in the elderly. They may also adversely alter glucose metabolism in diabetic patients, induce fluid retention and thus reduce control of hypertension and congestive heart failure, and aggravate cataracts and glaucoma. By suppressing adrenal activity, they also increase the elderly's vulnerability to stress. Prolonged steroid therapy will also increase the risk of infections, particularly respiratory infections. They can also unmask urinary tract, kidney, and bile duct infections. A negative nitrogen balance could also result from prolonged steroid therapy (Dordick 1956). Thus, if a clear and absolute need for steroid therapy has been established, they should only be given in low doses for short periods of time.

Osteoarthritis, also called degenerative joint disease and "wear-and-tear arthritis," is the most common form of arthritis. It is characterized mainly by degeneration of joint cartilage. Involved in the disease process are complex carbohydrate-protein substances known as proteoglycans and glycoproteins. Common symptoms are pain and stiffness. Osteoarthritis is more prevalent in women than in men, and women usually experience the first symptoms at the time of menopause. Treatment is directed at reduction of pain and disability, reduction of capsular inflammation, and reduction of muscle spasms. The same antiinflammatory agents as those used in treatment of rheumatoid arthritis are used for osteoarthritis, and they are also only of limited value. Skeletal muscle relaxants are often given in combination with the other drugs. Physical therapy and, if necessary, weight reduction and orthopedic measures are used.

Oxyphenbutazone and phenylbutazone are indicated for treatment of osteoarthritis of the hip. These drugs are also used in acute attacks of gout and pseudogout, in ankylosing spondylitis, tendinitis, and bursitis. Their use, as well as the use of indomethacin, must be carefully considered when treating elderly patients. They pose potential dangers to the elderly (indomethacin is possibly less dangerous). Indomethacin is also used for treatment of osteoarthritis of the hip, as well as for acute gout, and ankylosing spondylitis. All of these cause fluid retention and edema. Phenylbutazone could cause a significant plasma volume increase, which would be particularly undesirable in patients with cardiac disease. The risk of side effects is dose-related and increases with patient age and duration of treatment. Phenylbutazone should not be used at all in patients with hypertension and incipient heart failure (Prescott 1975). All these drugs can cause anorexia, nausea, vomiting, and abdominal pain. Hematopoietic reactions are the most serious toxic effects of these drugs and patients should be instructed to report immediately any fever, sore throat, oral lesions, or skin rash.

Relief of pain and prevention of recurrence is the goal of effective gout therapy. Colchicine is still the drug of choice in acute gouty attack, but must be used with caution in patients with impaired liver, kidney, or bone marrow function. If these functional decrements exist, half the normal dose is indicated (Bluhm et al 1977). For elderly patients, it may be safer to substitute such nonsteroidal, antiinflammatory agents as fenoprofen or naproxen. Ibuprofen also appears effective in the treatment of acute gouty arthritis, and may be an effective alternative to the standard colchicine therapy (Schweitz et al 1978).

Physical therapy is important in the management of joint stiffness and to preserve joint function. Physical measures may be used alone or, more often, they are used in combination with drugs. Both heat and cold are used. Application of heat or cold relieves pain by inhibiting peripheral sensation and reducing muscle spasms. Moist heat, applied by means of a hydrocollator pack, is most effective. It can be applied in the patient's home and can be followed by massage of the contracted muscles (McBeath 1978).

It is important that patients be instructed in the proper use of heat. Warmth may be provided by use of warm clothing during the day and a light electric blanket at night. If additional heat is desired, moist heat can be used, but must be used with care. The skin of elderly patients is particularly susceptible to burns, especially when circulation is impaired by varicose veins or partially occluded arteries. Thus, elderly patients might not perceive heat as readily as younger persons. Patients must be told to apply the heat source to the affected area and not to sit or lie on the source. Prolonged use, more than 20 to 30 minutes, may negate the beneficial, but temporary effect of the heat treatment. The use of heating pads should be discouraged because burns caused by improper use of heating pads are fairly common. These types of burns heal with difficulty in the elderly. If warm baths are recommended, care must be taken to avoid hyperthermia and dehydration. A bath should not exceed a 20-minute period and extra fluids should be administered after the bath.

Heat treatments should generally be followed by planned, therapeutic exercises, which are designed to yield early and progressive mobilization, to improve range of motion, and to strengthen the musculature. These exercises increase the circulation of synovial fluid in and out of cartilage and prevent joint contractures. An exercise program should only start after acute inflammation of the joint or surrounding area has subsided.

In addition to these supportive and adjunctive measures, various types of two-way elastic, stretch garments have been used, mainly to help control pain.

REFERENCES

Abrishami, M.A., and Thomas, J. Aspirin intolerance–a review. *Ann All.* 39:28, 1977.

Bayles, T.B. Salicylate therapy in rheumatoid arthritis. *Med Clin North Am.* 52:703, 1968.

Bienenstock, H., and Fernando, K.R. Arthritis in the elderly: an overview. *Med Clin North Am.* 60:1173, 1976.

Blau, S.P. All those joint pains may not be arthritis. *Drug Ther.* 6(11):144, 1976.

Blechman, W.J., Ehrlich, G.E., and Kaplan, H. Weighing drug options with arthritides. *Patient Care* 10(19):76, 1976.

Blechman, W.J., Ehrlich, G.E., and Kaplan, H. Update on anti-inflammatory agents. *Patient Care* 12(3):174, 1978.

Bluhm, G.B., McCarthy, D.J., and Wallace, S.L. "Live with it" is out for gout. *Patient Care* 11(6):18, 1977.

Brown, J.R., and Weir, A.B. Drug fever from tolmetin administration. *JAMA.* 239:24, 1978.

Chan, K., Kendall, M.J., Wells, W.D.E. et al. Factors influencing the excretion and relative physiological availability of pethidine in man. *J Pharm Pharmacol.* 27:235, 1975.

Cohen, A. A comparative blood salicylate study of two salicylate tablet formulations utilizing normal volunteers. *Curr Ther Res.* 23:772, 1978.

Cohen, A., and Garber, H.E. Comparison of choline magnesium trisalicylate and acetylsalicylic acid in relation to fecal blood loss. *Curr Ther Res.* 23:187, 1978.

Cohen, A., Thomas, G.B., and Cohen, E.B. Serum concentration, safety and tolerance of oral doses of choline magnesium trisilicate. *Curr Ther Res.* 23:358, 1978.

Craven, J., Craven, W., and Florence, S. Hospice care for dying patients. *Am J Nurs.* 75:1816, 1975.

Davison, W. Drug hazards in the elderly. Edited by L. Meyler, and H.M. Peck. In *Drug-Induced Diseases.* New York: Excerpta Medica Foundation, 1968.

Davison, W. Unwanted drug effects in the elderly. Edited by L. Meyler, and H.M. Peck. In *Drug-Induced Diseases.* Amsterdam: Exerpta Medica, 1972.

DiPalma, J.R. How you can prevent GI drug interactions. *RN* 40:63, 1977.

Ditunno, J., and Ehrlich, G.E. Care and training of elderly patients with rheumatoid arthritis. *Geratrics* 25:164, 1970.

Dordick, J.R. Rheumatoid arthritis in the elderly. *J Am Geriatr Soc.* 4:588, 1956.

Eastwood, H.D.H. Steroid therapy in the elderly. *Gerontol Clin.* 16:163, 1974.

Elliott, H.C. Salicylates: metabolism and biochemical effects: a review. *Ala J Med Sci.* 1:38, 1964.

Fordyce, W.E. Evaluating and managing chronic pain. *Geriatrics* 33(1):59, 1978.

Forrest, W.H., Brown, C.R., Mahler, D.L. et al. The evaluation of morphine and dexamphetamine combinations for analgesia. *Clin Pharmacol Ther.* 14:132, 1973.

Fritz, W.L., Paxinos, J., and Gall, E.P. Rational use of new non-steroid anti-inflammatory drugs. *Drug Ther.* 8(5):36, 1978.

Fye, K., and Talal, N. Cytotoxic drugs in the treatment of rheumatoid arthritis. *Rational Drug Ther.* 9(4):1, 1975.

Gifford, R.H. Corticosteroid therapy for rheumatoid arthritis. *Med Clin North Am.* 57:1179, 1973.

Greer, H.D. Chronic salicylate intoxication in adults. *JAMA.* 193:555, 1965.

Hopkinson, J.H., Blatt, G., Cooper, M. et al. Effective pain relief: comparative results with acetaminophen in a new dose formulation, propoxyphen napsylate-acetaminophen combination, and placebo. *Curr Ther Res.* 19:622, 1976.

Hunt, T.E. Management of chronic non-rheumatic pain in the elderly. *J Am Geriatr Soc.* 24:394, 1976.

Inaba, T., Steart, D.J., and Kalow, W. Metabolism of cocaine in man. *Clin Pharmacol Ther.* 23:547, 1978.

Kolodny, A.L., and Klipper, A.R. Bone and joint diseases in the elderly. *Hosp Practice.* 11(11):91, 1976.

Lasagna, L. Influence of age on analgesic pain relief. Letter to the Editor. *JAMA.* 218:1831, 1971.

LeShan, L. The world of the patient in severe pain of long duration. *J Chron Dis.* 17:119, 1964.

Lipman, A.G. Drug therapy in terminally ill patients. *Am J Hosp Pharm.* 32:270, 1975.

Maljovec, J.J., Nejman, J., and Etemad, B. An introduction to Brompton's cocktail. Presented at the 30th Annual Meeting of the Gerontology Society. San Francisco, 1977.

Marks, M.D., and Sachar, E.J. Undertreatment of medical in-patients with narcotic analgesics. *Ann Intern Med.* 78:173, 1973.

McBeath, A.A. Nonsurgical treatment of degenerative arthritis and tendinitis. *Drug Ther.* 8(5):41, 1978.

Medical Letter. Levodopa and related drugs. 15:21, 1973.

Melzack, R., Ofiesh, J.G., and Mount, B.M. The Brompton mixture: effects of pain in cancer patients. *Can Med Assoc J.* 115:125, 1976.

Melzack, R., and Taenzer, P. Concepts of pain perception and therapy. *Geriatrics* 32(11):44, 1977.

Mongan, E., Kelley, P., Nies, K. et al. Tinnitus as an indication of therapeutic serum salicylate levels. *JAMA.* 226:142, 1973.

Mount, B.M. The problem of caring for the dying in a general hospital: the palliative care unit as a possible solution. *Can Med Assoc J.* 115:119, 1976.

Mount, B.M., Ajemian, I., and Scott, J.F. Use of the Brompton mixture in treating the chronic pain of malignant disease. *Can Med Assoc J.* 115:122, 1976.

Multz, C.V., Bernhard, G.C., Blechman, W.C. et al. A comparison of intermediate-dose aspirin and placebo in rheumatoid arthritis. *Clin Pharmacol Ther.* 15:310, 1974.

National Commission on Arthritis and Related Musculoskeletal Diseases. *Report to the Congress of the United States, Volume I: The Arthritis Plan.* DHEW Publ. No. (NIH) 76-1150. Washington, D.C.: National Institutes of Health, 1976.

Pinsky, J.J. Chronic, intractable, benign pain: a syndrome and its treatment with intensive short-term group psychotherapy. *J Hum Stress.* 4(3):17, 1978.

Prescott, L.F. Anti-inflammatory analgesics and drugs used in the treatment of rheumatoid arthritis and gout. Edited by M.N.G. Dukes. In *Meyler's Side Effects of Drugs.* Amsterdam: Excerpta Medica, 1975.

Rainsford, K.D. The biochemical pathology of aspirin-induced gastric damage. *Agents Actions.* 5:326, 1975.

St. John, D.J.B., and McDermott, F.T. Influence of achlorhydria on aspirin-induced occult gastrointestinal blood loss: studies in addisonian pernicious anaemia. *Br Med J.* 2:450, 1970.

Sakai, J., and Joseph, M.W. Tolmetin and agranulocytosis. Letter to the Editor *N Engl J Med.* 298:1203, 1978.

Sale, L. Geriatrics: pharmacology in the aged. *J Missouri Med Assoc.* 49:476, 1952.

Saunders, C. *The Management of Terminal Illness.* London: London Hospital Medical Publications, 1967.

Schweitz, M.C., Nashel, D.J., and Alepa, P. Ibuprofen in the treatment of acute gouty arthritis. *JAMA.* 239:34, 1978.

Smith, M.T., Levin, H.M., Bare, W.M. et al. Acetaminophen extra-strength capsules versus propoxyphen compound-65 versus placebo: a double-blind study of effectiveness and safety. *Curr Ther Res.* 17:452, 1975.

Sternbach, R.A. Treatment of the chronic pain patient. *J Hum Stress.* 4(3):11, 1978.

Twycross, R.G. Euphoriant elixirs. *Br Med J.* 3:552, 1973.

Twycross, R.G. Clinical experience with diamorphine in advanced malignant disease. *Int J Clin Pharmacol.* 9:184, 1974a.

Twycross, R.G. Diamorphine and cocaine elixir. *BPC Pharm J.* 212:153, 1974b.

Twycross, R.G. Diseases of the central nervous system–relief of terminal pain. *Br Med J.* 1:212, 1975.

Twycross, R.G., Fray, D.E., and Wills, P.D. The alimentary absorption of diamorphine and morphine in man as indicated by urinary excretion studies. *Br J Clin Pharmacol.* 1:491, 1974.

Van Dyke, C., Jatlow, P., Ungerer, J. et al. Oral cocaine: plasma concentrations and central effects. *Science* 200:211, 1978.

Wallace, S., Whiting, B., and Runcie, J. Factors affecting drug binding in plasma of elderly patients. *Br J Clin Pharmacol.* 3:327, 1976.

Weintraub, M. Potentiation of narcotic analgesia. *Drug Ther.* 7(4):154, 1977.

17 Anticonvulsants

Epilepsy is relatively common in old age. In a substantial number of newly diagnosed, elderly epileptics, there may be potentially reversible causes, such as intermittent heartblock, drug-induced hypoglycemia, and raised levels of blood urea. Most often, epileptic seizures occur if cerebrovascular disease culminates in hemiplegia. Dementia is also a frequent cause of seizures in the elderly. After the age of 70, tumors become increasingly uncommon as the cause of seizures. Many elderly patients may suffer only from nocturnal seizures, which can be well controlled with anticonvulsant drugs.

The hydantoins and phenobarbital are probably the most frequently used anticonvulsants in the elderly, consistent, of course, with age of onset of first seizure and type of seizure. A question may be raised concerning the need for folic acid supplementation on long term use of these drugs. This has been suggested in order to prevent megaloblastic anemia. However, if folic acid is added to an already established therapeutic regimen, the number of seizures may increase. Thus, patients who receive this type of treatment must be carefully monitored.

Phenytoin doses often advised for the elderly are likely to be inadequate. Doses of less than 300 mg/day do not produce optimum serum concentrations for elderly patients. On the other hand, there is an age-related increase in serum concentrations on a fixed dose and an increase in clearance associated with a reduction in the degree of protein binding correlated with reduced serum albumin levels (Lambie and Caird 1977; Houghton et al 1975; Hayes et al 1975).

A reasonable dose would be 300 mg/day, as higher doses are likely to be toxic. Phenytoin also is known to interact with other drugs, among them furosemide which is absorbed less in the presence of phenytoin (Fine et al 1977). The many other potential interactions of phenytoin with other drugs have been listed (American Pharmaceutical Association 1976); the prescriber should be familiar with these.

The Food and Drug Administration plans to require important changes in prescribing directions for all oral phenytoin products. Apparently, there is new evidence that dissolution and absorption rates differ for different dosage forms, and in the case of phenytoin sodium capsules, between different brands.

No patient should be placed directly on a once-daily dosage therapy, as there appear to be two distinct forms of phenytoin: fast release for three or four times per day dosing, and slow release for once-a-day administration. New labeling for this class of products will advise physicians, in general, to keep patients on one dosage form and one manufacturer's product. When a change in dosage form or a change in brand of phenytoin sodium capsules involves Dilantin sodium capsules, physicians should check blood levels in patients as they switch from one product to another or from one dosage form to another (FDA Drug Bulletin 1978).

REFERENCES

American Pharmaceutical Association. *Evaluations of Drug Interactions.* Washington, D.C., 1976.

FDA Drug Bulletin. New prescribing directions for phenytoin. 8(4):27, 1978.

Fine, A., Henderson, I.S., Morgan, D.R. et al Malabsorption of furosemide caused by phenytoin. *Br Med J.* 4:1061, 1977.

Hayes, M.J., Langman, M.J.S., and Short, A.H. Changes in drug metabolism with increasing age. II. Phenytoin clearance and protein binding. *Br J Clin Pharmacol.* 2:73, 1975.

Houghton, G.W., Riches, A., and Leighton, M. Effect of age, height, weight, and sex on serum phenytoin concentrations in epileptic patients. *Br J Clin Pharmacol.* 2:251, 1975.

Lambie, D.C., and Caird, F.I. Phenytoin dosage in the elderly. *Age Ageing.* 6:133, 1977.

18 Antimicrobials

Elderly persons are less resistant to infectious diseases than are younger persons (Gladstone and Recco 1976). Major contributors to this decreased resistance are the declining immune system, important intercurrent diseases such as diabetes, and chemotherapeutic agents that can adversely affect the normal defense mechanism.

The Declining Immune System

Once an invading organism circumvents the body's primary defense mechanism, the serum immunoglobulins provide the major remaining defenses. A deterioration of B-lymphocyte function with advancing age leads to a variable fall in serum concentrations of IgA, IgG, IgD, and IgM, responsible for defense against infection by bacteria and viruses. There is less capacity to form primary antibody responses to various antigens. Furthermore, B-lymphocytes will not proliferate as easily as before. After the age of 60 years, T-lymphocyte function declines strikingly (Smith and Wiener 1978). Thus, the body's ability to mobilize cellular and antibody resistance to infectious disease decreases steadily with age. Particularly affected is the body's ability to respond to bacterial antigens (Hicks 1975). All this renders the elderly patient increasingly susceptible to infections (Buckley and Dorsey 1971), even to infections by the normal flora, such as *E. coli, Enterobacter, Klebsiella, Proteus,* and *Pseudomonas.*

Presentation of Infection

Infections in the elderly tend to be more latent and less acute. The signs are less overt. In bacteremia, for example, the elderly patient may merely manifest confusion, stupor, delirium, or agitation (McCabe 1973), instead of the classical signs of chills, fever, prostration, as well as occasional nausea and vomiting. Almost all serious infections are more severe in the elderly who may show only relatively few signs of inflammation.

Intercurrent Diseases and Conditions and Their Effects

The patient's nutritional state may affect and alter adversely the response to invading organisms. Protein-calorie malnutrition may cause a defect in cell-mediated immunity. Lack of certain vitamins can also be responsible for lack of normal immune responsiveness. For example, lack of vitamin A, pyridoxine, or riboflavin can inhibit this response.

Diabetes mellitus can cause a deterioration of the immune response. In diabetes mellitus, infections are very aggressive. Staphylococcal bacteremia is more frequently associated with diabetes mellitus in the elderly than in the young, probably because of the increased frequency of vascular disease in the elderly. There is a high incidence of coliform, candidal, and tubercular infections in the elderly diabetic. High glucose levels probably contribute to mycotic overgrowth. In elderly with infections, hyperglycemia must be strictly controlled, and it is probably best to use insulin rather than any of the oral hypoglycemic agents.

Intramuscular (IM) administration of antimicrobials in diabetic patients should not be considered. Intramuscular absorption of penicillin and polymyxin in elderly diabetics is impaired. Intravenous administration is favored, but caution must be exercised as dextrose overload and hyperglycemia and glucosuria can easily occur. Chloramphenicol and some sulfonamides may potentiate the action of the sulfonylureas. Furthermore, antimicrobials can yield false positive and negative results with urine sugar tests. Sulfonamides, for example, form a colorless complex with copper (Benedict's), and the cephalosporins, chloramphenicol, isoniazid, nitrofurans, and tetracyclines all interfere with the copper tests. There is no interference with the glucose oxidase test.

The elderly patient with arteriosclerotic cardiovascular disease or congestive heart failure may present a therapeutic problem when faced with infections.

Vascular disease makes an elderly patient vulnerable to infection or may complicate the treatment of the infection. Peripheral vascular disease, for example, predisposes a patient to cellulitis or pyelonephritis. In vascular disease, the decreased blood supply may reduce the ability of an antimicrobial to penetrate the target area (for example, in ischemic bowel disease), and the dose of the antimicrobial to be used may have to be increased to achieve higher blood levels. This, of course, can lead to greater toxicities. There is some evidence that the neurotoxicity of some antibiotics may increase in cardiovascular disease, particularly in patients who suffered cerebrovascular accidents (Moellering 1978). In the presence of hyponatremia and impaired renal function, the penicillins and cephalosporins can produce neuromuscular hyperexcitability and seizures. Cerebrovascular accidents also predispose a patient to decubitus ulcers, urinary tract infections, and aspiration pneumonia.

Coagulation disorders can be affected adversely by antibiotics. For example, carbenicillin, administered to patients with disorders of the clotting mechanisms, can lead to threatening degrees of bleeding (Weinstein 1977).

Pulmonary emboli or thrombophlebitis may be treated with coumarin anticoagulants. Several antimicrobials are known to interfere with the action of these anticoagulants, necessitating an adjustment of the established dose (Table 18-1).

Table 18-1
The Effects of Some Antimicrobials on Coumarin Anticoagulant Action

Drug	Effect	Action
Rifampin Griseofulvin	Induce microsomal activity	Increase anticoagulant dose
Ampicillin Tetracycline	Destroy gut flora and prothrombin formation	Decrease anticoagulant dose
Chloramphenicol	Inhibit microsomal enzyme activity	Decrease anticoagulant dose
Nalidixic acid Sulfonamides	Displacement from binding sites	Decrease anticoagulant dose

The patient with congestive heart failure most likely is treated with digitalis and a diuretic. Some data seem to indicate that neomycin may impair serum digoxin levels. A number of antimicrobials, such as carbenicillin, penicillin sodium, ticarcillin, and amphotericin B can cause hypokalemia, precipitating digitalis toxicity. Diuretics, in turn, can potentiate the ototoxic effects of cephalosporins, and there is some indication that furosemide and possibly ethacrynic acid may potentiate the nephrotoxicity of some antimicrobials.

Some antibiotics contain significant amounts of sodium, and their use could precipitate pulmonary edema in patients with congestive heart failure; therefore, they should be carefully considered before they are prescribed for the elderly patient with congestive heart failure.

While the elderly have often acquired immunity to certain infections, infections may often occur as complications of other diseases or of deteriorating organ function. Prostatic disease in elderly men and pelvic relaxation following multiparity and atrophy of the vaginal epithelium in older women can predispose the patient to infection of the genitourinary tract. Colonic diverticuli in older people can be the site of an infection, abscess formation, intestinal perforation, bacteremic shock, and peritonitis.

As mentioned, resistance to infection is lowered in older persons. Pneumococcal pneumonia is fairly common in the elderly. Elderly with chronic obstructive lung disease or emphysema are predisposed to bronchopulmonary infection and deterioration of respiratory function. As a result, pneumonia is the fourth leading cause of death among persons over 65 years of age (Clarke 1977).

Renal function is one of the most important determinants of the patient's potential response to antimicrobial agents. The patient's renal status will most likely play a major role in the choice of the drug to be used and the dose to be used. Elderly patients with renal insufficiency are likely to have a higher incidence of IgA deficiency, as well as an impaired primary antibody response, both of which tend to favor the infectious disease process.

In the older person, the efficiency of renal tubular secretion decreases. This is not always detectable as urea nitrogen and creatinine levels may remain normal. Thus, it is important for the prescriber to know the major excretory routes of the prescribed antibiotic (Table 18-2). In renal impairment, drugs that are potentially nephrotoxic should be avoided if at all possible. If this is not feasible, the patient who is to receive a potentially nephrotoxic drug should have a baseline and periodic measurements of renal function (BUN, creatinine, creatinine clearance). The loading dose of the prescribed antibiotic usually remains the same as the normal adult dose, but the maintenance dose must be adjusted in proportion to the degree of renal impairment (Smith and Wiener 1978).

Table 18-2
The Major Routes of Elimination of Some Antibiotics

Antibiotic	Eliminated by
Amikacin	Glomerular filtration
Ampicillin	Tubular secretion
Carbenicillin	Tubular secretion
Cefazolin	Tubular secretion
Cephalexin	Tubular secretion
Cephalothin	Tubular secretion
Cephradine	Tubular secretion
Chloramphenicol	Liver
Clindamycin	Glomerular filtration and liver
Colistimethate	Gomerular filtration
Erythromycin	Liver
Gentamicin	Glomerular filtration
Kanamycin	Glomerular filtration
Methicillin	Tubular secretion
Penicillin G	Tubular secretion
Polymyxin B	Glomerular filtration
Tetracycline	Glomerular filtration
Ticarcillin	Tubular secretion
Tobramycin	Glomerular filtration
Vancomycin	Glomerular filtration

The most consistently nephrotoxic drugs are the aminoglycosides, amphotericin, cephaloridine, and vancomycin (Hayes 1977). These drugs can impair their own excretion. Even the so-called soluble sulfonamides can precipitate in the renal collecting tubules and produce urinary tract obstruction. Thus, selection of an antibiotic for an elderly patient with impaired renal function, in particular, should be based on benefit/risk ratios (Appel and Neu 1977). Antibiotics may produce specific proximal and distal tubular defects which lead to electrolyte and acid-base imbalance, in addition to other toxic effects.

With the exception of the sulfonamides and the aminoglycoside antibiotics, antimicrobial drugs are largely excreted in the urine and do not have a narrow toxic-therapeutic ratio. Therefore, reduction in dosage of antibiotics in the elderly without uremia, despite reduction in glomerular filtration rates, is not as important as with most other drugs and is, therefore, often unnecessary (Department of Health, Education and Welfare 1978).

The elderly epileptic patient is at risk when the tetracyclines and nalidixic acid are used, which can cause benign intracranial hypertension (Hayes 1977). (This effect can also be seen in patients with parkinsonism and cerebrovascular insufficiency.) Chloramphenicol increases phenytoin blood levels by inhibiting microsomal activity, and the metabolism of phenytoin (Moellering 1978).

Isoniazid and cycloserine can cause toxic psychosis and seizures, which can be prevented, in the case of cycloserine, by administration of pyridoxine. Isoniazid, like chloramphenicol, will inhibit the metabolism of phenytoin and thus increase that drug's blood level. One other possible effect of antibiotic therapy in the elderly should be mentioned. Decreased acidity and achlorhydria are common among elderly patients, and, therefore, acid-unstable oral penicillin can be administered to those patients. This, of course, is also of economic advantage to the patient.

Immunosuppressive therapy The elderly often respond to infections in a compromised manner because of pre-existing immunosuppressive diseases or therapy. Malignancies or collagen vascular disease, for example, mandate the use of drugs that can adversely affect the patient's defense mechanism (Seneca 1970).

Response of the Elderly to Antimicrobials

Antimicrobials are designed to inhibit or destroy the infecting organisms. Thus, the target of the projected treatment is not the patient but the invading organism. Theoretically, at least, infection in older people should respond to antibiotic therapy like an infection in younger people. However, infections in the elderly are often of different etiology than those found in the general population. Also, in the elderly there is less body water and, therefore, the usual dose of an antibiotic could create higher blood levels and a greater incidence and severity of toxicities. Elderly patients will not respond as quickly to antimicrobial therapy as younger persons, because of reduced immunoglobulin levels. Even if an organism is reactive to the selected antibiotic, the response may not be anticipated if the patient's normal defenses do not function well (Das and Sharma 1971). Many of the common antimicrobials are bacteriostatic rather than bactericidal (Table 18-3). The use of the bacteriostatic antimicrobial requires that host defenses eliminate the infectious organisms. Since normal, immunologic functions decline with age, such therapy may be less than adequate in the elderly.

Broad-spectrum antibiotics, administered to elderly patients, may cause proliferation of different types of bacteria in the intestine,

Table 18-3
The Activities of Some Antibacterials

Bactericidal	Bacteriostatic
Aminoglycosides	Chloramphenicol
Cephalosporins	Cycloserine
Furantoins	Erythromycin
Penicillins	Lincomycin
Polymyxins	Sulfonamides
	Tetracyclines

Note: Reactions can vary with different strains of bacteria and dose.
Source: J.C. Tolhurst, G. Buckle, and S.W. Williams. Chemotherapy with antibiotics and allied drugs. Canberra: Australian Gov't Publ. Serv., 1972.

leading to gastrointestinal upset, and pruritus ani and vulvae. The pruritus tends to persist, possibly because of local skin atrophy.

Elderly patients immunosuppressed by disease or drugs are especially susceptible to suprainfections caused by antibiotic therapy. The spectrum of the drug and the duration of treatment contribute to the development of suprainfections.

The penicillins For most infections, except urinary tract infections and those that are penicillin-resistant, penicillin G is the choice of initial treatment. In case of penicillin-resistant infections, oxacillin, methicillin, or nafcillin are usually selected. Penicillin, in low doses to avoid risks of adverse reactions and suprainfections, is the drug of choice in treating pneumonia (Clarke 1977). All penicillins have essentially the same antibacterial action. Most are much more active against gram-positive than gram-negative bacteria. They probably exert less direct toxicity than any other antibiotics. About 10% to 15% of persons with a prior history of penicillin allergy will have an allergic reaction if penicillin is again administered. Allergy may occur as long as 7 to 12 days after initial administration of the drug.

After oral administration, only a small portion of the administered dose may be absorbed, depending on the pH of the stomach and the presence or absence of food. Penicillins should not be preceded by food for at least one hour or followed by food for about one to two hours.

In elderly patients, penicillin half-life is prolonged because of an age-dependent decrease in renal function, and creatinine clearance is a reliable index to penicillin clearance (Hayes 1977). Phenylbutazone, competing for active tubular transport, increases penicillin half-life.

A considerable sodium load can be administered if penicillin is given, which may cause electrolyte disorders, particularly in patients with congestive heart failure. The sodium content of some penicillins is listed in Table 18-4. In addition, when receiving drugs such as carbenicillin or ticarcillin, the patient should be closely monitored for signs of hypokalemia.

Table 18-4
Sodium Content of Some Penicillins

Drug	Sodium content
Sodium penicillin G	2.0 mEq/1 million U
Oxacillin	3.1 mEq/gm
Ampicillin	3.4 mEq/gm
Carbenicillin	4.7 mEq/gm

Several general reviews on antibiotic toxicity contain comments on iatrogenic psychiatric side effects of these agents. Toxic psychotic effects of penicillin have been described as far back as 1948. They may be associated either with an allergic-type reaction or, most commonly, are not of an allergic nature. Most often, these reactions follow intravenous administration of the drug.

If a psychotic reaction occurs and is severe, chlorpromazine and phenobarbital may be effective.

Mental confusion has also been reported following administration of chloramphenicol, cycloserine, isoniazid, and others. Neuropsychiatric side effects have also been noted following administration of aminoglycoside antibiotics.

The cephalosporins The cephalosporins are effective against some, but not all, gram-positive and gram-negative bacteria. There is a cross-resistance between the cephalosporins and beta-lactamase-resistant penicillins. Cephalothin, cephapirin, and cefamandole must be given parenterally, but cephalexin and cephradine are absorbed from the gut (Moellering and Swartz 1976).

Higher serum levels of cefazolin and cephradine have been observed in elderly patients (Simon et al 1976). The half-lives of these drugs are prolonged in elderly patients, probably because of impaired renal excretion and slower tissue perfusion. Specifically, the renal clearance of cefazolin was reduced from 83 ml/min to 43 ml/min, and that of cephradine from 378 ml/min to 152 ml/min. Cephaloridine is potentially nephrotoxic and should, therefore, be avoided in patients with renal failure.

The aminoglycosides The aminoglycosides are widely used in treating gram-negative infections. They share chemical, antimicrobial, pharmacologic, and toxic characteristics. All are thought to be more active at an alkaline than at an acid pH. All are potentially nephrotoxic and ototoxic, but to different degrees. All can accumulate in renal failure. Therefore, their use should be either avoided in renal failure or their dosage should be adjusted, either by prolonging the interval between dosing or by drastically reducing the dose.

Kanamycin and gentamicin are largely responsible for the adverse reactions of antibiotics in the elderly. In patients under 60 years of age, 2.5% of those receiving kanamycin and 4.8% of those receiving gentamicin experience adverse reactions. After the age of 60 years, 12.5% of patients receiving those drugs show evidence of adverse reactions (Department of Health, Education and Welfare 1978). The adverse reactions most frequently seen include renal failure, respiratory arrest, and candidiasis. Gentamicin, given to patients with progressive Parkinson disease, may lead to marked deterioration of their neurologic status (Holtzman 1976).

The principal risk posed by the aminoglycosides in the elderly is nephrotoxicity. The aminoglycosides can reduce renal function, even if blood levels remain in the desired therapeutic range. In the elderly, in whom renal functional reserve may already be marginal, uremia may be precipitated.

As a guide to avoid toxicities due to aminoglycosides, toxic blood levels have been suggested (Table 18-5). Thus, theoretically, dosage adjustment should avoid these levels. However, in establishing gentamicin dosage, for example, there is a poor correlation between the gentamicin elimination rate constant and creatinine clearance and between gentamicin dosage and creatinine. Therefore, methods to determine gentamicin dosage may not be reliable. Methods based on creatinine are less desirable than those based on creatinine clearance, as the latter are more responsive to changes in renal function.

In the elderly, there may be a physiologic loss of vestibular and cochlear hair cells and ganglia. This enhances risk of the elderly to ototoxic effects of many drugs, including the aminoglycosides. These drugs can produce both auditory and vestibular damage (Brummet et al 1972). Auditory toxicity can lead to hearing loss and vestibular toxicity causes dysfunctions in the vestibular apparatus, leading to dizziness and vertigo (Dorff 1978). The ototoxicity of aminoglycosides occurs because they attain high concentrations in the inner ear fluids

Table 18-5
Aminoglycosides: Toxic Blood Levels

	Toxic Level (mcg/ml)	
Drug	Peak	Trough
Amikacin	20	10
Gentamicin	10	2
Streptomycin	20–25	—
Tobramycin	10	2

Source: J.K. Smith, and S.L. Wiener. *Drug Ther.* (Hosp Ed), 3(4):19, 1978.

that are retained for prolonged periods of time. The aminoglycosides exert their ototoxic effect mainly at the labyrinth and the sensory (hair) cells, which suffer the most damage. Gentamicin and streptomycin cause mainly vestibular damage; amikacin, kanamycin, and neomycin cause auditory damage; and tobramycin can cause both auditory and vestibular damage. Drug-induced ototoxicity probably occurs in 13 of 1000 patients. The incidence of ototoxicity is probably lower with tobramycin than with other aminoglycosides, and about 50% less than with gentamicin.

Ototoxicity occurs most frequently in the elderly patient receiving potent diuretics, such as ethacrynic acid or furosemide, while also receiving one of these antibiotics (Dorff 1978).

URINARY TRACT INFECTIONS

Urinary tract infections occur when microorganisms proliferate in the urinary tract, causing a subsequent inflammatory reaction. Age is accompanied by physiologic changes in the urinary tract. In men, these changes most often are represented by a gradual enlargement of the prostate. Transurethral incision of the prostate has been advocated, which restores normal urination with minimal anatomic destruction (Orandi 1978). In women, cystoceles or a narrowing of the urethral meatus is most frequently seen. Urinary tract infections are the most common infections in women. By age 50 years, 5% to 10% of all women have some kind of urinary tract infection. Urinary tract infection, the most common type of renal disease in the elderly, is often caused by inadequate micturition from obstructive or neurologic bladder function disturbances. Urine retention may also be caused by drugs. Any drug with anticholinergic activity can cause urinary retention, including antidepressants, antiparkinsonism drugs, belladonna, atropine, propantheline, and others (Brocklehurst 1978).

The incidence of urinary tract infections increases with age, progressive disability, and dependency (Lye 1978). It rises sharply with institutionalization and urinary tract infections are the most common hospital-acquired infections (Warren et al 1978). The incidence of urinary tract infections is highest in long-term patients.

Bacteriuria will develop in approximately 50% of patients within 12 months of admission to a long-term care institution; the prevalence is considerably higher in women than in men. Individuals with mechanical obstructions to urine flow and those with neurogenic bladders are particularly at risk. There is no clear evidence that bacteriuria is associated with deteriorating renal function or with hypertension.

In men, increased incidence of urinary tract infections is often related to a loss of bactericidal prostatic secretions. Residual urine with ischemia of the bladder wall, recumbency, poor nutrition, and a decreased efficiency of the autoimmune system in elderly patients with chronic diseases contribute to the occurrence of urinary tract infections (Lye 1978).

Urinary catheterization, even if used only for a short period of time, predisposes a patient to bacteriuria. Catheterization causes acute complications like acute pyelonephritis and renal failure. Catheters are used to prevent skin breakdown of the perineum and buttocks from chronic urinary incontinence. As some degree of bladder instability is common in the elderly (Brocklehurst 1978), catheters are frequently used. Yet, the urinary catheter has long been associated with excess rates of morbidity and mortality, and urinary infections caused by catheterization are the most prominent source of nosocomial bacteremia caused by gram-negative rods. Urinary tract infections will most likely develop in 15% to 25% of patients with indwelling catheters (Cooper 1977a). Therefore, catheterization should not be performed routinely. In an effort to reduce the incidence of urinary tract infections caused by catheterization, the use of continuous antibacterial rinse of dilute neomycin-polymyxin has been recommended, but there is some indication that more organisms gain entry into an irrigated rather than a nonirrigated system and that use of this type of rinse may be counterproductive (Warren et al 1978).

Diagnosis

In many older patients, a urinary infection may be completely asymptomatic. For example, bacteriuria is often chronic and asymptomatic. It may, at times, also be difficult to recognize even acute urinary tract infections. In cystitis, for example, there may be just frequency and dysuria. Often, family physicians are not aware of urinary infections in their patients, and yet there is danger of renal destruction that might develop as a result of the silent disease.

Dysuria, frequency, rigors, fever, and pain strongly indicate urinary tract infection. Yet, it is often difficult to distinguish between lower urinary tract infections (cystitis and urethritis) and upper urinary tract infection (pyelonephritis). The latter is more serious and involves the kidney, and bacterial involvement of the kidney is more likely to cause serious sepsis and deterioration of function than bladder infection (Straffon 1974; Thomas et al 1974; Jones et al 1974; Kunin 1975b). Two urine cultures should be obtained, preferably one day apart, so significant organisms can be distinguished from contaminants. A febrile, urinary tract infection with the same organism isolated from both blood and urine suggests renal involvement. Furthermore, patients whose bacteria are coated with human globulin are likely to have a kidney infection.

Many women who complain of frequency or dysuria do not have bacteriuria. In most cases, symptoms will resolve spontaneously. Asymptomatic bacteriuria (when successive cultures show more than 10^5 bacteria/ml) should be suspected in diabetics with urologic abnormalities and in patients with indwelling catheters.

The Infecting Organisms

E. coli, originating in the gastrointestinal tract, is responsible for most upper and lower urinary tract infections. Acute symptomatic infections may also be caused by coagulase-negative staphylococci. In institutionalized patients, *E. coli* is still the primary causative agent in women, but *Proteus* is seen more frequently. In institutionalized males, *Proteus* is the major organism causing urinary tract infections. In patients with obstruction, *Proteus* and *Pseudomonas* are most often isolated as the causative organisms. About half the patients with indwelling catheters who develop infections will become infected with *E. coli,* but in chronically catheterized patients, other gram-negative organisms are seen more often.

Treatment

Failure to treat urinary tract infection can lead to the development of chronic pyelonephritis. Any patients who develop acute symptomatic urinary tract infection should receive prompt therapy, irrespective of the anatomic state of their urinary tract. Pyelonephritis and acute cystitis are such symptomatic infections. Acute, uncomplicated urinary tract infections can be treated and cured in up to 80% of patients. However, the recurrence rate following the first infection may be as high as 75% to 80%. Before the infecting organism is known, a soluble sulfonamide is usually selected (Kunin 1974; Brocklehurst 1971; Moore-Smith 1973; Gladstone and Recco 1976). Alternates are ampicillin or amoxicillin for *E. coli* or *Proteus mirabilis,* a cephalosporin for *Klebsiella,* and oral carbenicillin for *Proteus.* In patients with renal insufficiency the penicillins are preferred, the particular one selected on the basis of sensitivity testing. They can achieve high concentrations in the urine without causing toxicity. If symptoms are responsive to treatment, the patient should receive the drug for at least 10 days. If symptoms and urinary bacterial counts do not respond to the first drug selected, an alternate drug should be chosen based on sensitivity testing.

In case of chronic urinary tract infections, the recommendations, unfortunately, are not as clear-cut. There is still no consensus as to the best therapy for chronic urinary infections. Low dose antimicrobials, the methenamine salts, and specific antibiotic therapies have all been suggested and all have been effective to some degree (Smith and Martin 1966).

Chronic bacteriuria is often asymptomatic and unlikely to cause significant morbidity. However, complications can result, including acute and chronic pyelonephritis, bacteremia, renal failure, and death. The physician is faced with the decision to permit the persistence of a possible asymptomatic bacteriuria, or attempt to eradicate it. Even asymptomatic bacteriuria can lead to sudden acute pyelonephritis or bacteremia. On the other hand, if treated, even by prolonged antibacterial administration, only 20% to 30% of these infections will be cured. Of clinical significance is the fact that, in nonresponsive cases, resistant organisms often develop. Therefore, efforts to prevent chronic renal insufficiency should be directed toward patients with symptoms of sepsis and obstructive uropathy and not those with asymptomatic bacteriuria (Petersdorf and Plorda 1965; Kunin 1969; Alling et al 1975).

Concomitant diseases, common in older people, complicate the treatment of urinary tract infections. Among these are diabetes, impaired renal function, heart disease, and debilitation from arthritis. An aggressive treatment is necessary for patients with both diabetes and urinary tract infections because older diabetics lack the nephron compensatory mechanism. Diabetes also impairs mobilization of white cells, and possibly phagocytosis. Kidney damage may be irreversible, if not treated aggressively.

Recurrent or persistent infections are difficult to treat. They may either be relapses or reinfections. Relapses most often occur because of failure to complete an adequate course of therapy when the infections first occurred. The same organism will then cause reinfection.

Residual urine can lead to relapse, and it can also hinder treatment of the original infection. If the bladder does not function normally, higher doses of the selected antibacterial or more prolonged treatment is indicated. Mechanical problems, such as renal stones, can also cause relapse.

In women, relapse is often caused by migration and colonization of fecal bacteria on the vaginal vestibule, followed by retrograde entry into the urethra and bladder. Chronic bacterial prostatitis is probably the most common cause of relapsing urinary tract infections in men (Meares 1976). Chronic bacterial prostatitis is seldom, if ever, cured. Even when antibacterial agents are used for prolonged periods of time, most often they fail to achieve the desired results, as they do not diffuse into the prostatic fluid in sufficient concentration. Apparently though, the use of trimethoprim combined with a sulfonamide reduces the development of resistant strains significantly if used for prolonged periods of time. Treatment may have to be continued for as long as 12 weeks. Leukopenia, thrombocytopenia, other signs of bone marrow depression, and folic acid deficiency rule out this treatment. Complete blood and platelet counts should be ordered at least monthly. While this treatment may not always eradicate the infection, it often permits the patient to remain asymptomatic if treatment is continued with one tablet per day.

Antibacterial therapy is of no value in nonbacterial prostatitis. It has been suggested that symptoms can be relieved by periodic prostatic massage. Antiinflammatory agents and short courses of oral steroids have been tried.

Reinfections are recurrences caused by a different organism. These are usually lower urinary tract infections. In women, reinfections are much more common than are relapses. Individuals who suffer from symptomatic reinfections are not likely to benefit from prolonged intensive therapy. Each episode should be treated for 10 to 14 days. Frequently, recurring infections may be caused by resistant bacteria and, therefore, sensitivity testing should be done before any treatment is started.

If reinfections are frequent, suppressive therapy may be indicated. Prophylactic use of antimicrobials reduces the frequency of symptomatic urinary tract infections, even though therapy may only suppress and not eradicate the problem (Kunin 1975a). Either trimethoprim-sulfamethoxazole or nitrofurantoin is probably best for long-term prophylaxis, as they are least likely to cause emergence of resistant organisms (Meares 1975). One 50 mg tablet of nitrofurantoin daily or one-half tablet of the trimethoprim-sulfonamide combination are usually recommended. Alternatively, the methenamine salts are often used, which may have to be continued for prolonged periods of time, even years.

The importance of urinary pH Urinary levels of antibacterials determine treatment outcome of most urinary tract infections. The urinary pH, the total osmolarity of the urine, and the presence of individual solutes can inhibit the antibacterial action (Minuth et al 1976). In particular, urinary pH has a profound effect on the activity of some antibacterial agents. Adjustment of urinary pH to an alkaline pH can increase the activity of some antibiotics 100 times or more (Sabath et al 1970). This increased activity could then permit a lower dose, and thus expose the patient to less toxicity.

Erythromycin, kanamycin, neomycin, novobiocin, and penicillin all have increased activity at an alkaline pH. Gentamicin is 100 times more active at a urinary pH of 8.5 than 5.0. Therefore, only as little as 1% or less of the "usual" dose may be sufficient in patients who may safely be given alkalinizing medications.

The effectiveness of the nitrofurantoins does not seem to vary with different pH values, and sulfonamides seem to exhibit a variable response to altered urinary pH. On the other hand, the tetracyclines seem to be more active at an acid urinary pH, and the methenamine salts depend for optimal activity on as low a urinary pH as possible (Brumfitt and Percival 1962). In an effort to acidify the urine, cranberry juice has been used extensively, even though it produces only a slight and transient effect on urinary pH, and up to 4000 ml daily may be needed to produce this effect (Fellers et al 1933; Paps et al 1966; Kahn et al 1967). Most often, ascorbic acid, in tablet or liquid form, is used to acidify the urine. This has a highly variable effect and raises urinary pH in some patients. The urinary pH must be established whenever ascorbic acid is used (Naccarto et al 1979).

Methenamine Methenamine was first used in 1894. Its antibacterial action depends on its hydrolysis to formaldehyde. Both the mandelate and hippurate salts of methenamine require an acid urinary pH to be converted to formaldehyde. The optimal antibacterial action of methenamine is achieved at pH 5.5 or less, and its minimal inhibitory concentration against *E. coli* at pH 7.0 is double that at pH 4.9. If the urinary pH is greater than 6.5, methenamine cannot be hydrolized in the presence of urea-splitting organisms such as *Proteus*. Acetazolamide, the thiazide diuretics, and furosemide contribute to an alkaline urinary pH, as do the nonabsorbable antacids. Since the elderly frequently receive these drugs, it may be assumed that they have an alkaline urinary pH, which possibly negates action of the methenamine salts.

All bacteria, except the urea-splitting ones, are susceptible to the action of methenamine (Cooper 1977b). The drug is effective in the treatment of chronic urinary infections in noncatheterized patients. It is believed to eradicate bacteriuria in about 75% of elderly patients. Caution is advised when using the suspension, as it has caused lipid pneumonia in some senile hemiplegic patients (Timmerman and Schroeder 1973). Even moderate renal impairment precludes the use of methenamine. Concurrent use of alkalinizers must, of course, be avoided. Its use should also be avoided in patients with gout, as it may cause the formation of urinary urate crystals. The formaldehyde or the acidic urine may cause irritation of the urinary tract, dysuria, albuminuria, and hematuria.

The sulfonamides The sulfonamides (and other nonantibiotics) apparently do not cause suprainfections. Therefore, it has been recommended that infections of the lower urinary tract be treated with these drugs rather than with antibiotics. The sulfonamides are the treatment of choice for acute, uncomplicated, community-acquired urinary tract infections. They are not usually effective in chronic and recurrent infections or hospital-acquired infections (Kucers and Bennett 1974). Because the single entity sulfonamides are least expensive, they should be tried first.

They are not recommended, in general, if the patient's creatinine clearance is less than 50 ml per minute. In patients with good renal function, fluids should be forced. It is thought that an acid urine enhances their effectiveness, but it also enhances their propensity to cause crystalluria. The sulfonamides lose effectiveness with increasing duration of treatment and with decreasing intervals between infectious episodes.

For patients with recurrent sulfonamide-resistant infections, a good response is possible with long-term use of trimethoprim-sulfamethoxazole (Atkins and MacCannell 1978). Almost all urinary tract infections, including hospital-acquired infections, can be treated with this combination, except those caused by *Pseudomonas*. This combination appears to be more effective in chronic urinary tract infections than other agents (*Medical Letter* 1975). It increases the serum creatinine by 0.2 mg%, but has a fairly low order of toxicity. It cannot be used in high-risk patients; at least one fatal reaction, involving the kidneys, liver, lungs, skin, pancreas, and central nervous system has been reported in an elderly patient receiving this combination for bacteriuria (Brockner and Boisen 1978). The sulfonamides, of course, cannot be used in patients with known sulfonamide sensitivity. They may enhance the action of the sulfonylureas, and sulfamethizole may prolong the half-life of phenytoin.

The nitrofurans These drugs are effective in both acute and chronic urinary tract infections in patients with good renal function. In poor renal function, their concentration in the urine will be too low to be effective. Prophylaxis with nitrofurans seems adequate for less severe problems of reinfections. However, when bacteriuria occurs despite nitrofurantoin macrocrystal prophylaxis, the sulfonamide combination is usually indicated.

Acute hypersensitivity caused by the nitrofurans occurs more commonly in elderly than in young patients, and irreversible peripheral neuropathy occurs when toxic serum levels are reached.

The antibiotics The indications for the oral use of antibiotics are given in Table 18-6. If parenteral treatment is indicated, tobramycin or gentamicin are usually preferred, and sometimes kanamycin is used. Enterococcus is treated with ampicillin parenterally, and staphylococcus with penicillin G, oxacillin, or a cephalosporin. Impaired renal function mandates reduced doses of colistin, polymyxin, kanamycin, gentamicin, and vancomycin (Reidenberg 1971). Penicillin G can be given safely in large doses to patients with an impaired renal function. Renal insufficiency may also be responsible for relatively low concentrations of an antibiotic in the urine, eg, gentamicin (Riff and Jackson 1971). Because the effectiveness of drugs

Table 18-6
Oral Antibiotic Therapy for Urinary Tract Infections

Drug	Organism
Ampicillin	*Escherichia coli*
	Proteus mirabilis
	Enterococcus
Trimethoprim-sulfamethoxazole	*Enterobacteria*
	Proteus
Carbenicillin	*Pseudomonas aeruginosa*
Cephalosporin	*Klebsiella pneumoniae*
Penicillin V	*Staphylococcus aureus*

used in urinary tract infections depends on their concentration in urine rather than in the serum (Romankiewicz 1974), it is important to ascertain the drug levels in the urine.

The penicillins Penicillin G is effective, but the rate of recurrence of infection after use of penicillin G is relatively high (Hulbert 1972). Ampicillin is used extensively in the treatment of acute, uncomplicated urinary tract infections caused primarily by *E. coli*. If the infection is caused by *Pseudomonas,* ampicillin will not be effective. Use of this drug is questionable in the treatment of chronic or complicated urinary tract infections. In patients with poor renal function, rashes and pruritus occur relatively frequently.

Amoxicillin is probably as effective as ampicillin and can be used in lower doses with longer dosing intervals. Carbenicillin has some activity against *Pseudomonas.* In general, *Pseudomonas* infections are usually accompanied by underlying neurologic/structural abnormalities and are difficult to manage.

The cephalosporins These drugs are mainly used in infections resistant to sulfonamides or ampicillin.

Oxolinic acid This drug has been introduced for the treatment of initial or recurrent nonobstructive urinary tract infections, such as pyelonephritis, cystitis, and urethritis caused by susceptible gram-negative bacteria. Oxolinic acid, related structurally to nalidixic acid, is longer-acting than nalidixic acid and can be used in a twice-a-day schedule. However, it has a higher incidence of adverse effects, particularly a CNS stimulating action that is greatest in geriatric patients. The affected patient may suffer from dizziness, restlessness, nervousness, and insomnia. Because oxolinic acid is partially eliminated by the kidney, it should be used with caution in elderly patients with renal insufficiency. Similar to nalidixic acid, oxolinic acid may produce false positive results for a copper reduction urine glucose test like Clinitest, but does not affect the glucose oxidase tests such as Testape or Clinistix.

The aminoglycosides These are the drugs of choice for gram-negative sepsis or pyelonephritis caused by organisms resistant to less toxic drugs. Gentamicin is not indicated for the majority of urinary tract infections which usually respond to the safer, oral drugs. Gentamicin may, however, be valuable in the treatment of infections caused by *Pseudomonas*. In one study, tobramycin and gentamicin were found to be equally effective in eradicating urinary tract infections, although some patients needed a second course of treatment (Walker and Gentry 1976). Ototoxicity was not detected in any patient (mean age of 60 years), but gentamicin was responsible for more nephrotoxicity than tobramycin. Gentamicin and tobramycin are generally effective against all urinary tract infections except those caused by *S. faecalis*. Tobramycin may be effective against gentamicin-resistant *Pseudomonas* strains.

The effectiveness of gentamicin treatment depends both on the ability of gentamicin to exert its antibacterial effect in the urine and on the ability of the kidney to excrete gentamicin into the urine (Minuth et al 1976). Normal concentrations or electrolytes in the urine, such as magnesium and calcium, can interfere with the activity of gentamicin, possibly because of enhanced binding of bacteria by gentamicin in the presence of these ions. Furthermore, up to 40 times as much gentamicin may be needed to prevent growth of *E. coli* or *Pseudomonas aeruginosa* in concentrated acidic human urine.

The antibacterial activity of all aminoglycosides is decreased in an acid urinary medium and increased in an alkaline urine (Brumfitt 1962).

Urinary tract infections are difficult to treat. Treatment should be preceded by sensitivity testing and should be continued with a sufficient dose for a sufficient duration in order to prevent, as much as possible, recurrent infections.

REFERENCES

Alling, B., Brandberg, A., Seeberg, S. et al. Effect of consecutive antibacterial therapy on bacteriuria in hospitalized geriatric patients. *Scand J Infect Dis.* 7:201, 1975.

Appel, G.B., and Neu, H.C. The nephrotoxicity of antimicrobial agents. *N Engl J Med.* 296:663, 1977.

Atkins, E.L., and MacCannell, K.L. Long-term treatment of sulfa-resistant urinary tract infections with a sulfamethoxazole-trimethoprim combination. *J Clin Pharmacol.* 18:54, 1978.

Brocklehurst, J.C. The urinary tract. Edited by I. Rossman. In *Clinical Geriatrics*. Philadelphia: J.B. Lippincott Co., 1971.

Brocklehurst, J.C. Differential diagnosis of urinary incontinence. *Geriatrics* 33(4):36, 1978.

Brockner, J., and Boisen, E. Fatal multisystem toxicity after cotrimoxazole. *Lancet* 1:831, 1978.

Brumfitt, W. Adjustment of urine pH in the chemotherapy of urinary tract infections. *Lancet* 1:186, 1962.

Brumfitt, W., and Percival, A. Adjustment of urine pH in the chemotherapy of urinary tract infections. *Lancet* 1:136, 1962.

Brummett, R.E., Himes, D., Saine, B. et al. A comparative study of the ototoxicity of tobramycin and gentamicin. *Arch Otolaryngol.* 96:505, 1972.

Buckley, C.E., and Dorsey, F.C. Serum immunoglobulin levels throughout the lifespan of healthy man. *Ann Intern Med.* 75:673, 1971.

Clarke, J.T. Antibiotic therapy of pneumonia. *Geriatrics* 32(11):51, 1977.

Cooper, J.W. Urinary tract infections. I. Cause and prevention. *Hosp Formulary.* 12:106, 1977a.

Cooper, J.W. Urinary tract infections. II. Optimal drug therapy. *Hosp Formulary.* 12:175, 1977b.

Das, B.C., and Sharma, J.S. Linked cross-sectional study of age-related changes in human blood chemistry, hematology, and circulatory function. *Exp Gerontol.* 6:345, 1971.

Department of Health, Education and Welfare. Workshop on pharmacology and aging. DHEW Publ. No. (NIH) 78-353. Bethesda, Md.: National Institutes of Health, 1978.

Dorff, G.J. Avoiding aminoglycoside toxicity. *Drug Ther.* 8(1):153, 1978.

Fellers, C.R., Redmon, B.C., and Parrott, E.M. Effect of cranberries on urinary acidity and blood alkali reserve. *J Nutr.* 6:455, 1933.

Gladstone, J.L., and Recco, R. Host factors and infectious diseases in the elderly. *Med Clin North Am.* 60:1225, 1976.

Hayes, S.L. Safer use of antibiotics. *Drug Ther.* 7(3):67, 1977.

Hicks, R. Aging. *Pharm J.* 215:291, 1975.

Holtzman, J.L. Gentamicin and neuromuscular blockade. *Ann Intern Med.* 84:55, 1976.

Hulbert, J. Gram-negative urinary infections treated with oral penicillin. *Lancet* 2:1216, 1972.

Jones, S.R., Smith, J.W., and Sanford, J.P. Localization of urinary tract infection by detection of antibody-coated bacteria in urine sediment. *N Engl J Med.* 90:591, 1974.

Kahn, H.D., Panariello, V.A., Saeli, J. et al. Effect of cranberry juice on urine. *J Am Diet Assoc.* 51:251, 1967.

Kucers, A., and Bennett, N.M. *The Use of Antibiotics.* Philadelphia: J.B. Lippincott Co., 1974.

Kunin, C.M. Epidemiology of bacteriuria and its relation to pyelonephritis. *J Infect Dis.* 120:1, 1969.

Kunin, C.M. *Detection, Prevention and Management of Urinary Tract Infections.* Philadelphia: Lea & Febiger, 1974.

Kunin, C.M. Long-term therapy of urinary tract infections. *Ann Intern Med.* 83:273, 1975a.

Kunin, C.M. Developments in the diagnosis and treatment of urinary tract infections. *J Urol.* 113:585, 1975b.

Lye, M. Defining and treating urinary infections. *Geriatrics* 33(3):71, 1978.

McCabe, W.R. *Gram-Negative Bacteremia.* Chicago: Yearbook Medical Publishers, 1973.

Meares, E.M. Long-term therapy of chronic bacterial prostatitis with trimethoprim-sulfamethoxazole. *Can Med Assoc J.* 112:22S, 1975.

Meares, E.M. Prostatitis: diagnosis and treatment. *Drug Ther.* 6(10):111, 1976.

Medical Letter. Trimethoprim-sulfamethoxazole for treatment of urinary tract infections. 17:101, 1975.

Ninuth, J.M., Musher, D.M., and Thornsteinsson, S.B. Inhibition of the antibacterial activity of gentamicin by urine. *J Infect Dis.* 133:14, 1976.

Moellering, R.C. Factors influencing the clinical use of antimicrobial agents in elderly patients. *Geriatrics* 33(2):83, 1978.

Moellering, R.C., and Swartz, M.N. The newer cephalosporins. *N Engl J Med.* 294:24, 1976.

Moore-Smith, B. Urinary tract diseases. *Br Med J.* 3:686, 1973.

Naccarto, D.V., Bell, C.J., and Lamy, P.P. Appraisal of ascorbic acid for acidifying the urine of methenamine-treated geriatric patients. *J Am Geriatr Soc.* 27:34, 1979.

Orandi, A. New method for treating prostatic hypertrophy. *Geriatrics* 33(6):58, 1978.

Paps, P.N., Brush, C.A., and Ceresia, G.C. Cranberry juice in the treatment of urinary tract infections. *Southwest Med.* 47(1):17, 1966.

Petersdorf, R.G., and Plorda, J.J. Management of urinary tract infections in the elderly. *Geriatrics* 20:613, 1965.

Reidenberg, M.M. *Renal Function and Drug Action.* Philadelphia: W.B. Saunders Co., 1971.

Romankiewicz, J.A. Factors influencing renal distribution of antibiotics: a key to therapy of pyelonephritis. *Drug Intell Clin Pharm.* 8:512, 1974.

Riff, L.J., and Jackson, G.G. Pharmacology of gentamicin in man. *J Infect Dis* 124(suppl):S98, 1971.

Sabath, L.D., Gerstein, D.A., Leaf, C.D. et al. Increasing the usefulness of antibiotics: treatment of infections caused by gram-negative bacilli. *Clin Pharmacol Ther.* 11:161, 1970.

Seneca, H. Management of infections and infestations in the elderly. *J Am Geriatr Soc.* 18:798, 1970.

Simon, C., Malerczyk, V., Tenschert, B. et al. Die Geriatrische Pharmacologie von Cefazolin, Cefradin und Sulfisomidin. *Arzneimittel-Forsch.* 26:1377, 1976.

Smith, L., and Martin, W. Infections of the urinary tract. *Med Clin North Am.* 50:1127, 1966.

Smith, J.K., and Wiener, S.L. Life-threatening infections in the elderly: aging, immunity, and antibiotics. *Drug Ther.* Hosp Ed. 3(4):19, 1978.

Straffon, R.A. Urinary tract infections. *Med Clin North Am.* 58:545, 1974.

Timmerman, R.J., and Schroeder, J.A. Lipid pneumonia caused by methenamine mandelate suspension. *JAMA.* 225:1524, 1973.

Thomas, V., Shelokov, A., and Forland, J. Antibody-coated bacteria in the urine and the site of urinary tract infections. *N Engl J Med.* 290:588, 1974.

Walker, B.D., and Gentry, L.O. A randomized, comparative study of tobramycin and gentamicin in treatment of acute urinary tract infections. *J Infect Dis.* 134(suppl):S146, 1976.

Warren, J.W., Platt, R., Thomas, R.J. et al. Antibiotic irrigations and catheter-associated urinary tract infections. *N Engl J Med.* 299:570, 1978.

Weinstein, L. Some principles of antimicrobial therapy. *Rational Drug Ther.* 11(3):1, 1977.

19 Cardiovascular Drugs

Age-related changes occur in the heart and the peripheral vascular system. In the resting state, the duration of cardiac contraction and relaxation are prolonged. Peripheral vascular resistance is increased, cardiac output is lower, and impedance to left ventricular ejection is greater. Despite these changes, cardiovascular function is not altered significantly in the absence of stress. However, aging impairs the response to stress. Maximal heart rate, stroke volume, and A-V oxygen differences are all lowered with stress. The decline in maximal oxygen consumption parallels that during maximal work load. When the aged heart is stressed, there is a predisposition to the development of cardiac arrhythmias and failure, which has been termed presbycardia.

The decrease in cardiac contractility with age is paralleled by a decrease in functional reserve of other major organs. Thus, regional circulatory failure may precede symptoms of heart disease (Nejat and Greif 1976).

Chronic circulatory conditions increase with age (Table 19-1). In one sample institution, over 80% of those over 75 years of age had evidence of organic heart diseases, and 50% had some degree of failure (Department of Health, Education and Welfare, 1978a). Of the 21 million Americans 65 years and older, approximately one in four was hospitalized in 1972. Cardiovascular disease was the most frequent reason for hospitalization and cardiac disease alone accounted for more than 40% of all deaths in this age group (Gerstenblith et al 1976). Age-adjusted mortality from coronary heart disease increased 19% in the United States between 1950 and 1963. A decline in mortality from coronary heart disease started the year that the American Heart Association recommended a change in the general American diet, limiting intake of saturated fats and cholesterol. This decline has continued (Table 19-2). Cerebrovascular mortality began to decline in 1952, even before the advent of effective antihypertensive agents, and a major reduction in cerebrovascular deaths is now reported among patients treated for hypertension (Walker 1977).

Regardless of the intervention, cardiovascular mortality and morbidity increase with age. Fatalities from cerebrovascular disease are exceeded only by heart disease and cancer, and the death rate from heart disease in the aged is twice as high as that from stroke.

In 1975, the National Heart, Lung, and Blood Institute estimated that 1.3 million Americans would experience coronary disease. Coronary heart disease results from damage to the coronary arteries, and

Table 19-1
Chronic Circulatory Conditions*

Condition	All ages	45–64 years	65 years and older
Heart conditions	50	89	199
Hypertensive heart disease	11	20	53
Coronary heart disease	16	35	84
Other heart disease	2	4	7
Disorders of heart rhythm, unspecified	12	13	22
Heart trouble, unspecified	6	11	28
Hypertensive disease, other	60	127	199
Cerebrovascular disease	8	12	48
Arteriosclerosis, other	3	—	26
Varicose veins	37	74	94
Hemorrhoids	48	80	74
Phlebitis and thrombophlebitis	2	4	3
Poor circulation, unspecified	5	8	24

*Conditions per 1000 persons
Source: Prevalence of chronic circulatory conditions, U.S., 1972. DHEW Publ. No. (HRA) 75-1521. Rockville, Md.: National Center for Health Statistics, 1974.

Table 19-2
Decline in Cerebrovascular and Coronary Mortality 1963–1975

	Decline in Mortality (Percentage)	
Age (years)	Cerebro-vascular	Coronary
35–44	19.1	27.2
45–54	31.7	27.4
55–64	34.1	23.5
65–74	33.2	25.3
75–84	21.9	12.8
85+	29.4	19.3

Source: National Center for Health Statistics, 1977.

myocardial infarction is one of the most common forms of clinical coronary disease. It was further estimated that approximately 675,000 of the 1.3 million persons stricken would die, and 175,000 deaths would be premature, before the age of 65 years.

The majority of cardiac patients do not have excessive levels of serum cholesterol, only a small number are hypertensive, and even fewer are diabetic. The role of cholesterol in cardiac disease is disputed, as are other stress factors and risk factors.

Serum cholesterol levels apparently increase with age (Figure 19-1). Normally, low density lipoprotein (LDL) accounts for approximately 70% of total circulating cholesterol, high density lipoprotein (HDL) accounts for about 17%, and the very low density lipoprotein accounts for about 13%.

There are now reports that there is an inverse relationship between the level of cholesterol bound to the high density lipoprotein and the risk of developing coronary heart disease. Prevalence rates of coronary heart disease appear to decrease with increasing levels of cholesterol bound to high density lipoprotein. High density lipoprotein, it has been suggested, is protective, while low density lipoprotein is a major risk factor for the development of atherosclerosis. Moderate amounts of alcohol may shift the lipoprotein balance so that there is less LDL and more HDL, which might afford more protection against coronary disease (Castelli et al 1977).

It is not the purpose of this chapter to discuss risk factors and heart disease. In summary, stressful life events appear to be related to the risk of coronary disease, but it is by no means clear that obesity and/or lack of exercise increase the risk of heart disease. Others strongly feel that in the treatment of hypertension, greater emphasis should be placed on dietary therapy, including sodium restriction and return to "ideal" weight (Ames 1977).

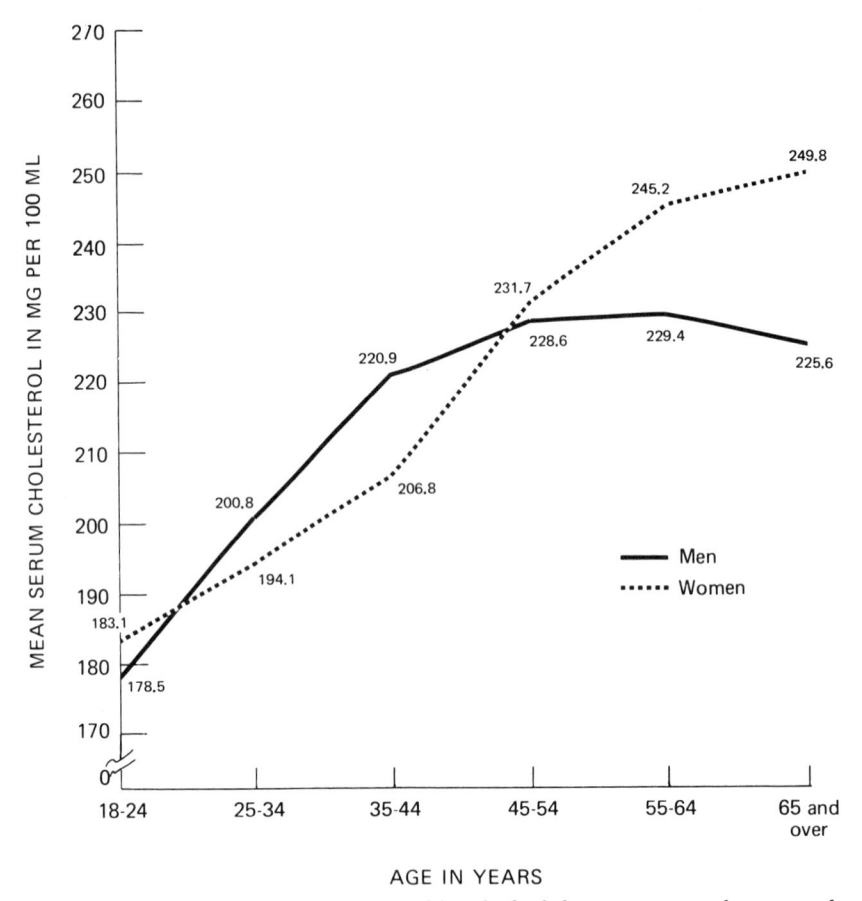

Figure 19-1 Mean serum cholesterol level of adults 18–74 years by age and sex: United States, 1971–1974.

Presenting symptoms of heart disease of the elderly may be confusing. The elderly commonly complain of shortness of breath. Acute dyspnea rather than chest pain may be the complaint in acute myocardial infarction. If chest pain is the presenting complaint, it could also be from angina pectoris, pneumonia, arthritis, a herniated disc, hiatus hernia, or a peptic ulcer. Cough and wheezing are frequent complaints of the elderly with heart disease.

In the elderly, heart disease may also cause vertigo, syncope, and acute mental confusion. The patient may complain of acute abdominal pain, anorexia, insomnia, fatigue, and nocturia. Infection, emotional stress, fever, and other factors are likely to cause heart failure in the elderly.

Cardiovascular drug therapy in the elderly aims primarily at three disease states: coronary artery insufficiency with the characteristic clinical picture of angina pectoris (ischemic heart disease), cardiac failure (congestive heart failure), and hypertension.

Essentially, drug treatment does not differ greatly from that used for younger patients. However, altered pharmacokinetics in the elderly may make drug treatment more difficult. For example, patients with congestive heart failure may exhibit decreased volumes of distribution for some drugs, which leads to higher than normal concentrations after normal dosage administration. Elderly patients with heart disease may also suffer from an impaired ability to excrete drugs as their kidney or liver may be inadequately perfused. This might lead to increased drug toxicities.

HEART DISEASES

Ischemic Heart Disease

This is the most important cardiovascular disease of the elderly. It is also the most common serious health problem of contemporary society. In the United States, 675,000 people die each year from ischemic heart disease and its complications. Ischemia is defined as a condition of oxygen deprivation secondary to reduced perfusion. In contrast, hypoxia is a condition of reduced oxygen supply despite adequate perfusion, while anoxia denotes the complete absence of oxygen despite adequate perfusion. Ischemic heart disease is almost always caused by atherosclerosis of the coronary arteries, which is a multifactorial disease. Angina pectoris is the result of localized ischemia.

Congestive Heart Disease

The prevalence of congestive heart failure (CHF) increases from less than one case per thousand persons under the age of 50 years to more than eight per thousand over the age of 70 years (Katzung 1974b). CHF may be caused by damage to the heart muscle, as a result of infarction or ischemia. Diastolic problems leading to underfilling of the ventricle can cause CHF, in addition to systolic problems that can cause an inefficient pump action.

Cardiac output in CHF patients decreases. The kidneys receive only 10% of the output instead of the normal 20% (Mason and Tonkon 1977).

CHF constitutes a significant cause of morbidity and mortality. The mortality rate is about 50% within five years of onset, even with good medical supervision. Fatigue, dyspnea, orthopnea, and edema are the classic signs and symptoms of CHF. Most cases of CHF are caused by hypertension or valvular disease.

Hypertension

Between 1971 and 1974, 23.2 million adults between the ages of 18 and 74 years were found to have hypertension, defined as a systolic pressure of at least 160 mm Hg or a diastolic pressure of 95 mm Hg or more. Between the ages of 18 and 54 years, hypertension is more prevalent among men than among women. Between the ages of 55 to 74 years, hypertension is more prevalent among women than men (Tables 19-3 and 19-4). Hypertension is substantially more prevalent among black adults than white adults in the United States. For example, 50% of black men but only 31% of white men between the ages of 55 and 64 years have hypertension (Department of Health, Education and Welfare 1978b). The figures for black and white women in the same age group were 55% and 32% (Figure 19-2).

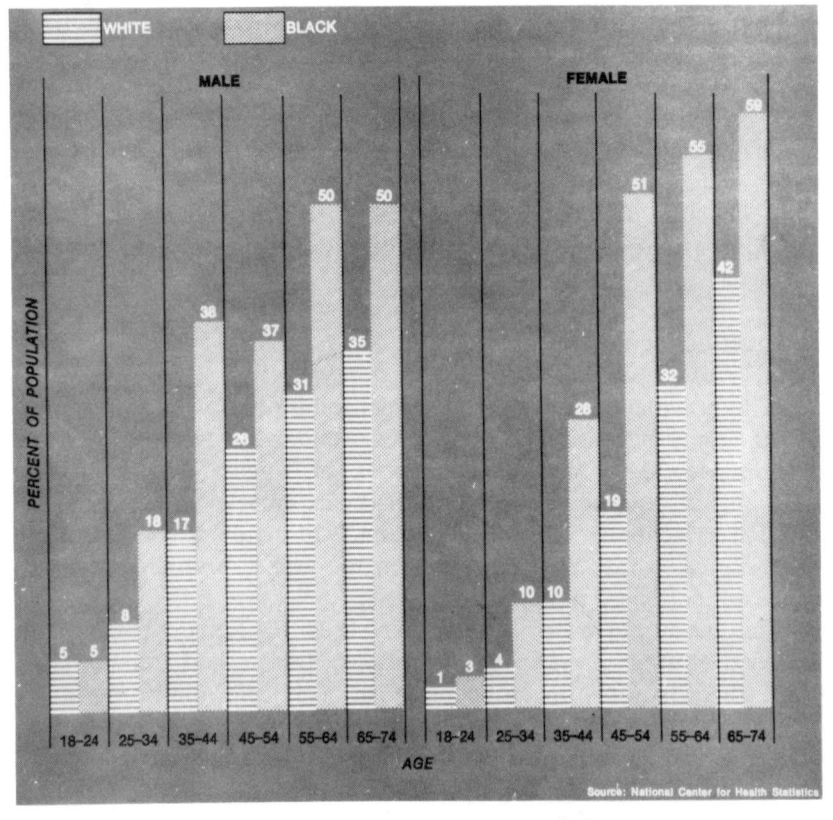

Figure 19-2 Hypertension by age, sex, and race—1971–1974.

Table 19-3
Hypertension: Summary of Prevalence Data[a] **(millions of persons)**

	Population Groups			Total Resident US Population	
	Under 18 years old, civilian, non-institutionalized	18–74 years old, civilian, non-institutionalized	75 years old and over, civilian and military, institutionalized (all ages)	1972	1977
Persons with definite high blood pressure, not adequately treated	0.5[b]	23.2[c]	3.7	27.3	28.4
Persons with borderline high blood pressure, not under medication	1.2[b]	21.0[c]	2.5	24.7	25.7
Persons with definite or borderline high blood pressure, controlled by medication	0.1	4.3[c]	0.7	5.1	5.3
Total with definite or borderline high blood pressure	1.8	48.5	6.9	57.1	59.3

Table 19-3 *(continued)*

	Population Groups			Total Resident US Population	
	Under 18 years old, civilian, non-institutionalized	18–74 years old, civilian, non-institutionalized	75 years old and over, civilian and military, institutionalized (all ages)	1972	1977
Total number of persons in population group	69.3	127.9	11.0	208.2	216.3

NOTES:

a. All figures are estimated from national sample data. Columns may not add due to rounding (to nearest 100,000). Sources: National Center for Health Statistics. Blood pressure of persons 6–74 years of age in the United States. *Adv Data.* No. 1, October 18, 1976. Roberts, J., and Maurer, K. Blood pressure levels of persons 6–74 years, United States, 1971–1974. *Vital and Health Statistics,* Series 11, Number 203, September 1977, National Center for Health Statistics, Washington, D.C., DHEW Publ. No. (HRA) 78-1648. Bureau of the Census. *Current Population Reports,* Table 2, Series P-25, No. 614, November, 1975.

b. Estimated by NHLBI from Health and Nutrition Examination Survey (HANES) data; negligible prevalence is assumed for persons under age 6. This survey collected data annually from 1971 to the present, based on surveys at between 30 and 35 sites nationally. Single blood pressure measurements were taken with the person seated, and an extensive interview was conducted. The resultant data constitute a national probability sample for civilian non-institutionalized adults between 18 and 74 years of age.

c. Based on HANES data.

Table 19-4
Hypertension: Influence of Sex and Age

	Percent	
Age (years)	*Male*	*Female*
All ages (18–74)	44	61
45–54	41	54
55–64	50	68
65–74	49	67

Source: Health Resources Administration. Health, United States, 1976–1977. DHEW Publ. No. (HRA) 77-1232. Hyattsville, Md.: National Center for Health Services Research, National Center for Health Statistics, 1977.

Systolic hypertension results from increased rigidity of the large arterial vessels. In this case, diastolic pressure tends to be low or normal, and pulse pressure will be increased (arteriosclerotic hypertension). Cerebral and coronary arteriosclerotic complications lead to enhanced mortality. The therapeutic goal would be to reduce pressure over a period of several weeks to prevent sudden reduction of blood pressure, which could be responsible for a significant decrease in cerebral blood flow and cerebral ischemia. Reduced flow in the presence of arteriosclerotic vessels predisposes the elderly patient to cerebrovascular thrombosis.

Diastolic hypertension is primarily caused by arteriolar constriction. In the elderly, diastolic hypertension may often be accompanied by an increase in systolic pressure caused by arterial rigidity. If untreated, renal function will decline, even in the aged, and complications will increase.

It is not true that older persons tolerate hypertension better than younger persons (Castelli 1976). Death rates from hypertension increase with age. The nonwhite population is more seriously affected than the white population (Table 19-5). There is a steady increment of risk at all pressure levels, both systolic and diastolic, even in the absence of symptoms. Hypertensive complications among the elderly

Table 19-5
Hypertension: Death Rates

Age	Nonwhite (A)	White (B)	A/B
45–54	115.3	13.8	8.36
55–64	204.3	42.7	4.78
65–74	428.0	117.9	3.63

Data are based on the National Vital Registration System. National Center for Health Statistics: Vital Statistics of the United States, Vol. II. Washington, D.C.: U.S. Government Printing Office, 1968.

usually manifest as cardiac insufficiency, or as an effect on coronary or cerebral vessels. Thus, hypertension should be controlled in the elderly.

Other Diseases

If cardiac failure is treated vigorously with diuretics, there will be an increase in blood viscosity and an increase in the likelihood of venous thromboembolic disease. A sedentary existence, bed rest, and CHF are important precipitating factors of this disease. For deep vein thrombosis, anticoagulants remain the treatment of choice. They prevent pulmonary embolism and preserve venous valvular function. Heparin is administered every four hours by the intermittent intravenous method, but continuous, carefully controlled intravenous infusion has also been recommended and seems to cause fewer hemorrhagic complications (Friedman 1976a).

Intermittent claudication is a common manifestation of degenerative arterial disease. It is the only symptom of skeletal muscle ischemia. Active patients with mild to moderate large vessel disease are likely to have symptoms when walking. While resting, sedentary persons will be faced with symptoms of this disease only when it is very advanced. As elderly persons often are sedentary, they may not experience claudication even with advanced disease. Nevertheless, they must avoid any trauma and must be taught rigid foot care (Friedman 1976b). Pain, discomfort, and tiredness are relieved by rest. There is no other effective treatment for intermittent claudication. There are no drugs which can selectively dilate only the peripheral arteries or arterioles, even if sclerotic vessels were capable of being dilated (*Medical Letter* 1978a). Thus, there is little evidence to support claims that drugs such as isoxsuprine or cyclandelate are useful for relieving the symptoms of ischemic peripheral arterial disease. Vasodilators simply do not increase blood muscle flow sufficiently to meet demands of normal walking.

The signs of thyrotoxic heart disease differ in older people. In apathetic thyrotoxicosis, the usual hyperkinetic signs are absent. The patient may complain of diminishing mobility, developing incontinence, loss of weight, anorexia, fatigue, or cardiac arrhythmia (Kennedy 1975). In hyperthyroidism, the circulation time is shortened, there are palpitations, and the patient will complain of shortness of breath and fatigue. Hypothyroidism is fairly common in the elderly. Characteristically, they will complain of weakness, cold intolerance, mental and physical slowness, dry skin, and a hoarse voice. This condition should be treated with levo-thyroxin, starting with no more than 0.05 mg daily, the dose being increased at slow, regular intervals.

Extreme caution is indicated in treating the elderly patient, as changes occur during transition from the hypothyroid to the euthyroid state that can burden the elderly heart (McConahey 1978). In hypothyroidism, oxygen consumption of the heart, cardiac output, and peripheral blood flow are diminished. Circulation time is prolonged and cardiac output increases with exercise.

The older patient with myocardial infarction must be cautiously approached (Rodstein and Rossman 1971). Passive and active exercises should be considered, as prolonged bedrest can lead to pneumonia and phlebothrombosis. The elderly's increased vascular fragility and susceptibility to bleeding makes use of anticoagulants highly questionable. Chest pain could be treated with small doses of narcotics, but sedatives that lead to depression should be avoided. Heart failure with congestion or pulmonary edema will require the use of diuretics. All arrhythmias should be treated promptly.

THERAPIES

Antianginal Therapy

When the existing circulation cannot meet increased oxygen demand, angina pectoris results. Systolic aortic pressure is a major determinant of myocardial oxygen demand, while diastolic aortic blood pressure primarily determines coronary flow. In general, oxygen supply and demand increases with increased pressure and diminishes with decreased pressure. An increase in cardiac rate also tends to increase myocardial oxygen demand (Levitt et al 1977). Diabetes, anxiety, tension, and severe psychosocial problems contribute to the development of angina pectoris, as can hypertension, obesity, anemia, hyperthyroidism, and arrhythmias. All are frequent in the elderly and part of the management of this syndrome is the control of these conditions (Harralson et al 1977). In the very old, reduced activity and greater collateral circulation reduces the incidence of angina pectoris. If angina persists or progresses in the very old, coronary thrombosis should be suspected. Angina pectoris in the elderly will most likely manifest with less pain but more dyspnea and congestive heart failure.

If patient is asymptomatic and if the syndrome is manifested by EKG changes only, medication is rarely required. Even if there is a grossly abnormal electrocardiogram, there may be no past history of cardiac pain. As a matter of fact, in the elderly there is often no history of pain, either on exertion or at rest (Kennedy 1975; Kitchin et al 1973). In case of cardiac pain, management aims at reduced frequency and severity of anginal attacks and includes avoidance of heavy meals, emotional upsets, strenuous physical action, and exposure to cold. Nocturnal or decubitus angina frequently respond to diuretics, but generally, the treatment of choice for angina is nitroglycerin, alone or in combination with a drug administered for beta-adrenergic blockade.

The nitrates reduce mean systemic arterial pressure, left ventricular filling pressure, systemic vascular resistance, and increase cardiac output (Franciosa et al 1978). Nitroglycerin has the capacity to influence heart rate, afterload, and preload, as well as the distribution of coronary flow (Levitt et al 1977), but does not act predominantly as a preload reducing agent. Nitroglycerin increases sinus node automaticity as manifested by an increase in sinus rate, and improves A-V node conduction as manifested by a reduction in the A-H interval and the A-V functional and effective refractory period (Gould et al 1977). In short, vasodilators such as nitroglycerin cause peripheral vasodilation and thus reduce venous return and the work of the heart by reducing cardiac output. The coronary dilators are only effective in those vessels that can still be dilated and may actually decrease blood supply to ischemic areas. The major differences in the various forms of nitrates is in their potency and duration of action.

Sublingual nitroglycerin produces a rapid and short-lived effect on the arterial and venous smooth muscle. The hemodynamic effect usually lasts for no more than 20 minutes (Cohn and Franciosa 1977). Nitroglycerin should be given within three minutes before exertion that would ordinarily produce angina (Graff 1974).

Sublingual nitroglycerin therapy is usually effective in the elderly. There are several reasons for treatment failure. It may be related to the fact that the patient suffers from xerostomia, as in Sjögren syndrome. There simply might not be enough saliva to wet the tablet adequately. Treatment failure may also be related to tablet deterioration. The patient must understand that deterioration of nitroglycerin tablets is hastened by light, heat, air, moisture, and time. The tablets should not be stored in plastic containers or containers stuffed with cotton, as the active ingredient will migrate into the plastic or the cotton.

Headaches are often encountered by patients on nitroglycerin therapy, but they are usually of short duration. There may be dizziness and syncopal episodes, which occur more frequently in the elderly, particularly those receiving concurrent therapy with other vasodilators. To prevent falls, the patient should be advised to sit or lie down.

Nitroglycerin ointment, applied topically to the skin, increases exercise capacity for at least three hours. It reduces ischemia and brings about beneficial hemodynamic changes (Harralson et al 1977). Others have put its duration of action at four to six hours (Cohn and Franciosa 1977). Its onset of action is about 30 minutes.

It is usually applied every three to four hours to the chest, after any residue from previous administrations has been carefully removed. It is applied in a thin layer. A polyethylene wrap improves the absorption of the active ingredient. It can be used in the prevention of recurrent angina attacks, especially to counteract nocturnal angina attacks. Nitroglycerin ointment may cause prolonged venodilation leading to venous pooling. In predisposed patients, this can lead to new or worsened peripheral edema (Lee 1978). This particular dosage form of the drug can be utilized to illuminate the need for the provider to go beyond the "usual" patient instructions, particularly when dealing with the elderly patient. It is not unreasonable to assume that many of the elderly who use this paste need help in applying it. Therefore, it is important to ascertain who will help the patient and warn that person that the paste should not be applied simply with an unprotected hand. Continuous contact with the paste by the "helper" may lead to absorption of the drug and side effects. Thus, the person applying the paste should use gauze or similar material, being careful that the paste comes in contact only with the patient's skin.

The long-acting nitrates are mainly used for prophylaxis of anginal pain and for the reduction of preload and afterload in patients with acute or chronic congestive failure (Reichek 1977). Their use can prevent angina if given in adequate doses, often two to four times greater than previously recommended. Patients using nitroglycerin daily for treatment of angina may be good candidates for long-acting nitrates (Amsterdam and Greenberg 1978).

Isosorbide dinitrate (ISDN) has qualitatively the same action as nitroglycerin. After sublingual administration, onset of action may occur between 45 seconds and five minutes. A single dose may be effective for four to six hours, and effective doses may range from 20 mg to 80 mg three or four times daily. This drug is also available in chewable form, but this mode of administration reduces its duration of action (Cohn and Franciosa 1977).

The long-acting nitrates may produce headaches and a drop in blood pressure. They have a high potential for causing postural hypotension and must, therefore, be used with caution. Patients may develop tolerance to its effect and the drug should be used with caution in patients with glaucoma. Patients with cerebral ischemia may be endangered by further reduction in blood flow to the brain. In those patients, the use of nitroglycerin is preferred.

The nitrates are usually used in treatment of acute episodes or in anticipation of stress, and propranolol is recommended for prophylaxis. It decreases myocardial contractility and heart rate, which leads to a decrease in myocardial oxygen consumption. It is probably most effective when combined with oral nitrates.

The regimen is usually started with 5 mg four times daily and is increased in 5 mg increments until symptoms are relieved or side effects appear. An upper limit of 160 mg/day is suggested.

Nausea, fatigue, and lightheadedness can occur. Because of its beta-adrenergic effect, it can cause heart failure in doses of 40 mg four times daily. Bradycardia, bronchospasms, and hypotension have been reported as side effects. Propranolol is contraindicated in all types of arterioventricular block, hyperactive carotid sinus, and sinus bradycardia (Graff 1974).

Accelerating or unstable angina is diagnosed when pain attacks occur with increasing frequency and duration, and when nitroglycerin becomes decreasingly effective. In this instance, aggressive therapy is needed. The patient should be sedated, and oxygen and morphine can be used to control pain. Lidocaine should be available. These patients are usually given propranolol, starting with 15 mg four times daily. Long-acting nitrates in adequate doses and nitroglycerin given hourly, is administered sublingually.

Drugs Used in the Treatment of CHF

The primary goal of any treatment regimen should be to correct the underlying cause of CHF, but in many patients that is impossible (Mason and Tonkon 1977). Many forms of CHF respond poorly, for example, CHF resulting from cardiomyopathy, which could be hypertrophic (with impaired diastolic compliance) or obliterative (secondary to obliteration of ventricular cavities). In general, treatment for elderly CHF patients does not differ from that of younger patients (Graff 1974), ie, the aim is to correct the hemodynamic imbalance so that the compensatory mechanism by which the body attempts to maintain cardiac output is no longer necessary. The treatment regimen of elderly CHF patients typically involves an attempt to enhance myocardial contractility, for which digitalis is used. Diuretics are used to control excessive fluid retention and, if necessary, bed rest and/or reduced activity is prescribed to reduce the workload placed on the heart. However, bed rest is undesirable in the elderly.

Drug use must be carefully tailored to the individual patient and, in general, the dosage should be lower than the usual doses. In the elderly, there is likely to be more renal and liver involvement, and this must be taken into account when selecting a particular drug. For example, a reduced glomerular filtration rate can lead to increased drug toxicity, particularly digitalis toxicity. Diuretics must be used more cautiously, and in patients with underlying lung disease dehydration may lead to inspissated secretions.

Many drugs to which the elderly are often exposed can precipitate or exacerbate CHF (Table 19-6). Methyldopa, guanethidine, and

Table 19-6
Drugs Which May Precipitate or Exacerbate Congestive Heart Failure

Drug	Effect
Androgens, estrogens	Sodium retention, edema
Corticosteroids	Sodium and water retention
Diazoxide	Sodium and water retention
Osmotic agents	Intravascular volume expansion
Phenylbutazone	Increased sodium reabsorption Plasma volume expansion
Propranolol	Blocks compensatory mechanism of increased sympathetic nervous system activity
Sodium-containing drugs	Water retention; expansion of extracellular fluid

aspirin in large doses tend to increase blood volume by causing salt and water retention (Gans 1977). Certain enemas may contain very large amounts of sodium of which more than 5% can be absorbed.

To treat the underlying cause and to improve myocardial contractility, cardiac glycosides are used. In mild cases, this is often all that is necessary. In CHF patients, digitalis has a positive inotropic effect exerted directly on the myocardium. It enhances the left ventricular pump action. Initially, the lowest dose should be used that will control the symptoms. The patient should become less dyspneic and treatment should enable the patient to start lying flat in bed. Increased urinary output and weight loss should occur. If renal function is normal, the patient should be started on an oral maintenance dose of digoxin. Digitoxin requires a loading dose, as a steady state would not be reached in a reasonable time because of its long half-life. Rapid digitalization should be reserved for very acute cases.

Digitalis has a very narrow therapeutic index, and can be potentially harmful to the electrical function of the cardiac cell membrane. An irritable myocardium mandates a slow approach to achieve steady state concentrations. Impaired renal excretion will enhance serum digoxin concentrations and toxicity can result if the maintenance dose is not adjusted. The digoxin half-life is usually 33 hours, but increases progressively as renal function decreases. A half-life of five days has been reported. Therefore, the maintenance dose should be one-half or even less that of younger patients (0.125 or 0.25 mg per day). Many older people may require only 0.0625 mg twice daily to maintain adequate cardiac output and control arrhythmia. The most frequently observed toxicities of digitalis therapy are listed in Table 19-7.

Table 19-7
Common Manifestations of Digitalis Toxicity

Symptoms	Effect
Gastrointestinal	Anorexia, nausea, vomiting
Cardiac	Development of aggravation of CHF, bradycardia
Neurologic	Headache, fatigue, insomnia, confusion, depression, vertigo
Visual	Color vision, green-yellow

The overriding dictum in digitalis therapy of the elderly is caution. Digitalis can be dangerous in the elderly, and when cardiac failure has been satisfactorily controlled, the need for continuous therapy must be reassessed. If patient response to digitalis therapy is not sufficient, diuretics may be used. The choice depends on clinical urgency but should be based on the consideration that excessive diuresis should be avoided as much as possible. Diuretics, which are second in effectiveness to digitalis in the treatment of CHF, act by reducing renal tubular reabsorption of salt and water, thereby increasing salt and water excretion, promoting urine formation and reduction of blood volume. Organ function is improved as fluid congestion is reduced in the lungs, heart, liver, kidney, bowel, and dependent areas. Overall, then, diuretics decrease the workload of the heart by reducing edema.

While diuretics may correct some imbalances, they may create others. A lowered blood volume may lead to a decreased cardiac output and an increased tendency toward electrolyte imbalance. Diuretic therapy must be balanced to remove sufficient fluid in order to relieve severe congestion, yet a substantial fall in cardiac output must be prevented.

In addition to the danger of hypovolemia, there is the danger of depletion of total body sodium to levels below normal. Hyponatremia will result if total body sodium falls below 125 mEq/liter. In the patient with edema, salt and water restriction are indicated, but in the patient without edema, diuretic therapy should be adjusted to less vigorous levels.

Potential potassium loss and potassium imbalance is always of concern. In mild CHF, there is only a minor potassium loss but, if permitted to continue for prolonged periods of time, this can become clinically significant. In more severe CHF, diuresis is accompanied by a more severe loss of potassium, and the patient's serum potassium should be monitored periodically.

Magnesium deficiency, induced by diuretic therapy, can result in arrhythmias that may be hard to treat, especially if the patient is receiving digitalis concurrently. A serious arrhythmia indicates discontinuance of digitalis and the diuretic. Antiarrhythmic drugs supplement the effects of potassium and phenytoin; lidocaine and propranolol have been found useful.

Both hypokalemia and hypomagnesemia enhance patient susceptibility to digitalis toxicity.

If brisk diuresis has been judged necessary (as in the case of acute left ventricular failure), a diuretic acting on the ascending limb of Henle's loop is selected, usually furosemide. This may exhaust the patient and lead to incontinence. Therefore, as soon as the acute phase has passed, there must be a reassessment of the diuretic need. In all other cases, diuretic therapy of CHF should be started with the milder oral diuretics, probably hydrochlorothiazide or chlorthalidone. Patients treated with chlorthalidone show an increase in serum cholesterol by 5% and serum triglyceride by about 26% (Ames 1977).

Furosemide is generally reserved for patients in whom the milder diuretics are not effective. The thiazides and loop diuretics both increase sodium and water flow to the distal tubules, resulting in an increased exchange of sodium for potassium, thus potassium levels become critical. It has been suggested that diuretics be used intermittently, alternating periods of diuresis with periods of rest, thus avoiding a too vigorous diuresis (Gans 1977).

Daily administration of diuretics also often inhibits the already restricted independence of elderly, who often complain that they cannot even go shopping on a strict diuretic therapy, as diuresis interferes significantly with freedom of movement.

The mercurial diuretics are not recommended, as they are too toxic. The carbonic anhydrase inhibitors are effective only for short periods of time, and ethacrynic acid is seldom used because of its potential ototoxic effect. The potassium-sparing diuretics are too weak to be used alone and, if used, are usually combined with other diuretics in case of hypokalemia.

CHF patients unresponsive to digitalis or diuretic therapy are now being widely treated with vasodilators, even though these drugs have not yet been approved by the Food and Drug Administration for that use (*Medical Letter* 1978b). Some properties of the oral vasodilators used in CHF are listed in Table 19-8. As yet there have not been reports of any large-scale controlled trials on the effectiveness of prolonged vasodilator treatment for patients with chronic heart failure.

Hydralazine usually does not change heart rate and may not relieve symptoms of pulmonary edema. It produces arterial vasodilation. Unlike patients with hypertension, patients with cardiac failure have little or no tachycardia when treated with this drug. Prazosin does not cause a change in heart rate. It causes a dilation of both the arteriolar and venous beds, decreasing the mean arterial pressure and systemic vascular resistance, and increasing the cardiac output and

Table 19-8
Some Properties of Oral Vasodilators

Drug	Site of action	Route of administration	Onset (minutes)	Duration (hours)	Cardiac output	Adverse reactions
Hydralazine	Arterial	Oral	within 60	4-6	Increase	Nausea, vomiting, headache, drug fever, skin rash
Isosorbide dinitrate	Venous	Oral	5-15	4-5	No change or decrease	Headache, postural hypotension, ascites, peripheral edema
		Sublingual	15	1-1½		
		Chewed	5	2		
Nitroglycerin	Venous	Sublingual	minutes	½	No change or decrease	Headache, postural hypotension
		Topical	15	4-6		
Prazosin	Arterial and venous	Oral	20-60	6	Increase	Dizziness, fatigue, palpitation, headache

cardiac index. It may be responsible for relief of pulmonary congestion. However, long-term treatment with this drug may induce tolerance to its effect. It should be used with extreme caution in patients with hypertension. Dizziness, vertigo, edema, and headache may occur.

The organic nitrate vasodilators, including nitroglycerin, are also used in the treatment of acute and chronic congestive heart failure (Mintz 1976). They act predominantly on the venous side with a lesser effect on the arterial side. In general, they do not induce any significant changes in heart rate. Nitroglycerin alone apparently alleviates symptoms of pulmonary congestion without change in cardiac output. Isosorbide dinitrate, given in adequate dosage, can apparently improve significantly symptoms of pulmonary congestion, and its oral administration can have a long-lasting effect (four to six hours), while sublingual administration will only yield an effect of up to 90 minutes. Use of nitrates can be limited by headaches and sometimes by gastrointestinal effects.

Some modifications of the principles governing CHF treatment are necessary in the case of the elderly. Dosage schedules frequently require adjustment because of reduced kidney and liver function. Precipitant factors such as concurrent drug treatment, pneumonia, or anemia should be identified and treated or eliminated.

It is important that the patient does not remain bedbound longer than absolutely necessary. Activity should be introduced as early as possible, but only gradually. This will minimize the danger of prolonged bed rest, including the appearance of bedsores.

The patient may well suffer from anxiety, restlessness, and insomnia. Thioridazine, 25 mg two to four times daily can be used to treat restlessness and confusion. Nitrazepam or flurazepam are useful for nocturnal sedation.

Elderly patients often suffer from diminished recognition of thirst. Therefore, except in cases of severe edema, water intake should not be severely restricted. In cases of refractory edema, salt restriction may be necessary, as well as severe fluid restriction. Aside from the side effects of diuretic therapy already mentioned, the elderly may frequently suffer from incontinence, and elderly men with prostatic hypertrophy should be closely watched for urinary retention.

Drugs Used in Hypertension

Approximately 40% of all people over the age of 60 years are estimated to have some form of hypertension. The importance of this has been addressed in over 200 citations on essential hypertension in elderly people, all of which appeared between 1973 and 1975 (Nowak

1975). However, what represents "normal" blood pressure in an adult may not represent an adequate standard for comparison for an elderly patient. The uncertainties of "normal" standards may result in inappropriate pharmacologic treatment of the elderly. Elderly may be treated with drugs originally developed for the purpose of lowering diastolic high blood pressure in younger individuals, even though little is known about the effectiveness of these drugs in the treatment of systolic high blood pressure that is common in old age. Characteristics of blood pressure in elderly patients differ from those in younger persons. For example, "labile hypertension" is four times more prevalent in patients under 50 years of age. Geriatric patients, who may be excessively sedentary, are subject to orthostatic hypotension.

Mean systolic blood pressure is generally believed to increase with age from approximately 103 mm Hg in children to 150 mm Hg among adults between the ages 65 and 74 years. Systolic pressure is higher among men than women through age 54, but then becomes higher for women than for men. In one study of healthy old people, the systolic pressure for men between 60 and 64 years of age was 151 mm Hg, and 173 mm Hg for people between 85 and 89 years of age. Comparable figures for women were 158 and 184 (Anderson and Cowan 1972). The upper limit of diastolic blood pressure for all ages and sexes in the same study was about 103 mm Hg. In general, it has been suggested that mean diastolic pressure is markedly higher among men than women until the age of 54 years. Pressure levels then slowly decrease among men, while for women they begin to level off at age 65. Both mean systolic and diastolic pressures are lowest in families with the highest income and the highest level of education.

Unquestionably, there are changes in blood pressure with increasing age. For an adult, a diastolic pressure over 90 mm Hg is undesirable and abnormal. A patient in the fifth or sixth decade could well have a systolic pressure as high as 150 mm Hg without any ill effect, as long as the diastolic pressure remains normal (Bravo et al 1977).

Some controversy about hypertension and the elderly still remains. Hypertension in the elderly is so prevalent that many clinicians still consider it a normal, if inevitable, concomitant of aging. Therefore, it remains untreated. Yet, the Framingham study has shown that the gradient of risk from hypertension increases with age (Kannel and Sorlie 1975). On average, the elderly tolerate high blood pressure less well than younger people. It is surprising that this simple fact is still not universally accepted, as the elderly are clearly more at risk because of the effects of aging on the normal physiologic functions. Hypertension, itself, can impair cerebral circulation, heart and kidney function, increase cardiac work, precipitate congestive failure, and aggravate arteriosclerosis. Hypertension is an even greater risk factor for stroke and intermittent claudication than it is for coronary artery disease.

Thus, high blood pressure is not a disease but a risk factor (Pickering 1968), a fact that is increasingly recognized (Colombo et al 1977). Risk increases with increasing pressure, and it has been suggested that life expectancy is inversely related to blood pressure. Untreated patients with benign essential hypertension (BEH) develop stroke (14%), heart disease (78%), and renal failure (8%).

Increasing blood glucose levels, frequently seen in the elderly, increase the risk of morbidity and mortality from hypertension, even if they are not in the diabetic range. Women are especially at risk. Left ventricular hypertrophy, as determined by an electrocardiogram, also places an individual in the high risk category (Castelli 1976). Proper treatment of hypertension can virtually eliminate strokes, heart failure, and renal failure as a consequence of hypertension. It can also lower the incidence of coronary heart disease (Vertes 1975). Antihypertensive treatment also seems to prevent secondary decline in cognitive ability with high blood pressure in later life (Wilkie and Eisdorfer 1971). This relationship is depicted in Figure 19-3 (Lamy et al 1977b).

The Veterans Administration studies (VA Cooperative Study 1967, 1970) and the Intervention Trial in Mild Hypertension from the Public Health Service Hospitals have provided the major basis for modern antihypertensive therapy. Both studies show the positive effects of lowering blood pressure, particularly on the rate of hypertensive events, such as stroke, hemorrhage, cardiomegaly and left ventricular hypertrophy, CHF, rising BUN, and hypertensive retinopathy. Neither

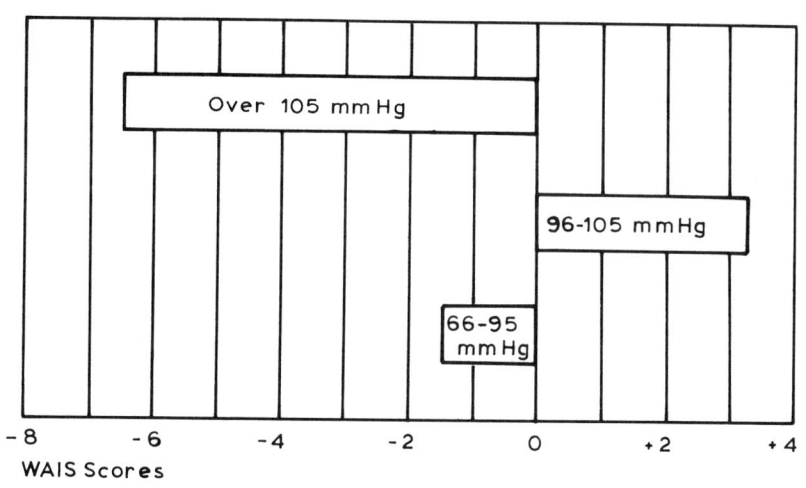

Figure 19-3 Relationship between blood pressure and intelligence scores in patients 60–69 years of age: a 10-year study. Adapted from Wilkie and Eisdorfer, 1971. From: P.P. Lamy et al. 1977. Reprinted with permission: E.R. Squibb and Sons, Inc.

Note: Bars represent diastolic pressure.

study found that antihypertensive therapy causes a significant reduction in the risk of atherosclerotic events, including myocardial infarction and sudden cardiac death. A small number of Swedish studies seem to indicate a different outcome. However, these studies involved the use of propranolol and the results may reflect the results of beta-blockade in high risk patients rather than a lowering of blood pressure.

There is general agreement as to the need for treatment in secondary hypertension, ie, hypertension resulting from a pre-existing disease. Accounting for about 15% of all cases of hypertension, these cases must be treated by addressing the underlying disease. Antihypertensives are usually not needed. A sudden rise in blood pressure may be caused by reactivation of chronic pyelonephritis, and appropriate treatment for the renal lesions is indicated (Kennedy 1975). Among other secondary causes of increased blood pressure are hyperthyroidism or pheochromocytoma, in addition to primary aldosteronism (Tuck 1978), which is manifested by muscle weakness, fatigue, and nocturia. Elevated plasma or urine aldosterone levels confirm diagnosis.

The value of treatment of essential hypertension in the elderly still remains a topic of dispute. A host of factors underscore this uncertainty, even though the risk of hypertension is readily recognized. For example, problems related to already reduced tissue perfusion and cerebral ischemia must be considered. There is some evidence that the hypertensive brain "resets" its autoregulation mechanism controlling the relationship between cerebral blood pressure and cerebral blood flow at a higher range than normal. Hypotensive therapy producing normal blood pressure may cause lowered cerebral perfusion (Strandgaard et al 1973). Severe cerebrovascular disease usually contraindicates energetic antihypertensive therapy in the elderly, and in persons with organic brain disease antihypertensive therapy may be contraindicated (Kennedy 1975). It may be hazardous to use antihypertensives in elderly with arteriosclerotic vessels which are unresponsive to therapy. Hypotension, reduced cardiac output, and cerebral and cardiac insufficiency can result (Keyes 1965). Sustained lowering of blood pressure to "normal" levels can increase mortality and morbidity rates in the elderly (Livesley 1975). The treatment of hypertension in the elderly is also difficult (Harris 1970), as many of the drugs used can cause iatrogenic symptoms. Many antihypertensive drugs and diuretics can cause postural (orthostatic) hypotension, which is particularly serious in the elderly. They may also be exposed to other drugs commonly causing orthostatic hypotension, such as the phenothiazines, and they are most at risk to trauma from resulting falls. The incidence rates for adverse antihypertensive drug reactions have been estimated at between 20% and 50%. Methyldopa alone is known to cause 58 different adverse effects. Sometimes overlooked is the fact that treatment of hypertension, particularly in the elderly, is a constantly changing treatment. Tolerance to certain drugs may develop, gout may appear, as well as hypoglycemia or hyperglycemia and other conditions. If the antihypertensive regimen is not adjusted accordingly, treatment outcome may well be judged insufficient. Recently, it has been suggested that elderly hypertensive patients should not be treated if the fundi (eyes), the kidneys, or the heart do not show any changes (Neurath 1978).

What seems to emerge from a careful consideration of all the arguments offered is that what is being disputed is the line at which the benefit of treatment outweighs the inconvenience and side effects of continuous medical treatment of hypertension. It is important to select patients and treatment according to the severity of the hypertension and the general condition of the patient. Thus, before selecting a particular antihypertensive agent, it is necessary to be familiar with the patient's possible concomitant pathologic and physiologic conditions (Fishback 1976). For example, a patient who has been receiving lithium therapy for a prolonged period of time may have consistently elevated blood pressure. Decreased glucose tolerance, decreased excretory function, irregular eating habits, and digitalization for CHF all cause increased side effects in the elderly. Decreased CNS regulation of blood flow, arteriosclerotic cardiovascular disease, and other comorbidities may lead to an increased incidence of orthostatic hypotension. Coronary artery disease, from which the elderly frequently suffer, mandates a more careful approach to antihypertensive therapy. Prostatic hypertrophy in elderly men may contraindicate use of certain antihypertensives (for example, the ganglionic blocking agents), and reserpine would be chosen only for an elderly, depressed patient if there is no response to any other agent. In short, instituting antihypertensive therapy in the elderly demands a careful benefit/risk approach. Specific therapy for elderly patients should be determined only after careful appraisal of many factors (Livesley 1975). Target-organ damage always mandates hypertension treatment.

The goal of hypertensive treatment should be to reduce pressure to at least 140/90 mm Hg. Drug treatment should not begin until other treatment modalities have been shown to be ineffective. Some elderly patients may respond well to reassurance and dietary restriction, such as reduced salt intake, aimed at weight reduction. This would definitely be the first choice in mild hypertension in the diastolic range of 90 mm Hg to 105 mm Hg. Hypertensive patients seem to exhibit greater preference for salt than do normotensive persons. It is important that they know the salt content of commonly used foods (Table 19-9). Relaxation therapy decreases sympathetic activity and, thus, may lower blood pressure. It has been shown to be effective in one series of studies. Regular, supervised exercise can lower blood

Table 19-9

Some Foods with High Salt Content		Some Foods with Low Salt Content
Bacon	Pizza	Avocado
Bouillon	Popcorn	Banana
Broth	Potato chips	Cantaloupe
Cheese	Pretzels	Honeydew melon
Corned beef	Relish	Nectarine
Corn chips	Sauerkraut	Raisins
Frankfurters	Sausage	Grapefruit juice
Ham	Soy sauce	Potatoes
Olives	Tunafish	
Oysters	Waffles	
Peanuts (salted)	Worcestershire sauce	
Pickles		

pressure in mild hypertension. Biofeedback has also been tried in a small number of patients (Benson 1977; Patel 1973, 1975; Kristt and Engel 1975; Boyer and Kasch 1970; Choquette and Ferguson 1973). While attempts at weight reduction, and other nondrug therapy should, of course, be considered, it is probably unrealistic that a patient in the seventh decade will either agree to or be successful in changing a life-long life-style.

The National Institutes of Health recommendations for treatment of hypertension have been released (National Institutes of Health 1978). They should only be viewed as guidelines:

1. Virtually all patients with a diastolic pressure of 105 mm Hg or greater should be treated with antihypertensive therapy
2. For persons with diastolic pressure of 90 to 104 mm Hg, treatment should be individualized with consideration given to other risk factors
3. The stepped-care approach is advocated as a cost-effective method of treating most patients
4. Treatment of patients with high blood pressure includes plans for facilitating long-term maintenance of blood pressure control.

Recommended actions are given in Tables 19-10 and 19-11. On looking at the recommendations as listed in Table 19-10, it appears that there is some distinction between hypertension in younger and older patients, as older patients "need" to be checked less frequently than younger patients. In face of the evidence that hypertension is just as great a risk

Table 19-10
Recommended Action for Initial Blood Pressure Measurement

Systolic/Diastolic (mm Hg)	Recommended action
Diastolic 120 or higher	All adults: prompt evaluation and treatment
160/96 or higher	All adults: confirm BP elevation within one month
140/90–160/95	Under age 50: BP check within two to three months
140/90–160/95	Age 50 or older: check within six to nine months

Source: National Institutes of Health. *Report of the Joint National Committee on Detection, Evaluation, and Treatment of High Blood Pressure.* DHEW Publ. No. (NIH) 77-1088, Bethesda, Md., 1978.

Table 19-11
Diastolic Blood Pressure and Treatment

Average Diastolic Blood Pressure (mm Hg)	Recommended action
120 or higher	Immediate evaluation and treatment indicated
105–119	Treatment indicated
90–104	Individualized treatment
Under 90	Remeasure BP at yearly intervals

Source: National Institutes of Health. *Report of the Joint National Committee on Detection, Evaluation, and Treatment of High Blood Pressure.* DHEW Publ. No. (NIH) 77-1088, Bethesda, Md., 1978.

factor in older as in younger patients, and in some instances even a greater risk factor, this recommendation is difficult to understand.*

On detection of hypertension and before treatment begins, it is important to obtain a serum electrolyte baseline. Recommended are a hematocrit, urinalysis for protein, blood, and glucose, determination of creatinine and/or BUN, serum potassium, and an electrocardiogram. Other tests which may be helpful include a chest x-ray, blood sugar, serum cholesterol, serum uric acid, microscopic urinalysis, and blood count.

As the mechanism of essential hypertension is not yet fully understood, an empirical approach to the prescribing of antihypertensives is still used. In general, the stepped-care approach is recommended and used, with the understanding that no one combination of

---

*A new *Statement on Hypertension in the Elderly* was released in September 1979.

drugs works in all patients. Particularly in the elderly, the selection of the drug to be used must take into account the possible side effects, as well as the patient's kidney and liver function. The possible effect of these are given in Table 19-12 (Garbus and Lamy 1976).

Following failure of dietary restrictions, weight reduction, or other attempts to lower blood pressure, drug treatment is indicated. Drugs most often used in the United States in the treatment of hypertension are listed in Tables 19-13 and 19-14. Drug treatment must be individualized. Some patients respond poorly to one drug and respond well to another. Drug treatment will most likely be of prolonged duration and will need constant supervision of the patient, both in the initial and maintenance stages. Usually, it will have to be adjusted with the passage of time. Rapid lowering of blood pressure is rarely indicated and most often contraindicated.

A typical, stepped-care approach involves the selection first of a diuretic, usually a thiazide type. If this is not effective, then another drug is added, usually methyldopa or propranolol. Alternatively, many clinicians still use a thiazide-reserpine combination. If a third step is needed, hydralazine is usually added to the regimen. As it can cause reflex tachycardia and increased cardiac output, the combination with propranolol is indicated, since propranolol will prevent side effects of hydralazine. In Great Britain, it is usual to start an antihypertensive

Table 19-12
Effect of Impaired Liver and Renal Function on Antihypertensive Drug Therapy

Drugs used with cardiovascular disease and/or hypertension	Implications of impaired liver function	Implications of impaired kidney function
Clonidine	No change	Use with caution
Digitoxin	Decreased dose	No change
Digoxin	No change	Decrease dose
Guanethidine	Not understood as yet	As renal function decreases, required dosage decreases
Hydralazine	95% metabolized in the liver. Monitor for signs of liver damage or toxicity.	Order no more than twice daily because of increased accumulation
Methyldopa	Will worsen condition of patient in end-stage disease	Reduce dose, expect exaggerated response
Reserpine/ Rauwolfia	Dose remains the same	Dose remains the same
Thiazide diuretics	Use with caution	Use with caution

Table 19-13
Drugs Used in Mild Hypertension
United States 1976

Drug	Percentage of total	Possible adverse effects
Thiazides	37.6	Hypokalemia, hyperuricemia, hyperglycemia, skin rashes
Methyldopa	29.4	Sedation, depression, orthostatic hypotension, fever, positive Coombs test
Rauwolfia and diuretics	24.0	Depression, nasal stuffiness, peptic ulcer
Propranolol	5.3	Heart failure, asthma
Clonidine	3.7	Drowsiness, dry mouth

Table 19-14
Drugs Used in Moderate and Severe Hypertension
United States 1976

Drug	Percentage of total	Possible adverse effects
Triamterene	29.5	Hyperkalemia, folic acid deficiency, anemia
Hydralazine	27.5	Increased sympathetic activity, sodium retention, dose-related lupus syndrome
Furosemide	18.0	Strong diuresis, hyperuricemia, hyperglycemia
Spironolactone	17.0	Hyperkalemia, gynecomastia, GI symptoms, impotence
Guanethidine	8.0	Orthostatic hypotension, bradycardia, diarrhea, sexual dysfunction

regimen with propranolol and add a thiazide, if necessary. In the elderly, in particular, this may not be indicated.

A recommended stepped-care approach is as follows:

Step 1 Drugs Initially, an easy-to-use and relatively inexpensive drug, such as a diuretic, should be selected, in preference to a second-step drug such as a beta-adrenergic blocker (Moser 1978). A diuretic alone can be expected to be effective in 30% to 50% of the patients with mild or moderate hypertension.

There is little difference in the effects of these drugs, although dose and duration may vary. These drugs produce a dose-dependent response, and once a plateau has been reached, a dosage increase will not cause increased response. The thiazides and related diuretics are the most commonly used drugs for treatment of mild hypertension, and, in conjunction with other agents, for treatment of moderate and severe hypertension. They are thought to be more effective in low rather than high renin patients. They exert their hypotensive effect by decreasing peripheral vascular resistance, possibly by depleting arteriolar wall sodium (Benowitz 1977). This action follows an initial decrease in plasma volume. In combination therapy, they counteract sodium retention that might be caused by other drugs. They are less potent but longer acting than the loop diuretics. Their action is not sufficient in severe sodium retention or impaired renal function (then the more potent loop diuretics are used).

The thiazides begin to exert their effect in three to four days and can produce a moderate reduction in blood pressure. Apparently they are particularly suited for long-term treatment of diastolic hypertension and are effective both in the supine and erect position. Resistance to their action rarely occurs.

Side effects with thiazides occur in the elderly with greater frequency than they do in younger patients. Elderly patients will exhibit a greater tendency toward blood glucose irregularities, and hyperglycemia is not uncommon. Hyperuricemia may also occur, and the frequency of acute gouty attacks may be doubled in patients with thiazide-induced hyperuricemia (Weinstein and Stason 1976).

If a diuretic lowers blood pressure insufficiently, the patient most likely has combined volume and vasoconstrictive hypertension. Both diuretics and vasodilators will be needed. If there is no response to diuretics, the patient probably has pure constrictive hypertension and diuretics will not be effective.

Step 2 Drugs When diuretics alone are not effective, a second drug is added to the regimen, usually a sympatholytic drug. They should be referred to as sympathoplegic drugs. Among those are the beta-adrenergic blocking agents (propranolol), the adrenergic neuron or postganglionic blocking agents (guanethidine), methyldopa, reserpine, and others.

Step 3 Drugs In patients with severe hypertension or those unresponsive to Step 1 or Step 2 treatment, a vasodilator is usually added to the regimen. Hydralazine remains the first choice vasodilator in the stepped-care approach. The effects of the diuretic and the other drugs will be additive. However, hydralazine has a short duration of action and may require multiple doses.

The nondiuretic antihypertensives cause the kidney to respond to decreased perfusion pressures by retaining sodium chloride and water. This leads to an expansion of plasma and extracellular fluid volumes, antagonizing the original decrease in blood pressure. Therefore, concomitant administration of diuretics is necessary (Onesti and Lowenthal 1977; Onesti 1978). Characteristics of the major antihypertensives are presented in Table 19-15.

Table 19-15
Antihypertensives

Name	Mode and site of action	Major side effects	Comments
Diuretics			
Thiazides	Initially, decrease blood volume and cardiac output. Long-term: Both return to previous levels and total peripheral resistance decreases: Vasodilation	Can produce hyperglycemia, hyperuricemia, and hypokalemia	Used to potentiate nondiuretic antihypertensives
Peripheral sympathetic blockers			
Guanethidine	Acts at sympathetic nerve ending. Depletes norepinephrine, prevents neurohumoral transmission	Fatigability and orthostatic hypotension frequent and severe	Use only if patient is non-responsive to other drugs. Response unpredictable
Rauwolfia alkaloids			
Reserpine	Depletes norepinephrine in post-gangliomic nerve endings. Decreases peripheral vascular resistance, reduces heart rate and cardiac output	Affects biogenic amines in brain, leading to behavioral changes. Also parasympathetic effect, ie, peptic ulcer. Nasal stuffiness	Upper dose limit of 0.25 mg

Table 19-15 (continued)

Name	Mode and site of action	Major side effects	Comments
Centrally acting vasodilators			
Methyldopa	Acts on vasomotor centers in medulla oblongata. Decreased sympathetic outflow. Peripheral sympathetic inhibition. Inhibition of renin release. Decrease in BP, preservation of cardiac output, decrease in peripheral vascular resistance. Cerebral and renal vascular resistance decreased	Postural hypotension, depression in elderly?	New data suggest possible once or twice daily administration
Clonidine	Centrally mediated decrease in sympathetic discharge. Vagal tone increased. Decrease in heart rate and cardiac output. Renal blood flow maintained. Decrease in renal vascular resistance	Sedation, constipation, dry mouth	Do not discontinue abruptly
Peripheral vasodilators			
Hydralazine	Peripheral vasodilation leads to baroreceptor stimulation. Increase in adrenergic discharge from vasomotor centers to heart and peripheral vessels. Increase in heart rate and cardiac output. Increase in renal blood flow and decrease in renal vascular resistance	Contraindicated in reflex tachycardia and increased cardiac output. Excessive cardiac stimulation	Blockade of cardiac beta-receptors, blocks cardiac response to hydralazine. Limit dose to 200 mg/day

Prazosin	Direct smooth-muscle relaxation. Inhibition of arteriolar contractile response. Direct postsynaptic alpha-adrenergic receptor blockade. Decrease of total peripheral vascular resistance, only minor changes in cardiac output	Acute orthostatic hypotension following first dose. Possible headaches and palpitations.	Lacks sedative effect. Should be combined with diuretic
Beta-adrenergic blockers			
Propranolol	Antagonizes beta-adrenergic action of catecholamines released from adrenergic nerve endings or adrenal medulla. Negative chronotropic and inotropic effect. Suppresses renin release. Decrease in cardiac output and heart rate	Contraindicated in patients with a history of bronchial asthma or chronic obstructive lung disease. Also in patients with myocardial decompensation, bradycardia, or atrioventricular conduction defects	Use with caution in diabetic patients. Causes no significant orthostatic or exercise hypotension

Treatment Failure An unsatisfactory response to antihypertensive drug therapy is often caused by poor compliance or an unrecognized drug interaction, such as the interaction between a tricyclic and guanethidine (Wollam and Vidt 1978a, 1978b). In the management of essential hypertension, patient compliance is one of the most difficult problems. Compliance can be increased by decreasing the total number of doses a patient must take. Reserpine, guanethidine, and the thiazides are usually given in a once-daily regimen. However, drugs such as methyldopa, propranolol, and hydralazine are still given in three or four daily doses. There are now indications that fewer administrations of these may be possible and effective (Gifford 1974; Smith 1974; McMahon 1975; Berglund et al 1973; Wilkinson et al 1974; Shand 1975; LeSher et al 1976; Wright et al 1976; Morgan 1976).

ANTIARRHYTHMICS

Auricular fibrillation and other arrhythmias are often found in the elderly receiving too much or too little digitalis, too high a dose of a diuretic, or not enough potassium. Elderly patients may be at high risk to potentially new arrhythmias when given barium enemas, possibly caused by dehydration produced by enema preparation procedures (Roeske et al 1975). Ventricular arrhythmias are frequent in patients with myocardial infarction, and they may contribute to increased mortality (Goldman and Ingelfinger 1978). Patients with acute, uncomplicated myocardial infarction apparently benefit from prophylactic administration of antiarrhythmics. It has recently been suggested that patients should be treated with drugs that would control abnormal heart rhythms for up to one year after a heart attack, to prevent premature ventricular contractions (PVCs). Untreated PVCs can lead to tachycardia, ventricular fibrillation, and sudden death.

PVCs may indicate underlying heart disease or coronary artery disease. Chronic obstructive lung disease may be responsible for PVCs, which may also be associated with digitalis intoxication resulting from hypokalemia. PVCs may also be caused by emotional stress and even some over-the-counter drugs. Bronchodilators, vasoconstrictors, and vasopressor sympathomimetics, the anticholinesterases, and the autonomic blocking agents can act as proarrhythmic drugs. Other such drugs include the cardioactive drugs, the antihypertensives and diuretics, and the neuroleptics (Aviado 1975).

All available antiarrhythmics (Table 19-16, disopyramide not listed) can have undesirable, even dangerous side effects. These effects are generally greatly increased in the presence of potassium concentrations of 5 mEq/liter or more. Cardioactive drugs can cause vertigo,

Table 19-16
Some Properties of Antiarrhythmic Drugs

Drug	Therapeutic serum concentration mcg/ml	Duration of action (hours)
Lidocaine (IV)	1–5	¼–½
Phenytoin (IV)	5–15	5–10
Procainamide	5–15	3–6
Propranolol (IV)	0.1–0.5	2–6
Quinidine For conversion of atrial fibrillation to normal sinus rhythm	3–8*	3–6
Maintenance	2–5	3–6

*A range of from 4–9 mcg/ml is also suggested.
Adapted from: Katzung, B. Action and interactions of antiarrhythmic drugs. *Therapeutics* 2(3):1, 1974.

tinnitus, diminished vision, and headache (the cinchonism syndrome). The action of the antiarrhythmics is poorly correlated with blood level data and is to some degree unpredictable. Therefore, the prescriber should use these drugs only after determining that the risk of using them is less than the risk of not using them. As these drugs must be given at precise intervals, poor clinical response often relates to lack of patient understanding of this necessity.

Digitalis Although not an antiarrhythmic in the strict sense of the word, it has important uses relating to cardiac arrhythmias. In patients with congestive heart failure, it is frequently used in combination with an antiarrhythmic agent to prevent arrhythmias. It is also administered to patients with arrhythmias before conversion with quinidine is attempted (Katzung 1974a).

Quinidine Quinidine is probably the drug of choice in the treatment of certain forms of cardiac arrhythmia and is the most reliable antiarrhythmic drug to use in ambulatory patients. It reduces excitability of myocardial tissue, depresses or eliminates ectopic pacemaker activity, and prolongs the effective refractory period of cardiac repolarization, during which impulses are suppressed. Clinically, it abolishes premature beats of atrioventricular and ventricular origin, as well as ventricular tachycardia (Aviado and Salem 1975). Cardioversion and successful correction of ventricular fibrillation is possible even in patients having had quinidine therapy.

For prophylaxis, blood levels between 2 and 5 mcg/ml are suggested. For conversion of atrial fibrillation to normal sinus rhythm, levels of 4 to 9 mcg/ml are usually optimal, and toxic levels range from

5 to 15 mcg/ml (Aviado and Salem 1975). It is immediately apparent that there is a significant overlap in these suggested levels. Following oral administration, peak plasma levels are reached in approximately 60 minutes. Peak levels can be reached faster and will be higher if the drug is administered on an empty stomach (Ueda et al 1976). Steady state levels are usually reached within three days.

Quinidine metabolites appear to contribute, sometimes significantly, to the effects of quinidine. Therefore, once steady state levels have been reached, patients with impaired renal function must be given smaller doses (Drayer et al 1978). Patient response is often erratic and in patients with heart disease, peak plasma levels develop slower than in patients without heart disease.

Quinidine exerts a highly toxic effect in as many as 30% of patients receiving it. Quinidine can dilate both the systemic and pulmonary circulation and, thus, provoke vasodilation. It must, therefore, be used with caution in patients on hypotensive medications. This action may be particularly dangerous in patients receiving nitroglycerin concurrently. These patients should be advised to sit down or lie down before taking a dose of nitroglycerin, to avoid the consequences of dizziness and, possibly, syncope.

Quinidine increases cardiac rate and reduces cardiac contractility; therefore, it reduces cardiac output. Based on this, it may be contraindicated in patients with CHF or a severely damaged myocardium. Its use is contraindicated in patients with greater than first degree A-V block, as it then may trigger cardiac arrest and ventricular fibrillation. Administration of quinidine can cause severe gastrointestinal symptoms, less with gluconate than with the sulfate salt.

Therapeutic doses of quinidine produce myocardial depression, especially in patients with impaired myocardial function (Orlando and Aronow 1976). High blood levels may cause profound depression of myocardial contractility, decreased systemic vascular resistance, hypotension or shock, and serious cardiac arrhythmias, including ventricular tachycardia, ventricular fibrillation, and ventricular asystole.

To test the patient for possible quinidine sensitivity, a test dose should be administered first. Side effects in sensitive patients will usually occur within two to three hours. The therapeutic dose varies with the individual. If PVCs are not caused by hypokalemia, a dose of 200 mg four times daily is suggested. This is usually given only during waking hours, even though, theoretically, the drug should be administered around the clock. Patients unresponsive to quinidine are sometimes given propranolol, in doses of 40 to 80 mg daily in divided doses, concurrently with quinidine. The totally unresponsive patient will most likely not respond to disopyramide or procainamide, either, although they should be given a trial. If necessary, the unresponsive patient will need to be hospitalized and treated with lidocaine.

Reabsorption of quinidine is increased in the presence of urine with an alkaline pH. This leads to elevation of serum quinidine levels and increased cardiotoxicity of the drug, if the dosage remains unadjusted. Elderly patients, who often receive chlorothiazide, antacids, or other drugs which tend to alkalinize the urine, are at risk to this interaction. Quinidine can also displace anticoagulants from their binding sites, thus increasing the action of coumarin drugs.

Finally, if quinidine is used concurrently with digitalis, the toxicity potential of digitalis is greatly increased. In a retrospective study, 25 of 27 patients exhibited an increased mean serum digoxin concentration during quinidine therapy (from 1.4 to 3.2 ng/ml). Anorexia and vomiting developed in more than one-half of the patients who had been stable before quinidine therapy was instituted. Gastrointestinal effects disappeared when digoxin dose was reduced. Another side effect was ventricular arrhythmias, and at least one fatality was ascribed to the combination therapy (Leahey et al 1978). Therefore, when quinidine is added to digoxin therapy, serum digoxin levels should be monitored, EEGs should be performed, and the patient should be followed closely. In case of digitalis intoxication, when reduction of digitalis is undesirable, phenytoin should be used. However, in case of underlying cardiac tissue damage, quinidine is the drug of choice.

Lidocaine Lidocaine is the drug of choice for treatment of ventricular premature beats and is preferred for initial treatment of ventricular tachycardia. For continued suppression of ventricular arrhythmias and long-term prevention of recurrences, procainamide or quinidine is used (*Medical Letter* 1977a). In patients with CHF, steady state lidocaine levels are significantly higher (more than double). Lidocaine clearance is reduced by almost two-thirds (Zito and Reid 1978).

Phenytoin Phenytoin sodium is used to suppress ventricular ectopic beats and atrial tachycardias caused by digitalis intoxication. It does not depress cardiac function. Phenytoin can significantly increase the liver metabolism of many drugs, particularly the anticoagulants. In turn, isoniazid increases its action.

Procainamide This drug has an action similar to that of quinidine. The same is true of its side effects and contraindications. However, it can be tolerated by patients who cannot tolerate quinidine at therapeutic levels. It is fast acting, and a daily dose of 2 gm to 3 gm should control PVCs. A test dose is recommended for patients who have not previously been treated with quinidine or who have reacted adversely to quinidine. The very high incidence of adverse effects caused by procainamide, it has been suggested, makes this drug unsuitable for long-term antiarrhythmic prophylaxis in most patients (Orlando et al 1976).

Propranolol The catecholamines may precipitate arrhythmias by interacting with cardiac beta-adrenergic receptors. The beta-blocking agents inhibit this interaction and, therefore, propranolol has an antiarrhythmic action. It also exerts a "quinidine-like," direct membrane-depressant effect on cardiac tissue, but at much higher doses than those used for beta blockade (Danahy and Aronow 1977). This drug causes far fewer side effects than other antiarrhythmics; however, its ability to cause beta-adrenergic blockade of the heart and the bronchi make this drug a difficult one to use in elderly patients. In patients already receiving propranolol for angina or hypertension, it may be possible to increase the dosage in an attempt to control arrhythmias. As propranolol reduces the heart rate and blood pressure, it must be used cautiously when added to a quinidine regimen or any regimen involving a cardiac depressant. Patients for whom propranolol is prescribed, in addition to quinidine should be cautioned to watch closely for early signs of congestive heart failure, such as a weight gain of one to three pounds within three to four days of the start of combination therapy. If the patient or a family member is taught pulse-taking, the presence of nonsymptomatic bradycardia can be detected. Congestive heart failure, poor myocardial contractility, severe valvular heart disease, or hypotension contraindicate the use of propranolol, as does obstructive lung disease with bronchospasms, severe peripheral arterial disease, and conditions predisposing a patient to hypoglycemia.

Disopyramide This drug has only recently (1977) been released and little has been published on its effect in the elderly. It has a quinidine-like action and appears to be effective for the treatment and prevention of ventricular arrhythmias. It shares the contraindications of quinidine and can precipitate or aggravate cardiac failure (*Medical Letter* 1977a). Urinary hesitancy and retention are often encountered, especially in men. It causes a burning sensation in the feet and sensorimotor neuropathy affecting the lower limbs (Dawkins and Gibson 1978). Because of its anticholinergic action, it must be used with caution in patients susceptible to glaucoma (Trope and Hind 1978). As is the case with quinidine and procainamide, QRS widening suggests toxicity. The recommended adult starting dose is 150 mg every six hours, but smaller doses must be given initially to patients with hepatic or renal insufficiency. The drug can be used concurrently with digitalis without the need to adjust the dose of digitalis downward.

ANTIHYPERTENSIVES

When an older patient presents with hypertension, the workup probably will not vary sharply from that for a younger patient. Following are some key points for the evaluation of the older patient:

1. In the aging patient, the EKG takes on added importance, particularly in view of the statistical chances for concomitant heart disease in the aging population.
2. The physical examination should attempt to identify any heart murmurs or other cardiac dysfunction. Check carefully for peripheral pulses. Ask about symptoms of intermittent claudication. Ask about symptoms of congestive heart failure: insomnia, paroxysmal nocturnal dyspnea, orthopnea, etc.
3. A careful neurologic examination should be conducted. Ask about symptoms of transient ischemic attacks and look for signs of weakness or other evidence of old stroke. Assess the patient's mental state in terms of both functional decline and organic disease. This is important since the patient will be expected to handle the management of the disease.
4. Look for possible chronic glomerulonephritis or other renal disease. It will affect management of the patient.
5. Evaluate potential drug risk to aging organs.

Successful treatment of hypertension, regardless of the patient's age, depends first on correct blood pressure measurements. To establish the systolic pressure, the first appearance of the Korotkoff sound on deflating of the blood pressure cuff is used. The issue of establishing diastolic pressure is somewhat confused. There is still substantial disagreement on whether or not the endpoint is muffling (Phase IV) or disappearance (Phase V) of the Korotkoff sound. The confusion probably stems from the fact that the American Heart Association now recommends muffling (Phase IV), while earlier, Phase V had been recommended and still earlier, Phase IV. Adding to the confusion is the fact that automatic devices record only Phase V. Of course, the appropriately-sized cuff should be used, and while muffling of the Korotkoff sound is often clearer in the left arm, the American Heart Association recommends the use of the arm that exhibits the higher pressure, usually the right arm.

Once the systolic and diastolic pressures are determined, it must be decided what constitutes hypertension. Persistent, multiple readings beyond the upper age-related normal limits establish hypertension.

As previously pointed out, there is still no complete agreement as to the value of treatment of hypertension in the elderly, although the preponderance of the evidence clearly indicates the beneficial effects of treatment. Thus, if the benefit/risk is carefully considered, in most instances treatment will be indicated. Perhaps, although the point is debatable, it is not particularly advantageous to employ drugs in order to treat hypertension caused by arteriosclerosis (high systolic and normal or slightly elevated diastolic pressures) but, as shown time and again, the value of treatment of hypertension in most instances is in the prevention or reduction of the concomitant morbidity.

Management of the aging hypertensive patient involves several different important steps (Table 19-17), of which drug use is only one part. Many different drugs are available for the treatment of hypertension. The hemodynamic effect of some of these is listed in Table 19-18 and the recommended dosages for some in Table 19-19.

The particular choice of a drug will depend on patient need. Cardiac function, arteriolar resistance, venous capacitance, and the blood volume regulated by the kidney are considered, as are the patient's renal and hepatic status. Moreover, the number of doses to be administered daily, which can influence compliance, will influence the choice of the particular agent. In any case, under the stepped-care

Table 19-17
Key Points for Managing the Aging Hypertensive

1. Establish and keep close personal contact with the patient.
2. In the diagnostic process, avoid invasive techniques as much as possible.
3. Diagnose and treat the patient, not the disease.
4. Set realistic goals for a lower blood pressure.
5. Establish a graduated exercise program as tolerated.
6. Establish a nutritional program.
7. Establish, if necessary, dietary restrictions:
   a. Salt: eliminate pretzels, table salt, etc.
   b. Foods high in cholesterol (eggs, milk, etc): restrictions are probably of limited value after age 65 for many patients.
8. Establish status of electrolyte balance.
9. Establish drug therapy:
   a. Use as few drugs as possible.
   b. Start with a lower than usual dose.
   c. Monitor patient's use of nonprescription drugs. Advise patient about sodium content of OTCs.
10. Involve the patient as much as possible in the therapeutic regimen:
    a. Use written instructions and brochures to explain the need for and correct use of each drug carefully.
    b. Keep in mind the possible effect on compliance of organic brain syndrome or forgetfulness.
    c. Consider combination therapy as an aid to compliance.
    d. Involve the patient's family in establishing a compliance pattern.
11. Consider possible economic and travel constraints.

Source: S.B. Garbus, and P.P. Lamy. Managing the aging hypertensive. *Patient Care*, Darien, Conn., 1976.

Table 19-18
Hemodynamic Effects of Some Antihypertensives

Drug	Change in peripheral resistance	Change in cardiac output	Change in heart rate
Clonidine	Slight decrease	Early: decrease LT*: No significant change	Decrease
Hydralazine	Decrease	Increase	Reflex tachycardia: Common
Methyldopa	No change or slight increase	Early: No significant change. LT: Decrease	No change
Prazosin	Decrease	No significant change	Reflex tachycardia: Uncommon
Thiazides	Moderate decrease	Early: Decrease LT: No decrease	No change

*LT: Long-term

approach, the mildest agent possible should be chosen first, with more potent agents added as need dictates. In general, these drugs can be divided into three categories, ie, those with peripheral sympathetic action (propranolol, reserpine, and guanethidine), those with central sympathetic action (methyldopa and clonidine), and the arteriolar dilators (hydralazine, prazosin, and minoxidil). In many instances, particularly with the newer drugs, information on their action in the elderly is very scarce, if available at all.

Traditionally, methyldopa or reserpine were used as Step 2 drugs. More recently, propranolol and clonidine have also been suggested as Step 2 drugs. Hydralazine still remains the drug of choice as Step 3 drug, and guanethidine is added only when absolutely necessary, as a Step 4 drug.

As malignant, rapidly progressing hypertension is not common in the aged, vigorous therapy is rarely required. If an older hypertensive patient does not respond to the simpler forms of antihypertensive therapy, the patient should first be evaluated for renal artery obstruction before drug dosages are increased or more powerful drugs are used. De novo hypertension in the older patient, especially if there is no previous family history, will probably be caused by involvement of the renin-angiotensin system, most likely the result of arteriosclerotic plaque formation.

Table 19-19
Dosage Suggestions for Some Antihypertensive Drugs in the Elderly

Agent	Starting dose in the aging	Range of usual daily maintenance dose	Onset of effectiveness	Duration of effectiveness
Clonidine	0.1 mg twice a day.* (Raise 0.2 mg every 7 days until control or intolerable side effects occur.)	0.2–0.8 mg	30–60 minutes	6–8 hours
Guanethidine	10 mg once daily. (Raise 10 mg every 14 days until control or intolerable side effects occur.) 5 mg if necessary.*	25–100 mg	48–72 hrs	10 days
Hydralazine	10–12.5 mg four times a day. (Raise 10–12.5 mg every 7 days until control or intolerable side effects occur.)	100–300 mg	3–5 hrs	6 hrs
Methyldopa	250 mg three times a day. (Raise 250 mg every 7 days until control or intolerable side effects occur.)	750 mg–2 gm	3–5 hrs	8 hrs
Rauwolfia/Reserpine	0.1 mg twice a day.	0.25 mg	3–6 days	2–6 weeks

*Tablets are scored, but are nonetheless difficult to break or cut; use half-tablets for lowest dose only if necessary.
Source: S.B. Garbus, and P.P. Lamy. Managing the aging hypertensive. *Patient Care*. Darien, Conn., 1976.

Once management of hypertension with drugs has been decided, all possible steps should be taken to enhance patient cooperation with the selected regimen:

1. Select drugs that permit the lowest number of tablets and daily administrations.
2. Talk over the regimen with both the patient and family members or other significant persons in the patient's life.
3. At each visit, review the medication schedules.
4. Share the blood pressure readings with the patient. This enables the patient to participate in the treatment and its effectiveness.

Reserpine Reserpine or other rauwolfia derivates were at one time the most widely used Step 2 drugs. Reserpine is still judged a safe and effective drug by many clinicians. Reserpine lowers blood pressure by depleting catecholamine storage sites in the CNS, heart, and peripheral neurons and blocks release of norepinephrine from peripheral sympathetic neurons. Its major advantage is the fact that it is relatively inexpensive and can be given in a once-daily regimen. Furthermore, its use causes little risk of postural hypotension.

If administered as the sole antihypertensive agent, reserpine will increase sodium and water retention. The drug's effect is cumulative and psychic depression is its most hazardous adverse effect. A patient history of depression presents an absolute contraindication for the use of this drug in the elderly. If depression occurs as a result of the use of reserpine, it may continue for months after the drug has been withdrawn. Reserpine also enhances parkinsonism symptoms, particularly in patients receiving levodopa, and should not be given to patients with peptic ulcer, as it increases gastric acidity. Side effects occur most often when high doses (0.5 mg daily or more) are used (Goodwin and Bunney 1971; Freis 1975). Increased dosage beyond the recommended 0.25 mg daily dose does not cause an increased therapeutic effect, as the drug has a plateau action. The recommended maximum dose of 0.25 mg daily is unlikely to cause depression, but it also makes the drug less effective than the thiazides. Therefore, it is most often used concurrently with a thiazide diuretic. Common rauwolfia-diuretic combinations, which are sometimes used to increase patient compliance once treatment with individual drug entities has brought the hypertension under control, are listed in Table 19-20 (Lamy et al 1977a).

Table 19-20
Some Rauwolfia-Diuretic Antihypertensive Combinations

Drug	Composition		Maximum maintenance dose in the elderly	Reserpine content
Ser-Ap-Es (Ciba)	Reserpine Hydralazine Hydrochlorothiazide	0.1 mg 25 mg 15 mg	1 tablet two or three times daily	0.20–0.30 mg
Hydropres-50 (MSD)	Reserpine Hydrochlorothiazide	0.125 mg 50 mg	1–2 tablets daily	0.125–0.250 mg
Regroton (USV)	Reserpine Chlorthalidone	0.25 mg 50 mg	½ to 1 tablet daily	0.125–0.250 mg
Rauzide (Squibb)	Rauwolfia Serpentina Bendroflumethiazide	50 mg* 4 mg	1–2 tablets daily	0.10–0.20 mg

*roughly equivalent to 0.1 mg Reserpine

Propranolol The safety and effectiveness of this drug used as an antihypertensive in elderly patients is difficult to evaluate. Increasingly, beta blockers are used as a first-step drug in Europe and similar recommendations have been made in the United States (Laragh 1976), although, in general, the thiazides are used as first-step drugs here. Several hospitals have developed hypertension treatment protocols that specifically mandate against the use of propranolol, at least as a first-step drug, in patients over 50 years of age. Yet, propranolol has much to recommend it as a hypotensive agent in old age (Raisfeld 1971), and, if patients with clinical signs of heart failure and those who cannot tolerate a minimal test dose of the drug are excluded, then propranolol is a much safer drug than usually assumed (Shand 1978).

Propranolol has been approved for use in hypertension, angina, cardiac arrhythmias, hypertrophic cardiomyopathy, and pheochromocytoma (Karch 1978). It may be of benefit to anxious patients with predominantly somatic complaints, including palpitations, shakiness, tremor, breathlessness, and hyperventilation. Acute pathologic states may also respond to propranolol (Heiser and DeFrancisco 1976), which is probably also useful in the treatment of senile tremors (Winkler and Young 1974).

Beta-receptor blockade represents a very significant advance in the treatment of hypertension (Ahlquist 1977). Blockade of beta receptors produces, in effect, cardiac sympathectomy. Propranolol is a nonselective beta blocker, blocking receptors in the myocardium as well as the bronchi and vascular smooth muscle (Anavekar 1978).

The drug decreases cardiac output by about 18% (Holland and Kaplan 1976), as it depresses myocardial contractility and probably venous return. It does not significantly increase total peripheral resistance or expand plasma volume. It also blocks the beta receptors in the kidney which mediate the release of renin. Overall, it produces a slow, relatively balanced reduction in elevated systolic and diastolic pressures.

The effectiveness of propranolol is related to its plasma concentration and not its dose. A major portion of the orally administered drug, as much as 50% to 70%, is lost to the first pass effect (Huffman et al 1976). Individual plasma levels vary widely with a given dose, and twentyfold differences in steady state plasma concentrations have been observed (Esler et al 1977). Therefore, patients with essential hypertension show widely differing sensitivities to the blood-pressure lowering effect of the drug. In the majority of patients, there is a minimal effect below plasma concentrations of 30 ng/ml and a peak effect is observed at 100 ng/ml.

The absorption rate seems to be slowed in elderly patients. The drug's half-life varies between three and six hours, and based on this, it is usually administered three or four times daily. However, the effects of physiologic beta blockage are apparently sustained for much longer and outlast propranolol's presence in the plasma, so that once or twice daily administration has been proposed. The maximum therapeutic effect with this drug should be expected within one week. For several reasons, this drug would be ideally suited for use in the elderly hypertensive. It is particularly useful in patients with angina pectoris. Its action is not blocked by the tricyclics, phenothiazines, or other antipsychotic agents, frequently used by the elderly. It is useful for patients with hyperuricemia and it has generally been recommended for patients for whom continued diuretic therapy is undesirable. Finally, and importantly, it does not cause postural hypotension, unlike many other antihypertensives, and does not appear to cause drowsiness. Although liver disease and kidney failure contribute to higher plasma levels (Greenblatt and Koch-Weser 1973), the drug seems safe and effective in hypertensive patients with pre-existing renal damage (Holland and Kaplan 1976).

Slightly more than 1% of patients receiving propranolol experience life-threatening adverse reactions, and almost 10% have some form of adverse reaction. It is important to note that these adverse reactions are not dose-dependent, and even more important to note that adverse reactions occur more commonly in uremic and in elderly patients (Shand 1978). In the elderly, propranolol can induce or worsen existing CHF.

Heart failure and bronchospasms can result even from very small doses. CHF occurs in some patients, as do bradyarrhythmias. Bronchospasms occur particularly in patients with asthma. Propranolol also deteriorates peripheral circulation in a significant number of patients. Cardiac insufficiency occurs more easily in patients in whom this drug reduces cardiac output without lowering blood pressure. Propranolol must be used with caution in patients on digitalis therapy, because of the danger that it may lead to excessive bradycardia. In patients with angina pectoris, sudden withdrawal can cause unstable or accelerated angina, arrhythmias, myocardial infarction, and death. Reflex vasoconstriction can lead to cold extremities, particularly in patients with severe peripheral arteriosclerosis. As the drug blocks the action of catecholamines on beta-receptors, it may suppress glucose release in response to epinephrine, causing an increased sensitivity to tolbutamide (Raisfeld 1971). Propranolol also blocks signs of impending hypoglycemia and potentiates insulin-induced reductions in blood sugar. Therefore, the drug is not usually recommended for use in insulin-dependent patients.

The drug crosses the blood-brain barrier and its neurologic effects are apparently not related to plasma level data, as they are sustained over much longer periods of time (Helson and Duque 1978). CNS side effects include insomnia, fatigue, bizarre dreams, hallucinations, paresthesia, and dizziness. Patients have been reported as psychotic after only a short course of propranolol therapy (Fraser and Carr 1976).

Thus, it would appear that this drug has much to offer in the treatment of hypertension, but whether or not it can or should be used in an elderly, hypertensive patient depends on many factors, including the patient's physical, physiologic, and mental status.

Metoprolol tartrate This drug, a beta-adrenergic blocking agent, has just been released. No data on its action in the elderly are as yet available. It seems to possess the same activity as propranolol in lowering both elevated systolic and diastolic blood pressures, but differs from propranolol in being a very weak inhibitor of the peripheral vasodilator effect of epinephrine. These two drugs may, therefore, produce differential hemodynamic effects in situations in which endogenous epinephrine contributes to cardiovascular control.

Guanethidine This is another drug with peripheral sympathetic action. It depletes the neurotransmitter norepinephrine at the sympathetic nerve endings, thus preventing neurohumoral transmission. It is probably the most potent oral antihypertensive agent available. It lowers blood pressure but reduces systolic blood pressure much more than diastolic pressure. It decreases cardiac output by decreasing adrenergic nerve stimulation and must, therefore, be used with caution in patients with limited cardiac reserve. Guanethidine does not cause any significant change in total peripheral resistance. It is a Step 4 drug which should be reserved for extremely severe hypertension in patients who cannot tolerate any other agent, or when other agents fail.

Guanethidine reduces renal plasma flow and the glomerular filtration rate while plasma volume is expanded. This leads to pseudotolerance to the drug which must, therefore, be given in conjunction with diuretics. Dose adjustment may be difficult as the drug is long-acting and has a slow onset of action (48 to 72 hours). Sodium restriction is usually necessary when this drug is used. The drug must be prescribed with caution for patients with cerebral vascular insufficiency, coronary artery disease, or angina pectoris. Its most significant side effect is severe postural and exertional hypotension, which can be aggravated by any agent or condition that causes vasodilation, such as hot weather or alcohol consumption. Hypotension is most severe after prolonged periods in the supine position. Elderly patients susceptible to postural hypotension should be instructed to:

1. Rise slowly from lying position. Sit on the side of bed for a few minutes before standing up.
2. Avoid bending over to tie shoe laces. It is best to use shoes without laces.
3. Sleep with the head in an elevated position.
4. Use support stockings, if necessary.

Guanethidine should not be used concurrently with tricyclics which block its action. Vasopressors, such as phenylephrine, can predispose the patient receiving this drug to cardiac arrhythmias.

Methyldopa This centrally-acting drug was at one time the most frequently used Step 2 drug. It decreases sympathetic tone, but does not inhibit reflex responses as completely as the peripherally-acting drugs. It probably replaces norepinephrine at the sympathetic neuro-effector junctions with alpha-methylnorepinephrine, which has a much lower pressor effect than norepinephrine. A moderately potent antihypertensive, methyldopa lowers blood pressure by reducing peripheral vascular resistance. It has little effect on cardiac output and renal blood flow is well maintained.

With this drug, the elderly experience a rather high incidence of hepatitis and drug fever. Lethargy and sedation are common side effects of this drug. In about 1% of patients treated with this drug, hypothermia occurs, to which the elderly are particularly susceptible. Psychic depression can also occur, but less so than with reserpine. Methyldopa can also cause amnesia-like episodes, difficulty with calculations, and inability to concentrate (Adler 1974), which is important in treating elderly patients who might be judged "senile" when they exhibit such symptoms. Both supine and postural hypotension occur, but less frequently than with guanethidine. The dosage for an elderly patient must be individualized, but usually starts with about 125 mg twice daily and is increased by about 125 mg every four days to no more than 2 gm/day or until control is achieved (Pomerance 1965). Higher doses are likely to precipitate depression or deepen existing depression in the elderly.

Clonidine This is a relatively new sympatholytic drug with central action. Similar to methyldopa in effect and adverse reactions, it lowers blood pressure by a direct effect on the vasomotor centers. It produces central alpha-adrenergic stimulation and leads to decreased sympathetic outflow from the brain, thus reducing sympathetic tone. There is reduction in heart rate and cardiac output, but no significant change in peripheral resistance. Renal blood flow and glomerular filtration rates are not altered. It is more effective when given together with a diuretic (as is true for methyldopa). Most often observed are drowsiness and dry mouth, restlessness, insomnia, irritability, and tremor. The dose-effect relationship does not plateau. Patients who are to be withdrawn from the drug must undergo planned withdrawl to avoid danger of rebound hypertension.

Hydralazine All arteriolar vasodilating agents are limited in their effectiveness by homeostatic compensatory mechanisms that increase cardiac output, plasma renin, and plasma volume. They are effective when used in combination with diuretics, an adrenergic blocking agent, or both. This has the added advantage that the three drugs would produce an additive effect on blood pressure. Vasodilators, such as hydralazine, are particularly useful in the treatment of essential hypertension if the hemodynamic defect is peripheral arteriolar vasoconstriction with increased total peripheral vascular resistance (Onesti 1976).

Until a relatively short time ago, hydralazine was the only vasodilator available and it remains the first-choice vasodilator in the stepped-care approach to hypertension (Benowitz 1977). It reduces arterial pressure by relaxing arterial smooth muscle which results in reduced peripheral resistance. Hydralazine increases cardiac rate, stroke volume, and cardiac output. It decreases diastolic and systolic pressures proportionally and causes little orthostatic hypotension.

Hydralazine induces sodium and water retention, thereby increasing plasma and extracellular fluid volumes and pseudotolerance to this drug. This is prevented by concurrent administration of a diuretic. The concurrent administration of propranolol has been suggested as that drug would suppress hydralazine side effects such as depression, fluid retention, and parkinsonism. It may cause anginal pain, particularly in patients with coronary artery insufficiency and other cardiac symptoms such as palpitations, EKG changes indicative of ischemia, in addition to flushing and headaches. Tachycardia is invariably associated with the subjective complaints of severe palpitations. These effects, too, can be overcome by concurrent administration of an adrenergic blocking agent. The maintenance dose is limited to 200 mg per day to avoid a lupus-like reaction. If hydralazine is used, it might be advisable to determine the patient's hepatic acetyltransferase activity. The dose required in slow acetylators is considerably lower than that needed for fast acetylators.

Prazosin A newly-marketed vasodilator, it, too, causes more frequent and severe side effects than the thiazides. Marketed as a "unique" vasodilator, it appears to act by blockade of post-synaptic alpha-adrenergic receptors and by direct relaxation of arteriolar smooth muscle. It is more potent than hydralazine and has a relative lack of cardiac stimulation. It must be used together with a diuretic and a beta-blocker, but even then the sodium-retaining properties may be too severe (Benowitz 1977). It does not consistently increase heart rate or cardiac output and causes less tachycardia than hydralazine. By itself, it is effective in mild to moderate hypertension, but is better used in combination with a diuretic. It lowers blood pressure more in the standing than in the supine position (*Medical Letter* 1977c).

Frequently, faintness and moderate to severe symptoms of postural hypotension occur after the first dose (Rosendorff 1976; Turner 1976). Syncope with sudden loss of consciousness has been observed after an excessive first dose.

The blood pressure lowering effect of prazosin is closely associated with its plasma concentration, which declines according to first order kinetics. The drug's half-life ranges from 2.5 to 4 hours. The drug is about 97% protein bound and its apparent volume of distribution is 75 liters. Its mean hepatic extraction rate is 448 ml/min. The treatment effect may be delayed by six to eight weeks and the hypotensive effect continues for a few weeks after the drug has been withdrawn (Brogden et al 1977). Prazosin does not increase serum uric acid or blood sugar levels and can, therefore, be used in diabetic patients and patients with gout.

Particular dosage suggestions for use in the elderly are not available. It is important to check dosage suggestions carefully. Much of the work on prazosin has been done outside the United States, using tablets. In the United States, only capsules are available and capsule formulations result in lower peak plasma levels.

Minoxidil An orally active vasodilating agent that is more powerful than hydralazine, this drug acts by reducing peripheral vascular resistance. Lowering of arterial pressure is accompanied by sharp, reflex-mediated increases in stroke volume, heart rate, and cardiac output. This limits the hypotensive effect of the reduced peripheral resistance. This drug, too, should be administered concurrently with a diuretic and propranolol, as it causes retention of sodium and water and increased plasma renin activity. It does not change glomerular filtration rate or effective renal plasma flow in hypertensive patients nor does it cause orthostatic hypotension. It has an onset of action of about two hours and a duration of action of about 12 hours, making twice-daily administration possible. No dosage recommendations for use in elderly patients are available.

Side effects and interactions Side effects of antihypertensives are common. Some are listed in Tables 19-21 and 19-22. Patient risk for adverse drug reactions increases with the number of concurrently administered drugs, and the elderly frequently receive a large number of drugs. The risk appears highest with antihypertensives; 12% of patients, on the average, suffer from adverse reactions (May et al 1977). About 44% of patients receiving antihypertensives may suffer from postural hypotension, 11% from excessive somnolence, about 10% from diarrhea, and about 7% from mental disturbances. The incidence among the elderly, more sensitive to drug actions, may be higher, although this has not been documented.

Interactions involving the cardiovascular agents are prominent among the clinically important interactions (Brater and Morrelli 1977b). They, of course, can change the relation between the dose administered and the expected drug effect. Some interactions are listed in Table 19-23. Both the pharmacokinetic and pharmacodynamic actions of a drug may be affected. For example, the phenothiazines and

Table 19-21
Common Side Effects of Sympatholytics

Drug	Side Effects	Incidence
Clonidine	Daytime sedation	In 40%-80%. Dose-related
	Dry mouth	At least as frequent as with methyldopa
	Orthostatic hypotension	Common, but less severe than with methyldopa or guanethidine.
Guanethidine	Postural hypotension	Almost every patient. Dose-related
	Gastrointestinal problems	Common
	Loss of blood pressure control	Not uncommon
Methyldopa	Decreased mental alertness, depression	Daytime sedation in 41%. Dose-related. May subside. Depression: 4%-13%
	Dry mouth	Very common
	Sodium and fluid retention	Very frequent. May be as high as 64%
Propranolol	Depression of heart rate and cardiac output	Variable
	Bronchospasm	In 2%-10% of non-asthmatic patients
	Effect on diabetic control	Rare, but can be severe
	Bradyarrhythmias	Depends on patient's cardiac status. Can be life-threatening. Potentiated by digitalis and antiarrhythmic agent.
Reserpine	Depression	20%, mostly at dose of 0.5 mg/day or more. Onset: 2-8 months. May be suicidal.
	Other CNS effects	Frequent, even at low dose. Onset: 1 week to several months
	Nasal stuffiness	Common. Onset: within one month
	Breast cancer	Not validated

the tricyclics have a quinidine-like effect on the conductivity and automaticity of the heart, and concurrent use of these drugs with quinidine or procainamide may, therefore, produce an additive effect (Williams and Sherter 1971). Over-the-counter drugs containing chlorpheniramine or phenylpropanolamine should be avoided in patients on guanethidine (Misage and McDonald 1970). Clinically important interactions caused by induction of hepatic microsomal enzymes can

Table 19-22
Common Side Effects of Hydralazine When Used as Vasodilator

Drug	Side Effect	Incidence
Hydralazine	Reflex tachycardia Increased cardiac output Loss of hypotensive effect Exacerbation of angina Exacerbation of CHF	All variable and dose-related
	Sodium and fluid retention	Edema in 4% of patients

Table 19-23
Some Interactions of Cardiovascular Agents

Drug	Interacting drug	Effect
Clonidine	Desipramine	Reduced antihypertensive activity
Guanethidine	Tricyclic antidepressants	Tricyclics will block antihypertensive action of guanethidine
	Chlorpromazine	Reversal of antihypertensive action over several days
Methyldopa	Phenothiazines Tricyclic antidepressants	Exacerbation of hypertension when added to regimen. No clear-cut evidence
	Lithium	Possible lithium toxicity
Spironolactone	Aspirin	Reduction (by 30%) of spironolactone-induced naturesis
	Digitalis	False elevation of serum digoxin as determined by radioimmunoassay

occur with phenytoin and quinidine (Hansen et al 1971). The interactions involving cardiovascular drugs have been reviewed extensively (Koch-Weser 1975; Dollery et al 1975; Crook and Nies 1978) and their preponderance underscores the need for the risk/benefit approach in hypertensive therapy.

ANTICOAGULANTS

Patients over 65 years of age should be "anticoagulated" to a lesser degree (eg, 8% to 13% by the Thrombotest method) than is usual for younger people (eg, 5% to 10%) (Loeliger 1968). The dispute regarding the use of anticoagulants for elderly patients continues unabated. Apparently, anticoagulants do not significantly reduce mortality or strokes in patients with transient ischemic heart attacks (Gotshall and Harker 1977) and their routine use for acute myocardial infarction is not justified (Rogel and Bassan 1976). It would appear, though, that warfarin does reduce the incidence of stroke and mortality in patients with cerebrovascular disease.

The effectiveness of heparin is diminished in the elderly (Brodows and Campbell 1972) and among the oral anticoagulants, phenindione is considered to have more harmful side effects than do the other ones. The kinetics of the oral anticoagulants are outlined in Table 19-24. According to its plasma half-life, phenindione must be administered in multiple daily doses. The clinical effect of dicoumarol is dose-dependent. A doubling of the dose will not, however, result in a predictable increase of its plasma level. Therefore, the clinical effect of an increased dose cannot be accurately predicted. Warfarin is 98% protein bound and has a relatively small volume of distribution. Therefore, even small changes in the degree of protein binding may lead to large changes in the concentration of free circulating drug.

Smaller doses of warfarin are usually required for females and the elderly. CHF contraindicates use of oral anticoagulants. Patients in cardiac failure are more likely to bleed, possibly as a result of liver dysfunction. There is an increased bleeding risk in elderly women, patients with heart failure, and patients with indwelling devices.

Genetic factors and liver function influence a patient's sensitivity to these agents. Elderly persons, in general, exhibit a greater sensitivity to anticoagulants than younger persons, as absorption of these agents in the elderly is slow and erratic. In addition, anticoagulant therapy is particularly risky in patients with vitamin K deficiency, frequently found in the elderly suffering from poor nutrition or chronic disease

Table 19-24
Pharmacokinetics of Oral Anticoagulants

Parameter	Warfarin	Dicoumarol	Phenindione
Absorption	Good	Poor	Good
Protein binding	98%	99%	97%
Plasma half-life	30–40 hrs	60–100 hrs	4–8 hrs
Kinetics	First order	Concentration dependent	First order

states (Hazell and Baloch 1970; *AMA Drug Evaluations* 1973). Seventy-five percent of geriatric admissions to a hospital showed evidence of vitamin K deficiency, which increases sensitivity to the action of anticoagulants (Hazell and Baloch 1970).

Up to 30% of elderly patients receiving anticoagulants may suffer from cerebral hemorrhage caused by these drugs, excessive hypoprothrombinemia can occur in about 25%, and gastrointestinal hemorrhage in about 21% of elderly patients (May et al 1977).

Greater sensitivity to warfarin is generally suggested for the elderly (O'Malley et al 1977), but whether this is caused by increased vessel fragility or by greater sensitivity to the pharmacologic effects of the drug has not been established. Even though elderly patients may be given smaller weight-related doses, their anticoagulant response to warfarin is greater than that exhibited by younger patients. The same plasma warfarin concentration causes greater vitamin K-dependent clotting factor synthesis in the elderly and, thus, the elderly seem to exhibit increased intrinsic sensitivity to warfarin (Shepherd et al 1977).

Thus, it is extremely important that the patient's dosage is carefully controlled, based on prothrombin times. Yet, even when prothrombin times are within therapeutic ranges, women with other associated serious medical problems are at risk to develop coumarin-associated soft-tissue lesions when treated with coumarin anticoagulants for thrombophlebitis or pulmonary embolism (Bahardi et al 1977).

For the patient on maintenance oral anticoagulant therapy, acute renal insults resulting in prolongation of prothrombin time are of potential clinical importance. Consideration must also be given to chronic care management of the patient and the effect on prothrombin time. For example, chlorpromazine and the salicylates may cause hypoprothrombinemia. It has been recommended that the initial dose of sodium warfarin be one-half the dose given to the average adult. There is a higher risk of bleeding because of heparin therapy, without a corresponding improvement in efficacy, in women over the age of 60 years. Of note is that the risk is appreciably lower in the elderly male population (Pomerance 1974). It has been suggested that the sooner the use of anticoagulants is discontinued in patients over 60 years of age, the better (Hazell and Baloch 1977).

Much of the risk of anticoagulant therapy, particularly to elderly patients, is related to the immense number of drugs which can interact with the oral anticoagulants (Lawson and Lowe 1977; Deykin 1970a, 1970b; Sigell and Flessa 1970; Koch-Weser and Sellers 1971a, 1971b). Some of these drugs are listed in Table 19-25. Often overlooked is the fact that foods can contain a significant amount of vitamin K which could interfere with the expected action of the anticoagulant (Table 19-26). Several mechanisms are involved in these interactions, such as reduced bacterial synthesis of vitamin K, reduced absorption of vitamin K, displacement of the anticoagulant from albumin binding sites, inhibition of liver metabolism and induction of microsomal enzyme activity, and competitive inhibition. For example, oral anticoagulants suppress the synthesis of vitamin K-dependent clotting factors in the liver. Quinidine and salicylates have the same action, thus potentiating the anticoagulant action. In contrast, estrogens stimulate the synthesis of these factors, decreasing anticoagulant action (Solomon et al 1971). Coadministration of aluminum hydroxide

Table 19-25
Drugs Which May Affect the Action of Oral Anticoagulants

Increase Action		Decrease Action
Alcohol	Methylphenidate	Barbiturates
Allopurinol	Metronidazole	Ethchlorvynol
Antibiotics	Mineral oil	Glutethimide
(broad spectrum)	Nalidixic acid	Griseofulvin
Chloral hydrate	Phenylbutazone	Rifampin
Chloramphenicol	Phenytoin	Spironolactone
Chloroquine	Probenecid	Vitamin K
Chlorpromazine	Quinidine	
Cholestyramine	Quinine	
Clofibrate	Reserpine	
Colchicine	Salicylates	
Diazoxide	Steroids, anabolic	
Ethacrynic acid	Sulfonamides	
Glucagon	Thyroxine	
Indomethacin	Tolbutamide	
Mefenamic acid	Tricyclics	

Table 19-26
Vitamin K Content of Some Foods*

Food Item	Vitamin K mcg/100 g
Green tea	712
Turnip greens	650
Broccoli	200
Cabbage	125
Beef liver	92
Lettuce	89
Spinach	89
Watercress	69
Asparagus	59
Coffee	38

*Normal intake of vitamin K varies between 300 and 500 mcg daily.

does not affect the absorption of either bishydroxycoumarin or warfarin, but 15 ml doses of magnesium hydroxide substantially increase absorption of bishydroxycoumarin (Ambre and Fischer 1973; Hurwitz and Schlozman 1974). The interaction of salicylates with oral anticoagulants is probably the best known anticoagulant interaction (Ascione 1977a, 1977b). Aspirin exerts a dose-dependent direct or indirect effect on the action of oral anticoagulants. With doses of 3 gm or less per day, there is usually no enhancement of the anticoagulant effect, but even slightly higher doses (3.9 gm/day) have precipitated hemorrhagic symptoms in patients (O'Reilly and Aggeler 1970; O'Reilly 1971). Acetaminophen appears to be a suitable alternative for analgesia and antipyresis, and tolmetin may be a suitable alternative to salicylates as an antiinflammatory drug.

CARDIAC GLYCOSIDES

The cardiac glycosides are most valuable in the treatment of recent atrial arrhythmia with rapid ventricular response and digitalis represents a rational choice in the pharmacologic management of CHF. In CHF, digitalis has a positive inotropic effect exerted directly on the myocardium. Transmembrane active transport of sodium and potassium is potently and specifically inhibited by digitalis, an action which is dose-related (Smith 1978). It increases the contractile force of the failing heart as well as cardiac output. As a result, the compensatory mechanisms begin to subside. Elevated venous pressure and pulmonary congestion should be alleviated. Digitalis is a complex drug with a very narrow therapeutic index. Furthermore, there is no sharp therapeutic endpoint for this drug, and subjective and objective improvement is the indication of successful therapy. This, of course, mandates very careful and close observation of the patient. Digitalis is frequently used in elderly patients, so much so that it has been suggested that its use is often unnecessary (Priddle and Rose 1966; Gibson and O'Hare 1968). Indeed, in several studies, elderly patients were withdrawn from digitalis therapy without detriment, even those who were in sinus rhythm (Dall 1970; Fonrose et al 1974; Hull and Mackintosh 1977). It is possible that a patient may have been treated for transient cardiac stress induced by an acute illness, from which the patient recovered, obviating the need for further digitalis therapy. Therefore, the need for digitalis therapy, particularly in the elderly, should be periodically re-assessed. Digitalis is overprescribed in patients whose signs and symptoms are caused primarily by an impairment of cardiac contractility or in whom increases in contractility could have a deleterious effect (Cohn 1974).

Digoxin is generally preferred over digitoxin, as it has a much shorter duration of action (Davison 1972), but the half-life of digoxin can be significantly prolonged in elderly patients (Ewy et al 1968a). Yet the popularity of digoxin is difficult to understand (Cattell 1978). Digitoxin in contrast to digoxin, is completely absorbed. Changes in intestinal motility do not affect digitoxin, in contrast to digoxin. Formulation differences do not appear to affect digitoxin as seriously as digoxin. On the other hand, it is consistently believed that longer-acting digitoxin is more difficult to regulate, as it is metabolized by the liver. Age-related reduction in hepatic function as well as interference with enterohepatic reabsorption could alter the action of the drug, as could concurrent administration of many drugs that could stimulate microsomal enzyme activity. Efficient therapy with cardiac glycosides is often uncertain in face of unknown or uncertain absorption and elimination rates and formulation effects (Schwarzfischer 1976). The pharmacokinetic characteristics of digoxin and digitoxin are presented in Table 19-27.

The main route of excretion of digoxin is via the kidneys, and the increased half-life (which could reach 72 hours) is probably caused by a decreased clearance of the drug. Thus, unquestionably, the elderly are not more susceptible to the toxic effects of the drug and it is not age, but renal function which determines toxicity. Other factors, such as a decreased volume of distribution, may also contribute. Diminished excretion can quickly lead to serious side effects and the incidence of digitalis toxicity is high, estimated at between 23% and 30% (Dall 1965; Soffer 1961; MacGregor 1965; Ewy et al 1968b; Riccitelli and Hirschfeld 1961; Hermann 1966; Doherty and Kane 1973).

In an effort to establish circulating steady state levels of digoxin to monitor clinical effectiveness and prevent toxicity, several pharmacokinetic models have been proposed. Digoxin excretion rates and serum concentrations are needed to characterize digoxin disposition accurately (Koup et al 1975). In general, for patients with renal impairment, creatinine clearance is used to adjust dosage regimens of drugs excreted partially or completely by the kidney, such as digoxin. This is not convenient and the method is not routinely used (Lott and Hayton 1978). Creatinine clearance is, therefore, estimated based on serum creatinine levels. Declining renal blood flow and the consequent reduction in the glomerular filtration rate are correlated with the decline in creatinine excretion rate, so that serum creatinine levels are relatively unaffected by age (Cockroft and Gault 1976). Therefore, normal serum creatinine does not indicate the same level of renal function in young and older subjects. In addition, liver disease or any disease causing loss of muscle tissue, may affect creatinine production. Therefore, while steady state digoxin levels can be sufficiently predicted based on serum data (Paulson and Welling 1976), serum digoxin levels do not correlate well with the patient's clinical state of digitalization

Table 19-27
Pharmacokinetics of Cardiac Glycosides

	Gastrointestinal Absorption	Peak Effect	Average Half-life	Excretory Pathway	Maintenance Dose
Digoxin Tablet Elixir	60%–80% 85%–95%	1.5–5 hrs	36 hrs	Renal (gastrointestinal)	0.125–0.5 mg
Digitoxin	90%–100%	4–12 hrs	4–6 days	Hepatic Renal Metabolism	0.1 mg

(Dimant and Merrit 1978), cannot be relied on as a test of digitalis toxicity (Ingelfinger and Goldman 1976), and pharmacokinetic models to estimate levels of digoxin in geriatric patients cannot be relied on (Simonson and Stennett 1978). Knowledge of the digitalis dosage, renal function, serum potassium concentration, and cardiac status are all essential to successful monitoring of the patient.

Digitalis toxicity can occur even if the drug is given in doses usually judged to be nontoxic (Ingelfinger and Goldman 1976), to patients with normal serum creatinine or blood urea nitrogen (BUN) values (Ewy et al 1969). Toxicity is most likely caused by advanced heart disease (Kabelitz 1975) and diminished renal clearance (leads to higher blood levels), as well as a reduction of lean body mass and a smaller volume of distribution caused by smaller body size (Ingelfinger and Goldman 1976; Ewy et al 1969). Pulmonary disease increases the risk of toxicity. Patients with acute or chronic respiratory disease face increased risk to digitalis toxicity, probably caused by enhanced sensitivity to the arrhythmogenic effects of digitalis (Green and Smith 1977). There are significantly higher levels of serum digoxin in patients with hypothyroidism and lower levels in those with hyperthyroidism, calling for appropriate dose adjustment of digoxin (Croxson and Ibbertson 1975). Thyroid disease also modifies the response of the myocardium to digitalis. Anemia, rheumatic carditis, or subacute bacterial endocarditis cause resistance to the action of digitalis, as can hypocalcemia. In contrast, hypercalcemia increases the effect of digitalis on the heart (Mason 1974). Patients with arrhythmias may exhibit higher steady state levels of digoxin (1.2 to 0.7 ng/ml) than those without (0.7 to 0.2 ng/ml) (Manninen et al 1976).

Toxic effects of digitalis in the elderly differ from those in younger patients. Digitalis therapy may lead to a worsening of CHF. Responding to this, an increased dosage may be prescribed leading to increased toxicity. What is needed is a decreased dosage. Sometimes, toxicity may manifest only as confusion or by a slow onset of apparent dementia. Importantly, the elderly are likely to develop asymptomatic digitalis toxicity and must, therefore, be monitored closely. Very often, intoxicated elderly patients present only with arrhythmia. The most potentially harmful effect of digitalis therapy in the elderly involves the electrical function of the cardiac cell membrane. Cardiac glycosides promote automaticity in Purkinje tissue by evoking a depolarizing after-potential, which follows the normal action potential. An ectopic beat can result (Cranefield 1977). In addition, inhibition of sodium transport increases intracellular sodium and consequently enhances the contractile calcium pool (Smith 1978). Thus, in patients with a very irritable myocardium, there should be a very slow and careful approach to steady state concentrations. Serious arrhythmias indicate immediate withdrawal of digitalis and diuretics. Cardiac arrhythmias in the elderly often affect other end organs.

Dizziness, syncope, and transient ischemia may result from tachycardia or bradyarrhythmias.

Common noncardiac symptoms of toxicity in the elderly include fatigue, muscular weakness, and difficulty in walking or raising the arms. Anorexia is often present instead of nausea and vomiting. Muddy vision is less prevalent. Also observed are mental symptoms such as restlessness, insomnia, apathy, and drowsiness (Doherty and Kane 1973).

Some infrequent physiologic manifestations of digitalis therapy, such as gynecomastia, occur more frequently in the elderly (Davison 1972). The treatment of intercurrent diseases may also interfere with digitalis therapy. Digoxin absorption is impaired in patients with malabsorption syndrome due to hypermotility, which may be caused by laxative use. Antibiotic therapy may induce a decreased transit time, mandating a higher maintenance dose. When the antibiotic is withdrawn, the maintenance dose must be lowered (Bigger and Strauss 1972). In patients on maintenance digoxin therapy, propantheline increases digoxin concentrations, as would any drug which decreases gastrointestinal motility (Manninen et al 1973). Ingestion of food decreases the rate, but not the extent of digoxin absorption. Initially, therefore, the plasma concentration would tend to be lower, but this would not affect maintenance therapy (Johnson et al 1978).

Thus, digitalis is a valuable and very necessary drug in the treatment of elderly patients. However, effective digoxin therapy demands recognition of the possible effects of reduced renal function, the possible effects of intercurrent diseases, and the likely interaction with drugs concurrently administered. The dosage must be adjusted with these factors in mind, and particular attention must be paid to signs of developing toxicity, which may present differently in elderly than in young patients. Treatment failure in the elderly is often associated with the possibility that the cardiac reserve may have been reduced too far by a long-standing disease. Peripheral oxygen demand may be increased and cardiac output may not be reduced and, finally, oxygen transport capacity may be decreased, rather than cardiac output. Importantly, patient noncompliance with an established regimen may be the true cause of treatment failure; as many as 30% of patients may not comply (Johnston et al 1978; Weintraub et al 1973).

Potassium The body contains about 4000 mEq of potassium. Normally, 80% to 90% of the daily intake is excreted in the urine. Serum or plasma potassium levels may be deceptive; they are not necessarily indicative of the intracellular concentration.

External potassium homeostasis controls total body potassium content, which results from the difference in intake and excretion (Cox et al 1978). Renal excretion usually determines this balance, but diarrhea or malabsorption may lead to large potassium losses. The distribution of potassium between the extracellular and intracellular fluid compartments is controlled by the internal balance. It is critical in the control of the plasma potassium concentration. Only about 2% of total body potassium is contained in the extracellular fluid. Therefore, shifts of relatively small amounts of potassium in or out of the extracellular fluid can produce major changes in the plasma concentration.

Serum potassium levels and incidence of digitalis toxicity are inversely related. A reduction of serum potassium levels, even from elevated to normal levels, may unmask digitalis toxicity or cause digitalis toxicity even at low doses. The incidence of digitalis toxicity in patients receiving both digitalis and diuretics increases significantly when measured against the incidence in patients receiving only digitalis (Wade 1972). The most important reason for the rapid increase in digitalis toxicity is the use of more vigorous diuretics (Steiness 1973). The elderly, whose diet is often poor, are especially at risk, as their potassium levels may be low even before the start of therapy.

Hypokalemia may result from excessive potassium loss via the kidneys or gastrointestinal tract, or by redistribution of extracellular potassium into intracellular space. All diuretics, except spironolactone and triamterene, cause hypokalemia through kaluresis. Excessive use of laxatives and drugs which can cause diarrhea, such as neomycin or quinidine, can also cause excessive gastrointestinal loss of potassium.

Diuretics which lower plasma potassium may enhance the myocardial response to digitalis because potassium ions and digitalis compete for the same binding sites on the sodium/potassium-dependent ATPase. If the extracellular concentration of potassium falls too low to compete effectively, more digitalis will be bound to the enzyme, increasing myocardial contractility, (Ascione 1977b). There is an additive effect of the toxicity of digitalis and abnormal ratios of potassium concentrations inside and outside the cardiac cell (Brater and Morrelli 1977a). Patients treated with prednisone or the methylxanthines are often hypokalemic.

In view of the clear relationship between digitalis toxicity and hypokalemia, the use of potassium supplements has been frequently discussed. Neither potassium-sparing diuretics nor potassium supplements should be given routinely to patients (Kassirer and Harrongton 1977). Even long-term furosemide therapy does not automatically call for potassium supplementation, unless there is preexisting potassium depletion or cardiac failure, liver disease, or nephrotic syndrome (Dargie et al 1974). While the therapeutic efficacy of potassium administration is well recognized, so is the hazard of hyperkalemia. A possible exception to the caution against automatic potassium supplementation is the patient with renal insufficiency where electrolyte disturbances can be expected.

Potassium levels must be checked initially, and rechecked every one to two months. When a stable potassium level is present, it should be rechecked every four to six months.

If potassium supplementation is chosen, it should be carefully controlled to avoid hyperkalemia. Patients receiving potassium-sparing diuretics, who suffer from renal insufficiency, are particularly at risk. Paresthesia of fingers, diarrhea, nausea, weakness, muscle cramps, and muscle pains are indicators of hyperkalemia, which can be confirmed by an EKG.

Potassium supplementation and patient compliance with it is extremely hard to achieve, because of the bitter taste of the available formulations. Therefore, from time to time, notes appear on how to make potassium more palatable. One that continues to reappear is the suggestion that a plain potassium chloride solution be mixed with tomato juice (Corash 1977). In the early 1970s, a similar approach was suggested in the *New England Journal of Medicine,* which was quickly followed with other notices that this would most certainly solve the taste problem, but would expose the patient to high sodium loads, most likely undesirable. The usual type of tomato juice contains about 500 mg of sodium per eight ounces.

In order to overcome the bitter taste of potassium, which so often leads to patient noncompliance, there were developed enteric-coated tablets, which were later withdrawn from the market as they caused a high incidence of adverse effects. A newer product is represented by slow-release potassium tablets. When originally marketed, there were warnings that their use should be avoided in patients with problems of stasis, obstruction, or delayed intestinal transit time. More recent reports address their ability to cause small bowel ulceration and stricture. Ulceration of the esophagus caused by these tablets has also been reported. It has now been suggested that slow release potassium chloride tablets are potentially hazardous and should not be used as a source of potassium supplementation (Sopko and Freeman 1977; Katholi and Levitin 1977; Howie and Strachan 1975; McCall 1975; Hefferman and Murphy 1975; Peters 1976).

Liquid potassium chloride preparations are usually the treatment of choice. The chloride ion is essential. While it will not increase absorption of potassium, it will act to retain it. Potassium will neither move into cells nor be retained in the absence of chloride ions. Thus, organic potassium salts are unsuited for potassium replacement therapy. Potassium gluconate, acetate, bicarbonate, or citrate can be used, though, for patients who are not on a low salt diet, as they take in sufficient chloride ions (Heineman et al 1976a).

Appropriate salt substitutes may provide an excellent alternative to potassium chloride use. Testing a number of these, it was found that Neocurtasal and Featherweight "K" Salt Substitute were most salty, while Morton Salt Substitute was least bitter (Sopko and Freeman 1977).

In summary, clinically significant hypokalemia is uncommon in patients without heart failure. Potassium supplements should not be used automatically for elderly patients, even those receiving digitalis and diuretics concurrently. They should be used with caution, as hyperkalemia following their use is not infrequent and elderly and uremic patients are particularly at risk to adverse reactions to potassium chloride (Lawson 1974). The use of potassium-rich foods to replace potassium deficiency is questionable. A four ounce glass of orange juice adds 55 calories to the diet, but only 6.7 mEq of potassium. One banana provides 130 calories, but only 13 mEq of potassium. Since patients with diuretic-induced hypokalemia must be treated with at least 60 mEq of potassium, foods, on the average, cannot meet this deficit.

THE DIURETICS

The oral diuretics are used both for diuresis and hypertension (Schwartz 1977). Diuretics, used in hypertensive therapy, initially diminish the vasoconstrictor response to norepinephrine, preventing compensatory re-elevation of the blood pressure. As blood pressure is reduced, cardiac output is lowered and total peripheral resistance is increased. With long-term therapy, plasma volume remains depressed, the cardiac output returns to normal, and peripheral resistance is modestly decreased. The latter effect contributes to the decreased vascular response to sympathetic stimulation (Beyer 1978). In CHF, there is an abnormal sodium and water retention in response to a diminished effective blood volume. When edema in CHF does not respond to digitalis and sodium restriction, diuretics are added to the regimen, particularly when edema leads to pulmonary congestion, venous stasis, and thrombosis of the extremities. A hazard of vigorous diuretic therapy is excessive depletion of the intravascular volume, diminished venous return, and, ultimately, decreased cardiac output. Therefore, intermittent dosing has been recommended, either in the form of every other day therapy, single dose therapy, or therapy for several days followed by rest periods (Kelit et al 1970). In CHF, there is no standard therapy schedule. Patient and physician must use weight gain as a guide (Heineman et al 1976b). Before starting long-term diuretic therapy, the physician should obtain a baseline serum uric acid, blood glucose, and serum potassium.

Treatment failure with diuretics may be caused by excessive sodium intake. Drinking water may contain as much as 200 mg/liter and OTC drugs may be another source of excessive sodium intake. The sodium content of drinking water may be substantially increased when the patient has a water softener attached to the faucet. Caution: diuretics make the elderly more prone to heat injury, and exposure of old people on diuretic therapy to high ambient temperatures can, therefore, be dangerous, particularly when humidity is high (Hall 1972).

It is important for the prescriber to know the site of action of the individual diuretics, both in case patient response to a diuretic chosen is poor or if combination therapy is inidicated. These sites are listed, in general, in Table 19-28 and, specifically for each drug in Table 19-29.

The diuretics acting primarily on the proximal tubule, such as carbonic anhydrase inhibitors, are not useful in the treatment of hypertension (Vidt 1978) unlike those that act secondarily distal to the proximal tubule. Among them are the thiazides, furosemide, and metolazone. Furosemide and ethacrynic acid both act at the ascending limb of the loop of Henle, and, appropriately, they are named loop diuretics. The organomercurials also act at this site, but are not effective in treating CHF. They are generally reserved to treat either severe edema or acute situations, such as severe volume overload or hypertension with concomitant renal failure. The major site of action of the thiazide diuretics is the cortical diluting segment and the so-called potassium-sparing diuretics, spironolactone and triamterene, act at the distal convoluted tubule (Vidt 1978).

The characteristics of some oral diuretics are given in Table 19-30, some common side effects in Table 19-31 and suggested dosages in Table 19-32.

The thiazides Thiazide diuretics are the drugs of choice in nonazotemic patients. The thiazides inhibit reabsorption of sodium in the proximal tubules of the nephron. They are strict saluretic drugs and do not increase bicarbonate excretion. They do not affect the sodium concentrating mechanism of the loop of Henle (Beyer 1977). Hydrochlorothiazide is the drug of choice both for initial and maintenance therapy as it is much better absorbed than chlorothiazide. Some clinicians feel that its action is too short to be suitable for maintenance therapy, but this could be overcome by twice-daily administration. If necessary, a second diuretic of different potency and site of action could be added to the thiazide regimen.

The major side effects encountered with thiazides are hypokalemia, hyperuricemia, and hyperglycemia (Riddiough 1977). Actually, these diuretics interfere with the action of insulin on the cell membrane. An optimum antihypertensive dose for the thiazides has not yet been clearly determined, but doses in excess of 100 mg/24 hours will

Table 19-28
The Diuretics

Diuretic	Site of action	Primary action(s)	Most common side effects
Thiazides	Proximal tubule	Inhibit reabsorption of sodium. Saluretic. Decrease blood volume and peripheral vascular resistance. Do not affect the sodium concentrating mechanism of loop of Henle	Hypokalemia, hyperglycemia, hyperuricemia
Loop	Ascending limb of loop of Henle	Inhibit transport of sodium and chloride from lumen to interstitium. Saluretic. Kaliuretic. Greater and more rapid decrease in blood volume. Furosemide also inhibits carbonic anhydrase.	More severe hypokalemia. Hyperuricemia equal to or more than thiazides. Hypoglycemic potential is mild. Increased calcium loss. Possible hearing loss which is reversible
Potassium-sparing	Distal convoluted tubule	Interfere with exchange of sodium for potassium	Hyperkalemia, gynecomastia, mastodynia

Table 19-29
Site of Action of Diuretics

Name	Site of Action
Acetazolamide	Proximal convoluted tubule
Bendroflumethiazide	Cortical section of the ascending distal tubule
Benzthiazide	Cortical section of the ascending distal tubule
Chlorothiazide	Cortical section of the ascending distal tubule
Chlorthalidone	Cortical section of the ascending distal tubule
Cyclothiazide	Cortical section of the ascending distal tubule
Ethacrynic acid	Medullary diluting segment; loop of Henle
Furosemide	Medullary diluting segment; loop of Henle
Hydrochlorothiazide	Cortical section of the ascending distal tubule
Hydroflumethiazide	Cortical section of the ascending distal tubule
Mercaptomerin sodium	Proximal tubule
Methyclothiazide	Cortical section of the ascending distal tubule
Metolazone	Cortical section of the ascending distal tubule
Polythiazide	Cortical section of the ascending distal tubule
Quinethazone	Cortical section of the ascending distal tubule
Spironolactone	Primarily the aldosterone dependent sodium-potassium exchange site in the convoluted renal tubule
Triamterene	Segment of distal tubule under the control of the adrenal mineralocorticoids, especially aldosterone
Trichlormethiazide	Cortical section of the ascending distal tubule

probably cause acute electrolyte losses and diuresis, without decreasing hypertension further (Schwartz 1977). Almost all patients on thiazide therapy will have reduced potassium stores, which sensitizes the patient to digitalis effects (*Medical Letter* 1977b). Subjective symptoms of hypokalemia are weakness and muscle fatigue which, if prolonged, can lead to arrhythmias and, occasionally, sudden death.

Table 19-30
Characteristics of Some Oral Diuretics

	Onset of action (hours)	Peak effect (hours)	Duration (hours)
Chlorothiazide	1	4	6–12
Chlorthalidone	2	6	24
Ethacrynic acid	½	2	6–8
Furosemide	1	1–2	6
Hydrochlorothiazide	2	4	12 or more
Spironolactone	gradual	2–3 days	2–3 days after withdrawal of drug
Triamterene	2	6–8	12–16
Trichlormethiazide	2	6	24

Potassium depletion caused by chronic thiazide diuretic administration may result in extracellular fluid volume contraction, with subsequent stimulation of ADH release by activation of volume receptors (Moses and Miller 1974). Response to the thiazides decreases with decreasing glomerular filtration rate and, therefore, in cases of advanced renal insufficiency, the thiazides cannot be used.

Chlorthalidone This drug is comparable to the thiazides in antihypertensive activity. It has a more prolonged duration of action and, therefore, needs to be administered less often. Chlorthalidone, as well as the thiazides, can induce inappropriate secretion of the antidiuretic hormone when a patient has an excessive water intake (Luboshitzky et al 1978).

Carbonic anhydrase inhibitors Acetazolamide may be the drug of choice in the hypertensive patient with glaucoma. It may cause metabolic acidosis.

Triamterene The drug does not consistently lower blood pressure. It increases the excretion of sodium moderately by inhibiting its reabsorption in exchange for potassium in the distal portion of the tubule. Although it has only a modest natriuretic effect, it is sometimes preferred because of its longer duration of action. Its antikaliuretic effect is produced by a direct action on the renal tubules that is independent of mineralocorticoids. Patients on triamterene should be watched for signs of hyperkalemia.

Spironolactone This drug should be ideal for long-term treatment of mild or moderate hypertension. It does not induce hypokalemia or alter the carbohydrate metabolism. Neither does it induce hyperuricemia. However, it is not used widely, as it is not as effective as the thiazides. Spironolactone is an aldosterone antagonist

Table 19-31
Some Common Side Effects of Diuretics

Drug	Side effects	Incidence
Thiazides	Hypokalemia	In 10% to 40% receiving 50 mg to 100 mg hydrochlorothiazide daily. Incidence may increase with heavy salt intake, patient perspiration
	Hyperglycemia	Incidence not known. Onset: 2 to 4 weeks. Mostly in known or latent diabetics
	Hyperuricemia	Predisposed patients may develop clinical gout. Critical serum level: 9 mg/100 ml
Furosemide and ethacrynic acid	Hypokalemia	Probably as frequent as with thiazides
	Hyperglycemia	Less diabetogenic than the thiazides
	Hyperuricemia	Same as thiazides
Spironolactone	Hyperkalemia	3% in patients with normal renal function not receiving potassium. 42% in azotemic patients receiving potassium. Dose-related (400 mg/daily) Muscular weakness: 43% Nausea: 20%
	Gynecomastia	Not uncommon

Table 19-32
Common Thiazide Diuretic/Antihypertensives

Thiazides and related diuretics	Starting dose in the aging	Range of usual daily maintenance dose (mg)	Onset of effectiveness (hours)	Duration of effectiveness (hours)
Bendroflumethiazide	5 mg once daily in AM	2.5–15	2	18–24
Benzthiazide	25 mg bid after meals	50–100	2	12–18
Chlorothiazide	250 mg bid after meals	500–1000	2	6–12
Cyclothiazide	1 mg once daily in AM	1–2	2	18–24
Hydrochlorothiazide	12.5 mg bid after meals 25 mg bid if necessary	25–100	2	6–12
Hydroflumethiazide	50 mg once daily in AM	50–100	2	18–24
Methylclothiazide	2.5 mg once daily in AM	2.5–5	2	24

Table 19-32 *(continued)*
Common Thiazide Diuretic/Antihypertensives

Thiazides and related diuretics	Starting dose in the aging	Range of usual daily maintenance dose (mg)	Onset of effectiveness (hours)	Duration of effectiveness (hours)
Polythiazide	1 mg once daily in AM	2.5–5	2	24–48
Trichlormethiazide	2 mg bid after meals	2–4	2	24
Chlorthalidone	50 mg once daily in AM	50–100	2	48–72
Quinethazone	50 mg once daily in AM	50–100	2	18–24

and it exerts its effect on sodium/potassium exchange indirectly, by inhibiting the aldosterone effect on potassium excretion by the distal convoluted tubule. Spironolactone blocks the kaliuretic activity of aldosterone by competing with the endogenous mineralocorticoids for renal receptors. The drug is most frequently used for fluid retention caused by hepatic cirrhosis and in CHF; it is seldom used in hypertension. About 20% of patients receiving spironolactone suffer adverse effects; the percentage doubles in patients on potassium supplementation. If BUN reaches 50 mg/100 ml, hyperkalemia occurs frequently.

Loop diuretics   The loop diuretics, furosemide and ethacrynic acid, are short-acting and produce rapid swings in fluid and electrolyte balance. As they are very potent diuretics, they should be reserved for instances in which thiazides do not elicit the desired response. For reasons that are somewhat unclear, however, they are more and more the diuretics of choice.

They are not suitable for long-term treatment of hypertension (Chrysant 1976), but they may be needed when there is a significant degree of renal failure (serum creatinine 3 to 8 mg%). They are substantially useful and the drugs of choice in the treatment of hypertension associated with frank renal insufficiency, as they are renal vasodilators and their effects are dose related. The dose must be titrated in an ascending order until therapeutic blood pressure control is achieved. In general, the loop diuretics offer no advantage over the thiazides in the treatment of patients with mild or moderate hypertension.

These two drugs are saluretic agents that inhibit the transport of sodium and chloride ions from the lumen to the interstitium by the ascending limb of the loop of Henle. As they can inhibit as much as 20% to 25% of sodium and chloride reabsorption, they are sometimes called "high-ceiling" diuretics (Williamson 1977). The extrarenal effects of the loop diuretics, primarily venodilation, occur before diuresis and result in diminished venous return, a fall in pulmonary artery pressure, and an improvement of gas exchange (Heineman 1978). The renal effects bring about diuresis, a reduction of intravascular volume, and mobilization of edema fluid. However, these effects can also lead to a fall in blood pressure and cardiac output, to hyponatremia, prerenal azotemia, and extracellular bicarbonate excess. The major danger involving the use of these diuretics is excess diuresis and consequent dehydration. Elderly men with heart disease often present with urinary retention within one week of initial administration.

Potassium loss is directly related to sodium loss. Furosemide, because of its sulfamyl group, also inhibits carbonic anhydrase, unlike ethacrynic acid. When used for prolonged periods of time, both drugs can cause systemic alkalosis. Furosemide is usually preferred to the use of ethacrynic acid as it has fewer side effects and less potential to cause ototoxicity (Wollam and Vidt 1978a, 1978b). Furosemide is frequently prescribed in the treatment of nephropathies, arterial hypertension, CHF, and ascites associated with chronic liver disease. It has a good therapeutic index in cardiovascular disease, is less safe in renal insufficiency, and has to be closely monitored in patients with liver cirrhosis (Naranjo et al 1978).

Apparently, many clinicians like to use furosemide as a first-step drug in hypertension, for diverse reasons. It has been suggested that even with long-term use, the drug does not easily disrupt the electrolyte balance and that its use rarely provokes hypokalemia. Clinicians seem to feel that the use of furosemide, rather than thiazides, permits the patient more freedom of movement. The drug, taken two hours before bedtime or two hours before a patient wishes to begin a certain activity, will have induced its major diuretic effect by bedtime or the time that the activity is scheduled to take place, thus not interfering with sleep or the activity.

REFERENCES

Adler, S. Methyldopa-induced decrease in mental activity. *JAMA.* 230:1428, 1974.

Ahlquist, R.P. Propranolol in hypertension. *J Clin Pharmacol.* 17:93, 1977.

American Medical Association. *AMA Drug Evaluations,* 2nd Ed. Acton, Mass.: Publishing Sciences Group, 1973.

Ambre, J.J., and Fischer, L.J. Effect of coadministration of aluminum and magnesium hydroxides on absorption of anticoagulants in man. *Clin Pharmacol Ther.* 14:231, 1973.

Ames, R.P. Serum lipid response to antihypertensives. *Drug Ther.* 7(8):101, 1977.

Amsterdam, E.A., Greenberg, B. Try long-acting nitrates for angina. *Patient Care* 12(3):212, 1978.

Anavekar, S.N. Propranolol in the management of hypertension. *Drug Ther.* 8(2):99, 1978.

Anderson, W.F., and Cowan, N.R. Arterial blood pressure in healthy old people. *Gerontol Clin.* 14:129, 1972.

Ascione, F.J. Digitalis preparations and diuretics. *Drug Ther.* 7(2):31, 1977a.

Ascione, F.J. Digitalis glycosides with potassium-depleting diuretics. *Drug Ther.* 7(1):106, 1977b.

Aviado, D.M. Drug action, reaction, and interaction. II. Iatrogenic cardiopathics. *J Clin Pharmacol.* 15:641, 1975.

Aviado, D.M., and Salem, H. Drug action, reaction, and interaction. I. Quinidine for cardiac arrhythmias. *J Clin Pharmacol.* 15:477, 1975.

Bahardi, I., James, E.C., and Fedde, C.W. Soft tissue necrosis and gangrene complicating treatment with the coumarin derivatives. *Surg Gynecol Obstet.* 145:497, 1977.

Benowitz, N.L. New antihypertensive drugs: promise and problems. *Hosp Formulary.* 12:767, 1977.

Benson, H. Systemic hypertension and the relaxation response. *N Engl J Med.* 296:1152, 1977.

Berglund, G., Anderson, D., Hansson, L. et al. Propranolol given twice daily in hypertension. *Acta Med Scand.* 194:513, 1973.

Beyer, K.H. Diuretics in perspective. *J Clin Pharmacol.* 17:618, 1977.

Beyer, K.H. The pharmacological basis for modern diuretic therapy. *Rational Drug Ther.* 12(2):1, 1978.

Bigger, J.T., and Strauss, H.C. Digitalis toxicity: drug interactions promoting toxicity and the management of toxicity. *Semin Drug Treat.* 2(2):142, 1972.

Boyer, J.L., and Kasch, F.W. Exercise therapy in hypertensive men. *JAMA.* 211:1668, 1970.

Brater, D.C., and Morrelli, J.F. Digoxin toxicity in patients with normokalemic potassium depletion. *Clin Pharmcol Ther.* 22:21, 1977a.

Brater, D.C., and Morrelli, J.F. Cardiovascular drug interactions. *Ann Rev Pharmacol Toxicol.* 17:293, 1977b.

Bravo, E., Chrysant, S., Harris, T.R. et al. Hypertension: doctrine vs doctoring. *Patient Care* 11(15):20, 1977.

Brodows, R.G., and Campbell, R.G. Effect of age on post-heparin lipase. *N Engl J Med.* 287:969, 1972.

Brogden, R.N., Heel, R.C., Speight, T.M. et al. Prazosin: a review of its pharmacologic properties and therapeutic efficacy in hypertension. *Drugs* 14:163, 1977.

Castelli, W.P. CHD risk factors in the elderly. *Hosp Practice.* 11(10):113, 1976.

Castelli, W.P., Doyle, J.T., Gordon, T. et al. Alcohol and blood lipids. *Lancet* 2:153, 1977.

Cattell, M. Bioavailability of digitalis glycosides. Editorial *J Clin Pharmacol.* 18:375, 1978.

Choquette, C., and Ferguson, R.J. Blood pressure reduction in "borderline" hypertensives following physical training. *Can Med Assoc J.* 108:699, 1973.

Chrysant, S.G. Effects of antihypertensive agents. *Drug Ther.* 1(12):22, 1976.

Cockroft, D.W., and Gault, M.H. Prediction of creatinine clearance from serum creatinine. *Nephron* 16:31, 1976.

Cohn, J.N. Indications for digitalis therapy: a new look. *JAMA.* 229:1911, 1974.

Cohn, J.N., and Franciosa, J.A. Vasodilator therapy in cardiac failure. *N Engl J Med.* 297:27, 1977.

Colombo, F., Shapiro, S., Slone, D. et al (eds). *Epidemiological Evaluation of Drugs.* Littleton, Mass.: PSG Publishing Co., Inc., 1977.

Corash, L. "Mix your own" K supplements. *Patient Care* 11(14):66, 1977.

Cox, M., Sterns, R.H., and Singer, I. The defense against hyperkalemia: the roles of insulin and aldosterone. *N Engl J Med.* 299:525, 1978.

Cranefield, P.F. Action potential, afterpotentials, and arrhythmias. *Circ Res.* 41:415, 1977.

Crook, J.E., and Nies, A.S. Drug interactions with antihypertensive drugs. *New Ethic Med Prog.* 15(2):81, 1978.

Croxson, M.S., and Ibbertson, H.K. Serum digoxin in patients with thyroid disease. *Br Med J.* 2:566, 1975.

Dall, J.L.C. Digitalis intoxication in elderly patients. *Lancet* 1:194, 1965.

Dall, J.L.C. Maintenance digoxin in elderly patients. *Br Med J.* 2:705, 1970.

Danahy, D.T., and Aronow, W.S. Assessing antiarrhythmic actions. III. Propranolol. *Drug Ther.* 7(1):127, 1977.

Dargie, H.J., Boddy, K., Kennedy, A.C. et al. Total body potassium in long-term furosemide therapy: is potassium supplementation necessary? *Br Med J.* 4:316, 1974.

Davison, W. Unwanted drug effects in the elderly. Edited by L. Meyler, and M. Peck. In *Drug-Induced Diseases.* Amsterdam: Excerpta Medica, 1972.

Dawkins, K.D., and Gibson, J. Peripheral neuropathy with disopyramide. *Lancet* 1:329, 1978.

Department of Health, Education and Welfare. Workshop on pharmacology and aging, DHEW Publ. No. (NIH) 78-353. Bethesda, Md.: National Institutes of Health, 1978a.

Department of Health, Education and Welfare. *Health, United States, 1976–1977.* DHEW Publ. No. (HRA) 77-1233. Hyattsville, Md.: National Center Health Service Research, 1978b.

Deykin, D. Warfarin therapy, Part I. *N Engl J Med.* 283:691, 1970a.

Deykin D. Warfarin therapy, Part II. *N Engl J Med.* 283:801, 1970b.

Dimant, J., and Merrit, W. Serum digoxin levels in elderly nursing home patients: appraisal of routine periodic measurements. *J Am Geriatr Soc.* 26:378, 1978.

Doherty, J.E., and Kane, J.J. Clinical pharmacology and therapeutic use of digitalis glycosides. *Drugs* 6:182, 1973.

Dollery, C.T., George, C.T., and L'E Orme, M. Drug interactions affecting cardiovascular therapy. Edited by L.E. Cluff, and J.C. Petrie. In *Clinical Effects of Interaction Between Drugs.* Amsterdam: Excerpta Medica, 1975.

Drayer, D.E., Lowenthal, D.T., Restivo, K.M. et al. Steady-state serum levels of quinidine and active metabolites in cardiac patients with varying degrees of renal function. *Clin Pharmacol Ther.* 24:31, 1978.

Esler, M., Zweifler, A., Randall, O. et al. Pathophysiologic and pharmacokinetic determinants of the antihypertensive response to propranolol. *Clin Pharmacol Ther.* 22:299, 1977.

Ewy, G.A., Kapadia, G.G., Yao, L. et al. Digoxin metabolism in the elderly. *Circulation* 38(suppl 6):74, 1968a.

Ewy, G.A., Marcus, F.I., and Kapadia, G.G. Digoxin metabolism in the elderly. *Clin Res.* 16:27, 1968b.

Ewy, G.A., Kapadia, G.G., Yao, L. et al. Digoxin metabolism in the elderly. *Circulation* 39:449, 1969.

Fishback, D.B. An approach to the treatment of hypertension in the aged. *Angiology* 27:212, 1976.

Fonrose, H.A., Ahlbaum, N., Bugatch, E. et al. The efficiency of digitalis withdrawal in an institutional aged population. *J Am Geriatr Soc.* 22:208, 1974.

Franciosa, J.A., Blank, R.C., and Cohn, J.N. Nitrate effects on cardiac output and left ventricular outflow resistance in chronic congestive heart failure. *Am J Med.* 64:207, 1978.

Fraser, H.S., and Carr, A.C. Propranolol psychosis. Letter to the Editor *Br J Psychiatry.* 129:508, 1976.

Freis, E.D. Reserpine in hypertension: present status. *Am Fam Physician.* 11:120, 1975.

Friedman, S.A. Venous disease and its complications. *Med Clin North Am.* 6:1093, 1976a.

Friedman, S.A. Common manifestations of degenerative arterial disease. *Med Clin North Am.* 6:1979, 1976b.

Gans, J.A. Congestive heart failure. *Environ Pharm.* 3(6):13, 1977.

Garbus, S.B., and Lamy, P.P. Managing the aging hypertensive. *Patient Care,* 1976.

Gerstenblith, G., Lakatta, E.G., and Weisfeldt, M.L. Age changes in myocardial function and exercise response. *Prog Cardiovasc Dis.* 19(1):1, 1976.

Gibson, I.I., and O'Hare, M.O. Prescription drugs for old people at home. *Gerontol Clin.* 10:271, 1968.

Gifford, R.W. A standard approach to therapy. *Postgrad Med.* 56:20, 1974.

Goldman, P., and Ingelfinger, J.A. Therapy with antiarrhythmic drugs. Editorial *N Engl J Med.* 298:1193, 1978.

Goodwin, F.K., and Bunney, W.E. Depression following reserpine: a reevaluation. *Semin Psychiatry.* 3:435, 1971.

Gotshall, R.A., and Harker, L.A. Using antithrombotic therapy in ischemic cerebrovascular disease. *Geriatrics* 32(11):101, 1977.

Gould, L., Reddy, C.V.R., Chua, W. et al. Electrophysiologic properties of nitroglycerin in man. *Am Heart J.* 94:341, 1977.

Graff, A.C. Drug therapy of cardiovascular disease. *Geriatrics* 29:51, 1974.

Green, L.H., and Smith, T.W. The use of digitalis in patients with pulmonary disease. *Ann Intern Med.* 87:459, 1977.

Greenblatt, D.J., and Koch-Weser, J. Adverse reactions to propranolol in hospitalized medical patients. *Am Heart J.* 86:478, 1973.

Hall, M.R.P. Drugs and the elderly. *Adv Drug Reaction Bull.* 35:108, 1972.

Hansen, J.M., Siersbaek-Nielsen, K., and Skovsted, L. Carbamazepine-induced acceleration of diphenylhydantoin and warfarin metabolism in man. *Clin Pharmacol Ther.* 12:539, 1971.

Harralson, A., Chow, M., and Deglin, S.M. Angina pectoris: update on therapy. *US Pharm.* 2(8):44, 1977.

Harris, R. *The Management of Geriatric Cardiovascular Disease.* Philadelphia: J.B. Lippincott, 1970.

Hazell, K., and Baloch, K.H. Vitamin K deficiency in the elderly. *Gerontol Clin.* 12:10, 1970.

Hefferman, S.J., and Murphy, J.J. Ulceration of small intestine and slow-release potassium tablets. *Br Med J.* 2:746, 1975.

Heineman, H.O. Right-sided heart failure and the use of diuretics. *Am J Med.* 64:367, 1978.

Heineman, H.O., Hines, C., Lothian, G. et al. Using diuretics over the long term. *Patient Care.* 10(13):150, 1976a.

Heineman, H.O., Hines, C., Lothian, G. et al. Using diuretics over the long term. *Patient Care* 10(13):120, 1976b.

Heiser, J.F., and DeFrancisco, D. The treatment of pathological panic states with propranolol. *Am J Psychiatry.* 133:1389, 1976.

Helson, L., and Duque, L. Acute brain syndrome after propranolol. *Lancet* 1:98, 1978.

Hermann, G.R. Digitoxicity in the aged. Recognition, frequency, and management. *Geriatrics* 21:109, 1966.

Holland, O.B., and Kaplan, N.M. Propranolol in the treatment of hypertension. *N Engl J Med.* 294:930, 1976.

Howie, A.D., and Strachan, R.W. Slow-release potassium chloride treatment. *Br Med J.* 2:176, 1975.

Huffman, D.H., Azarnoff, D.L., Shoeman, D.W. et al. The interaction between halofenate and propranolol. *Clin Pharmacol Ther.* 19:807, 1976.

Hull, S.M., and Mackintosh, A. Discontinuation of maintenance digoxin therapy in general practice. *Lancet* 2:1054, 1977.

Hurwitz, A., Schlozman, D.L. Effects of antacids on gastrointestinal absorption of isoniazid in rat and man. *Am Rev Respir Dis.* 109:41, 1974.

Ingelfinger, J., and Goldman, P. The serum digitalis concentration—does it diagnose digitalis toxicity? *N Engl J Med.* 294:867, 1976.

Johnson, B.F., O'Grady, J., Sabey, G.A. et al. Effect of a standard breakfast on digoxin absorption in normal subjects. *Clin Pharmacol Ther.* 23:315, 1978.

Johnston, G.D., Kelley, J.G., and McDevitt, D.G. Do patients take digoxin? *Br Heart J.* 40:1, 1978.

Kabelitz, H.J. Die Therapie bei Dekompensierten Altersherzen und Klappenfehlern. *Z Ther.* 13(2):71, 1975.

Kannel, W.B., and Sorlie, P. Hypertension in Framingham. Edited by O. Paul. In *Epidemiology and Control of Hypertension.* New York: Stratton Intercontinental Medical Book Corp., 1975.

Karch, F.E. Propranolol: something for everyone. *Drug Ther.* 8(7):89, 1978.

Kassirer, J.P., and Harrongton, J.T. Diuretics and potassium metabolism: a reassessment of the need, effectiveness, and safety of potassium therapy. *Kidney Int.* 11(6):1, 1977.

Katholi, R.E., and Levitin, P.M. Letter to the Editor *N Engl J Med.* 296:112, 1977.

Katzung, B.G. The rational use of digitalis in congestive heart failure. *Drug Ther.* 4(10):75, 1974a.

Katzung, B.G. Action and interactions of antiarrhythmic drugs. *Therapeutics* 2(3):1, 1974b.

Kelit, S.A., Hamburger, R.J., Martz, B.L. et al. Diuretic therapy: current status. *Am Heart J.* 79:700, 1970.

Kennedy, R.D. Drug therapy for cardiovascular disease in the aged. *J Am Geriatr Soc.* 23:113, 1975.

Keyes, J.W. Problems in drug management in cerebrovascular disorders. *J Am Geriatr Soc.* 13:118, 1965.

Kitchin, A.H., Lowther, C.P., and Milne, J.S. Prevalence of clinical and electrocardiographic evidence of ischaemic heart disease in the older population. *Br Heart J.* 35:946, 1973.

Koch-Weser, J. Drug interactions in cardiovascular therapy. *Am Heart J.* 90:93, 1975.

Koch-Weser, J., and Sellers, E.M. Drug interactions with coumarin anticoagulants, Part I. *N Engl J Med.* 285:487, 1971a.

Koch-Weser, J., and Sellers, E.M. Drug interactions with coumarin anticoagulants, Part II. *N Engl J Med.* 285:547, 1971b.

Koup, J.R., Jusko, W.J., Elwood, C.M. et al. Digoxin pharmacokinetics: role of renal failure in dosage regimen design. *Clin Pharmacol Ther.* 19:9, 1975.

Kristt, D.A., and Engel, B.T. Learned control of blood pressure in patients with high blood pressure. *Circulation* 51:370, 1975.

Lamy, P.P., Eisdorfer, C., Kassel, V. et al. *The Aging Brain.* Princeton, N.J.: E.R. Squibb and Sons, 1977a.

Lamy, P.P., Filiatrault, L., Harris, R. et al. *The Aging Cardiovascular System.* Princeton, N.J.: E.R. Squibb and Sons, 1977b.

Laragh, J.H. Modern system for treating high blood pressure based on renin profiling and vasoconstriction-volume analysis: a primary role for beta blocking drugs. *Am J Med.* 61:797, 1976.

Lawson, D.H. Adverse reactions to potassium chloride. *Q J Med.* 43:433, 1974.

Lawson, D.H., and Lowe, G.D.O. Drug therapy reviews: clinical uses of anticoagulant drugs. *Am J Hosp Pharm.* 34:1225, 1977.

Leahey, E.B., Reiffel, J.A., Drusin, R.E. et al. Interaction between quinidine and digoxin. *JAMA.* 240:533, 1978.

Lee, S.G.T. Nitroglycerin ointment therapy and leg edema. *Am Heart J.*

95:273, 1978.

LeSher, P.A., Harris, L., and Hawkinson, R.W. Comparison of BID vs QID hydralazine dosage regimens in hypertensive patients on multiple-drug therapy. *Clin Pharmacol Ther.* 19:110, 1976.

Levitt, B., Cagin, N., Kleid, J. et al. Anti-anginal therapy: a physiologic approach. *Hosp Formulary.* 12:659, 1977.

Livesley, B. Management of hypertension in the elderly. *Update* 11:1343, 1975.

Loeliger, E.A. Anticoagulant drugs. Edited by L. Meyler, and A. Herxheimer. In *Side Effects of Drugs.* Amsterdam: Excerpta Medica, 1968.

Lott, R.S., and Hayton, W.L. Estimation of creatinine clearance from serum creatinine concentration–a review. *Drug Intell Clin Pharm.* 12:140, 1978.

Luboshitzky, R., Tal-Or, Z., and Barzilai, D. Chlorthalidone-induced syndrome of inappropriate secretion of antidiuretic hormone. *J Clin Pharmacol.* 18:336, 1978.

MacGregor, A.G. Review of points at which drugs can interact. *Proc R Soc Med.* 58:943, 1965.

Manninen, V., Melin, J., Apajalahti, A. et al. Altered absorption of digoxin in patients given propantheline and metaclopramide. *Lancet* 1:398, 1973.

Manninen, V., Reissell, P., and Paukkala, E. Transient cardiac arrhythmias after single daily maintenance doses of digoxin. *Clin Pharmacol Ther.* 20:266, 1976.

Mason, D.T. Digitalis pharmacology and therapeutics: recent advances. *Ann Intern Med.* 80:520, 1974.

Mason, D.T., and Tonkon, M.J. *Management of Fluid and Electrolyte Disturbances in Congestive Heart Failure.* San Juan, Puerto Rico: Searle and Co., 1977.

May, F.E., Stewart, R.B., and Cluff, L.E. Drug interactions and multiple drug administration. *Clin Pharmacol Ther.* 22:323, 1977.

McCall, A.J. Slow K ulceration of oesophagus with aneurysmal left atrium. *Br Med J.* 3:230, 1975.

McConahey, W.M. Diagnosing and treating myxedema and myxedema coma. *Geriatrics* 33(3):61, 1978.

McMahon, F. Efficacy of an antihypertensive agent: comparison of methyldopa and hydrochlorothiazide in combination or singly. *JAMA.* 231:155, 1975.

Medical Letter. Disopyramide (Norpace) for ventricular arrhythmias. 19:101, 1977a.

Medical Letter. Drugs for hypertension. 19:21, 1977b.

Medical Letter. Prazosin (Minipress) for hypertension. 19:1, 1977c.

Medical Letter. Drugs for ischemic peripheral arterial disease. 20:11, 1978a.

Medical Letter. Use of vasodilator drugs in congestive heart failure. 20:89, 1978b.

Mintz, G.S. Newer applications of organic nitrate vasodilator therapy. *Drug Ther.* 1(12):5, 1976.

Misage, J.R., and McDonald, R.H. Antagonism of hypotensive action of bethadine by "common cold" remedy. *Br Med J.* 4:347, 1970.

Morgan, T. Once-daily treatment of hypertension. *Br Med J.* 2:235, 1976.

Moser, M. Physician adherence in hypertension management. *Drug Ther.* 8(12):30, 1978.

Moses, A.M., and Miller, M. Drug-induced dilutional hyponatremia. *N Engl J Med.* 201:1234, 1974.

Naranjo, C.A., Busto, U., and Cassis, L. Furosemide-induced adverse reactions during hospitalization. *Am J Hosp Pharm.* 35:974, 1978.

National Institutes of Health. *Report of the Joint National Committee on*

Detection, Evaluation, and Treatment of High Blood Pressure. DHEW Publ. No. (NIH) 77-1088. Bethesda, Md., 1978.

Nejat, M., and Greif, E. The aging heart: a clinical review. *Med Clin North Am.* 60:1059, 1976.

Neurath, O. Cardiovascular changes in/of old age. *J Am Geriatr Soc.* 26:286, 1978.

Nowak, G.D. *Hypertension in the Elderly.* Bethesda, Md.: National Library of Medicine, 1975.

O'Malley, K., Stevenson, I.H., Ward, C. et al. Determinants of anticoagulant control in patients receiving warfarin. *Br J Clin Pharmacol.* 4:309, 1977.

Onesti, G. Antihypertensive agents as seen by the clinician. Edited by E.L. Engelhardt. In *Antihypertensive Agents.* Washington, D.C.: American Chemistry Society, 1976.

Onesti, G. Antihypertensives and their modes of action. *Drug Ther.* 8(2):35, 1978.

Onesti, G., and Lowenthal, D.T. (Eds.). *The Spectrum of Antihypertensive Drug Therapy.* New York: Biomedical Information Corp., 1977.

O'Reilly, R.A. Impact of aspirin and chlorthalidone on the pharmacodynamics of oral anticoagulant drugs in man. *Ann NY Acad Sci.* 179:173, 1971.

O'Reilly, R.A., and Aggeler, P.M., Determinants of the response to oral anticoagulant drugs in man. *Pharmacol Rev.* 22:35, 1970.

Orlando, J., and Aronow, W.S. Assessing antiarrhythmic actions. II. Quinidine and procainamide. *Drug Ther.* 1(12):32, 1976.

Patel, C.H. Yoga and bio-feedback in the management of hypertension. *Lancet* 2:1053, 1973.

Patel, C.H. Twelve-month follow-up of yoga and bio-feedback in the management of hypertension. *Lancet* 1:62, 1975.

Paulson, M.F., and Welling, P.G. Calculation of serum digoxin levels in patients with normal and impaired renal function. *J Clin Pharmacol.* 16:660, 1976.

Peters, J.L. Benign oesophageal stricture following oral potassium chloride therapy. *Br J Surg.* 63:698, 1976.

Pickering, G.W. *High Blood Pressure.* London: J and A Churchill, Ltd., 1968.

Pomerance, A. Pathology of the heart with and without cardiac failure in the aged. *Br Heart J.* 27:697, 1965.

Priddle, W.W., and Rose, M. Curtailing therapy in a home for the aged, with special reference to digitalis, diuretics and low-sodium diet. *J Am Geriatr Soc.* 14:731, 1966.

Raisfeld, I.H. Drug interactions in the therapy of cardiovascular disorders. *Am Heart J.* 81:709, 1971.

Reichek, N. Potential uses of long-acting nitrates. *Drug Ther.* 7(12):78, 1977.

Riccitelli, M.L., and Hirschfeld, H. Digitalis allergy: a study of 1720 skin tests on 430 patients. *J Am Geriatr Soc.* 9:277, 1961.

Riddiough, M.A. Preventing, detecting and managing adverse reactions to antihypertensive agents in ambulant patients with essential hypertension. *Am J Hosp Pharm.* 34:465, 1977.

Rodstein, M., and Rossman, I. (Eds.). *Clinical Geriatrics.* Philadelphia: J.B. Lippincott Co., 1971.

Roeske, W.R., Higgins, C., Karlinger, J.S. et al. Incidence of arrhythmias and ST-segment changes in elderly patients during barium enema studies. *Am Heart J.* 90:688, 1975.

Rogel, S., and Bassan, M. Anticoagulants in ischemic heart disease. *Arch Intern Med.* 136:1229, 1976.

Rosendorff, C. Prazosin: severe side effects are dose-dependent. *Br Med J.* 2:508, 1976.

Schwartz, A.B. Diuretics in the treatment of hypertension. *Drug Ther.* 7(1):158, 1977.

Schwarzfischer, P. Serumglykosid Spiegel im Alter: Problem der Verlaufskontrolle bei Glykosid Therapie. *Fortschr Med.* 94:841, 1976.

Shand, D.G. Propranolol. *N Engl J Med.* 293:80, 1975.

Shand, D.G. Propranolol, resolving problems in usage. *Drug Ther.* 8(7):53, 1978.

Shepherd, A.M.M., Hewick, D.S., Moreland, T.A. et al. Age as a determinant of sensitivity to warfarin. *Br J Clin Pharmacol.* 4:315, 1977.

Sigell, L.T., and Flessa, H.C. Drug interactions with anticoagulants. *JAMA.* 214:2035, 1970.

Simonson, W., and Stennett, D.J. Estimation of serum digoxin levels in geriatric patients. *Am J Hosp Pharm.* 35:943, 1978.

Smith, A.J. Hypertension. *Practitioner* 215:327, 1974.

Smith, T.W. Digitalis: ions, inotropy, and toxicity. *N Engl J Med.* 299:545, 1978.

Soffer, A. The changing clinical picture of digitalis intoxication. *Arch Intern Med.* 107:681, 1961.

Solomon, H.M., Barakat, M.J., and Ashley, C.J. Meigs' syndrome or Meigs' salmon. Letter to the Editor *JAMA.* 216:1036, 1971.

Sopko, J.A., and Freeman, R.M. Salt substitutes as a source of potassium. *JAMA.* 238:608, 1977.

Steiness, E. Incidence of electrolyte disturbance on the effects of digitalis. *Acta Cardiol.* 17(suppl):145, 1973.

Strandgaard, S., Olsen, J., Skinhoj, E. et al. Autoregulation of brain evaluation in severe arterial hypertension. *Br Med J.* 1:507, 1973.

Trope, G.E., and Hind, V.M.D. Closed-angle glaucoma in patients with disopyramide. *Lancet* 1:329, 1978.

Tuck, M. The role of adrenal mineralocorticoids in hypertension. *Geriatrics* 33(1):77, 1978.

Turner, A.S. Prazosin in hypertension. Letter to the Editor *Br Med J.* 2:1257, 1976.

Ueda, C.T., Williamson, B.J., and Dzindzio, B.S. Absolute quinidine bioavailability. *Clin Pharmacol Ther.* 20:260, 1976.

Vertes, V. *Management of Fluid and Electrolyte Disturbance In Hypertension.* San Juan, Puerto Rico: Searle and Co., 1975.

Veterans Administration Cooperative Study Group on Antihypertensive Agents. Effects of treatment on morbidity in hypertension. Results in patients with diastolic blood pressures averaging 115 through 129 mm Hg. *JAMA.* 202:1028, 1967.

Veterans Administration Cooperative Study Group on Antihypertensive Agents. Effects of treatment on morbidity in hypertension. Results in patients with diastolic blood pressures averaging 90 through 114 mm Hg. *JAMA.* 213:1143, 1970.

Vidt, D.G. Combination therapy in hypertension: a rational approach. *Drug Ther.* 3(8):33, 1978.

Wade, O.L. Drug therapy in the elderly. *Age Ageing.* 1(2):1972.

Walker, W.J. Changing United States life-style and declining vascular mortality: cause or coincidence? *N Engl J Med.* 297:163, 1977.

Weinstein, M.C., and Stason, W.B. *Hypertension: A Policy Perspective.* Cambridge, Mass.: Harvard University Press, 1976.

Weintraub, M., Au, W.Y.W., and Lasagna, L. Compliance as a determinant of serum digoxin concentration. *JAMA.* 224:481, 1973.

Wilkie, F., and Eisdorfer, C. Intelligence and blood pressure in the aged. *Science* 172:959, 1971.

Wilkinson, P.R., Dixon, N., and Hunter, K.R. Twice-daily propranolol treatment for hypertension. *J Int Med Res.* 2:220, 1974.

Williams, R.B., and Sherter, C. Cardiac complications of tricyclic antidepressant therapy. *Ann Intern Med.* 74:395, 1971.

Williamson, H.E. Furosemide and ethacrynic acid. *J Clin Pharmacol.* 17:663, 1977.

Winkler, G.F., and Young, R.R. Efficacy of chronic propranolol therapy in action tremors of the familial, senile or essential varieties. *N Engl J Med.* 290:984, 1974.

Wollam, G.L., and Vidt, D.G. The patient with resistant hypertension. *Drug Ther.* 3(2):36, 1978a.

Wollam, G.L., and Vidt, D.G. The patient with resistant hypertension. *Drug Ther.* 8(2):72, 1978b.

Wright, J.M., McLeod, P.J., and McCullough, W. Antihypertensive efficacy of a single bedtime dose of methyldopa. *Clin Pharmacol Ther.* 20:733, 1976.

Zito, R.A., and Reid, P.R. Lidocaine kinetics predicted by indocyanine green clearance. *N Engl J Med.* 298:1160, 1978.

20 Diabetes and Its Management in the Elderly

Diabetes mellitus is a chronic disease which is rapidly increasing in importance as a major health problem. Since 1950, the number of diabetics in the United States has increased 300%, while the general population has increased by only 50% (Maugh 1975). According to the National Commission on Diabetes, the number of diabetics will double every 15 years at the current rate of increase (Maugh 1976). Diabetes is now the third leading cause of death by disease, ranking only behind heart disease and cancer. It has also been cited as the second leading cause of blindness in the United States.

Diabetes mellitus is largely a disease of middle age. Of the over 4.5 million estimated diabetics in this country, about 80% are 45 years of age or older and almost 60% are 65 years or older (Kumble 1974). The incidence and prevalence rates of diabetes mellitus increase with age (Table 20-1). Over 80% of newly diagnosed diabetics are significantly overweight.

Table 20-1
Diabetes Mellitus

Age (years)	Incidence per 1000 persons
All ages	20
55–64	43.7
65–74	64.4
75 and over	57.9

Source: Department of Health, Education and Welfare, 1969.

For the most part, the cause of diabetes is unknown. However, its pathogenesis is probably attributable to some inheritable trait and it is estimated that 25% of the American population carry the defective genetic material.

Essentially, diabetes is a metabolic disorder in which the metabolism of carbohydrates is impaired and that of fats and proteins is enhanced because of a relative or absolute deficiency of insulin secretion. Certain symptoms are characteristic of the diabetic state. These include frequent urination, excessive thirst, increased appetite, weight loss, visual disturbances, and slow healing of cuts and scratches (Khachadurian and Detzkin 1975; Kryston and Shaw 1975). Not all diabetic patients, particularly the elderly, will experience these symptoms. Some will have several while others apparently have none.

Failure to control the diabetic state may lead to serious, acute manifestations of the disease, such as acidosis and coma. Even when the symptoms are apparently controlled, many long-term complications may arise. These may manifest as impaired coronary or cerebral circulation caused by accelerated atherosclerosis. Thickening of the basement membrane of the microvasculature is responsible for impaired peripheral circulation which can lead to retinal damage, ulceration, poor wound healing, and increased susceptibility to infections. Peripheral nerve dysfunction is a common complication of diabetes mellitus.

DIABETES AND THE ELDERLY

In people of advanced age, there is an increase in circulating insulin levels and islet cell adenomatosis is more prevalent in older than in younger persons. No doubt with advancing age the carbohydrate homeostasis becomes disordered, a condition called diabetes senilis. The aged pancreas maintains carbohydrate metabolism but is functionally deficient in case of stress. Insulin is less efficient in older people and they also respond qualitatively in a different fashion to insulin than do younger persons. However, there are indications that insulin degradation and peripheral utilization do not change with age (Barbagallo-Sangiorgi 1970; Streeten 1965; Giarnieri and Lumia 1961). It is generally agreed that plasma insulin response to glucose tends to increase with age, that elderly persons are either insulin-deficient or insulin-resistant, and that the progressive rise in glucose levels with age is associated with obesity (Kimmerling et al 1977; O'Sullivan 1974).

In any case, fasting and postprandial blood glucose values appear to increase with age. After middle age, response to a standard oral glucose load increases by about 10 mg% per decade for males and 13 mg% for females. At least 50% of those over 60 years of age manifest abnormal blood glucose responses in relation to standard curves. The diminished carbohydrate tolerance that is associated with aging contributes to the increased prevalence of diabetes in older people (Tubbs and Tubbs 1971; Davidowicz 1968; Kingsbury 1968).

Thus, with aging, there is generally a progressive loss of glucose tolerance, but there is also a rise in sensitivity to exogenously supplied insulin and a decline in the reactive capacity of tissues to insulin action (Shagan 1976).

All the accumulated evidence by numerous studies, though, has not yet yielded a clear answer to some of the most nagging questions facing a geriatrician: is the normally higher blood sugar in the elderly normal from a pathophysiologic point of view? Can this higher level be related to the chronic complications of diabetes? In short, using the norms established for younger persons indicates that many elderly are diabetics—but are they? (Andres 1971).

Diagnosis

It is obvious that normal levels that indicate diabetes in younger persons might not be applicable to older persons. A determination of blood sugar levels alone does not provide a sufficient basis for diagnosis of diabetes in the elderly. Certainly, if there is hyperglycemia with glucosuria, polyuria, polydipsia, weight loss, and polyphagia, the diagnosis is clear. But the elderly most likely will not present with the classical symptoms of the disease. Many may be hyperglycemic but not glucosuric, even with blood sugars of 300 mg%.

Elderly patients, in general, have less glucosuria for a given blood sugar than do younger diabetics. The elderly have lower glomerular filtration rates and a higher threshold for glucose. Symptoms related to glucosuria may not manifest until blood sugars are quite elevated. Therefore, in the elderly, diagnosis must depend on a good correlation of laboratory tests with clinical findings. In addition, the patient's family history should be very carefully reviewed.

Maturity-onset diabetes is characterized by a persistently elevated fasting glucose level, with or without glucosuria (Palumbo 1977). The most distinctive disease characteristic in the elderly is mild abnormality of carbohydrate metabolism. Early disease symptoms include fatigue, physical depression, emotional instability, prolonged wound healing, visual disturbances, and dulled perception to pain and temperature, especially in the lower extremities (Karam 1977; Thomas and Jones 1976). Most of these symptoms can be easily confused with normal aging changes.

On the other hand, older people likely will manifest symptoms of the "complications" of disease before any signs of metabolic disturbance become apparent. These may involve cardiovascular disease, neuropathies, and nephropathies (which are not peculiar to elderly patients). Peripheral vascular disease affecting the lower extremities tend to appear early in the disease, as the skin of the elderly bruises more easily.

All patients with furuncles, carbuncles, cellulitis, and superficial gangrene of the toe or heel should be tested for diabetes before a treatment regimen is selected. Transient nocturnal pain in the leg muscles may also be a sign of uncontrolled diabetes, and osteomyelitis of the bones of the feet is a common complication of neglected superficial foot infections in the diabetic.

All patients with the classical signs of the disease would, of course, be diagnosed as diabetic. Patients with peripheral complications should also be so diagnosed, regardless of their blood sugar level, as should patients who develop hyperglycemia and symptoms when given diuretics.

The Diabetic Patient

Diabetics are usually classified by the etiology of hyperglycemia. Those in whom hyperglycemia is caused by insufficient insulin are usually referred to as insulinopenic, while the insulin-plethoric diabetics suffer from hyperglycemia in the presence of normal or even above normal insulin concentrations, most likely caused by impaired response of the target organ to insulin.

Fully 75% of patients with acute myocardial infarction manifest marked glucose intolerance. Even several weeks after the attack, about 15% of the patients still exhibit this intolerance. Among patients with myocardial infarction, obese diabetic women have a death rate eight times that of obese diabetic men, twice that of other diabetics, and three times that of nondiabetics (Tansey et al 1977).

About 20% to 30% of patients with maturity-onset diabetes may have peripheral arteriosclerotic disease. Mortality in patients with poor diabetic control is significantly higher than in those with good control (Brownlee 1978). Apparently, there is a definite correlation between the incidence of retinopathy and both the duration of the disease and the degree of control of blood glucose (Goodkin 1975). There does not appear to be any correlation between the incidence of complications and the severity of the disease.

Many additional patient complaints stem from uncontrolled diabetes. For example, hyperglycemia may cause myopia which results from an increased refractive index of the lens. The patient may also complain of dry throat. The pharynx may be inflamed and the tonsils may be enlarged. The development of atherosclerosis is accelerated in diabetes. Coronary artery disease is seven times more common in diabetic than in other women.

Severe postural hypotension can occur and cause syncope, cardiac arrhythmias, and anginal pain. Patients with uncontrolled diabetes are also frequently predisposed to chronic respiratory diseases and they may also complain of epigastric discomfort, anorexia, and nausea. One-fourth of all patients with pancreatic carcinoma have frank diabetes mellitus.

Often, a patient may try to control polyuria by restricting fluid intake. This may lead to constipation and large, hard stools, rectal fissures, and prolapsed hemorrhoids. Glucosuria and fungus may cause pruritus ani, which seems to occur more frequently in women than in men. Diabetic women also frequently suffer from pruritus vulvae with or without vulvo-vaginitis.

Finally, the diabetic elderly may also complain of nocturnal diarrhea and disturbed micturition. Sorbitol, present as a sweetening agent in many dietetic foods, such as ice cream, may produce a laxative effect and diabetic patients who suffer from diabetic diarrhea should be counseled against use of these foods (Lamy and Kitler 1970).

TREATMENT OF DIABETES

Current trends in diabetic therapy are based on findings that restoration of normoglycemia may halt or even reverse the progression of the complications of the disease. The primary methods to achieve normoglycemia include dietary control, the use of hypoglycemic agents, and the regulation of exercise. After the physician chooses the appropriate combination of these modalities, successful management depends largely on the patient. Control of diabetes, once a treatment regimen has been established, is a function of the patient's successful inclusion of the required self-care activities (Table 20-2) in the established daily routine (Backscheider 1974; Powell and Lamy 1977).

Table 20-2
The Most Important Self-Care Activities of the Diabetic Patient

Activity	Purpose
Dietary control	Regulation of caloric intake and weight control; delay of vascular complications.
Exercise regulation	Avoidance of unnecessary swings in blood glucose levels caused by irregular exercise.
Medication (insulin or oral hypoglycemics)	Regulate blood glucose; prevent vascular, neurologic, renal, ocular complications.
Urine testing	Monitor control of blood glucose; monitor effects of other diseases on control.
Foot care	Prevention of injuries; detection of unnoticed injuries, avoid infections.
Oral hygiene	Maintenance of the integrity of the gingiva; detection of abscesses.

The degree of control achieved will depend, in part at least, on the patient's willingness to rotate injection sites, care for instruments, use correct methods of urine testing, and exercise dietary control.

Yet many studies have shown that compliance with these procedures is very poor among diabetic patients, and it cannot be anticipated that elderly patients would necessarily play a more active and positive role in self-care.

A series of studies showed that 59% of diabetic patients erred by at least two units when preparing an insulin injection, 35% made potentially serious errors (greater than 15% in dose administered), only 23% performed urine tests as instructed, only 28% followed the dietary regimen, less than 50% performed acceptable footcare, and only 20% employed acceptable insulin equipment practices (Watkins et al 1967). It is quite apparent, therefore, that elderly patients, who may have difficulty in following instructions, must be made aware of all necessary procedures for any regimen to be successful (Shangraw and Lamy 1969). On the other hand, the regimen should be selected so that it will place minimal restrictions on the elderly patient, who may already be restricted in day-to-day living by other diseases or conditions. For example, the patient should understand clearly that it will not be necessary to buy special foods, which may also be economically undesirable, and that regular foods will be entirely satisfactory.

It may be difficult to set the desired treatment goal. Generally, in diabetic patients it is important to maintain the blood glucose level in the "normal" fasting range of 70 mg% to 100 mg%. This is necessary as the brain depends on glucose as its major energy source (Service 1977).

Many elderly patients, though, may manifest clinical features of neuroglycopenia when the blood sugar is lowered to an apparently normal range, and for these, blood sugars in the 150 mg% to 250 mg% range may be acceptable (Marks 1966). The aging brain tolerates hypoglycemia much less readily than it does hyperglycemia. Apparently "good" control of blood sugar in the elderly can lead to depressed intellectual function, confusion, bizarre behavior, amnesia, and blurred vision. Irreversible brain damage can result, as can hypothermia and death. By far the most common cause of hypoglycemia in the elderly is the use of hypoglycemic drugs.

The Dietary Regimen

In both men and women, mortality from diabetes appears to be highest in insulin-dependent patients, second highest in those treated with oral hypoglycemic drugs, and lowest in those patients who can be managed with a purely dietary regimen (Kent 1978). In the elderly, diabetes is normally stable and not too difficult to manage. Most elderly patients should be managed by dietary restriction only. Particularly, if the fasting glucose level is less than 200 mg%, the patient, who is usually asymptomatic, does not require more than dietary restrictions. The diet should be carefully designed to meet certain requirements:

1. It should consist of readily available, commonly consumed, and generally acceptable foods.
2. It should take into consideration the patient's ethnic background and economic status.
3. It should interfere as little as possible with the patient's daily activity.
4. It should be flexible.

In 1971, the American Diabetes Association issued a statement formulated by its Committee on Food and Nutrition. Essentially, it stated that there no longer appears to be any need to restrict disproportionally the intake of carbohydrates in the diet of most diabetic patients. Apparently, in subjects with normal fasting plasma glucose levels, fasting levels decrease and oral glucose tolerance improves with high carbohydrate meals. Concurrently, increased carbohydrate intake reduces intake of fats, leading to better weight control. An increase in sugar consumption in most diabetics stimulates enzyme systems of several body tissues to increase direct utilization of sugar as a source of energy (Bierman and Nelson 1975).

According to these suggestions, then, as much as 60% of calories can be derived from cereal grains and starchy vegetables, ie, complex carbohydrates. If diabetes is moderately severe, simple sugars still should be avoided, since they easily produce hyperglycemic peaks and a transient increase in glucosuria (Bierman 1977).

Regulation of the size and frequency of meals helps protect the patient from symptomatic hyperglycemia and hypoglycemia (Albrink and Davidson 1971). Perhaps, more importantly, control of caloric intake helps the diabetic patient to achieve and maintain ideal body weight (Tunebride and Wetherill 1970), as obesity tends to increase the incidence of the complications of the disease (West and Kalbfleisch 1970). Reduction of overweight, on the other hand, decreases hyperglycemia and glucose intolerance. In obese patients insulin cannot induce the movement of glucose from the blood into the body's cells. A weight loss often restores tissue sensitivity to insulin. Thus, weight reduction is highly desirable from several points of view.

If an elderly patient is maintained only by dietary control, a sudden loss of control may not be caused by a lack of dietary compliance. Upper respiratory or urinary tract infections, as well as certain drugs, could be responsible.

The Oral Hypoglycemic Agents

In maturity-onset diabetes, most patients are not insulin-dependent and maturity-onset diabetes is no longer viewed as an insulin deficiency disease. However, there may be a delayed response to glucose stimulus, but the most important abnormality may be a peripheral resistance to insulin utilization associated with a defect in cell surface hormone receptors. In elderly patients with elevated sugar or diagnostic diabetes, drug treatment should not start until such symptoms appear. In this regard, spilling of sugar is not viewed as a symptom of diabetes.

The oral hypoglycemics, ie, the sulfonylureas, are still widely used for the elderly with adult-onset diabetes, ie, those who still have some endogenous insulin production.

Severe criticism has been directed toward the use of oral hypoglycemics. However, there is no question that hypoglycemic therapy is necessary when dietary management alone is not sufficient to control a patient's blood sugar level. Furthermore, much of the criticism of oral hypoglycemics may be applicable to younger patients. In the case of older patients, though, other considerations predominate. The oral hypoglycemics may well be the drugs of choice simply because the use of insulin presents a multitude of problems which may be most difficult to overcome for the elderly, if they can be overcome at all. For example, the elderly may have extreme problems in handling insulin and insulin syringes and the parenteral administration of insulin. Nevertheless, if an oral hypoglycemic agent is chosen in view of these considerations, the need for its continued administration should be periodically re-evaluated.

Tolbutamide is the drug of choice initially. It is extensively metabolized in the liver and should not be given to patients with liver impairment. Improper excessive use and presence of renal disease may cause hypoglycemia in patients receiving tolbutamide. Despite the voluminous literature on alcohol interaction with the oral hypoglycemics, these interactions usually occur only in alcoholic patients. Those who restrict their alcoholic intake to small amounts only in social circumstances are probably not at risk to significant side effects due to this interaction (Seltzer 1972).

The initial recommended dose for tolbutamide in the elderly is 0.5 gm twice daily (the patient must clearly understand that this does not mean one at 10 AM and one at 11 AM. The elderly are likely to select this dosage regimen so as "not to forget" to take their tablets. Both verbal and label instructions should clearly state the time that the tablet should be taken). The maximum recommended dose is 2 gm per day. The duration of action of tolbutamide is six to eight hours, and its hypoglycemic effect can be intensified by aspirin, bishydroxycoumarin, phenylbutazone, probenecid, and sulfonamides, all drugs frequently used in the treatment of the multiple diseases of the elderly.

Chlorpropamide Chlorpropamide is a very long acting drug, of particular hazard to elderly diabetics. Its duration of action, in the elderly, may be as long as four or five days. One aspect of its hazard to elderly patients is that conventional methods to treat symptomatic hypoglycemic episodes are most likely ineffective. Administration of sugar or orange juice may help, but their effect will be felt only for a short period of time, after which symptomatic hypoglycemia will reappear because of the drug's long action.

Chlorpropamide and the other oral hypoglycemics are principally excreted by the kidney (Department of Health, Education and Welfare 1969). It is easily apparent, then, that a patient's renal status can importantly affect the pharmacokinetics of these drugs. They are likely to accumulate in patients with impaired renal function. Chlorpropamide, which has a half-life of 36 hours, or seven times that of tolbutamide, is often associated with sulfonylurea-induced hypoglycemia.

It has been suggested that the oral hypoglycemics not be given to elderly patients living alone and in isolation. An environment which permits the patient's observation by friends or family members is essential to use of these drugs. It is of utmost importance that those in closest contact with the elderly patient receiving hypoglycemic therapy should be instructed about the signs and symptoms of hypoglycemia and its immediate treatment (Table 20-3). Four to eight

Table 20-3
Diabetic Acidosis and Hypoglycemia

Diabetic Acidosis

Symptoms—general malaise, weakness, pains in abdomen, aches and pains elsewhere, drowsiness, anorexia, nausea, vomiting, prostration, unconsciousness, signs of shock, odor of acetone on breath, dryness of mouth and skin, labored breathing, soft eyeballs

Laboratory findings—hyperglycemia, glycosuria, ketonuria, reduced carbon-dioxide combining power

Causes—
1. neglect of treatment, particularly omission of needed insulin
2. aggravation of diabetes resulting from complications, such as acute infections, thyrotoxicosis, and surgical operations

Treatment—in acidosis and circulatory collapse
1. continuous nursing care is imperative
2. insulin—administer unmodified insulin subcutaneously repeating dose hourly until blood sugar falls
3. fluids—administer electrolyte solutions (sodium r-lactate and/or sodium chloride), 1000 to 5000 ml, intravenously
4. glucose—administer 5% glucose intravenously after blood sugar falls
5. watch for signs of hypokalemia after four to six hours of treatment (flaccidity, weakness, absence of reflexes and rapid, shallow breathing replacing Kussmaul's respiration) and treat with potassium-containing foods, beverages, or solutions

Hypoglycemia

Symptoms—faintness, palpitations, headache, double vision, emotional instability, unconsciousness, hunger, excessive perspiration, trembling, nausea and vomiting (rare), convulsion (rare), unsteadiness of gait—think of a hypoglycemic reaction whenever a patient receiving insulin complains of an unusual sensation or behaves in an unusual manner

Causes—
1. overdose of insulin
2. delay in eating
3. failure to eat entire meal
4. undue physical exercise
5. decrease in need for insulin after control of glycosuria or following recovery from complications which temporarily had caused an increased requirement

Treatment—sugar or glucagon—
1. if patient is able to swallow, give readily absorbable carbohydrate—for example, orange juice, cola beverages, candy, corn syrup, honey, or a lump of sugar
2. if oral administration of carbohydrate is not possible or response is inadequate, administer glucagon by the subcutaneous, intramuscular, or intravenous route and repeat dose in 20 minutes if necessary (seldom used except in treatment of juvenile diabetes)
3. if the patient fails to respond to two injections of glucagon, glucose (10 to 20 gm) must be given intravenously and in severe cases, this may be repeated over periods of several hours as indicated by frequent laboratory estimations of the blood glucose level
4. when the patient responds, give supplemental carbohydrate to restore liver glycogen and prevent recurrence of hypoglycemia

fluid ounces of orange juice or a sugar-containing soft drink can be helpful for immediate response to hypoglycemia, as can candy, honey, or plain sugar.

The Insulins

The insulins currently marketed and available are listed in Table 20-4.

A note of caution must be added to the data in Table 20-4, which depict some pharmocokinetic characteristics. It is known, for example, that the peak level of NPH in elderly is delayed, and probably occurs in 12 hours, not in 8 hours. This may have serious implications because that particular insulin may reach its peak action well after the patient has been given the evening meal. During the night no food will be ingested by the patient, so hypoglycemic episodes may occur.

The overall action of insulin is thought to enhance the incorporation of amino acids into muscle protein and the transport of some, but not all, amino acids into the muscle cell, while it suppresses the rate of protein catabolism (Lamy 1974). The postulated action of insulin, which itself is an anabolic hormone, can be summarized to include: a) transport of glucose, ions, and amino acids, b) glycogen formation, c) glucose conversion to triglycerides, d) nucleic acid synthesis, e) protein synthesis.

Insulin is indicated whenever a patient is ketoacidosis-prone. In other words, insulin must be given whenever a patient does not have any natural insulin or if insulin is critically deficient. Very careful consideration must be given in all other cases. The prescribing of insulin may lead to drastic changes in the elderly patient's lifestyle. Outside supervision may be necessary and the patient will likely lose more of the already restricted independence. Furthermore, the elderly patient may likely exhibit mild cognitive disturbance. This may lead to forgetfulness, either in eating or in administration of insulin. Economic constraints may force the patient to eat less, and all these factors may be cumulative.

For all these reasons, insulin is probably the greatest cause of hypoglycemia in the elderly. Its action will most likely be influenced by fluctuations in activity and eating habits, which are expected with elderly patients. Therefore, from a risk-benefit consideration, since there is still no clear evidence that insulin treatment abates, delays, or aborts the chronic complications of diabetes in the elderly, the indications for insulin use must be very clear and not simply based on sugar spillage.

Age does not change insulin therapy. The starting dose is usually recommended to be 10 to 15 units of NPH or Lente insulin. This is adjusted until late afternoon sugar is 250 mg%. It has also been suggested that the initial dose be based on body weight, using 0.2 units per kilogram of body weight. The maintenance dose usually will be between 0.5 to one unit/kg of body weight. Crystalline zinc insulin may

Table 20-4
Types of Insulin Available in the United States

	Regular crystalline*	Semilente†	Globin	NPH	Lente†	Protamine zinc	Ultralente†
Appearance	clear	turbid	clear to pale amber	turbid	turbid	turbid	turbid
Action	rapid	rapid	intermediate	intermediate	intermediate	prolonged	prolonged
Duration (hours)	5-7	12-16	18-24	24-28	24-28	36+	36+
Peak activity (hours)	2-3	5-11	6-12	10-20	10-20	16-24	18-30
pH	3.0	7.0	3.6	7.2	7.0	7.2	7.0
Buffer	none	acetate	none	phosphate	acetate	phosphate	acetate
Preservative	phenol and m-cresol	methyl paraben	phenol	phenol and m-cresol	methyl paraben	phenol	methyl paraben
Isotonicity agent	glycerin	NaCl	glycerin	glycerin	NaCl	glycerin	NaCl
Animal source	beef, pork, beef-pork mixed	beef, beef-pork mixed	beef-pork mixed	beef, pork, beef-pork mixed	beef, pork, beef-pork mixed	beef, pork, beef-pork mixed	beef, beef-pork mixed
Zinc content	0.016-0.04	0.2-0.25	0.25-0.35	0.016-0.04	0.2-0.25	0.2-0.25	0.2-0.25
Protein and concentration mg/100 units	none	none	globin 3.8	protamine 0.5	none	protamine 1.25	none

*Only insulin preparation which can be given intravenously. If self-administered, all other given subcutaneously only. May be given IM on physician's order.
†The terms Lente, Semilente, and Ultralente are registered trademarks of the Novo Industri A/S of Copenhagen and should not be used as generic terms.
Note: All commercially available insulins are now "single-peak" insulins. Insulin now has a potency of 26 to 27 units/mg and consists of 99% insulin and pro-insulin-like substances and 1% non-insulin material.
Note: The concentrations of U=40 and U=80 are to be phased out in the near future.

be added to the morning dose of the intermediate acting insulin to improve daytime control of hyperglycemia. Some clinicians feel that multiple dose injections control the appearance of retinopathy and nephropathy better than a single-dose administration of long-acting insulin (Johnson 1960).

Other considerations concerning insulin Many factors may combine to negate the effects of a carefully developed treatment regimen. There is, for example, the recurrent question of insulin storage. This is important not only from a stability point of view, but it has been suggested that patients should not administer cold insulin. The United States Public Health Service has suggested the maximum time that insulin can be kept unrefrigerated without deleterious effect (Table 20-5). Therefore, the patient should be advised to keep the bottle in use at room temperature and the other bottles refrigerated, but not frozen.

Table 20-5
Maximum Time Limit for Keeping Insulin Unrefrigerated*

Product	Time limit (days)
Insulin injection, Isophane, USP	7
Insulin injection, USP	7
Insulin, protamine zinc, injection, USP	10
Insulin zinc suspension	7

*Temperature must neither exceed 95°F nor fall below freezing.

The mixing of insulins, if required, may be a difficult procedure, for the patient. The aim of all insulin mixtures is to combine the various types to meet an individual patient's need. Mixtures of Lente and Ultralente are used particularly in transient responders, while mixtures of Lente and Semilente are used primarily for delayed responders.

Regular insulin and NPH:

Any combination is possible. Mixing must be done immediately before use.

Regular insulin and Lente:

The amount of regular insulin should not exceed 50% of the mixture, or pH differences may cause changes that would make the time activity unpredictable. Must be mixed immediately prior to use.

Regular insulin and PZI:

Mixture should not contain less than 50% of regular insulin, or the resulting mixture will have the activity of PZI itself. A ratio of two parts of regular insulin to one part of PZI yields an effective mixture, with the same onset and duration of action as

NPH. Mixtures of these two insulins may be used at any time after preparation.

Lente mixture:

May be combined in any desired ratio. May be mixed at any time which means that a person other than the patient can prepare the mixture prior to dispensing it.

At times, the physician may wish to dilute a commercially available insulin. Eli Lilly and Company makes available, free of charge, insulin diluting fluids for regular, NPH, Lente, and protamine zinc insulins. These sterile fluids contain the same ingredients as described in the official monographs of insulin products, of course omitting the insulin and any modifying materials.

In skin testing and desensitization, diluted regular insulin is used. The diluent can be isotonic saline solution, but if the solution is to be kept longer than eight hours, the regular diluting fluid should be used. Empty, sterile 20 ml vials, labeled "Sterilized Bottle for Insulin Mixtures" are also available.

Poor patient compliance and poor diabetic control have often been associated with the elderly patient's inability to use syringes correctly. Dead space volume, that is the volume of insulin contained in the hub of the syringe and the needle, has also been cited as a potential source of dosage error (Dube 1962). One manufacturer's disposable syringes were shown to vary by as much as eight units in delivering insulin. A hypodermic syringe, which can be preset for self-use by visually impaired patients is now available through the American Foundation for the Blind.* Sold only to physicians or registered nurses, the syringe can be disassembled for sterilization without disturbing the setting of the stop which controls the amount of insulin to be drawn up.

Urine Testing

Urine testing for glucose is used by patients and physicians to monitor control of blood glucose levels. Several different urine tests, based either on copper reduction or glucose oxidase reactions, are available. Copper reduction methods, such as Clinitest, are not specific for glucose while those based on the glucose oxidase system are. However, Clinitest is generally considered the method of choice for monitoring insulin therapy because glucose oxidase tests, such as Testape or Clinistix, are quantitative only when the amount of glucose in the urine is less than 0.25%. The glucose oxidase methods are often preferred for monitoring most cases of adult-onset diabetes, because of their simplicity, specificity, and ability to detect minute amounts of sugar in the urine.

---

*15 West 16th Street, New York, N.Y. 10011

These tests, though, may present difficulties to the elderly, visually impaired patient, as they demand that the patient be able to differentiate between shades of green or brown.

Many drugs can interfere with the results of these tests (Tables 20-6 and 20-7). Aspirin, ascorbic acid, levodopa, and methyldopa can produce false negative readings if a patient uses Testape. The copper-reduction test method (Clinitest) can yield false positive results if patient receives concurrently levodopa, ascorbic acid, nalidixic acid, cephalosporins, or probenecid.

It must also be remembered that a patient should be impressed with the need not to switch arbitrarily from one test method to another, as one color in one system may indicate a positive reading (Clinistix), but the same color will indicate a negative reading in another test system (Testape). Furthermore, the five-drop method must be used differently than the two-drop method, which can lead to erroneous results and loss of control. Finally, all test tablets and strips are sensitive to moisture and should be stored in tightly closed containers.

The physician, faced with a patient lacking control, must also be aware that reimbursement policies have changed. In many instances, these test materials are now considered nonprescription items and are thus the patient's responsibility. In other words, the patient will not

Table 20-6
Drugs Which Might Affect Test Values of the Glucose (Benedict's) Test*

Amino acids	Indomethacin
Aminosalicylic acid	Isoniazid
Ascorbic acid	Metaproterenol
Aspidium oleoresin (if absorbed)	Metaxalone
Bismuth (glucosuria)	Nalidixic acid
Cephalothin	Nicotinic acid
Chloral hydrate	Nuceloproteins
Chloramphenicol	Oxalic acid
Chloroform	Oxytetracycline
Chlortetracycline	Penicillin
Corticosteroids	Phenols
Corticotropin	Probenecid
Creatinine	Protein
Edathamil	Pyrazolone derivatives (aminopyrine)
Ephedrine (large doses)	Quinethazone (glucosuria)
Ethacrynic acid	Salicylates
Formaldehyde	Streptomycin
Gluconates	Sulfonamides
Hippuric acid	Tetracyclines (degraded)
Homogentisic acid	Thiazide diuretics
Hydrogen peroxide	Trioxazine
Hypochlorites	Uric acid

*All of these would cause an elevated or false positive value.

**Table 20-7
Drugs Which Might Affect the Diagnostic Test
For Diabetes Mellitus (Fasting Glucose)**

Drug	Effect of Drug Elevated or false positive	Effect of Drug Decreased or false negative
Acetohexamide (overdose)		+
Corticotropin (ACTH)	+	
Corticosteroids	+	
Chlorpropamide (overdose)		+
Carbutamide		+
Chlorthalidone	+	
Epinephrine	+	
Ethacrynic acid	+	
Furosemide (in diabetic)	+	
Indomethacin	+	
Insulin (overdose)		+
Isoniazid (excessive dose)	+	
Metformin (overdose)		+
Pargyline		+
Phenformin		+
Phenytoin	+	
Phosphorous (toxicity)		+
Physostigmine	+	
Potassium chloride		+
Potassium oxalate		+
Potassium para-amino benzoate (extended use)		+
Progestin-estrogen combination (oral contraceptives)	+	
Quinethazone	+	
Salicylates		+
Sulfaphenazole		+
Tolazamide		+
Thiabendazole	+	
Thiazide diuretics	+	
Trioxazine	+	

be reimbursed for them, and it has been suggested that therefore, many patients, particularly the elderly, economically disadvantaged patients, simply do not purchase these items.

Drug Interactions

Many drugs have been shown to have the potential to interact with either insulin or the oral hypoglycemic agents. These are listed in Table 20-8. Table 20-9 lists the specific results of possible interactions in terms of hypoglycemia or hyperglycemia. In addition, the hypoglycemic agents can interfere with a large number of laboratory test values (Table 20-10).

Table 20-8
Interactions of Hypoglycemic Agents with Other Drugs

Hypoglycemic Agent	Drug	Interaction

Insulin
Phenformin
Sulfonylureas
  Acetohexamide
  Chlorpropamide
  Tolazamide
  Tolbutamide
	Corticosteroids
	Dextrothyroxine
	Diuretics
	  Thiazides
	  Chlorthalidone
	  Ethacrynic acid
	  Furosemide
	Estrogens
	Nicotinic acid
	Oral contraceptives
		These agents can cause an increase in blood glucose levels. Increased doses of the hypoglycemic agent may be necessary.

	Alcohol	Response is unpredictable. Disulfiram-like reactions have been reported with the sulfonylureas. Increased metabolism of tolbutamide in alcoholic patients has been reported. Response probably depends on the amount of alcohol taken and other factors.
	Monoamine oxidase inhibitors	Enhances hypoglycemic effect.
	Propranolol	May cause hypoglycemia. Potential danger may be increased because propranolol may prevent the premonitory signs and symptoms of acute hypoglycemia.
Sulfonylureas	Oral anticoagulants	The coumarin anticoagulants have been shown to enhance the hypoglycemic effect of the sulfonylureas caused by inhibition of metabolism.
	Barbiturates (and other sedatives and hypnotics)	Sulfonylureas may prolong the effect of these CNS depressants.
	Insulin	Enhanced hypoglycemic effect.

Oxyphenbutazone Phenylbutazone	Enhanced hypoglycemic effect. Phenylbutazone has been reported to interfere with the excretion of the active metabolite of acetohexamide. Protein displacement may also be involved in these interactions.
Phenformin	Enhanced hypoglycemic effect.
Phenyramidol	May enhance the hypoglycemic response due to inhibition of metabolism.
Probenecid	Enhanced hypoglycemic response has been reported. One study indicates that probenecid has little effect on the metabolism of tolbutamide.
Salicylates	May enhance hypoglycemic response, due, in part, to displacement from protein binding sites.
Sulfinpyrazone	Hypoglycemic effect may be enhanced.
Sulfonamides	May enhance hypoglycemic response, possibly caused by displacement from protein binding sites. The most conclusive studies have involved the use of sulfaphenazole and tolbutamide.

Table 20-9
Possible Interactions of Hypoglycemic Agents

Drugs	Interacting drugs	Effect
Insulin Oral hypoglycemics	Salicylates, beta blockers Adrenergic blockers MAO inhibitors	Hypoglycemia potentiated
	Diuretics Glucocorticoids Barbiturates Sympathomimetics	Hypoglycemia antagonized
Sulfonylureas	Coumarins MAO inhibitors (enzyme inhibitors)	Hypoglycemia potentiated
	Clofibrate Phenylbutazone Sulfonamides (displacement from binding sites)	Hypoglycemia potentiated

All of the widely used thiazide diuretics can cause hyperglycemia and abnormal glucose tolerance. The elderly patient with latent diabetes is at greatest risk to these effects. Much discussion has centered around the possible effect of propranolol. It masks the clinical manifestations of hypoglycemia and can produce severe hypoglycemia in normal or diabetic subjects after insulin administration, exercise, or severe fasting. This effect is considered especially dangerous as patients so affected often lack the usual signs and symptoms of hypoglycemia.

Therefore, the use of propranolol in insulin-dependent patients has been discouraged (Greenblatt and Koch-Weser 1974). Some patients receiving propranolol show a dramatically enhanced diaphoretic response to insulin-induced hypoglycemia, probably because of a change in alpha-adrenergic receptor activity during beta-adrenergic blockade (Molnar and Read 1973). Therefore, as the lack of symptoms of hypoglycemia was the foremost factor causing concern, it might be that the dangers of concurrent administration of propranolol and insulin have been overestimated (Strom 1978). The use of ACTH in the elderly poses a particular hazard (Lovell 1970); it increases the patient's susceptibility to diabetes. In general, patients receiving sulfonylureas concurrently with barbiturates or diuretics have much less diabetic control than those receiving insulin.

Table 20-10
The Effect of Hypoglycemic Agents on Some Laboratory Test Values

Hypoglycemic Agent	Laboratory Test	Specific Effect *Elevated or false positive*	Specific Effect *Decreased or false negative*
Acetohexamide	Bilirubin and Icteric index in serum	+	
	BUN	+	
	Leukocytes		+
	Thrombocytes		+
Chlorpropamide	Alkaline phosphatase in serum	+	
	Cephalin flocculation	+	
	Thymol turbidity	+	
	Leukocytes	+ (eosinophilia)	+
Insulin	Amino acids	+	
	Calcium in serum		+
	Phosphate (inorganic) in serum		+
Phenformin	Acetone in urine	+	
	Bicarbonate in serum		+
	Potassium in serum	+	
Sulfonylureas	Erythrocyte count and/or hemoglobin	+	
	Leukocytes		+
	Thrombocytes		+
Tolazamide	Alkaline phosphatase in serum	+	
Tolbutamide	Protein in urine	+	
	Alkaline phosphatase in serum	+	
	BSP retention	+	
	Cephalin flocculation	+	
	Thymol turbidity	+	

PERSONAL HYGIENE

Skin Care

In general, diabetic patients are more susceptible to bacterial and fungal, especially monilial, infestations than the general population (Maugh 1975). Impaired peripheral circulation, especially in elderly diabetic patients, reduces the patient's resistance to infection (Dobson 1974). Neuropathies experienced by these patients, can produce insensitivity to pain. As a result, blisters and simple cuts can become infected before they are noticed. Since the skin, particularly of the hands, is very likely to carry infectious material, the patient should wash frequently with warm water. Use of a bland powder, possibly baby powder, is advocated to prevent irritation of skin surfaces. It is important to prevent chapping of the hands by thorough drying and use of a bland cream.*

Foot Care

Proper foot care is immensely important and neglected by the elderly diabetic patient. The older diabetic is likely to present with arteriosclerosis obliterans (ASO), particularly the elderly patient with mild maturity-onset diabetes mellitus. Frequently, it might be the first manifestation of diabetes. Intermittent claudication usually occurs in the calf muscles but can also occur in the arch of the foot, the thigh, and the buttocks. Proper foot care is most important in the management of ASO.

The elderly diabetic patient is likely to complain of icy or burning feet and suffer from a decreased sensation in the extremities. This prevents the usual sensation of heat and cold, and the patient may not feel small objects that may have lodged in shoes. This lack of sensation in the extremities, particularly the feet, is likely to change a casual infection to a serious one. Since the patient is already predisposed to skin infections, the diabetic patient must be taught correct foot care, which can prevent almost all foot problems:

1. Look at feet daily, using a mirror if necessary. It is usually easy to see an infected area, often easier than feeling it.
2. Wash feet twice daily with warm water and soap, avoid hot water. Dry feet carefully (to avoid fungal infections) by a blotting motion, rather than by rubbing or pressure.
3. Use a vaseline or lanolin-type cream to prevent dry, scaly skin, which is liable to infections. If skin is moist, use rubbing alcohol.
4. Special attention must be paid to toe nails. Cut toe nails straight across.
5. Avoid irritating antiseptics such as iodine, unguentine, and others. Also, avoid corn cures. Athlete's foot, corns, bunions, and calluses should be treated by a physician or

---

*Eucerin, Beiersdorf, Inc., South Norwalk, Conn. 06854. A water-in-oil emulsion, it is based on petrolatum.

a podiatrist. Simple cuts and broken blisters can be treated with a gauze dressing, moistened with 70% alcohol. This dressing should be alternated with a dry dressing every 12 hours.
6. Except for electric blankets, do not use any means to apply heat to feet, such as hot water bottles or electric heating pads.
7. Avoid garters, constricting bandages or anything that might impair circulation. Remember that crossing the legs while sitting will also do that.
8. Never walk barefoot.

Fragmented care poses the greatest danger to the elderly diabetic patient, who may be treated for congestive heart failure at one place, for urinary tract infection at another, and may self-administer cold preparations containing sympathomimetics. Establishment of good control is important, as some of the conditions that afflict the elderly, such as cataracts or glaucoma, can be worsened by diabetes.

The cumulative and progressive losses of advancing age may lead to sadness and depression in the elderly patient. In turn, this can lead to changes in food intake. Emotional stresses, which the elderly are poorly equipped to overcome, can elevate blood sugar levels.

A prolonged and careful process may be necessary to establish control in the elderly diabetic patient. Hypoglycemic agents should only be used once it has been established that the patient cannot be controlled by diet. Exercises support dietary control, and, if conducted according to a predetermined schedule, can permit the use of a less restrictive diet.

REFERENCES

Albrink, M.J., and Davidson, P.C. Dietary therapy and prophylaxis of vascular disease in diabetics. *Med Clin North Am.* 55:877, 1971.

Andres, R. Aging and diabetes. *Med Clin North Am.* 55:835, 1971.

Backscheider, J.E. Self-care requirements, self-care capabilities and nursing systems in the diabetic nurse management clinics. *Am J Public Health.* 64:1138, 1974.

Barbagallo-Sangiorgi, G. The pancreatic beta cell response to intravenous administration of glucose in elderly subjects. *J Am Geriatr Soc.* 18:529, 1970.

Bierman, E.L. Bring adult-onset diabetes under control. *Drug Ther.* 7(9):27, 1977.

Bierman, E.L., and Nelson, R. Carbohydrates, diabetes, and blood lipids. *World Rev Nutr Diet.* 22:280, 1975.

Brownlee, M. Normoglycemia as a therapeutic goal in insulin-dependent diabetes. *Drug Ther.* 3(7):13, 1978.

Davidowicz, A. Disorder of carbohydrate homeostasis in old people (diabetes senilis) in the light of the mutation theory of aging. *Diabetologia* 4:387, 1968.

Department of Health, Education and Welfare. *Diabetes Source Book.* PHS Publ. No. 1168. Washington, D.C.: U.S. Government Printing Office, 1969.

Dobson, H.L. *The Older Diabetic.* Kalamazoo, Mich.: The Upjohn Co., 1974.

Dube, A.H. Diabetes teaching manual for patients and hospital personnel. *NY State J Med.* 62:3754, 1962.

Giarnieri, D., and Lumia, V. Action of insulin on blood diphosphothiamine (DPT) in young and aged diabetics. *Clin Chim Acta.* 6:144, 1961.

Goodkin, G. Mortality factors in diabetes: a 20-year mortality study. *J Occup Med.* 17:716, 1975.

Greenblatt, D.J., and Koch-Weser, J. Adverse reactions to beta-adrenergic-blocking drugs. *Drugs* 7:118, 1974.

Johnson, S. Retinopathy and nephropathy in diabetes mellitus: comparison of the effects of two forms of treatment. *Diabetes* 9:1, 1960.

Karam, J.H. Diabetes mellitus, hypoglycemia, and lipid disorders. Edited by M.A. Krupp, and M.J. Chatton. In *Current Medical Diagnosis and Treatment.* 16th Ed. Los Altos, Calif.: Lange Medical Publications, 1977.

Kent, S. Reevaluating the dietary treatment of diabetes. *Geriatrics* 33(5):99, 1978.

Khachadurian, A.K., and Detzkin, M.D. Diabetes in concept and in fact. *Drug Ther.* 5(3):137, 1975.

Kimmerling, G. Javorski, W.C., and Reaven, G.M. Aging and insulin resistance in a group of nonobese male volunteers. *J Am Geriatr Soc.* 25:349, 1977.

Kingsbury, K.J. Glucose tolerance, age and vascular disease. *Diabetologia* 4:377, 1968.

Kryston, L.J., and Shaw, R.A. Lessening the swings of diabetes. *Drug Ther.* 5(3):150, 1975.

Kumble, M.A. Diabetes. *J Am Pharm Assoc.* NS14:80, 1974.

Lamy, P.P. A review of insulin and insulin preparations. *Md Pharmacol.* 50(8):10, 1974.

Lamy, P.P., and Kitler, M.E. The pharmacist and diabetes. *J Am Pharm Assoc.* NS10:608, 1970.

Lovell, R.G. Problems in allergy with advancing age. *Geriatrics* 25:101, 1970.

Marks, V. Spontaneous hypoglycemia. *Hosp Med.* 1:118, 1966.

Maugh, T.H. Diabetes: epidemiology suggests a viral connection. *Science* 188:347, 1975.

Maugh, T.H. Diabetes commission: problems severe, therapy inadequate. *Science* 1919:272, 1976.

Molnar, G.W., and Read, R.C. Propranolol enhancement of hypoglycemic sweating. *Clin Pharmacol Ther.* 15:490, 1973.

O'Sullivan, J.B. Age gradient in blood glucose levels: magnitude and clinical implications. *Diabetes* 23:713, 1974.

Palumbo, P.J. How to treat maturity-onset diabetes mellitus. *Geriatrics* 32(12):57, 1977.

Powell, M.F., and Lamy, P.P. Compliance obstacles to the insulin-dependent diabetic. *Md Pharmacol.* 53(3):10, 1977.

Seltzer, H.S. Drug-induced hypoglycemia. *Diabetes* 21:955, 1972.

Service, F.J. Hypoglycemia. *Contemp Nutr.* 2(7):1, 1977.

Shagan, B.P. Diabetes in the elderly patient. *Med Clin North Am.* 60:1191, 1976.

Shangraw, R.F., and Lamy, P.P. Pharmacuetical aspects of the treatment of diabetes mellitus. *J Am Pharm Assoc.* NS9:117, 1969.

Streeten, D. Reduced glucose tolerance in elderly human subjects. *Diabetes* 14:579, 1965.

Strom, L. Propranolol in insulin-dependent diabetes. *N Engl J Med.* 299:487, 1978.

Tansey, M.J.B., Kennelly, B.M., and Opie, L.H. High mortality in obese women diabetics with acute myocardial infarction. *Br Med J.* 1:1624, 1977.

Thomas, J.A., and Jones, J.E. Insulin, hypoglycemic drugs, and glucagon. Edited by J.A. Bevan. In *Essentials of Pharmacology.* 2nd Ed. Hagerstown, Md.: Harper and Row, Inc., 1976.

Tubbs, H.A., and Tubbs, J.E. The oral glucose tolerance test in adults of various ages. *J Am Geriatr Soc.* 19:264, 1971.

Tunebride, E., and Wetherill, J.H. Reliability and costs of diabetic diets. *Br Med J.* 2:78, 1970.

Watkins, J.D., Robert, E.E., Williams, T.F. et al. Observations of medication errors made by diabetic patients in the home. *Diabetes* 16:882, 1967.

West, K.M., and Kalbfleisch, J.M. Diabetes in Central America. *Diabetes* 19:656, 1970.

21 Ophthalmic Drugs

Many systemic drugs can have adverse effects on the eyes, as can topically applied drugs. Ocular side effects have special importance to those caring for the elderly. Patients are likely to receive drugs on a chronic basis, and if the dosage is not age-adjusted, it may result in an overdose; both factors favor the development of ocular side effects of drugs. The elderly also suffer from a high incidence of ocular disease and conditions which make them more vulnerable to these side effects.

Drugs implicated are the anticholinergic drugs, the antidepressants, the cardiovascular drugs, and the phenothiazines. The vision, lens, retina, conjunctiva, lid, iris, and cornea can also be affected. Table 21-1 lists some of the drugs known to cause ocular side effects. The listing is not intended to be exhaustive and does not necessarily indicate the incidence or severity of these effects. It is simply designed to alert the practitioner that many drugs, used particularly frequently in the chronic care of the elderly, may cause undesired ocular effects (Fraunfelder 1976).

Table 21-1
Sources Which Might Cause Ocular Effects

Alcohol	Gonadotrophic agents
Analgesics	Heavy metals
Anesthetics	Hormones
Anthelmintics	Hypocholesterolemic agents
Antiarrythmics	Hypotensives
Antibacterials	Monoamine oxidase inhibitors
Anticholinesterases	Neuromuscular-blocking agents
Anticonvulsants	Parasympatholytics
Antidepressants	Parasympathomimetics
Antifungal agents	Radiodiagnostic agents
Antimalarials	Sedatives
Antitubercular agents	Smooth muscle relaxants
Carbonic anhydrase inhibitors	Sympathomimetics
Cardiac glycosides	Tranquilizers
Chelating agents	Vasopressors
Demulcents	Vitamins
Diuretics	

Ophthalmic Changes with Advancing Age

The aging process creates unique eye problems for which ophthalmic medications are frequently indicated. Their use, however, is not without possible adverse effects. By being aware of the physiologic and anatomic changes in the aging eye and the possible harmful effects of the various drugs used for treatment of ocular conditions, visual well-being, so important to the older patient, can be protected (Means and Lamy 1975). As one becomes older, certain changes take place in the eye, both physiologic and pathologic (Streiff 1967), which can lead to structural and functional alterations (Bell 1968).

The tissues of the eyelids and surrounding area undergo changes with age mainly because of dehydration of the skin and ocular muscles, atrophy of fat tissue, and a loss of skin elasticity and fibrous tissue. The skin of the lids wrinkles, leading to the "baggy" eyes so common in older people. Lower lid pouches and sagging folds in the upper eyelids occur, as well as small wart-like lesions, and one may expect atrophy of the sebaceous glands, which often leaves the lid margins dry and scaly.

As the elastic and fibrous tissues of the eyelids atrophy and sag, the lower lid may fall away from the eyeball (senile ectropion), leaving it unprotected and allowing tears to accumulate. Eversion of the eyelid margins or ectropion exposes the conjunctiva to chronic infection (Kornzweig 1977). As the conjunctiva becomes thin and increasingly more sensitive to irritants with age, conjunctivitis is a common geriatric problem. It is not unusual to find the conjunctiva and eyelid margins congested and inflamed. Senile entropion (inversion of the lid margin) occurs when the eyelashes turn in towards the cornea, causing irritation of both the lower cornea and the bulbar conjunctiva. Patients complain of feeling foreign bodies in the eye. Temporary measures, such as adhesive tape, may help for a while, but surgery may ultimately be indicated. The corneal endothelium can undergo degenerative changes (Graham 1971). A degenerated endothelium can become edematous, decreasing the optical efficiency of the cornea. Symptoms are usually experienced in the morning upon awakening and disappear later. As one ages, the cornea also increases its curvature, producing astigmatism, and may be partially circumscribed by infiltration of lipids into the periphery of the cornea, a condition known as arcus senilis.

The corneoscleral trabeculae become denser because of tissue sclerosis and hyalinization, thus reducing the iridocorneal angle and increasing resistance to the outflow of aqueous humor (Streiff 1967).

The vitreous body changes with age (Newell 1965). Two of the most common symptoms resulting from these changes are "floaters" or floating bodies which the patient sees when looking at a bright field or light surfaces. The patient may also experience light flashes (photopsia) when the eyes are moved while the lids are closed. Fine fibers or cellular aggregates are responsible for the floaters. They become more visible as the vitreous gel liquefies. The photopsia is thought to be caused by traction as the contracting vitreous body pulls away from the retina.

The part of the eye displaying the most obvious changes from age is the lens (Anderson 1971; Kornzweig 1971). The lens continues to grow throughout life. New fibers are formed and superimposed on the old, which become smaller, dehydrated, denser, and less flexible. Eventually, the lens becomes so hard and inflexible that it is limited in its ability to accommodate (focus objects clearly on the retina), and corrective lenses will be required. The lens also becomes less transparent, resulting in a decreased amount of light that reaches the retina (Bell 1968). Lessening in lens clarity is referred to as a cataract. Cataracts are the most common disability in the aged eye (Fischer 1947; Kornzweig et al 1957). Little can be done to prevent cataract formation and almost all people 80 years and older have some degree of opacity. Everyone would experience cataracts given a long enough lifespan (Beehler 1968). Cataracts pose one of the two most common threats to the vision of the elderly (glaucoma is the other), and one of the most common causes of blindness in the aging patient (Fox 1968).

These cataracts can be ascribed to physiologic changes associated with the gradual loss of transparency caused by an increased number of dense fibers, or pathologic changes. The etiology of pathologic cataracts still has not been elucidated (Anderson 1971), but certain drugs have been implicated (Paterson 1971; Pietsch et al 1972).

Among the systemic drugs implicated are the corticosteroids and the phenothiazines. The lens opacities associated with steroid therapy start in the posterior subcapsulary region and are referred to as posterior subcapsulary cataracts (PSCC). Although PSCC are not only caused by steroids, there is a higher incidence in the older patient and especially in patients on long-term corticosteroid therapy. Almost 21% of those patients showed evidence of PSCC, as opposed to an incidence of 0.2% in the general population (Spaeth and van Sallman 1966). The cataractogenic properties of steroids appear to be age- and dose-related (Black et al 1960; Giles et al 1962; Crews 1963). PSCC did not develop when patients were treated with less than 10 mg of prednisone per day, but did develop in about 75% of those receiving over 16 mg of the drug daily. It is unclear whether or not different corticosteroids have different cataractogenic properties.

Chlorpromazine causes lens changes in patients on chronic therapy (Howard et al 1969). As little as 300 mg chlorpromazine daily, administered for several years, can cause changes, and in patients receiving a total of 250 gm, about 90% experience lens opacities (Mathaline 1965; Delong et al 1965). Other phenothiazines may also cause lens changes (Siddall 1965).

Once a cataract has occurred, surgery, in general, should not be withheld because of patient age. Unfortunately, cataract in only one eye cannot be corrected with glasses. Glasses magnify vision by 35%. The patient with the other lens still intact, cannot fuse the resulting two different pictures and will suffer from blurred and double vision. Most often, an eye patch will have to be worn over the operated eye. With the advent of contact lenses, this patient might be helped because these lenses cause only a 1% magnification.

Efforts are being made to find new devices for the 400,000 yearly postcataract patients, but there is still no therapy safer than eyeglasses.

Intraocular lenses have been used to replace the natural lens of the human eye after surgical removal. These lenses came into widespread use before adequate tests were completed, and they pose safety questions. Infections have been reported with intraocular lenses, particularly those sterilized with sodium hydroxide as a sterilant and sodium bicarbonate as a neutralizing solution. Intraocular acrylic lenses may increase the endothelial cell death rate so that the cornea may be clouded irreversibly. Thus, medically, this system is not yet an acceptable alternative to eyeglasses. The FDA has not approved intraocular lenses, and applications for approval will have to meet the intraocular lens investigational device regulation.

As an alternative to the intraocular lens transplant, extended wear soft lenses have been recommended for correction of aphakia. To date, extended wear soft lenses, less likely to cause complications, have been tested in 12 medical institutions. It is hoped that these lenses can be worn for periods of up to three months, although reports from

England suggest that they can be worn for as long as two years. However, the lenses present certain drawbacks. They are difficult to fit and must, initially at least, be checked several times per day. In addition, they should be suggested only when the patient has immediate access to skilled help and advice, since the patient should not handle the lenses.

Macular degeneration affects about 30% of those over 65 years of age. It involves a gradual loss of central vision, but peripheral vision is not affected. Since the macula is that part of the retina responsible for visual acuity, these older persons complain about an inability to read or recognize faces. This condition will not result in blindness. Hypertension, diabetes, nephritis, central nervous system disorders, and vascular thrombosis can affect the macula.

Glaucoma is the second most important eye problem in the elderly. Different studies report its prevalence in persons over the age of 40 years to range from 0.65% to 9% (Foote and Boyce 1955; Feldstein et al 1959; Schneider et al 1959). Glaucoma may occur as a primary disease entity or as a result of other intraocular pathology. It is always characterized by increased intraocular tension, which, in turn, will be responsible for changes in the optic disk and loss of the visual field (Schwartz 1978).

There are primary and secondary glaucomas. Both angle-closure glaucoma, in which the iris blocks access to the canal of Schlemm, and open-angle glaucoma, in which there is no obstruction, are primary glaucomas. Most common is the primary open-angle glaucoma, followed by angle-closure and secondary glaucomas. The intraocular pressure associated with the glaucomas causes cupping and atrophy of the optic nerve, which results in progressive and irreversible loss of peripheral vision. Normally, intraocular pressure remains constant because of a decrease in aqueous humor production that matches the increased resistance to flow from the anterior chamber. When the resistance increases to the point that the intraocular pressure rises above normal levels, however, a person is said to have open-angle glaucoma. It develops slowly and insidiously over a period of years and is not characterized by pain until much of the peripheral vision has been lost. Primary open-angle glaucoma is most common, and one eye may be more involved than the other (Phelps 1977). Medical treatment is preferred for this type glaucoma, using the parasympathomimetics (both cholinergic and anticholinesterase agents) such as pilocarpine, epinephrine, and carbonic anhydrase inhibitors. It has now been suggested that the beta blockers hold great promise in the treatment of glaucoma. Preliminary reports on timolol indicate that it is a most effective drug.

Accurate prevalence data are not available. There is a question about patients with ocular hypertension with pressure in the middle 20s (mm Hg) who may or may not be diagnosed as having primary open-angle glaucoma. Ocular hypertension, defined as ocular pressure equal to or greater than 21 mm Hg increases sharply with age, from 5% in those between the ages of 40 and 44 years, to 10% between 55 and 59 years, and 15% in those aged 70 to 75 years. These data cannot be correlated well with a prevalence of primary open-angle glaucoma, as the increased ocular pressure may not be associated with loss of visual field. Primary open-angle glaucoma is thought to occur in 0.5% of those aged 60 to 64 years and 1.3% in those 70 to 74 years.

Angle-closure (narrow-angle) glaucoma occurs primarily in the fifth and sixth decade, more often in women than in men. It appears to occur mainly in persons anatomically predisposed to the condition by a shallow anterior chamber, especially those with hyperopia (farsightedness). It is probably more prevalent in those over 50 years of age because of the increasing size of the lens, which continues to grow throughout life, decreasing the depth of the anterior chamber (Pollack 1968). All glaucomas require early diagnosis and proper treatment in order to preserve vision.

There are reports of various drugs adversely affecting the patient's eye by increasing intraocular pressure (Table 21-2). It is impossible to construct an all-inclusive list; the patient with angle-closure glaucoma is probably most vulnerable to their effects. The anticholinergic and sympathomimetic drugs probably present a significant danger to persons with a narrow anterior chamber regardless of the presence of glaucoma (Lund 1972; Willetts and Hopkins 1972). The risk to the patient with a narrow anterior chamber is probably proportional to the dilating effect of the drug.

The anticholinergics are of particular concern when caring for the elderly, as many of the drugs they receive on a chronic basis have anticholinergic properties. Among these are the phenothiazines, the tricyclics, the antiparkinsonism drugs, and the antihistamines. Although it has been speculated that significant increases in intraocular pressure on administration of atropine would occur only in a small minority of patients with open-angle glaucoma (Lazenby et al 1970), the elderly are likely to take several drugs with anticholinergic properties concurrently and, thus, there may be a cumulative effect. Drugs commonly used to treat parkinsonism should be used with caution in patients with glaucoma.

The topical vasoconstrictors, eg, phenylephrine and tetrahydrazoline, are to be used with caution in patients with angle-closure glaucoma. Xerophthalmia or keratoconjunctivitis sicca, commonly known as dry eye, may be caused by either a mucinous or aqueous deficiency. This predisposes the patient to disease, and patients complain about a burning or sandy feeling. Systemic medications such as antihypertensives, antihistamines, anticholinergics, or sympatholytics may contribute to the development of dry eye, which can cause loss of vision.

**Table 21-2
Drugs Labeled as Contraindicated or to be Used
With Caution in Patients With Glaucoma**

Amitriptyline	Erythrityl tetranitrate	Oxyphenonium
Amphetamines	Ethopropazine	Papaverine
Amyl nitrite	Flavoxate	Pentapiperide
Anisotropine	Fluphenazine	Pentaerythritol
Atropine	Glycopyrrolate	tetranitrate
Belladonna	Hexocyclium	Penthienate
Benzphetamine	Homatropine	Phendimetrazine
Benztropine	Imipramine	Phenelzine
Biperiden	Isocarboxazid	Phenmetrazine
Carbamazepine	Isopropamide	Phentermine
Chlorphenoxamine	Isosorbide dinitrate	Pipenzolate
Chlorphentermine	Levodopa	Piperidolate
Chlorprothixene	Mepenzolate	Poldine
Cycrimine	Methamphetamine	Procyclidine
Cyproheptadine	Methantheline	Propantheline
Desipramine	Methixene	Protriptyline
Dextroamphetamine	Methscopolamine	Tricyclamol
Diethylpropion	Methylatropine	Tridihexethyl
Dimethindene	Methylphenidate	Trihexyphenidyl
Diphemanil	Nialamide	Triprolidine
Diphenidol	Nitroglycerine	Trolnitrate
Doxepin	Nortriptyline	
	Orphenadrine	
	Oxyphencyclimine	

While persons of all ages are susceptible to eye inflammation, certain conditions are more frequent in the geriatric patient. The corners of the eye (canthi) in the older patient are particularly prone to infection. Wrinkled and loose skin has a tendency to retain tears, which are an ideal site for an infection. The elderly are also particularly susceptible to inflammation of the conjunctiva and the eyelids. In case of red eye, one must differentiate between an acute and chronic disorder, which is determined by the duration of the complaint. In addition, crusting or a discharge indicates a bacterial infection, while a small pupil suggests acute angle-closure glaucoma (Ehrlich and Keates 1978).

Excessive tearing may be a problem in the old, especially on exposure to cold, wind, dust, and air pollution. Tearing of the eye will not cause loss of vision but will be a source of irritation and embarrassment. It may be caused either by excess lacrimation or by defective tear drainage. It may also be caused by cholinergic drugs.

Treatment of Eye Problems in the Aged

The treatment of pathologic ocular conditions in the elderly is relatively specific. Cataracts are a surgical problem, the indication for surgery based largely on the degree of vision impairment and the needs of the patient. This surgical procedure is almost always safe and successful.

Macular degeneration, which causes older patients to lose central visual acuity, cannot be treated. The patient is reassured that the condition will not result in blindness and encouraged to participate in activities that rely more on peripheral vision.

Glaucoma generally responds to drug therapy. An acute attack of angle-closure glaucoma is treated with miotics and, if necessary, with systemic drugs. Mannitol or urea can be given intravenously, and glycerine, in a 50% to 70% solution, can be administered orally. These drugs lower intraocular pressure by making the blood hyperosmolar in comparison to the aqueous humor of the eye. Glaucoma is generally cured by surgery.

The chronic open-angle glaucoma may be more dangerous than the acute type because of its insidious nature. Chronic open-angle glaucoma can usually be controlled by ophthalmic drugs and the tendency is to use surgery only as a last resort (Kornzweig 1971).

Cholinergics such as pilocarpine and carbachol have been used to treat glaucoma. Pilocarpine is first tried in a weak strength (0.5%) up to every six hours. The strength may then be increased until an adequate response is obtained. Carbachol may be used in patients allergic to pilocarpine. These drugs facilitate the movement of the aqueous humor from the anterior chamber through the trabecular network.

Epinephrine, for some time, had fallen into disuse as its use had been associated with attacks of acute closed-angle glaucoma. It is thought to have a dual mechanism of action. It decreases the production of aqueous humor and also increases the rate of filtration of fluid out of the anterior chamber (Lazenby et al 1970). It is not uncommon to see pilocarpine and epinephrine used concurrently. The organophosphate cholinesterase inhibitors are also useful in the treatment of open-angle glaucoma. They frequently maintain normal intraocular pressure when the more commonly used miotics are not successful. Echothiophate iodide is probably one of the more well known products of this type.

There has been some concern that the cholinesterase inhibitors can cause lens opacities (Pietsch et al 1972; Paterson 1971). Lens changes have been shown to occur in some patients after only four months of echothiophate therapy (Pietsch et al 1972), and isoflurophate and demecarium bromide have also been implicated (Schaffer and Heatherington 1966). While oral anticholinesterases do not appear to be cataractogenic (Lieberman et al 1971), the topically applied ones apparently have a dose- and age-related cataractogenic activity. Thus, there is, for example, little rationale for using echothiophate in concentrations above 0.06% (Harris 1971).

Dry eye is a problem prevalent among older patients and may be treated with topically administered agents. The tear film is a three-part structure (Lemp et al 1971). There is a thin superficial lipid layer, a thicker aqueous layer, and an innermost mucoid layer. The mucin layer may be inadequate in diseases causing vitamin A deficiency or scarring of the conjunctiva.

The cornea is a hydrophobic structure. The conjunctival mucus is produced in the conjunctival goblet cells and mechanically spread over the cornea by blinking, which provides a hydrophilic surface for the tears. If this hydrophilic, mucus layer is not present, the tear film breaks up prematurely. Either a decrease in tear production or a decrease in the amount of mucus adsorbed on the cornea could be responsible for dry eye.

Many agents have been promoted for the treatment of dry eye. Among these are agents to increase tear viscosity (eg, methylcellulose) and agents to produce a film-like corneal covering (eg, polyvinyl alcohol) (Lemp 1972). Methylcellulose solutions are available in concentrations of 0.5% to 5%, and polyvinyl alcohol is used as a 1.4% solution.

A disadvantage of methylcellulose is that, as the solution evaporates, a flaky residue is left that combines with any mucus to cause a decrease in vision and comfort. Patients may, therefore, prefer polyvinyl alcohol (Sabiston 1969). The chief disadvantage of either methylcellulose or polyvinyl alcohol is their short duration of action (Barsam et al 1972), and mucoid-like polymers prevent tear breakup longer than any other agents. Thus, dry eye can be treated with artificial tears, but they must be applied frequently, and treatment failure is often caused by lack of frequent administration. Mucolytic agents such as acetylcysteine are also recommended (Ehrlich and Keates 1978).

Antiinfective and/or antiinflammatory drugs are available in many ophthalmic preparations, singly or combined. They are probably overused, particularly in nursing homes, and should not be refilled automatically. An examination of the patient should precede any order. Long-term use of steroid-antibiotic combinations is frequent, as the elderly eye is particularly susceptible to infections and inflammations. However, the use of topical steroids, used either alone or in combination with antibiotics or sulfonamides is dangerous to the elderly patient. There is ample documentation that topical steroids, used for prolonged periods of time, increase intraocular pressure (Kitazawa 1970) and that these drugs exhibit cataractogenic properties (Paterson 1971). Increased intraocular pressure occurs in at least one-third of patients treated with these drugs if they are used longer than four to six weeks (Theodore 1975). Considering that nursing home residents may not be seen by a physician for a two-month period, this time span can be easily exceeded. Long-term use of steroid-antibiotic mixtures increases the patient's susceptibility to bacterial, fungal, and virus infections, especially herpes simplex, and loss of vision may result (Theodore 1975). Thus, bacterial conjunctivitis should be treated with a sulfonamide or a combination antibiotic, but not with a steroid or antibiotic-steroid mixture (Ehrlich and Keates 1978).

In nursing homes, the antihistamine-decongestants also appear to be relatively frequently used, most often for tired, red eyes. Most of these preparations contain phenylephrine or some other vasoconstrictor. It is recommended that these drugs be used with caution in patients with angle-closure glaucoma. In the geriatric population, both in the community and the nursing home, it is likely that there will be persons disposed to angle-closure glaucoma, which has not yet been diagnosed. It would make sense, therefore, to use ocular lubricants or artificial tears, rather than products containing vasoconstrictors to avoid the possibility of precipitating an angle-closure glaucoma attack.

REFERENCES

Anderson, B. The aging eye. *Postgrad Med.* 50:235, 1971.

Barsam, P., Sampson, W., and Feldman, G. The treatment of the dry eye and related problems. *Ann Ophthalmol.* 4:120, 1972.

Beehler, C.C. Ocular problems of the elderly. *J Florida Med Assoc.* 55:912, 1968.

Bell, B. Maintenance therapy in vision and hearing for geriatric patients. Edited by J.L. Rudd, and R.J. Margolin. In *Maintenance Therapy for the Geriatric Patients.* Springfield, Ill.: Charles C Thomas, 1968.

Black, R.L., Oglesby, R.B., von Sallman, L. et al. Posterior subcapsular cataracts induced by corticosteroids in patients with rheumatoid arthritis. *JAMA.* 174:166, 1960.

Crews, S.J. Posterior subcapsular lens opacities in patients on long-term corticosteroid therapy. *Br Med J.* 1:1644, 1963.

DeLong, S.L., Poley, B.J., and McFarlane, J.R. Ocular changes associated with long-term chlorpromazine therapy. *Arch Ophthalmol.* 73:611, 1965.

Ehrlich, D.R., and Keates, R.H. What to do when the elderly patient complains of external eye problems. *Geriatrics* 33(7):34, 1978.

Feldstein, M., Kornzweig, A.L., and Schneider, J. Ocular surgery in the elderly. *JAMA.* 170:1261, 1959.

Fischer, F. Senescence of the eye. In *Modern Trends in Ophthalmology.* New York: Hoeber, 1947.

Foote, F.M., and Boyce, V.S. Screening for glaucoma. *J Chronic Dis.* 2:387, 1955.

Fox, S.L. The eye in the aging patient. *J Maryland Optom Assoc.* 1(2):19, 1968.

Fraunfelder, F.T. *Drug-Induced Ocular Effects and Drug Interactions.* Philadelphia: Lea & Febiger, 1976.

Giles, C.L., Mason, G.L., Duff, I.F. et al. The association of cataract formation and systemic corticosteroid therapy. *JAMA.* 182:719, 1962.

Graham, P.A. Geriatrics and the special senses. *Gerontol Clin.* 13:321, 1971.

Harris, L.S. Dose-response analysis of echothiophate iodide. *Arch*

Ophthalmol. 86:502, 1971.

Howard, R.O., McDonald, C.J., Dunn, B. et al. Experimental chlorpromazine cataracts. *Invest Ophthalmol.* 8:413, 1969.

Kitazawa, Y. Primary angle-closure glaucoma, corticosteroid responsiveness. *Arch Ophthalmol.* 84:724, 1970.

Kornzweig, A.L. The eye in old age. Edited by I.R. Rossman. In *Clinical Geriatrics.* Philadelphia: J.B. Lippincott Co., 1971.

Kornzweig, A.L. Visual loss in the elderly. *Hosp Practice.* 12(7):51, 1977.

Kornzweig, A.L., Feldstein, M., and Schneider, J. The eye in old age. IV. Ocular survey of over one thousand aged persons with special reference to normal and disturbed visual function. *Am J Ophthalmol.* 44:29, 1957.

Lazenby, G.W., Reed, J.W., and Grant, W.M. Anticholinergic medication in open-angle glaucoma. *Arch Ophthalmol.* 84:719, 1970.

Lemp, M.A. Ophthalmic polymers as ocular wetting agents. *Ann Ophthalmol.* 4:15, 1972.

Lemp, M.A., Dohlman, C.H., Kuwabara, T. et al. Dry eye secondary to mucus deficiency. *Trans Am Acad Ophthalmol Otolaryngol.* 75:1223, 1971.

Lieberman, T.W., Leopold, J.H., and Osserman, K.E. Lens findings in patients with myasthenia gravis on long-term treatment with oral anticholinesterases. *Mt Sinai J Med.* 38:324, 1971.

Lund, O.E. Second round table on medical therapy of glaucoma. *Doc Ophthalmol.* 33(1):244, 1972.

Mathaline, M.B.R. Oculocutaneous effects of chlorpromazine. *Lancet* 2:111, 1965.

Means, B.J., and Lamy, P.P. Ophthalmic drugs for the geriatric patient. *Clin Med.* 82(10):30, 1975.

Newell, T.W. *Ophthalmology, Principles and Concepts.* St. Louis: C.V. Mosby Co., 1965.

Paterson, C.A. Effects of drugs on the lens. Edited by P.P. Ellis. In *International Ophthalmology Clinic.* Vol. 11. Boston: Little, Brown and Co., 1971.

Phelps, C.D. The treatment of open-angle glaucoma. *Drug Ther.* 7(4):68, 1977.

Pietsch, R.L., Bobo, B.B., Finklea, J.F. et al. Lens opacities and organophosphate cholinesterase-inhibiting agents. *Am J Ophthalmol.* 73:236, 1972.

Pollack, I.R. The challenge of glaucoma screening. *Surv Ophthalmol.* 13:4, 1968.

Sabiston, D. The dry eye. *Trans Ophthalmol Soc NZ.* 21:96, 1969.

Schaffer, R.N., and Heatherington, J. Comparison of cataract incidence in normal and glaucomatous population. *Am J Ophthalmol.* 62:613, 1966.

Schneider, J., Feldstein, M., and Kornzweig, A.L. Scleral rigidity and tonometry in the aged. *Am J Ophthalmol.* 48:643, 1959.

Schwartz, B. The glaucomas. *N Engl J Med.* 299:182, 1978.

Siddall, J.R. The ocular toxic findings with prolonged and high-dose chlorpromazine intake. *Arch Ophthalmol.* 74:460, 1965.

Spaeth, G.L., and von Sallman, L. Corticosteroids and cataracts. *Int Ophthalmol Clin.* 6:915, 1966.

Streiff, E.B. Gerontology and geriatrics of the eye. *Surv Ophthalmol.* 12:311, 1967.

Theodore, F.H. External eye problems in the elderly. *Geriatrics* 30(4):69, 1975.

Willetts, G.S., and Hopkins, D.J. Systemic therapeutic agents and glaucoma. *Practitioner* 209:27, 1972.

22 Psychopharmacologic Drugs

Impaired intellectual function is not a concomitant of normal aging. The elderly probably fear loss or impairment of brain function more than death itself.

Yet the prevalence of brain failure, acute or organic, and functional disorders (affective, paranoid, neurologic) increases with age (Ariea 1973). The reasons for this increase are still poorly understood, as is the treatment. Yet, as the number of old-old, those over the age of 75, increases, one can assume an increase in these disorders and, thus, it is important that more intense efforts be directed toward solving the many unanswered questions regarding intellectual impairment in old age.

Accurate statistics are difficult, if at all obtainable. On one hand, waste basket diagnoses such as senility, depression, and schizophrenia are too often and all too easily made (Rosenhan 1975). Particularly in the case of the institutionalized elderly, such a diagnosis, once made, is often permanently retained. The patient so labeled is then not infrequently judged to be "untreatable." On the other hand, much has been made of the reduction in the number of patients in mental hospitals with the appearance of powerful and effective psychoactive drugs (Figure 22-1).

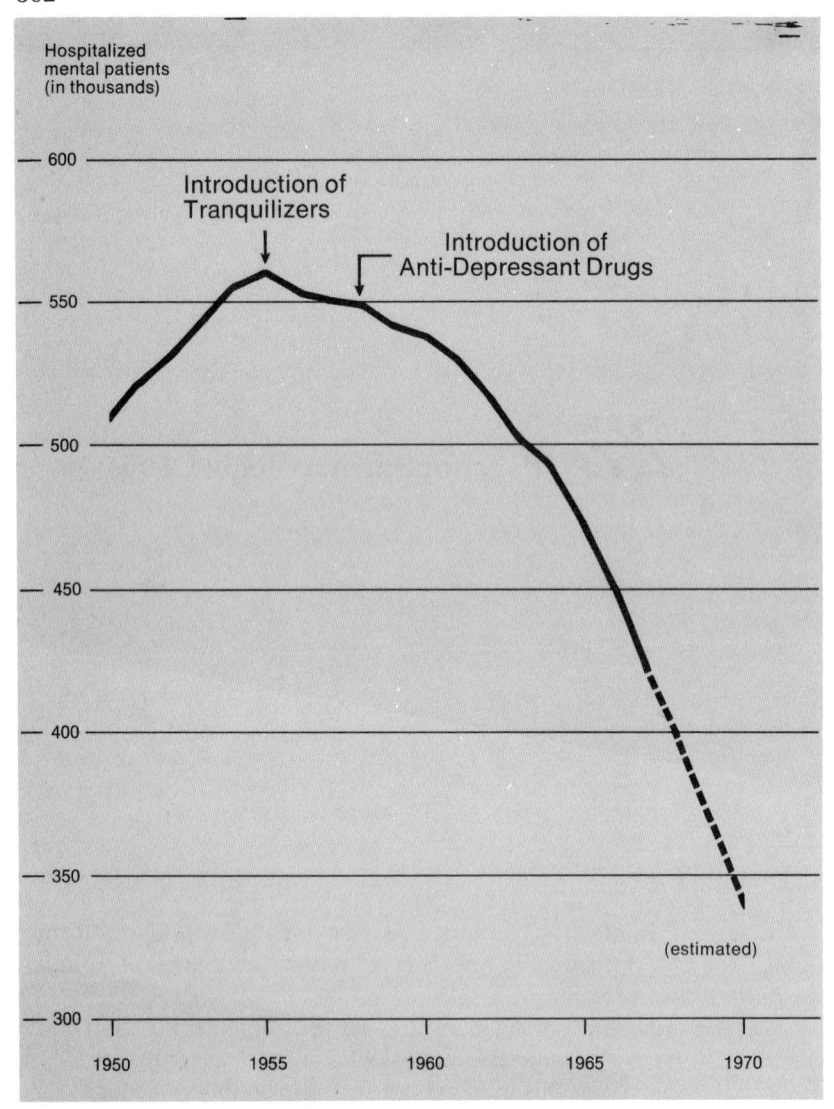

Figure 22-1 The hospitalization equation... new drugs/less hospital time. Annual patient load in mental hospitals. Reprinted with permission of Roche Laboratories.

There can be no argument that the psychoactive drugs, particularly the newer ones, are effective in many instances. However, unquestioning acceptance of such statistics overlooks the well-known "dumping syndrome." Many patients, being "controlled" with these drugs, are simply transferred from state mental hospitals to nursing homes.

The statistics available are thought-provoking. The proportion of psychiatric inpatients over 65 years of age has risen from 31% in 1954 to 44% in 1971 in England (Pasker et al 1976). About one-half million of the elderly residing in nursing homes have some degree of organic brain disease. Care of these patients costs six billion dollars annually, which does not include the devastating cost to individuals and their families both in economic terms and in terms of quality of life (Butler 1978). Those living in the community do not fare much better. One-fifth to one-third of all patients seen in general practice have some element of psychological disturbance (Blackwell 1973). Ten percent of people over 65 years of age and 30% of those over 80 years of age have measurable cognitive impairment and 50% to 75% have some type of function-disturbing impairment. Overall, it has been estimated that about three million of the elderly are so afflicted, two-thirds of whom live in the community and not in nursing homes. Still other statistics estimate that of those over 65 years of age, about one in six has some manifestation of organic brain syndrome but as many as 25% to 30% may have some type of functional disorder, such as depression or neurosis.

Thus, intellectual impairment among the elderly is a major public health problem which will increase in magnitude as a progressively larger proportion of the population reaches advanced age, unless more research efforts are devoted to the identification of the causes and more decisive and effective intervention methods are developed than are currently available. It must be realized that mental disorders in the elderly more often than not have multifactorial causes, and equal attention must be given to social and psychotherapeutic as well as medical measures (Kanowski and Paur 1976). Particularly important are good diagnostic procedures.

Hypochondriasis is mainly a disease of youth and middle age. If older patients complain, particularly if they complain about nonspecific symptoms, intensive diagnostic efforts are indicated. Hypochondriasis is poorly understood. It is a psychopathologic disorder characterized by a constant concern with health and a tendency to feel ill (Goldstein and Birnbom 1976). Hypochondriasis occurs more often among the economically disadvantaged as they face higher social stress and have fewer social opportunities (Busse 1976). The disease can become chronic if social stress persists and these patients can easily become dependent on medical services. Thus, these patients are difficult to treat and based on a relatively poor prognosis, extreme care should be exercised not to label elderly patients too readily as hypochondriacs. The elderly with anxiety and depression often present with hypochondriasis, irritability, and agitation (Brodie et al 1975), and unless the underlying illness is treated, all therapeutic efforts are doomed to failure. Other so-called hypochondriac symptoms, such as intractable pain in the back or chest wall, abdominal discomforts, visual difficulties, and obession about constipation may signal an organic brain syndrome (Walsh 1976).

Brain Failure

The diagnosis of "senility" in the elderly is a diagnostic waste basket. It is insidious and hazardous to the patient, as it often leads to an irreversible compromise of the patient's quality of life. The term "brain failure" was introduced in the latter part of the 19th century in England and has recently been revived in this country. It includes all intellectual impairments. Organic mental disorder is an equivalent term. It is hoped that this type of designation will lead to a more intense diagnostic effort and the realization that the prognosis may not necessarily be hopeless. Treatment, if not actually able to reverse the disease process, can well maintain existing functions and/or maintain or increase the patient's quality of life.

Yet, often, an array of presenting symptoms of behavioral, perceptual, and emotional disorders is automatically categorized as evidence of chronic brain syndrome, if the patient happens to be over 65 years of age (Ernst et al 1977a), precluding any treatment effort. At a recent conference on treatable brain diseases in the elderly, held at the National Institutes of Health, it was stated that some 300,000 elderly Americans who have been labeled "demented" or "senile" could have been restored to a useful life with proper evaluation and treatment.

Quite apparently, proper evaluation is the key. Yet American physicians formulate the diagnosis of "organic brain syndrome" for the aged far more often than do their British counterparts (Zarit et al 1978) possibly because a full evaluation of the patient is not undertaken. Brain failure is a syndrome characterized by impaired social functioning. There is an inability to learn because of a decline of intellect associated with impaired memory. The patient fails to fulfill social norms (Livesley 1976). However, the type and severity of the mental symptoms are not necessarily directly proportional to the extent of the physiologic disturbance (Post 1951).

Diagnosis is difficult and time consuming. It is not a one-time determination but a continuous process of assessment which is likely to change with time. A full diagnosis of brain failure involves clinical, social, psychologic, and psychiatric assessments (Williamson 1977). Every patient and every situation requires a detailed individual assessment, with particular emphasis on developing organic diseases that might necessitate extra support.

The accurate and early diagnosis of brain failure is crucial. Acute disorders, if untreated, may be followed much later with development of altered brain function. In addition, minor memory disturbances show a high correlation with death four years after first being observed (Zarit et al 1978). Thus, brain failure is a significant factor in increasing mortality in the aged, mortality rates increasing when poor physical health is present concurrently (Kay 1962; Peck et al 1978). Full evaluation is mandatory also because of the high proportion of treatable causes often encountered (Harrison and Marsden 1977). From 20% to 30% of patients may have disorders which are potentially treatable either by medical or surgical intervention (Marsden and Harrison 1972; Freemon 1976). It must be recognized that the diagnostic process is made more difficult by the fact that all organic brain syndromes are found in combination with a functional (emotional) component not related to the cause of the organic brain syndrome.

Classification of Brain Failure

The terms "acute" and "organic" brain syndrome are no longer used. What used to be called acute organic brain syndrome is now referred to as acute confusional state or, more precisely, as delirium. It is common, denotes a global impairment and is treatable. Sometimes, it is divided into brain failure due to a variety of reversible factors, and depression, due to a series of disorders.

The disorder formerly referred to as organic brain syndrome is now called dementia. Dementia denotes disturbances of a single or of a few functions. Cognitive impairment or senile dementia is not a specific disease. It is, rather, a symptom or syndrome, each having its own differential diagnosis. Dementia has also been called senile dementia, senility, and hardening of the arteries. Dementia and organic brain syndrome are equivalent terms indicating loss of brain function as measured by degree of impairment of memory, orientation, judgment, and ability to perform tasks. Organic brain syndrome and senile dementia should not be used interchangeably. Senile dementia is a disease of unknown origin and only one of the diseases which used to be classified as organic brain syndromes (Cohen 1978).

Presenile dementia (Alzheimer) and senile dementia were, at one time, thought to be two different diseases. It is now recognized that histochemically and electromicroscopically, they do not differ. Senile dementia of the Alzheimer variety is also referred to as primary neuronal degeneration, while senile dementia due to cardiovascular disease is referred to as multi-infarct dementia. Alzheimer disease (Wolstenholme and O'Connor 1970) is responsible for the majority of cases of presenile and senile dementias (Wells 1978). Identification of the different types of brain failure is often difficult. Elderly depressed patients may present with demented symptoms (pseudodementia), but the expected guilt complex is often missing.

The initial picture of delirium and dementia may be the same. There may be, initially at least, impaired memory, disorientation to person, place, or time in both, and impaired calculation and judgment abilities.

In both, behavioral changes may include agitation, hostility or excitement, lethargy, apathy, or somnolence (Cameron et al 1977). Therefore, a precise separation of delirium and dementia can often not be made.

In any case, though, the more recent the onset of the disturbance, the more likely is treatment success. Therefore, a mental examination must be conducted which is reliable, comprehensive, and repeated over time.

Delirium Delirium or acute confusional states may occur in an elderly person who prior to the confusional episode has functioned normally. An acute confusional state has an easily definable recent onset of confusion, disorientation, and excitement. The patient may exhibit a diminished attention span, change in the quality of sleep, change in memory, and a perception deficit. After the original symptoms appear, the condition may not progress.

The symptoms of confusion, disorientation, agitation, or disturbances in levels of consciousness may be related to underlying organic diseases such as pneumonia, myocardial infarction, renal infection, or head trauma (Bayne 1978). Hypokalemia or dehydration should also be suspected. It is most important to suspect drug toxicity as a possible cause of the confusional state (Cameron et al 1977; Glickman and Friedman 1976; Reichel 1978; Joffe 1978). Confusional states may also arise as a result of hypoxia, fever, or drug withdrawal (Judge 1977).

Delirium is a very common, nonspecific cause of secondary dementia. It is frequently superimposed on dementia and can, therefore, be missed in the diagnostic process. In the case of organic disease, treatment is directed toward that disease. It is important to provide a supportive environment, as any change can further confuse the patient. A psychotropic drug may have to be used for the first few days, given early in the evening and repeated, if necessary. This type of regimen, therefore, addresses the cause and provides, initially, symptomatic relief.

As mentioned previously, drug toxicity is often the cause of a confusional state. The elderly, possibly exposed to the effects of reduced kidney and liver function, may experience reduced drug excretion and increased drug toxicity and, thus, impaired mental function.

Many commonly prescribed drugs are likely to cause delirium in the elderly. Among those may be digitalis, phenytoin, the so-called fast-acting antidepressants, L-dopa, the steroids, lidocaine, and propranolol (Glickman and Friedman 1976). Cimetidine is currently frequently mentioned as a drug that is likely to cause mental confusion in the elderly (Delaney and Ravey 1977). More than 5% of patients admitted to one hospital for an acute drug crisis ranged in age from 50 to 80 (Peterson and Thomas 1975). Psychiatric side effects of non-psychiatric drugs probably occur in as many as 3% of patients, not necessarily only elderly (Boston Collaborative Drug Surveillance Program 1971). Prednisone, isoniazid, methyldopa, NPH and regular insulin, and furosemide were found to be most frequently involved.

If drug toxicity is suspected, as many drugs as possible should be withdrawn from the patient's regimen. Beneficial results should occur within two weeks (Cameron et al 1977).

Dementia Dementia is life-shortening. Its incidence increases with increasing age. Crude values (Table 22-1) indicate that women are more frequently affected than men, but that may simply be a statistical aberration as men do not live as long as women. The rate, which does not include those living in the community, rises abruptly after the age of 85 years. However, even though the probability for appearance of the syndrome increases drastically with the very advanced age, only about 50% of those over 90 years of age have some kind of involvement. Even if not associated with a specific disease, senility or senile dementia increases mortality significantly.

Dementia is probably the fourth leading cause of death in the United States, and it is estimated that about 100,000 to 120,000 Americans die each year of some kind of Alzheimer disease. The statistics are uncertain, as this disease is not listed by the United States Vital Statistics. The death certificate would usually show the immediate or precipitating cause, which may be cardiovascular disease, for example, but the underlying, long-term cause might have been Alzheimer disease. There is, further, some doubt on the accuracy of the statistics of cognitive impairment and dementia. Statistics, of course, list only those patients making contact with the health care system. Therefore, utilization data, on which statistics are based, may yield false results.

Table 22-1
Specific Incidence of Dementia in Nursing Homes

Age	Male	Female
65–74	0.54	0.61
75–84	2.53	4.44
85+	12.27	19.21

Source: National Nursing Home Survey. Nursing Homes in the United States: 1973–1974. DHEW Publ. No. (HRA) 78-1812. Hyattsville, Md.: National Center for Health Statistics, 1977.

In any case, most older people are not senile, but the problem of senility is becoming increasingly important. It is not quite clear whether the incidence of senility is increasing or whether or not there are more senile patients because there are more older people. It is vital, therefore, that reversible causes of dementia be identified as soon as possible. If left untreated, even reversible dementia can become irreversible.

It may well be that the diagnostic process is not pursued as vigorously as it might be as 70% to 80% of the elderly demented patients probably suffer from irreversible dementia (Table 22-2). As Table 22-2 shows, Alzheimer disease and the vascular diseases, both of which are irreversible with currently available management methods, predominate. Table 22-3 lists the "treatable" dementias in more detail. It is important to stress that up to 30% of patients have been identified to have reversible dementias, often caused by drug toxicities (Heilman

Table 22-2
Some Causes of Progressive Intellectual Deterioration

Alzheimer, including presenile and senile dementias, simple cerebral atrophy	50%

Vascular disease
  Carotid occlusive disease
  Hyperlipidemic dementia
  Low cardiac output
  Multiple (large) cerebral infarcts
  Multiple lacunar (small) infarcts*
	20%

Resectable mass lesions
  Benign tumors
  Cysts
  Subdurals	

Normal pressure hydrocephalus	

Vitamin and mineral deficiency
  B-12
  Folate
  Niacin
  Thiamine	

Metabolic-toxic
  Alcohol dementia
  Carbon monoxide poisoning
  Drug intoxication
  Heavy metal poisoning
  Hepatic, renal, and pulmonary failure
  Hypercalcemia
  Hypoglycemia
  Hypothyroidism and hyperthyroidism	

Depression (pseudodementia)	

*Multiple infarct disease is now referred to as Repeated infarct disease, apparently more precisely indicating a series of events over time.

Table 22-3
Some Treatable Causes of Dementia

Vascular
  Multiple infarcts
  Emboli, subacute bacterial endocarditis, fat
  Decreased cardiac output
  Myocardial infarction, heart failure
  Collagen vascular diseases
    lupus, polyarteritis
  Increased viscosity

Metabolic and Endocrine
  Hypothyroidism
  Hyperparathyroidism
  Pituitary insufficiency
  Repeated hypoglycemia
  Respiratory acidosis
  Uremia
  Hepatic encephalopathy
  Porphyria
  Wilson's disease

Nutrition
  Pernicious anemia
  Alcoholics and thiamine deficiency
  Pellagra

Toxicity
  Bromides
  Mercury
  Others

Infections
  General paresis
  Cryptococcal meningitis
  Encephalitis
  Sarcoid
  Postinfectious encephalomyelitis

Mass Effect
  Lymphoma and leukemia (with or without pathologic change)
  Intracranial tumor–subfrontal meningioma
  Subdural hematoma

Subclinical Seizures

Demyelinating Disease

Low-Pressure Hydrocephalus

and Fisher 1974; Gilbert 1977; Adler 1974). Drug-induced brain failure may be caused by hypotension (Powell 1977). The hazard of lowered cerebral perfusion is very real in the elderly treated with antihypertensives or vasodilators. The butyrophenones, phenothiazines, and tricyclics may also be responsible, as may diuretics, antiparkinsonism agents, and sedatives. Vitamin and mineral deficiency can lead to dementia, especially a deficit in vitamin B-12. This is often overlooked as vitamin B-12 deficiency may not have any hematologic indices. To

Table 22-4
Reversible Causes of Dementia

D —drugs
E —emotional disorders
M —metabolic or endocrine disorders
E —eye and ear deficit
N —nutritional deficiencies
      normal-pressure hydrocephalus (ataxic gait, urinary incontinence, mild dementia)
T —tumor and trauma
I —infections
A —arteriosclerotic complications

help identify reversible causes of dementia, the mnemonic in Table 22-4 has been suggested.

Thus, a thoughtful and careful diagnostic process is mandatory. It can lead to the discovery of 15% of disorders which are correctable, and another 20% to 25% which require specific therapeutic intervention (Wells 1978). It is a difficult diagnosis; senile dementia can be confused with depression and the diagnosis may be clouded by alcoholism. It is also one of the most far-reaching and serious diagnostic processes in medicine. Many conditions can mimic senility. The prognosis of senile dementia is very serious. Once labeled "demented," a patient may experience withdrawal of the support system at a time when it is needed most. This may lead to further but artificial deterioration of the patient's mental status.

Every patient diagnosed as "demented" should have a comprehensive physical examination, including a rectal, pelvic, and genital evaluation, in addition to neurologic and mental evaluations. The physical examination is necessary to rule out any condition or event whose symptoms or side effects can mimic irreversible dementia. It has been suggested that, in addition to these examinations, the physician should obtain chest and skull x-rays, EKG, EEG, urinalysis, SMA 12, T_3 and T_4, CBC, VDRL, serum creatinine, electrolytes, serum B-12, and serum folate. Vision and hearing evaluations are mandatory (Cameron et al 1977).

Computerized axial tomography has also been suggested as a diagnostic tool, as it permits an anti-mortem examination of the brain. Most of the irreversible dementias are caused by Alzheimer disease (50% to 60%) and multiinfarct dementia (about 35%), which was formerly called cerebrovascular arteriosclerosis and is caused by small focal infarcts of brain tissue. Irreversible dementia may also be due to Creutzfeldt-Jakob disease, Huntington chorea, and parkinsonism. Still others, uncertain as to cause, are labeled progressive idiopathic dementias. An unambiguous diagnosis of brain senility is difficult to obtain (Obrist 1972).

Some clinicians feel that there is no good evidence that senile dementia and dementia caused by cerebrovascular disease can be differentiated. Others have suggested that senile dementia of the Alzheimer type (SDAT) has an insidious onset, a slow progressive course, and no focal neurologic symptoms. Dementia of the cerebrovascular type is characterized by an abrupt onset, remissions and exacerbations, stuttering progression, and focal neurologic symptoms and signs (Wells 1978).

In multiple infarct disease, development is incremental, ie, there is a step progression. Initially, a patient can improve and, indeed, recovery can be complete. However, with repetition, there is less and less chance of improvement. Multiinfarct disease is similar to both core and associated symptoms of organic brain disease.

It should be noted that "irreversible" dementia is not necessarily synonymous with "deteriorating" dementia. If dementia is caused by reversible causes, it need not be deteriorating or irreversible. If an organic brain syndrome is caused by senile dementia, on the other hand, there will be a course of deterioration. However, some patients will deteriorate, some may deteriorate and then stabilize, and still others may have a nonprogressive disorder. It is extremely difficult to differentiate between progressive and nonprogressive disorders. The differentiation is important, though, because it is particularly the patient with the nonprogressive disorder who may gain substantially from good therapeutic management.

In assessing the patient's cognitive function, it is important that the patient not feel threatened and feel comfortable. It is of utmost importance, furthermore, that questions be tailored to the patient's particular circumstances. The Wechsler Deterioration Quotient has traditionally been used as an index of intellectual impairment (Wechsler 1944). It is based on the premise that certain intellectual functions "hold" with age, whereas others do not. The vocabulary, for example, is thought to hold, both in normal and secondary aging. However, it appears that verbal abilities remain relatively constant with age only when the initial level of ability was high. Thus, some of the assumptions on which the effectiveness of this evaluative instrument are based have come under increasing criticism (Bureau of Drugs 1976). In assessing disorientation to time, for example, it must first be determined whether or not a particular patient has any reason to know what day it is. Is it reasonable, for example, to expect a resident of a nursing home, faced with the overly protective and nondemanding atmosphere so often found in nursing homes, to remember the day? Quite possibly, elderly patients may, on the other hand, remember very clearly "bingo day," as this is something they look forward to and which demands their involvement. Similarly, loss of an ability to do simple arithmetic problems may not be correctly identified by asking the amount of change which will remain after spending a certain amount of money. A nursing home resident may not have been faced with this type of decision-making for a long time. Conversely, it is quite possible that the elderly woman is quite certain as to the tip to be given to the hair dresser in order to receive the best service possible.

What causes dementia? Why and how brain deficit occurs is still not known. It is thought that there is not a loss in intelligence per se. Rather, it has been suggested that intelligence is composed of two parts. Crystallized intelligence represents a body of knowledge, and it is remarkably persistent. On the other hand, fluidized intelligence deteriorates. Many patients who show mental decline often have normal blood vessels, so that mental decline in aging is not only related to arteriosclerosis of brain vessels (Peress et al 1973). As a matter of fact, arteriosclerotic changes are found only in about one-third of organic brain syndromes of old age. They contribute substantially to the pathologic condition in only about 10% of the cases (Hollister 1973). However, it has also been suggested that arteriosclerotic dementia may be much more prevalent than is thought. Carotid and other large vessel disease may also be much more prevalent than thought and should be considered potentially operable in all elderly patients with dementia.

Senile dementia of the Alzheimer type is now believed to be causally related to organic disease of nerve cells. In healthy elderly persons, significant reduction in brain weight does not begin until about 70 years of age. There is probably some decline in neuronal population in specific areas of the brain, but only minor changes in cerebral blood flow and glucose consumption (Bowen 1976; Meier-Ruge et al 1975). Older research results indicated that cerebral blood flow, oxygen consumption, and glucose metabolism decline with age. Newer, more sophisticated research methods seem to indicate that this may not hold true for all brain areas.

Loss of brain neurons occurs unevenly, seemingly affecting the frontal and temporal lobes more than other brain areas. These areas play key roles in verbalization and hearing. Degenerative changes such as senile plaques and neurofibrillar tangles, granulovacuolar degeneration, and lipofuscin granules appear in the normal aging brain. In senile dementia, they are more marked, particularly in the grey matter, including the hippocampus. Senile plaques apparently correlate with the degree of dementia, as do neurofibrillar tangles of the Alzheimer type. In contrast, granulovacuolar degenerations occur with equal frequency in senile demented patients and normal elderly individuals.

Certain neurologic conditions (at one time considered degenerative) are actually viral infections, possibly caused by the so-called "slow" viruses, also called unconventional viruses, as they do not create an antibody response (Alter and Rosenberg 1977).

Age is an important determinant of the levels of neurotransmitters and their associated enzymes and metabolites in certain regions of the brain (Samorajski 1977). Behavioral events alter neurochemical function and, in turn, neurochemical function can change behavior. Both neurotransmitters and neuromodulators, together termed neuroregulators, are involved. Thus, it has been suggested that cholineacetyltransferase (CHAT) decreases significantly in certain brain regions and that this decrease can be correlated with high regional concentrations of tangles.

In summary, the chronic organic brain syndrome is most likely a group of manifestations secondary to pathologic changes in the cerebral tissue, possibly linked to changes in brain neuroregulators.

Patient Presentation

Dementia syndromes develop slowly and have an uncertain time of onset. The demented patient is often vague, less focused than the depressed patient, and less able to give specific information. Dementia is characterized by an extreme impoverishment of mental resources.

Intellectual function, last acquired, is lost first. The next cognitive function to be lost is memory, starting with the most recent. The patient may be unable to remember the name of acquaintances or to recall recent events. This stage may or may not progress, but if it progresses, loss of orientation for time, place, and person would probably follow in that order, resulting in a profound loss of contact with the environment and other people. Depression, if it occurs, is likely to be a reaction to memory loss.

Carelessness in dress and personal habits occurs. The patient may become loud and obscene and long-standing personality characteristics may become magnified. There is loss of adaptability, an increasing rigidity of response and, finally, complete helplessness, total dependency, and loss of all intellectual and manual skills. In short, as the organ of adaptation (the brain) ceases to adapt, the patient's physiologic adaptive capacity is lost. The patient will become bedridden and there is loss of sphincter control. Bronchopneumonia is the most common cause of death.

On the other hand, the patient is likely to retain social skills and graces. This can be very deceptive. There is likely to be a denial of memory deficit, avoidance, jocularity, and confabulation, primarily in unfamiliar settings. The core symptoms of clinical senile dementia are summarized in Table 22-5.

Patient Management

A certain level of cerebral damage must be reached before deterioration associated with multiinfarct dementia (MID) or Alzheimer disease (AD) becomes apparent. It has been reasoned, but not yet shown, that

Table 22-5
Core Symptoms of Clinical Senile Dementia

Early:	Manifestations are subtle and onset is very gradual.
	Depression, listlessness, anxiety, agitation, loss of concentration. Irritability and petulance.
	Some patients are aware that something is wrong. There may be sudden panic. Then coping mechanism takes over. Self-esteem may be eroded.
Full:	Common disorientation to time and place. Then disorientation to persons.
	Instructions are quickly forgotten. Can lead to gross errors in medication administration.
	Altered sleep patterns. Carelessness in personal appearance.
	Note: Late-onset dementias seem to stabilize and in some cases, may even show some improvement.

therapeutic intervention early enough should prevent the "threshold effect" and prevent irreversible damage (Jarvik 1975).

Both MID and AD syndromes cause irreversible damage to the nervous system and therefore, treatment is directed toward prevention of future damage, rather than to repair past damage. Treatment is also directed toward strengthening the remaining functions and supporting the patient in general. Thus, a diagnosis of either MID or AD should not preclude the use of available treatment modalities (Ernst et al 1977b). Treatment, which should be very thoughtful (Wershow 1977), should revolve around the following principles (Glickman and Friedman 1976):

1. Select an appropriate target symptom.
2. Select the one which is most dangerous, disabling, or unacceptable to the patient.
3. Begin with a low dose and increase slowly.
4. If another target symptom is to be treated, add another drug after the original target symptom has been controlled.

Of course, there is no one best treatment. Many antipsychotic drugs are acceptable for relieving severe agitation, anxiety and restlessness, delusions, and hallucinations. Thioridazine is the choice of many clinicians and has been labeled the drug of choice for everyday use (Judge 1977). Its side effects appear to be predictable and relatively mild. It should not be used for patients with poor cardiac status. Haloperidol appears to be useful, starting with 0.5 to 2.0 mg two or three times daily, but it is probably best used in emergencies, as it causes rigidity (Judge 1977). In general, antipsychotics should be used only during crises requiring medications for a short time only.

Antidepressants can be used in cases of severe depression. Also, a therapeutic trial with antidepressants may be indicated for apparently demented patients with no obvious cause for the dementia. The antidepressants, and all other drugs with an anticholinergic action, should be used with extreme caution, as they can cause confusion or aggravate existing confusion. Therefore, for severely demented patients with Parkinson disease, amantadine should be used initially and only later should an attempt be made to switch to levodopa. The patient and the patient's family should be warned against using any nonprescription drug without first contacting the physician. Particularly dangerous are the scopolamine-containing drugs for insomnia.

If a patient is not severely demented, a trial with Hydergine may be indicated. This drug is receiving increasing attention. Most often, the drug seems to be able to improve the patient's mood and personal care, rather than the cognitive performance. If used, the trial must last for a sufficient time. Recently, treatment of patients with precursor amino acids of the neurotransmitters, dopamine and serotonin, seems to have shown some promise (Meyer et al 1977).

Drug treatment, therefore, is directed mainly toward the control of the most troublesome manifestations of behavior disturbances, such as restlessness, night wandering, and sleeplessness, which is disturbing not only to the patient but also to those caring for the patient. It is most important, though, that these disorders should not just be treated with drugs. The management of these dementias primarily involves an effort at environmental manipulation to maintain cognitive functioning.

Even if the elderly are physically disabled, it is important to maintain as much of their functional capacity as possible. The feedback effect of the autonomic nervous system on brain activity and vice versa must be carefully borne in mind. Particular attention must be paid to causes of functional decline, such as sensory deprivation caused by impairment of hearing or sight, nutritional factors, and social stress. Attention to supportive care involving adequate nutrition, vitamin intake, and the use of night lights or a clock radio for sundowning is most important.

FUNCTIONAL DISORDERS

Affective Disorders

Depression Depression is the most common functional disorder in the geriatric age group (*British Medical Journal* 1976). Depression in the elderly varies both in depth and intensity. It is too often overlooked as its symptoms may be regarded as being consistent with aging (Epstein 1978), and may also be confused with various organic states (Roth 1977; Cohen 1977). Ten percent to 65% of elderly, both institutionalized and in the community, may suffer from affective disorders, including depression (Butler 1975). There is a significant relationship between poverty and depressive symptomatology (Mon et al 1976). Unfortunately, particularly as depression in the elderly is frequently reversible with appropriate treatment (Epstein 1976), many elderly may not seek help when suffering from depressive states; they may feel that this is a normal part of the aging process.

The reason for the relatively high incidence rate of depression among the elderly (more women seem to be affected than men) is explained by the fact that the elderly face a high level of psychosocial and physical stress. To cope successfully with these demands, an increasing level of psychological reactions is needed, as well as a high degree of adaptation at a time when capacities for these functions diminish. Furthermore, there is an interdependence of physical and mental illness which becomes more prominent at these age levels.

Depression is an affective state reflecting a variety of reasons, not necessarily diseases. Depression may be idiopathic and it is then referred to as a primary depression (Biggs 1978). A primary depression may have some cognitive dysfunction which can be resolved. Depression can also arise secondarily to some serious medical or psychiatric illness, or be caused by some traumatic event (Biggs 1978). Depressions are now also classified as unipolar and bipolar (Grauer 1977). Unipolar depression describes patients with recurrent depressive episodes without evidence of mania or hypomania. Bipolar depression, conversely, describes patients who have depressive and manic episodes. Most often, though, the terms reactive and endogenous depression are still used (Table 22-6).

Reactive depression can be experienced by anyone; it is a characteristic response to certain life events. It is a self-limiting condition and may require only time and reassurance. In severe cases, psychotherapy may be indicated, but antidepressants are usually not required. Reactive depression in the elderly is usually associated with a physical disability, social isolation, or loneliness.

The appearance of endogenous depression is independent of life events. It is a result of decreased cerebral function, largely caused by a shortage in the brain of neurotransmitters that facilitate conduction of nerve impulses across the synaptic gap between neurons (Diamond et al 1977). The precise cause of endogenous depression can often not be identified. Endogenous depression has been subdivided into a number of different disorders.

Retardive depression is the most common of the endogenous ones. There will be excessive but nonproductive activity by the patient, inhibition of psychomotor activity, low and monosyllabic speech and slowness in initiation and execution of tasks. Patients with retardive depression usually respond well to tricyclics.

Table 22-6
Depression

Type	Description	Signs/Symptoms	Treatment
Reactive	Normal grief response to loss. Should not last longer than 3 months. For correct diagnosis, there must have been a concrete loss. In early stage, may not be able to differentiate from endogenous depression	Brooding, insomnia, loss of appetite, sadness	Small doses of anti-anxiety agent for a few days. Need reassurance and support
Psychoneurotic	Maladaptive coping with normal life situations. Requires authoritative evaluation	Signs of maladaptive coping such as alcoholism, stimulant or sedative abuse, hypochondriasis. Patient may feel sad but not look sad. Weeping, preoccupied with loss, emotional liability, histrionic behavior, complaining, irritability, anger, dependency, pessimism, self-pity, anxiety, possible suicide threat	Comparatively nonresponsive to tricyclics
Endogenous	Disordered brain physiology, presumably of biochemical nature. Diagnosis can be missed if depression expressed primarily by somatic symptoms. Symptoms are in themselves destructive	Patient may look sad but deny feeling sad. Patient dislikes symptoms. Inappropriate fatigue, musculoskeletal malaise, "nerves," GI and sleep disturbances, weight loss, inability to concentrate, sadness, guilt feelings, inability to experience pleasure, suicidal thoughts. Patient may feel worse in the morning than evening. Early awakening is primary clue	Tricyclics. Risks of inappropriate treatment small compared to benefits of appropriate treatment. Patient needs reassurance and support

The patient with agitated depression usually presents with hand-wringing, pacing, and expression of psychic pain, and may be helped by antipsychotics.

Involutional depression is most often found in later years and may occur because the patient has difficulties in adjusting to lifestyle changes. It is usually characterized by guilt feelings, anxiety, and agitation. These patients usually respond well to tricyclics.

Finally, endogenous depression has also been classified as psychotic or neurotic. In psychotic endogenous depression, the patient's thought processes are impaired, and these patients may respond to an antipsychotic.

Depression may be the first symptom of a serious medical disease. It may also be caused or aggravated by many drugs used chronically in the elderly.

The decreased motility in idiopathic Parkinson disease may resemble the physical signs of retarded depression (Salzman and Shader 1978a). The patient may exhibit lassitude, weakness, and slowness. Mask-like facies may be mistaken for depression. In Parkinson disease, 40% to 90% of the patients may have depression. Brain tumors, small silent strokes, REM sleep deprivation, and bacterial infections may be associated with depression. The severity of depression depends on the organ system involved and its role in the maintenance of life. For example, cardiac illness or cancer almost always produces severe depressive illness.

Pernicious anemia commonly produces depression in the elderly, as may an altered electrolyte balance secondary to impaired renal function. Apathy is fairly common in uremia. Endocrine abnormalities can alter the affective state. For example, depression was common in one group of hypothyroid patients (Bahemuka and Hodkinson 1975), but regular screening for thyroid abnormalities is thought to be unnecessary (Henschke and Pain 1977). Depression associated with guilt and shame is common in elderly patients who have lost a body part or function.

The elderly are also particularly at risk for iatrogenic illness secondary to direct or indirect drug action. The overuse or incorrect use of drugs has been cited as one of the major causes of depression in the elderly. Depression, as a matter of fact, may have been caused or exacerbated by any one of such diverse drugs as digitalis, anticancer drugs, corticosteroids, the psychotropics, propranolol, procainamide, or phenobarbital. The price of lowering blood pressure is often mental depression and antihypertensives are very likely to induce true mood depression (Hollister 1972; Lewis 1971). As many as 50% to 70% of patients receiving antihypertensives may exhibit sadness, apathy, agitation, and insomnia. Older persons are more likely to experience such depression. Depression associated with reserpine administration probably occurs as the drug depletes the CNS adrenergic neurons of norepinephrine, serotonin, and dopamine (Faucett et al 1957). Patients over the age of 70 years are particularly at risk to psychiatric reactions when treated with L-dopa (Winkelman and DiPalma 1971). Thus, unquestionably, depression in the elderly could well be caused by drugs and this should be taken into consideration in the differential diagnosis (Salzman and Shader 1978b).

About one-half of depressed patients present initially with somatic complaints such as insomnia, anorexia, weight loss, aches and pains, or gastrointestinal disorders. If a medical workup is negative, the problem is likely to be an affective disorder (Murphy 1977). Depression is usually diagnosed if a patient presents with depressed mood and if four or five of the associated symptoms in Table 22-7 are present. Depressed mood is usually characterized by any or all of the following: feeling of sadness, down in the dumps, being discouraged, feeling blue, despondent, hopeless, or gloomy (Bureau of Drugs 1976). Of greatest importance is the determination of a possible change from the patient's previous state.

Depression often masquerades as dementia and/or overlaps it. Poor concentration, difficulties in solving everyday problems, indecisiveness, and impaired memory (Kahn et al 1975) easily mimic dementia. To differentiate between the two disorders or to determine coexistence, subjective observations must be used extensively. Clinical impressions, patient response to cognitive function tests, and neurologic findings must all be used.

The diagnostic process must take into account that depression is often atypical in older age (Kelly et al 1977). "Learned" helplessness may be present (Seligman 1975) and the somatic equivalent may differ. There is a significant increase of complaints about fatigue, insomnia,

Table 22-7
Associated Symptoms of Depression

Depressed mood
Anhedonia—inability to experience pleasure
Poor appetite or weight loss
Sleep difficulty (insomnia or hypersomnia)
Loss of energy; fatigue; lethargy
Agitation
Retardation
Decrease in libido
Loss of interest in work and usual activities
Feelings of self-reproach or guilt
Diminished ability to think or concentrate, such as slowed thinking or mixed-up thoughts
Thoughts of death and/or suicide attempts
Feelings of helplessness and hopelessness
Anxiety or tension
Bodily complaints

anxiety, and "low spirits" with increasing age (Gurland 1976). As previously noted, in the elderly, depressive illness can also cause brain decompensation eliciting signs of organic brain syndrome (Goldfarb 1967). In the very early stages of depression, there may be sudden changes in odor perception and taste, and dry and burning mouth may be present. In the elderly patient, who frequently suffers from impaired smell and taste and from dry and burning mouth, these indications would not be helpful. Elderly patients often overestimate their memory impairment and, in the elderly, depression frequently presents as anxiety.

It is still suggested that depression, and particularly mild depression, need not be treated. Treatment, it has been suggested, may well suppress the patient's own coping mechanism. However, the risks of inappropriate treatment are small, compared to the benefits that can be gained and the risk of no treatment (Talley 1977). The greatest risk, particularly among the severely depressed elderly, is their fear that there is no help, which can lead to suicide attempts. While suicide attempts are more frequent in younger age, successful suicide attempts are more frequent in older age. An older person attempting suicide is genuinely serious about it (Dublin 1963). Twenty-five percent of all suicides in the United States occur in the group 65 years and older (Butler and Lewis 1973). Psychoactive drugs are often used in suicide attempts (Ghodse 1977) and there is a strong correlation with alcoholism (Joffe 1976). The general suicide rate in the United States is 10 to 11 per 100,000 population, which increases to 150 per 100,000 for elderly, divorced, white males in their seventh decade (Pfeiffer and Busse 1975; Schmidt 1974). Depression should be treated.

Depression is the most treatable emotional disorder of old age. It is generally accepted that a combination of psychotherapy and drug therapy is more effective than either of the modalities alone. If possible, the patient's family should be included in the treatment process. Psychogeriatric sessions are usually fewer, shorter, but closer together. Elderly patients with depression generally respond well to psychotherapy or counseling.

The monoamine oxidase (MAO) inhibitors are excellent antidepressants, but should not be used in the elderly unless all other modalities and treatment approaches have failed. It is simply too difficult to control an elderly's diet sufficiently to prevent severe adverse reactions caused by dietary-drug interactions.

Combinations of antidepressants and anxiolytic agents have been suggested (Brodie et al 1975) and combinations of phenothiazines and tricyclics are often used. This combination is not recommended because the anticholinergic effects of both drugs are additive and can be incapacitating.

The tricyclics are the drugs of choice. They seem to be most effective in severe, abrupt-onset depression, but chronically depressed patients are much less likely to respond. The overall benefit/risk ratio of the tricyclics is favorable. They cause comparatively few severe, adverse factors, but have numerous unpleasant side effects. The physiologic effects can be very disturbing and the patient must be prepared for them. Correct use of the tricyclics involves a certain amount of trial and error, as patients respond in variable fashion (Biggs 1978; Diamond et al 1977; Epstein 1978). In agitated patients, thioridazine may be useful (Cameron et al 1977).

Anxiety This era has been labeled "the age of anxiety." Mental illness, psychiatric problems, stress illness, and functional disorders are some of the names given to psychologic dysfunction associated with many elderly patients. The elderly are particularly susceptible to psychophysiologic vulnerability as they often face a high incidence of chronic illness, reduced financial resources, social isolation, loneliness, and various losses.

Anxiety reactions are common in older persons. They probably present a lesser disturbance than true depression. Thus, anxiety is often viewed as a relatively minor behavioral syndrome in the elderly. Yet, anxiety can be a fearful emotion accompanied by certain physical symptoms and a painful dread of certain life situations (Rickels 1977). It may mimic a number of organic diseases, such as adrenal insufficiency, anemia, hypoglycemia, and cerebral arteriosclerosis (Langsley and Martin 1973).

There is a wide range of symptom complexes which may be associated with anxiety (Table 22-8) which are restated in Table 22-9 (Bureau of Drugs 1976).

Table 22-8
Anxiety: A Constellation of Physical Complaints

System	Symptoms
Cardiovascular	Chest pain, pounding heartbeat, tachycardia
CNS	Tremors, tics, twitching, trembling, restlessness and increased psychomotor activity, profuse sweating, tingling in hands and feet, cold and clammy hands, headaches, dizziness, lightheadedness, sleep disorders, difficulty in concentrating and/or with memory, change in appetite
Gastrointestinal	Constipation or diarrhea, indigestion, distension, nausea
Genitourinary	Change in urinary frequency
Musculoskeletal	Tense, aching muscles
Respiratory	Choking, dyspnea, hyperventilation, lump in throat

Table 22-9
Symptoms of Anxiety

Feeling nervous, jittery, jumpy
Feeling fearful, apprehensive, anxious, panicky
Fears of fainting, screaming, losing control, crowds, places, disaster, death
Avoiding certain places, things, or activities because of fear
Feeling tense or keyed up

Muscular or motor phenomena
  Tense muscles, aches
  Trembling, shaking
  Restlessness, fidgeting

Autonomic phenomena
  Heart beating fast or pounding; chest pain
  Trouble catching breath, air hunger, smothering, lump in throat, choking
  Sweating, especially armpits, palms, soles of feet
  Cold, clammy hands
  Dry mouth
  Dizziness, faintness, lightheadedness, weakness
  Tingling feelings in hands or feet
  Stomach gas, nausea, upset stomach
  Wanting to use the toilet often (urine or bowels)

It is important to elicit the patient's present life situation, family or other support systems, current interests, and concurrent medical problems (Goldstein and Brauger 1971). In assessing the patient with anxiety, it is important to differentiate anxiety as a personality trait from anxiety as a neurotic reaction. The former patient may require constant reassurance and may be unable to cope with ordinary life problems. The latter patient, on the other hand, is usually confident and self-reliant (Abuzzahab 1976) and, therefore, therapeutic management of these patients will differ.

As anxiety, much like other behavioral or psychiatric disturbances, does not present a single target symptom as an infection would, for example, it is not surprising that a large number of drugs have been used and continue to be used in the treatment of anxiety (Table 22-10). Of all, the benzodiazepines are the preferred drugs. They are effective, relatively safe, and useful adjuncts in nondrug management of anxiety.

Specifically, they are almost suicide-proof, do not interfere with the metabolism of other drugs, and their action is long enough so that a once-a-day dose is sufficient. The benzodiazepines are less likely to produce physical dependence than drugs like phenobarbital or meprobamate, and they cause relatively little change in normal sleep patterns. Some factors have now been suggested which can be used to predict a positive response to these antianxiety drugs.

When prescribing any one of the benzodiazepines for an elderly patient, the physician should never write an open-ended prescription. This practice, all too common, is never justified.

Table 22-10
Some Antianxiety and Hypnotic Drugs

Antianxiety	
Benzodiazepines	As a group, the benzodiazepines are less sedating and cause less mental clouding than either the barbiturates or hypnotics
Chlordiazepoxide	Relatively short duration of action
Clorazepate	Moderate duration of action
Diazepam	Moderate duration of action
Oxazepam	Less sedating than diazepam; short duration of action
Lorazepam	Relatively short duration of action
Prazepam	More sedating than diazepam; long duration of action
Propanediols	
Meprobamate	High potential for addiction; not as sedating as diazepam; relatively short duration of action
Tybamate	Less addictive than meprobamate, but not as therapeutically effective
Barbiturates	
Amobarbital	Moderate duration of action
Pentobarbital sodium	Onset of action in 15–30 minutes; moderate duration
Phenobarbital	Long duration of action
Secobarbital sodium	Moderate duration of action
Others	
Chlormezanone	Not as well tolerated as the benzodiazepines
Hypnotics	
Benzodiazepine	
Flurazepam	Safest of the hypnotics; long duration of action
Others	
Chloral hydrate	Short duration of action
Ethchlorvynol	Short duration of action
Ethinamate	Short duration of action; rapid onset
Glutethimide	Does not cause respiratory depression in therapeutic dosages; overdosage can be life-threatening; short duration of action
Methaqualone	Drowsiness ensues within 10–20 minutes; moderate duration of action
Methyprylon	Short duration of action
Triclofos sodium	Short duration of action

Insomnia Sleep and insomnia are still not well understood. It is known that dreams occur during REM (rapid eye movement) sleep and that REM and non-REM sleep differ as to heart rate, respiration rate, muscle tone, cerebral blood flow, and rate of secretion of various hormones (Johns 1972). With aging, REM sleep and Stage 4 slow-wave sleep are decreased (Raskin and Eisdorfer 1977). At the same time, the duration of physiologic sleep decreases with advancing age. A newborn child sleeps more than 16 hours per day, while an elderly person may sleep only five or six hours, indicating that both the quality and quantity of sleep change with age (Blunk and Gross 1971; Koeller and Levin 1973; Jovanovic 1974). However, beyond a certain minimum, the quality of sleep is more important than is its duration (Johns 1972).

A general relationship has been established between age, sex, and sleep (Lasagna 1972). Women in general tend to have more sleep problems than do men.

Unquestionably, the elderly suffer from increased sleep disturbances. While in general it is believed that sleep time tends to decrease with age, it seems clear that most insomniac patients underestimate their actual sleeping time (Regenstein 1976). Total duration of sleep probably does not change with age, but there is a significant increase in the number of wake periods and a significant lengthening in the duration of the wake periods during sleep. Nocturnal wake periods normally increase from less than 5% of time in bed at age 20 to more than 20% at age 85 (Feinberg and Carlson 1968). To the elderly, the most distressing change in sleep pattern may be the increase in nocturnal awakenings.

The normal elderly person also sleeps "lighter" than younger persons, and many of the elderly focus on sleep problems to avoid facing an underlying condition (Kales and Kales 1973). With advancing age, patients complain increasingly that they sleep badly, not long enough, or not at all. The type of sleep problem most often encountered, ie, problems with falling asleep, staying asleep, or early awakening indeed, seems to be related to age rather than to psychopathology.

Psychiatric illnesses often are the cause of sleep disturbances in the elderly. Depression, often seen in the elderly, is often accompanied by changed sleep patterns and changes are especially pronounced in patients with senile dementia. The psycho-organic deficiency syndrome of the elderly is responsible for a characteristic increase in the frequency and duration of wake periods between sleep, and emotional reactions to any disease may also cause insomnia. Uncomfortable and painful conditions, such as arthritis and other pain syndromes, dyspnea, endocrine disorders, congestive heart failure, and fever also may impair normal sleep. Inadequate regulation of blood sugar may lead to glycosuria and nocturia in the elderly, again disturbing sleep. On the other hand, hypoglycemic episodes, which can mimic anxiety attacks with sympathetic hyperactivity, can be the cause of sleep disturbances.

Many sleep disorders of the elderly may be caused by nutritional deficiencies. When protein intake is deficient, there will be a concurrent deficiency in amino acids, which are important in the regulation of sleep.

Many drugs are known to cause insomnia. Among these are the centrally-acting adrenergic blockers and the hypnotics. The rapidly-acting diuretics, if given late in the day or in the evening, also can worsen sleep.

Finally, daytime naps interfere with nighttime sleep, as do many environmental factors such as noise, temperature, and humidity. The elderly who complain of sleep disorders should be cautioned to avoid coffee and other stimulants.

The differential diagnosis should establish whether the patient has difficulty in falling asleep or remaining asleep, as well as possible early morning awakening. The total sleep time should be established, if possible, including daytime naps. It is important to establish how long the patient has been troubled by insomnia and whether or not its onset coincided with some external or internal change.

Careful attention should be paid to the specific etiology of insomnia. Stress, pain, melancholia, poorly timed diuretics, and other conditions causing insomnia may call for different treatment strategies. In other words, primary sleep disorders, ie, those in which disordered sleep is the only sign and symptom of abnormality, would be treated differently from a secondary sleep disorder, where the underlying condition must be treated (Williams and Karacan 1973).

Therefore, the patient should be carefully checked for organic diseases such as heart or respiratory failure. A neurologic examination should identify the presence or absence of any diseases which could give rise to pain or discomforts, such as restless legs. The possibility of mental disorders and diseases should be considered, as well as cerebrovascular insufficiency.

Indeed, particular sleep disturbance can indicate the underlying disease or disorder. For example, painful conditions, anxiety, or apprehension can cause a patient difficulty in falling asleep. They are also responsible for frequent awakenings and restless sleep. Depression, though, which is an extremely frequent cause of insomnia in the elderly, causes early morning awakening. Metabolic abnormalities and tension anxieties are usually responsible for a patient's difficulty in remaining asleep (Hartman 1977; Kahn and Fisher 1969; Feinberg 1968).

The key to the selection of treatment modality for insomnia in the elderly is a thoughtful consideration of the question: Should this particular sleep disturbance be treated with drugs? Hypnotics, in general, should not be used until and unless every other treatment modality has been tried and found to be unsuccessful.

If the differential diagnosis identified certain environmental factors as causes, then every effort should be made to eliminate those. Daytime naps are, of course, highly undesirable, but increased interest in daytime activities, exercise, or any increased physical activity will improve sleep. Quite often, treatment of insomnia in the elderly will revolve around treatment of an underlying disease. When depression is suspected, for example, a tricyclic antidepressant may be indicated, possibly amitriptyline or doxepin, in a single bedtime dose. At other times, control of hypoglycemia or hyperglycemia is indicated, or the use of a benzodiazepine for anxious patients may be considered. When a hypnotic seems to be indicated, a number of considerations should enter into the prescribing process. Long-term use of hypnotics is rarely indicated and often undesirable. Hypnotic use, if essential, should be occasional and not habitual.

Clinical evidence indicates that the elderly are more susceptible to the effects of these drugs than the general population. This may be caused by a difference in the sensitivity of drug receptors with advancing age or to age-related changes in pharmacokinetic factors or a combination of both. These drugs may cause lethargy, slurred speech, tremor, and insomnia. With the possible exception of the benzodiazepines, there is no hypnotic that cannot be used successfully for suicidal purposes. Therefore, only small amounts should be prescribed at a time. The elderly may respond to hypnotics with a paradoxical excitement related to a decrease in sensory cues that occurs in darkness.

Finally, use of hypnotics can lead to aggravation of chronic clinical syndromes of certain diseases during sleep. Cardiovascular, respiratory, and neuromuscular disorders can all be aggravated by prolonged sleep. The elderly are susceptible to nocturnal pseudohemiplegia, a numbness and immobility of one arm or side of the body. Night cramps and abnormally wide swings in blood sugar concentrations can also occur with prolongation of sleep (Williams and Karacan 1973). The hypnotic selected should induce sleep rapidly, not disturb normal sleep, reduce the number of awakenings, and have few daytime after-effects. Most importantly, the drug should not induce tolerance and habituation, which many elderly fear, and should not be able to be used in suicide attempts. Of all drugs currently available, flurazepam probably best meets these requirements (Hartman 1977). If the patient has particular difficulty in falling asleep, chloral hydrate or oxazepam is most often recommended.

Paranoid Disorders

Paranoid ideation occurs in the elderly of both sexes, but it occurs more often in men than in women. Loss of hearing ability, impairment of visual acuity, or other physical deficiencies combine to lead to misinterpretations of incidents. Poorly heard conversations are transformed and there is confusion with reality.

Neurologic Disorders

The central nervous system is a dynamic system which has enormous reserves. Morphologic changes do not parallel chronologic progression of neurologic disorders and physiologic aberrations are often independent of anatomical changes.

Parkinson disease Parkinson disease is a progressive neurologic disorder that affects the brain centers controlling movement. It was formerly called "shaking palsy." It occurs insidiously in older persons, and produces a slowly increasing movement disability (Bianchine 1976). The idiopathic type (paralysis agitans) is associated with diffuse cortical atrophy, especially in the frontal lobes. Other forms are also recognized, such as arteriosclerotic Parkinson disease, caused by multiple cerebrovascular accidents, and postencephalitic Parkinson disease.

Coordinated muscle control depends upon a balance between the cholinergic and dopaminergic systems. Parkinson disease probably develops if one or the other of these two systems develops either overactivity or underactivity. Currently, parkinsonism is considered a striatal dopamine deficiency syndrome. In the elderly, there is a significant reduction of dopamine and its metabolites and in glutamic acid dehydrogenase, the enzyme which decarboxylates glutamic acid to form gamma amino butyric acid. There may also be changes in the receptor sites for these neurotransmitters (Beasley and Ford 1976). Parkinson disease consists of the clinical tetrad of akinesia (poverty of spontaneous movements, mask-like facies), rigidity of muscular tone, a characteristic tremor in repose, and an aberration of postural mechanisms (flexed position of stance, difficulty in turning, hurried gait) (Cohen and Scheife 1977).

Parkinson disease affects the brain center involved in the control and regulation of movement. Because of disordered control of movement, rigidity of muscles develops, accompanied by uncontrollable trembling of the extremities, stooped posture, loss of facial expression, and difficulty in walking, talking, or any activity requiring a high degree of muscular coordination. Slowness of movement accompanies rigidity, and movements become very deliberate, abbreviated, and stiff. In advanced stages, there may be impairment of postural reflexes, reduced blinking, microphagia, and microphonia (Bianchine 1976). The tremor of Parkinson disease, usually five or six cycles per second, tends to decrease or disappear on purposeful movements. It is increased by excitement, self-consciousness, fatigue, or cold. It disappears during sleep.

Symptoms may also be caused, and indeed are not infrequently caused in the elderly by drugs which decrease CNS dopamine, such as the butyrophenones, thioxanthenes, and phenothiazines. In drug-induced parkinsonism, akinesia and rigidity predominate, while tremors are less prominent. Drugs with strong anticholinergic action rarely cause the symptoms of parkinsonism, while those with little or no anticholinergic activity can be expected to cause them on prolonged use.

Treatment of Parkinson disease is at best uncertain, unsatisfactory, and, in the long run, unsuccessful. In clinical practice, antiparkinsonism drugs are still often used when antipsychotics are chronically administered. It was believed that the antiparkinsonism drugs would "prevent" the occurrence of Parkinson disease. It is now generally agreed that there is no foundation for this belief and that concurrent administration of these drugs should not be used, as it exposes the elderly patient to increased adverse effects. If these drugs must be used, they should be used only for a short course of therapy.

Treatment, in general, involves the manipulation of the dopamine-acetylcholine system. It may involve augmentation of the synthesis of brain dopamine, using levodopa. It may also involve an attempt to stimulate dopamine receptors directly. Bromocriptine shows considerable promise, although the drug has not yet been approved for this use. Amantadine, which may be effective in about 60% of patients receiving it, is used to stimulate dopamine release, while the tricyclic antidepressants are sometimes used in an effort to decrease dopamine re-uptake by presynaptic sites.

PSYCHOPHARMACOLOGIC DRUGS

The elderly do not receive a fair share of mental health services (Special Committee on Aging 1971). One of the reasons might be an apparent over-reliance on drug use. Psychopharmacologic drugs alter perception, intellectual function, mood, behavior, and consciousness. Unquestionably, the use of psychoactive drugs to regulate personal and interpersonal processes is increasing (Lennard et al 1970), as a result of efforts to treat societal needs with drugs (Lennard and Bernstein 1974; Lennard et al 1971). While these drugs can be powerful and effective tools in the management of mental disorders of the elderly, their use should not and cannot take the place of an overall treatment program. Their use constitutes only one part of such a program. If possible, it is best to avoid drug therapy (Bergmann 1974) and drug use should be preceded and paralleled by a continuous physical and social evaluation of the patient. Before prescribing a psychotropic drug, the physician must remember that those over 65 years of age are twice as likely to receive a prescription after a physician-patient encounter than are younger patients. Those over 65 years of age receive three times as many prescriptions as do younger patients and women receive twice as many as men. If an adverse effect occurs, the elderly are more likely to be vulnerable to these effects and more than likely will take twice as long to recover from them as will younger patients. Furthermore, use of psychotropic drugs is difficult. Most other drugs are used to treat a specific disease or problem, and drug specificity is one of the major achievements of modern drug development. Psychotropic drugs, on the other hand, produce a wide range of physiologic responses, many of them undesirable. This frequently will necessitate the addition of another drug to a psychotropic drug regimen to control the nonspecific actions of the first drug (Lennard et al 1970).

Long-term treatment of intellectual disorders of the elderly is similar to chronic treatment of medical diseases. In many instances, unfortunately, treatment does not cure but is relatively effective in improving the patient's quality of life (Verwoerdt 1976; Klerman 1978). While at one hand there have been widespread concerns with and claims of overuse and misuse of these drugs, particularly among the elderly, it is also true that to ignore the use of these drugs would constitute neglect of an important therapeutic element. It has even been suggested that in many instances physicians may be hesitant to use these drugs thus withholding from patients therapy which could be extremely helpful and necessary. What is needed is thoughtful and rational use of these drugs, based on an appreciation of the relationship between somatic, psychologic, and interpersonal alterations brought about by aging and disease (Salzman et al 1976).

For elderly patients, psychotropic drugs are commonly prescribed for behavior disorders, depression, anxiety and apprehension, cognitive and memory impairment, and sleep disturbance. Therapy is aimed at altering abnormal behavior and at the restoration of mental and emotional equilibrium. Use of these drugs, however, should not be expected to resolve conflicts, affect personal or social attitudes, or eliminate undesirable mental habits (Berger 1976b).

Overuse (Barton and Hurst 1966) and misuse of these drugs is thought to be common, possibly because of a lack of knowledge of the physiology, pharmacology, pharmacokinetics, and toxicology of psychotropic drugs (Gottlieb et al 1978). Misprescribing of psychotropic drugs often stems from lack of certainty as to their indications and unfamiliarity with all their incompatibilities and side effects. There may be a missed diagnosis and somatic complaints may be attributed to side effects of these medications. An underdose or failure to wait an appropriate time to elicit a desired effect could lead to treatment failure. Abrupt discontinuance of medication can lead to severe undesirable effects. Failure to know and respond to side effects may cause a patient to discontinue a drug. Drug-drug interactions involving these drugs are common, as may be drug-disease interactions. For example, caution is indicated when psychotropic drugs are used in dementia, as these drugs may worsen the patient's mental disturbance. Their use can also lead to chronic oversedation which in turn can be responsible for such complications as pneumonia, bedsores, or dehydration. In short, adverse reactions to psychotropic drugs occur frequently in the elderly (Hall 1974). One side effect frequently overlooked is the peripheral anticholinergic action of most antipsychotics and antidepressants. It is particularly threatening to the elderly who are likely to receive several drugs with an anticholinergic effect, which can be worsened by the use of certain nonprescription drugs such as the antihistamines. The anticholinergic potency of some drugs is given in Table 22-10a. Constipation is common in geropsychiatric patients (Van der Kolk et al 1978) but is even more frequent in patients receiving potent anticholinergics. Chronic drug-induced constipation may lead to dilatation of the intestine, which is most frequently seen associated with the use of the tricyclics or the aliphatic and piperidine phenothiazines. Anticholinergic drugs can also decrease salivary flow, already diminished in the elderly, and provoke dental caries and undesirable changes in nutritional intake. Urinary retention, particularly in the elderly male with a prostatic involvement, has been reported with the tricyclics, the phenothiazines, and the butyrophenones. This happens when antipsychotics are combined with antiparkinsonism drugs.

The cholinergic stimulation of the sphincter muscle of the iris and the ciliary muscle of the lens can be blocked by anticholinergic drugs, leading to mydriasis and cycloplegia. Finally, these drugs, through a central effect to which the elderly are apparently more susceptible than are younger patients, also may produce anxiety, delirium, agitation, visual and auditory hallucinations, and convulsions. It is easy to see that some of these side effects may be mistaken for intellectual disturbances and may be treated with increased doses of psychotropic drugs.

Certain patient characteristics apparently also influence use of psychotropic drugs. It seems that anxiety, low mental status, and unfriendliness influence their use (Milliren 1977), and that women are more likely to receive these drugs than men (Cooperstock 1971). Apparently, women are more likely than men to report symptoms of mental disturbance and seek treatment for it. It has also been suggested that health care providers presume emotional instability in women more so than in men and, therefore, tend to prescribe more mood-altering drugs for women (Cooperstock 1971).

Table 22-10a
Anticholinergic Potency (%)

Atropine, scopolamine	100
Benztropine, trihexyphenidyl	20–50
Amitriptyline	10
Thioridazine	1
Imipramine	0.8

Classification of Psychopharmacologic Drugs

There are many psychopharmacologic drugs (Table 22-11) and various terms have been used to describe different classes of these drugs (Eisdorfer 1975). Possibly, much of the uncertainty about these drugs is based on the profusion of terms that have been applied to them.

It was common, at one time, to divide these drugs into major and minor tranquilizers, indicating that large doses of a minor tranquilizer may possibly equal the effects of a normal dose of a major tranquilizer. This is inappropriate and it has been suggested that these terms no longer be used. Nevertheless, they are still frequently used. The antipsychotics were at one time termed neuroleptics, as their effects can mimic the effects of neurologic disease. It has also been suggested that the psychopharmacologic drugs can be divided into the psychotropic

Table 22-11
Some Geropsychiatric Drugs

Antipsychotic Agents	Antianxiety Agents	Antidepressant Agents
Phenothiazines	Barbiturates	Tricyclic derivatives
Aliphatic derivatives	Phenobarbital	Amitriptyline
Chlorpromazine		Desipramine
Promazine	Dibenzoxepines	Doxepin
	Chlordiazepoxide	Imipramine
Piperazine derivatives	Diazepam	Nortriptyline
Perphenazine	Oxazepam	Protriptyline
Trifluoperazine	Clorazepate	
Prochlorperazine	Lorazepam	
Acetophenazine		
	Others	
Piperadine derivatives	Hydroxyzine	
Thioridazine	Meprobamate	
Mesoridazine		
Dibenzoxazepine		
Loxapine		
Butyrophenone		
Haloperidol		
Dihydroindolone		
Molidone		
Thioxanthenes		
Thiothixene		
Chlorprothixene		
Rauwolfia alkaloid		
Reserpine		

drugs, ie, those drugs used to treat psychiatric diseases, and the psychoactive drugs, ie, those drugs used for nontherapeutic purposes such as personal enjoyment. Of late, there seems to be a tendency to classify all psychopharmacologic drugs as psychoactive drugs, as all can alter perception, intellectual function, mood, behavior, and consciousness.

Psychotropic drugs can also be divided into the psychotherapeutic drugs (antipsychotics, antianxiety agents, antidepressants, and stimulants) and the psychotomimetic drugs, ie, those drugs that can induce psychosis-like symptoms (Cooper et al 1978). The antipsychotics would be those drugs which have been variously called ataractics, neuroleptics, and major tranquilizers. The antidepressants have also been called thymoleptics, and the antianxiety agents are frequently referred to as anxiolytics, relaxants, or minor tranquilizers.

Probably the clinically most useful classification divides the psychotropic drugs into the antipsychotics, the antidepressives, the antimanics, the antianxiety agents, and the cognitive-acting drugs (Hollister 1973). However, this classification does not include the sedative-hypnotics.

Final Considerations

Before prescribing psychopharmacologic drugs for an elderly patient, the physician should be familiar with the important seven points outlined in Table 22-12, (deGrott 1974) and should remember that use of psychopharmacologic drugs will be followed by numerous adverse effects (Stotsky 1970), which are outlined in general form in Table 22-13.

Table 22-12
Considerations for the Clinical Use of Psychotherapeutic Drugs in the Elderly

Know pharmacologic action of drug
Know metabolic and excretion processes
Use lowest effective dose; accomplish this by titrating patient
Use minimum number of drugs
Avoid symptomatic treatment with drugs
Do not withhold medication because a patient is "too old"
Do not use drug longer than necessary

The Antipsychotics

These drugs were once termed "tranquilizers." This is a misnomer. They do not simply sedate or reduce anxiety, but appear to have unique antipsychotic properties (Baldessarini 1977).

Table 22-13
Possible Adverse Effects of Psychopharmacologic Drugs in the Elderly

---

Expect therapeutic effects at lower initial dose

Expect toxic side effects, even at lower dose, particularly neurologic and cardiovascular effects; watch for severe jaundice, anemia, dermatologic reactions

Watch for long-term side effects; psychotropic agents may cause changes in pigmentation, tardive dyskinesia

CNS side effects are not uncommon, such as dyskinesia and parkinsonism-like effects

There may be hypotension, arrhythmias, and congestive failure

Agitation, insomnia, and excitement (paradoxical reactions) occur often following administration of phenobarbital and chloral hydrate

Expect severe adverse reactions at night; drugs that increase confusion or decrease cognitive control may heighten symptoms patient experiences at night, such as hallucinations or delusional behavior

---

Before the use of an antipsychotic is considered as part of patient management, any possibility that the patient's symptoms are drug-induced should be eliminated. Symptoms of confusion, disorientation, agitation, or disturbances in level of consciousness in the elderly may have a basis in physical disease or drug toxicity. In anticipating treatment outcome, it must be considered that many drugs may interact with the antipsychotics. In some patients, this kind of interaction can lead to acutely psychotic states, while in others a regressive state may result. Physically ill patients and patients with dementia require much lower doses than do patients with functional psychoses who are physically well.

While the initial dose for antipsychotics for elderly patients is usually recommended to be one-quarter to one-third of the usual adult dose, it is often overlooked that inadequate dosages of these drugs may lead to increased confusion and emotional disturbances.

In general, drug therapy dominates the psychiatric treatment of behavior disorders. The efficacy of these drugs is limited by their inherent toxicities and their possible misuse. Variability in drug responsiveness also increases with age. Nevertheless, the use of psychotherapeutic agents increases significantly with increasing patient age, as does length of therapy. It is exceedingly disturbing to note that, contrary to expectations, the doses used for these drugs in the elderly are usually higher than recommended (Friedel 1978). In general, the value of therapy with antipsychotic drugs declines with patient age and with the chronicity of the disease. Social therapy then becomes more and more important. There is no indication that a combination of antipsychotic drugs or a combination of an antipsychotic agent and a tricyclic will yield better results than the use of an antipsychotic drug alone (Charalampous 1978).

Classification The antipsychotics do not constitute a homogeneous group of drugs, either chemically, pharmacologically, or psychopharmacologically (Bignami 1978). While the exact mechanism of their action is still not fully understood, all antipsychotics have a strong antidopaminergic action, which presumably accounts for their effects on psychotic symptoms. All, except the rauwolfia derivatives, block central dopaminergic transmission. Reserpine decreases the level of biogenic brain amines, particularly dopamine. The following classes of antipsychotics are available:

1. Phenothiazine derivatives of the chlorpromazine type with aliphatic side chains (chlorpromazine), with piperidyl side chains (thioridazine), or with piperazinyl side chains (fluphenazine).
2. Thioxanthene derivatives, which resemble the phenothiazine derivatives structurally and in their pharmacologic and therapeutic action.
3. The tricyclic psychopharmacologic agents, in which category the dibenzodiazepine derivatives, such as clozapine, and the azaphenothiazines are listed. The tricyclic piperazine, loxapine, is one of the newer drugs.
4. The butyrophenones, of which haloperidol is the outstanding example.
5. The indole derivatives, such as reserpine, which are no longer of any significance for practical antipsychotic therapy. Molindone is one of the newer indole derivates which shows certain promise.

Indications for antipsychotics The antipsychotics are specific remedies acting on the basic processes responsible for the manifestations of the schizophrenic state (Freeman 1967).

Most importantly, the antipsychotics are used in psychotic excitement and all other syndromes associated with psychomotor disturbances and in psychotic states with symptoms of mental derangement delusions, schizophrenic ego disorders, and disturbances of the formal thinking process. However, the therapeutic range of these drugs is not strictly limited to the schizophrenic psychoses.

These drugs are sometimes used in managing affective (manic or depressive) disorders and even organic psychoses. They are also of value in various types of paranoid illnesses. Some patients with mild or moderate dementia who function well during the daytime may exhibit the sundown syndrome. The confusional state responds fairly well to thioridazine or chlorpromazine. Others, like haloperidol and perphenazine also appear to be effective and have less anticholinergic and cardiovascular toxicity. In dementia, these drugs cannot restore mental faculties of elderly patients, but, paralleled by social and occupational intervention, they can increase the patient's quality of life. Small doses of the less-sedating phenothiazines or haloperidol may help agitation, but patients with intercurrent parkinsonism should probably be treated with thioridazine (Gardos and Cole 1976).

Drug of choice The antipsychotics are the single most effective aspect of the management of acute or active psychoses (Baldessarini and Lipinski 1973). Yet, their use is not indispensable and, more importantly, their use is not without serious risks, particularly in the elderly. It is also important to note that the difference between those patients treated with drugs and those not treated with drugs decreases with time (Crane 1973a). These drugs are still selected on an empirical basis, as clinically, the antipsychotics are equally effective. Their relative potencies are given in Table 22-14. For reasons not clear, some patients will respond better to one drug than another. There is still no reliable index to predict which patient will respond in an optimal manner to a particular drug. Therefore, a particular drug is often chosen based on the expected quality and intensity of side effects and the patient's capacity to tolerate them. In short, the physician prescribing an antipsychotic will select a drug by considering side effects such as sedation, hypotension, or parkinsonian symptoms. An effort must be made to obtain an optimal balance between therapeutic and side effects (Frazer and Winokur 1977).

Table 22-14
Equivalency of Oral Antipsychotic Drugs

Name	Approximate Equivalent (mg)
Fluphenazine	1.0
Haloperidol	1.0
Thiothixene	2.0
Trifluoperazine	2.5
Molindone	5.0
Perphenazine	5.0
Loxapine	5.0
Butaperazine	5.0
Piperacetazine	5.5
Prochlorperazine	7.5
Acetophenazine	10.0
Carphenazine	12.5
Triflupromazine	14.0
Mesoridazine	28.0
Chlorprothixene	50.0
Chlorpromazine	50.0
Thioridazine	50.0
Promazine	100.0

Thioridazine is widely assumed to be the drug of choice, although it does cause electrocardiographic changes and gynecologic and genitourinary symptoms. Many clinicians feel that haloperidol is probably as effective and produces no more serious side effects, although studies to document effectiveness are singularly lacking (Cole and Stotsky 1974).

The key factor to effective treatment is the dosage selected. In many elderly, an almost homeopathic dose should be used initially, for example 10 to 25 mg of thioridazine or 0.25 mg of haloperidol, keeping in mind that the vigorous elderly will need a different dose than the frail elderly. The danger inherent in this approach is undertreatment. Thus, for optimum effect, a low starting dose should be selected, the patient should be carefully monitored, and the dose increased, if necessary, after the low dose has been retained for one or two weeks.

While these theoretical considerations are fairly clear, even when a reasonably homogeneous group of patients is observed, one finds little uniformity in the dosage of antipsychotics prescribed. It is of interest to note that those patients receiving large doses for prolonged periods of time present the most serious management problems (Crane 1973a).

In general, the maintenance dose must be based on clinical observations, which includes the possible development of tolerance both to the side effects and the therapeutic effects. Currently, the monitoring of plasma concentrations does not offer any advantage to the clinician, as there are large variations in blood levels in reponse to a given dose of any of these drugs and as there are no guidelines available as yet as to optimum levels.

Consensus, at one time, indicated the need for continuation of antipsychotic therapy, as a significant number of patients seem to depend on it for continued existence in the community. Thus, it was suggested continued therapy was needed to prevent relapse. However, it has now been suggested that a re-examination of this belief is needed because of the serious and sometimes irreversible complications of prolonged antipsychotic therapy. It appears that the majority of patients who relapse after withdrawal of an antipsychotic recompensate fairly rapidly once drug administration is resumed (Gardos and Cole 1976). Many studies have shown that long-term phenothiazines could be withdrawn from patients without any adverse effects (Pathy 1977).

Utilization data are practically nonexistent. In one large survey, it was found that of 1276 psychiatric patients 60 years and older, 61% were receiving psychopharmacologic drugs (Prien 1975; Prien et al 1975). Forty-five percent of the patients were treated with a single drug, and thioridazine was most frequently prescribed. With increasing age, there was a decreasing use of antianxiety agents, antipsychotics, and antidepressant drugs, but an increasing use of drugs such as dihydroergotoxine. In general, history of cardiovascular disease or stroke or a serious threat from hypotension indicates the use of a piperazine phenothiazine or haloperidol. Haloperidol is also often preferred when the patient has a compromised hepatic function (Charalampous 1978). If sedation is unacceptable, a phenothiazine such as perphenazine or haloperidol would probably be selected, which also may help in agitation, given in small doses. Patients with intercurrent Parkinson disease probably respond best to thioridazine (Gardos and Cole 1976).

Loxapine differs chemically from the phenothiazines, the thioxanthenes, and the butyrophenones. One-half of an oral dose is excreted within 24 hours. Up to 70% is excreted through the kidney and almost 20% through the gastrointestinal tract. Peak serum levels occur within two hours and range from 0.006 to 0.0013 mg/ml. Its major metabolite is 8-hydroxyloxapine. The drug has a sedating effect, causes initially transient drowsiness and causes extrapyramidal reactions. Most studies on loxapine so far have involved patients previously treated with other antipsychotics. Thus, the prognosis for these patients would be poor, as prolonged duration of a psychosis impoverishes the patient's affect and only a poor therapeutic response would be expected. However, loxapine is reported to have had good antipsychotic effects even in those patients (Fann and Wheless 1978).

Molindone is an indole derivate which produces its effects without muscle relaxation or incoordination. Peak blood levels are reached one hour after administration and its duration of action is about 36 hours after a single oral dose. The drug is rapidly metabolized by the liver, 90% of it being excreted within 24 hours. The therapeutic dose in geriatric patients may be as low as 1 mg. Side effects are similar to and occur to the same degree as with phenothiazines. Elderly patients are more likely than young patients to develop parkinsonian symptoms. To achieve sedation, the drug must be coadministered with a hypnotic or a sedative phenothiazine (Ayd 1974).

The phenothiazines, in general, act specifically on agitation, violent and irrational behavior, and perceptual disturbances. They still remain the first choice in most elderly patients showing disturbed behavior due to clouding of consciousness (Bergmann 1974). Apparently, the phenothiazines are of no value in the memory deficit of geriatric patients, but they may have some effect in anxious states. Nevertheless, the antianxiety drugs are preferred, as the phenothiazines may also decrease the patient's activity. Thioridazine may sometimes be effective in anxious depression, while chlorpromazine may be effective in agitated depression. Treatment of elderly schizophrenics should probably be started with a high-potency drug (Branchey et al 1978). The phenothiazines often have unpredictable effects. A paradoxical response to phenothiazines can easily be misinterpreted as treatment failure and be responded to by an increase, rather than the necessary decrease in dose (Pathy 1977).

Similarly, patients receiving fluphenazine or haloperidol can develop a syndrome marked by features of catatonia, which may easily be confused with a worsening of schizophrenic symptoms and be responded to with an increase in dose rather than the necessary withdrawal of the drug (Gelenberg and Mandel 1977). If drug withdrawal is undesirable, the patient may respond to amantadine or an anticholinergic drug. Treatment is often difficult as the therapeutic end points of these drugs are often not clear and the signs and symptoms are often vague.

High dosage regimens are probably of very limited value in elderly chronic patients. Starting doses of drugs such as chlorpromazine or thioridazine should not exceed 30 mg per day and often should be even lower. For other drugs, such as perphenazine or trifluoperazine, the initial dose should not exceed 2 mg twice or three times daily (Joffe 1978).

The phenothiazines differ mainly in their potencies and the nature of their toxicities (Rivera-Calimlim 1977). It is most often suggested that the specific phenothiazine to be chosen should be selected on the basis of its expected side effects, which are most often simply an extension of their therapeutic actions (Table 22-15). Some are believed to be more sedating and others more activating. It has been questioned whether that differentiation is really of benefit, as sedation in most instances is short-lived and the stimulation caused by the more potent piperazine phenothiazines is more in the form of restlessness than useful psychomotor activation (Cole 1976). When sedation is required, thioridazine is probably the best choice. It causes extrapyramidal symptoms (EPS) infrequently, though it causes pigmentary retinopathy (Gardos and Cole 1976). Hypotension and sedation are less likely with perphenazine, fluphenazine, trifluoperazine, or haloperidol, but they all can cause parkinsonism-like syndromes.

Table 22-15
Relative Side Effects of Phenothiazines

Name	Sedation	Hypotension	Extra-pyramidal symptoms
Chlorpromazine	Marked	Occasional	Occasional
Thioridazine	Moderate	Moderate	Infrequent
Acetophenazine	Mild	Mild	Occasional
Trifluoperazine	Minimal	Minimal	Frequent

The difficulties inherent in the use of antipsychotic drugs in the elderly can be illustrated using chlorpromazine as an example. This drug has 168 possible metabolites of which 70 have so far been identified (Rivera-Calimlim et al 1976; Rivera-Calimlim 1977). It can cause sedation and postural hypotension, but tolerance to these effects may develop within a few weeks. This may be a metabolic tolerance, in that the drug may induce its own metabolism, thus lowering plasma levels. It may also be a tissue tolerance. The drug potentiates the effects of alcohol, sedatives, and narcotics. Trihexyphenidyl, an anticholinergic often given in association with the drug, antagonizes the therapeutic effect of chlorpromazine, which in turn inhibits the metabolism of the tricyclics, increasing their plasma levels. Lithium also reduces chlorpromazine blood levels and oral antacids may interfere with the bioavailability of chlorpromazine. The drug should be used with caution in patients receiving antihypertensive medications. Of 566 patients treated with chlorpromazine, 12.2% had adverse reactions and in 1.2% the adverse reaction was considered life-threatening. Adverse reactions apparently occur more frequently with high doses and the parenteral route of administration (Swett 1975b).

Side and adverse effects of antipsychotics Many of the adverse reactions involving the antipsychotics are due to drug interactions. The incidence of these interactions increases with age, and mesoridazine and chlorpromazine are most often implicated (Ayd 1975a). Interactions can occur very quickly in the elderly. For example, an elderly patient may receive a phenothiazine for agitation. The phenothiazine has an anticholinergic effect and may well be the cause of extrapyramidal symptoms. These symptoms may be treated with an antiparkinson drug, which also may have an anticholinergic action. If the patient then purchases one or two nonprescription drugs, such as a sleep medication and possibly a cold preparation containing an antihistamine, the anticholinergic effects may aggravate glaucoma, or cause xerostomia, ileus, hypotension, urinary retention, and cardiac irregularities. Urinary retention caused by antipsychotics is dose-related and can be treated with bethanechol or diphenhydramine. The combination of all these drugs with anticholinergic action may produce the so-called "central anticholinergic syndrome," in which an atropine-like psychosis is superimposed on the primary psychiatric disorder. The psychotic symptoms will worsen and there will be disturbance of immediate memory, disorientation, visual hallucinations, and peripheral anticholinergic signs (Ayd 1975).

Anticholinergics can also reduce the plasma levels of the antipsychotics, reducing their therapeutic effectiveness and, thus, antagonizing their antiavoidance action (Hanson et al 1970).

Barbiturates and lithium can also decrease their plasma levels, while the tricyclics and estrogens may increase them. Most antihypertensives will increase the hypotensive effects of the antipsychotics. Chlorpromazine may potentiate the action of the warfarin anticoagulants. However, the single most common interaction involves the simultaneous administration of alcohol and the antipsychotics, where alcohol will potentiate the action of these drugs. The phenothiazines can also enhance the activity of analgesics and central depressant drugs and cause some tolerance but not dependence. Bizarre withdrawal effects can occur.

The risk of side effects of the antipsychotics increases with age and seems to be greatest in elderly patients on high doses, particularly females. Most of the side effects of these drugs are predictable (Eisdorfer 1975).

In a small number of patients, the antipsychotics will cause cardiovascular side effects. These dose-dependent effects occur most often with aliphatic and piperadine phenothiazine derivatives. Patients particularly at risk are those who receive these drugs for a prolonged period of time and who are susceptible to or have cardiovascular disease (Hollister 1973). In some patients agranulocytosis may develop. The elderly, who are particularly at risk, face an increased risk if they are obese or suffering from chronic physical disability (Cole et al 1976). Patients receiving these medications should, therefore, be strongly advised to report immediately any sore throat or fever.

The antipsychotic (neuroleptic) drugs can produce five different reversible extrapyramidal side effects, usually in the early weeks of treatment. Recognition of these effects in the early stages is important as it serves to differentiate them from the signs of tardive dyskinesia (TD), which occurs much later in the course of treatment and is usually irreversible (DiMascio and Sovner 1976). The reversible extrapyramidal symptoms (EPS), listed in Table 22-16, characteristically disappear during sleep and are exacerbated by strong emotions. In general, the phenothiazines, which are more potent on a milligram basis, produce more side effects.

The mechanisms by which these drugs elicit EPS are not clear. It is believed that the antipsychotics interfere with the actions of dopamine as a synaptic neurotransmitter in the brain. Some of the side effects may also be caused by antagonism of dopamine. Abnormal movement disorders occur because of a disturbance of the theoretical neurotransmitter balance between dopamine and acetylcholine (Leopold 1977). Excessive dopamine activity presents clinically as hyperkinesia, as will reduced cholinergic activity. In contrast, reduced dopamine or excessive cholinergic activity produces hypokinesia, which is one of the major manifestations of parkinsonism. It has similarly been proposed that EPS may be inversely proportional to the drug's affinity for the muscarinic receptor (Snyder et al 1974). Drugs

Table 22-16
Extrapyramidal Symptoms Which May Be Caused by Antipsychotic Drugs

Symptoms	Time Sequence (weeks)		
	Onset	*Peak*	*Decline of symptoms*
Pseudoparkinsonism			
Akinesia: (hypokinesia, bradykinesia) diminished muscular movements, joint and muscle pain, muscular weakness and numbness	0–2	1	3–4
Rigidity: abnormally high muscle tone or tension, greater resistance to movement with stiffness and slowness, unchanging blank facial expression, stiff and mechanical gait, slow monotonous speech, stooped posture	1½–2	2–4	5–10
Tremor: alternating rapid contractions especially of arm muscles, pill rolling, tremor of hands and fingers, rhythmic resting tremor, could involve head or lower extremities	1½–2	2–6	8–16
Autonomic Nervous System: drooling, sialorrhea, heart intolerance			
Akathisia	2–4	6–10	12–16
Feeling of restlessness, compulsion to walk about, marked inability to sit still, shifting of weight while standing, insomnia, poorly tolerated			
Acute Dystonic Reactions			
Dystonias: uncoordinated spastic movements of neck, face, eyes, tongue, oculogyric crisis, torticollis	0–1	1	2
Dyskinesias: involuntary muscle spasms, tics, contractions			

such as thioridazine apparently owe their low incidence of EPS to anticholinergic properties that compensate for their intrinsic extrapyramidal effects (Table 22-17). Perhaps trifluoperazine elicits a high incidence of these side effects because it is a very weak muscarinic anticholinergic and can thus not counteract its own propensity to produce EPS.

Table 22-17
Muscarinic Affinity of Antipsychotics Relative to Their Extrapyramidal Effects

Drug Class	Muscarinic Affinity*	Frequency of EPS
Dibenzodiazepine	1*	5
Piperidine phenothiazine	2	4
Alkylamino-phenothiazine	3	3
Piperazine phenothiazine	4	2
Butyrophenone	5	1

*Highest incidence or highest affinity
Adapted from Snyder, S., Greenberg, D., and Yamamura, H.I. Antischizophrenic drugs and brain cholinergic receptors–affinity for muscarinic sites predicts extrapyramidal effects. *Arch Gen Psychiatry.* 31:58, 1974.

Only a minority of patients (about 30%) develop extrapyramidal symptoms (DiMascio and Demirgian 1970). Akathisia seems to occur most often, followed by pseudoparkinsonism and the dystonic reactions (Ayd 1961).

Drug-induced extrapyramidal syndromes are usually clinically indistinguishable from their noniatrogenic counterparts (Lader 1970). The clinical features of drug-induced parkinsonism, called pseudoparkinsonism, closely resemble those of idiopathic parkinsonism.

However, treatment of the idiopathic and the drug-induced symptoms differ. Levodopa is not effective in drug-induced parkinsonian symptoms as there is no dopamine deficiency but a dopamine blockade with an increase in cholinergic activity. Therefore, anticholinergics or antihistamines must be used in the drug-induced syndrome. Akinesia can be produced by antipsychotics which depress the action of catecholamine brain systems. It is possible that many patients on maintenance antipsychotics suffer from akinesia which has been diagnosed as psychopathology unresponsive to drug therapy (Rifkin et al 1975). Akinesia is also a prominent symptom of parkinsonism, which has been related to the destruction of cells and depletion of catecholamines in the nigrostriatal system. Anticholinergics do not counteract akinesia (Schallert et al 1978).

Akathisia may be misdiagnosed as an exacerbation of the psychosis for which the antipsychotic was originally prescribed. Therefore, the dose might be raised instead of lowered (Lader 1970).

Acute dystonic reactions or acute dyskinesias are the most dramatic of the extrapyramidal syndromes. They may be misdiagnosed as hysteria. Dystonias occur most often among patients receiving haloperidol and the long-acting injectable fluphenazine (Swett 1975a). In general, dystonias are more common in men and in younger patients.

Treatment of drug-induced EPS Antiparkinsonism drugs have many adverse clinical effects and are not harmless. Their use should be considered only after all other techniques for managing EPS have been tried (DiMascio and Sovner 1976).

As a first step, a lowering of the daily dose of the antipsychotic should be considered. This is often effective. It is important to note that there may be a tendency to increase the dose of the antipsychotic if a patient exhibits exacerbated psychotic symptomatology, which will only increase the EPS. A rescheduling of the administration time is sometimes advantageous. EPS may be most severe several hours after administration of the antipsychotic. Since some of the EPS disappear during sleep, appropriate rescheduling might help. In akathisia the patient may be able to tolerate its effects better while active, so the antipsychotic should be tried in the morning.

For many patients, a two- or three-day holiday each week from antipsychotic administration may also be tried. When properly used, total drug intake is reduced and side effects decreased without appreciably worsening the disease state. These holidays would also serve simultaneously to unmask first signs of tardive dyskinesia.

In the past, prophylactic and maintenance use of antiparkinsonism drugs were widely favored for patients receiving antipsychotic drugs. It is now felt that the majority of patients receiving antipsychotics rarely require prophylatic administration of antiparkinsonism drugs, as EPS occur only in the minority of patients and there is no reason to expose the majority of patients to the risk of the effects of these drugs. On the other hand, if these drugs are needed, they should be used only for a short period of time (DiMascio and Demirgian 1970). As the data in Table 22-16 show, the EPS disappear mostly three to four months after the start of antipsychotic therapy, and there is therefore no need for prolonged administration of antiparkinsonism drugs. If discontinued after this period of time, only a very small number of patients may require them again. Thus, these drugs should be administered only for a short-term therapy. Yet, studies show that patients have received them for as long as 21 months, some for more than seven years (Raleigh 1977). Recently, it has been argued that there are serious questions about the common opinion that antiparkinsonism drugs are not necessary for prophylaxis (Rifkin et al 1977).

Whatever choice is made, it must be remembered that the antiparkinsonism drugs (Table 22-18), given for a prolonged period of time, can cause blurred vision, dry mouth, decreased gastric motility, constipation, tachycardia, and dizziness. More importantly, these drugs may be responsible for decreased bladder or bowel function,

Table 22-18
Antiparkinsonism Drugs

Drugs acting primarily on dopaminergic system
  Levodopa
  Levodopa-Carbidopa
  Amantadine

Drugs acting primarily on cholinergic system
  Benztropine
  Biperiden
  Chlorphenoxamine
  Cycrimine
  Diethazine
  Diphenhydramine
  Ethopropazine
  Orphenadrine
  Procyclidine
  Trihexyphenidyl

Experimental
  Bromocriptine

---

altered cardiac rhythm, aggravation of glaucoma, and prostatic hypertrophy. They may also increase the incidence and severity of tachycardia. Suggestions for treatment of drug-induced EPS are presented in Table 22-19.

The anticholinergics resemble belladonna in pharmacologic action and side effects. They are no longer the drugs of choice in the treatment of parkinsonism, although they may be tried in drug-induced EPS before more powerful drugs are used. In general, anticholinergics produce only limited improvement and symptoms tend to progress despite continued drug use. Of the available anticholinergics, none is consistently superior to another (Cohen and Schiefe 1977). These drugs are used as adjuncts to levodopa therapy, as sole therapy for patients with mild impairment, for patients who cannot tolerate levodopa, and in drug-induced EPS in which levodopa is ineffective. They block the effect of acetylcholine, decrease salivation, and improve muscular control. However, they may not decrease tremors, which might be expected according to the dopamine theory. On prolonged use, these drugs may become ineffective.

A saliva-stimulating chewing gum, called Quench, has now been marketed. It claims to relieve thirst and is suggested for patients receiving anticholinergics who often suffer from dry mouth.

Of the antihistamines, diphenhydramine is most often used, either as an adjunct to more potent drugs or for patients with relatively mild EPS who cannot tolerate the more potent drugs. The elderly seem to

Table 22-19
Suggested Treatment of Drug-Induced EPS

Symptom	Treatment
Akinesia (Hypokinesia)	Probably caused by phenothiazine or haloperidol, which reduce central dopaminergic activity, partly by blocking dopaminergic uptake at the postsynaptic receptor site. Raise central dopamine activity or lower central cholinergic activity. Use anticholinergics or amantadine where anticholinergics are contraindicated. Reassess need for continuous use early.
Hyperkinesia Tremors at rest (patterned type) of choreoathetosis (non-patterned type)	Reduce central dopamine activity. Use a neuroleptic, such as haloperidol. If anxiety is present, add a benzodiazepine such as chlordiazepoxide to regimen.
Rigidity	Lower dose of antipsychotic drug
Akathisia	Treatment with antiparkinsonism drug not very effective
Dystonia	Use antiparkinsonism drug for several days to treat acute reaction, then discontinue.

tolerate the antihistamines well and may obtain slightly better relief from tremor when antihistamines are prescribed (Yahr 1972). The sedative effect of the antihistamines may be beneficial in insomnia. Patients receiving these drugs may exhibit side effects similar to those of the anticholinergics (the antihistamines have an anticholinergic effect) and may also manifest euphoria, hypotension, headache, weakness, and tingling and heaviness of hands.

Amantadine may increase available dopamine by increasing synthesis, augmenting release, and inhibiting cellular re-uptake (Parkes 1974). Amantadine is less potent than levodopa but may be more potent than the anticholinergics. It is as effective as benztropine in the treatment of drug-induced EPS, except for rigidity, which seems to be better controlled by benztropine (DiMascio et al 1977; Greenblatt et al 1977). Amantadine apparently produces fewer side effects than benztropine. The usual adult dose (up to 200 mg/day) reduces the severity of symptoms and improves functional capacity, but not in all patients. Amantadine is probably effective in 60% of patients and its action is enhanced in the presence of levodopa (Fah and Isgree 1975). It exerts its maximum effect within a few days, but loses its efficacy, at least partially, within six to eight weeks. It is, therefore, primarily used for short-term administration of two to three weeks when a patient needs additional therapeutic assistance. The side effects of amantadine are similar to those of the anticholinergics and may also manifest as depression, orthostatic hypotension, ankle edema, CHF, and peripheral vascular mottling of the extremities, which is benign and completely reversible. Intoxication with amantadine can occur either from an overdose or impaired renal function. There is no specific antidote (Postman and Van Tilburg 1975).

Bromocriptine, a synthetic ergot alkaloid, acts as a dopamine agonist. It has a direct action on the dopamine receptors and, unlike levodopa, does not require the presence of the enzyme amino acid decarboxylase for effective action. Bromocriptine can sometimes achieve effects comparable to those of levodopa in relieving the effects of Parkinson disease and may be useful for patients who do not respond to levodopa. Bromocriptine has a significantly longer half-life than levodopa and may be especially useful in patients with tremor (Kartzinel et al 1976). Used in conjunction with levodopa, it may reduce the frequency of the "on-off" reaction. Adverse reactions are supposedly similar to those seen with levodopa and there may be a significant increase in adverse mental changes and orthostatic hypotension with bromocriptine compared with levodopa. The FDA has not yet cleared this drug for use in Parkinson disease (Calne 1976; Grøn 1977; Godwin-Austen and Smith 1977; Kristensen and Hansen 1977; *Medical Letter* 1977b).

Levodopa is often the drug of choice for treating Parkinson disease. Idiopathic Parkinson disease is associated with pathological changes in the substantia nigra, the globus pallidus, and the cortical fibers that project to them. Elderly patients often lack classical, pathologic changes. Therapy is directed toward replacing dopamine (Bianchine 1976). Levodopa is an amino acid which can pass the blood brain barrier if taken in large amounts. In the brain, it is decarboxylated to dopamine, the deficient neurotransmitter (Sweet and McDowell 1975).

Patients with Parkinson disease have a higher death rate than people representing the general population, probably as a result of their immobility. Apparently, levodopa has a positive effect on the process of aging and can increase a parkinsonian patient's survival time (Cotzias et al 1977). Therefore, levodopa should be used for all patients with important functional disability caused by Parkinson disease. The administration of levodopa, even to patients with heart disease, is relatively safe, although patients over 70 years of age with a history of myocardial infarction exhibit a higher incidence of clinically significant hypotension upon levodopa administration (Werner et al 1976). In patients with senile dementia, levodopa apparently can improve intellectual function (Lewis et al 1978). Levodopa reduces the tremor and rigidity associated with parkinsonism, but it has an unpredictable effect on abnormal movements. Most importantly, it is effective in reducing akinesia, the inability to perform voluntary movements, which is the most devastating effect of the disease.

About one-third of patients on levodopa show a 75% improvement and more than one-half improve at least 50%. Antacids increase the absorption of unchanged levodopa by hastening the gastric emptying time, thus decreasing contact time and deactivation of the drug. Slow emptying and hyperactivity may interfere with the drug's bioavailability (Bianchine and Sunyaprikadul 1974).

The severity of the disease at onset of treatment does not affect treatment outcome. Levodopa does not arrest the progression of Parkinson disease. On prolonged treatment, most patients will deteriorate seriously. Initial improvement in speech and sialorrhea are lost, but improvement in rigidity may be maintained. In any case, most patients will retain some improvement over baseline data. Posture and mentation will probably deteriorate most. The decline in responsiveness to the drug and the deterioration have been related to the fact that, as the disease progresses, the activities of the enyzmes required to synthesize dopamine decrease (Lloyd et al 1970). The best improvement from levodopa treatment is expected to last from six months (when full benefits of treatment are usually manifested) to two years.

Levodopa should be used with caution in patients with renal, hepatic, or endocrine disorders, as well as those with pulmonary disease, bronchial asthma, and patients with psychoses. It is contraindicated in patients with narrow angle glaucoma, hemolytic anemia, G-6-PD deficiency, severe angina, or a history of melanoma.

The drug can cause a high incidence of adverse reactions, among them nausea, vomiting, anorexia, cardiac irregularities, or orthostatic hypotension. Often, patients will develop tolerance to the hypotensive effect. If orthostatic hypotension persists in severity and if a patient's medical status permits, oral administration of 0.05 mg to 0.2 mg of fludrocortisone acetate may reduce hypotension. Elastic stockings may help (Hoehn 1975). Nausea and anorexia peak at about six months and then decrease. Adventitious movements increase with time and are dose-related. Sinus tachycardia and premature ventricular systole are the most common cardiac arrhythmias induced by levodopa. Levodopa may also cause an enormous increase in libido in elderly men. It has been suggested that large doses of ascorbic acid may ameliorate such side effects of high levodopa dosages as nausea and excess salivation, but ascorbic acid should be used with great caution in diabetics and those with a tendency to form urate stones (Dettman 1976). The most well-known shortcoming of levodopa therapy is the "on-off" phenomenon, also called akinesia paradoxica (Willington and Vance

1977; Claveria et al 1973). This is usually observed after prolonged therapy and in patients who have done well with therapy at high doses (Yahr 1974). The patient will suddenly be in a state of akinesia, masked facies, and stooped posture. This may rapidly alternate with a phase of dyskinetic movements. Attacks can be profound and distressing. The "off" periods are usually associated with lowered levodopa plasma levels. Treatment may consist of lowering the levodopa dose (Klawans 1973a), increasing the dose, temporarily withdrawing the drug, use of adjunctive medication, or the use of a high protein diet, because other amino acids, competing for the same absorption mechanism, would decrease absorption of levodopa. As the "on-off" phenomenon occurs most often at higher doses, an arbitrary upper dose limit of four grams per day is suggested (Claveria et al 1973).

Many drugs negate the effect of levodopa (Table 22-20). Reserpine, the phenothiazines, butyrophenones and thioxanthenes, including haloperidol, phenytoin, and possibly papaverine, appear to reduce the effec-

Table 22-20
Possible Interactions of Levodopa with Other Drugs

Drug	Recommended Action
Anticholinergics	The usual dose of each drug may need to be reduced
Antihistamines	May exert a peripheral anticholinergic effect. The usual dose of each drug may need to be reduced
Antihypertensives	As levodopa may cause postural hypotensive episodes, it may be necessary to adjust the dose of guanethidine, methyldopa, or rauwolfia derivatives
Monoamine oxidase inhibitors	The concomitant use of MAO inhibitors and levodopa could result in a hypertensive crisis. MAO must be discontinued two weeks prior to initiating levodopa therapy
Phenothiazines	The phenothiazines most likely block the uptake of dopamine. The phenothiazines may also cause parkinsonian-like symptoms which are usually resistant to levodopa. Avoid combination.
Sympathomimetic amines	Accumulation of sympathomimetic catecholamines may occur
Vitamin B-6 (pyridoxine)	Oral doses of more than 10 mg as found in therapeutic vitamins rapidly reverse the antiparkinsonian effects of levodopa. Use only vitamin preparations that do not contain pyridoxine.

tiveness of levodopa (Hausner 1976). Pyridoxine-deficient diets are not needed. Only if pyridoxine is administered to patients in the form of multiple vitamins containing more than 10 mg of pyridoxine is interference with levodopa activity encountered (Yahr and Duvoisin 1972).

Large doses of levodopa are necessary, as much of it, after oral administration, is metabolized peripherally to dopamine, which is largely responsible for the drug's side effects. The induction phase lasts usually from six to eight weeks. Initially, a dose of 250 mg three times daily with meals is used, which is increased gradually to two to four grams daily.

In order to reduce side effects and increase the effectiveness of levodopa, the drug has been combined with carbidopa, which is a decarboxylase inhibitor. Carbidopa does not pass the blood brain barrier and will diminish the peripheral decarboxylation of levodopa. Therefore, more of levodopa can enter the brain, and the levodopa dose can be reduced by 75%. It also reduces the induction phase considerably. A patient would usually be started with 400 mg levodopa and 40 mg carbidopa. The full therapeutic effect should be reached within six to seven days. During that time, the patient is titrated so that the maintenance dose should probably be three to six tablets a day (1.5 gm levodopa and 150 mg carbidopa). No more than eight tablets per day should be given. The advantage of this combination therapy rests with a reduction in dosage of levodopa and a concurrent reduction of such side effects as nausea, vomiting, and the "on-off" phenomenon. However, abnormal involuntary movements may appear more rapidly and frequently as more levodopa reaches the brain. This might include oral-facial dyskinesia, turning of head, and choreoathetoid movements of limbs and trunk. This effect limits the dose of the combination that a patient can receive. The combination should be used for all patients who are to be started on therapy for Parkinson disease.

When a patient is to be switched from levodopa to combination therapy, the usual daily schedule should be completed, but the usual evening dose should be omitted. The regimen should then be started in the morning, with a 75% reduction in dose.

Tardive dyskinesia (TD) is considered the most common serious adverse effect of antipsychotic therapy. TD has also been called terminal extrapyramidal insufficiency, persistent dyskinesia and complex dyskinesia (Byck 1975; Donlon and Stenson 1976; Mehta et al 1977).

TD is distinct from the early extrapyramidal reactions in late onset, unresponsiveness to anticholinergics, and lack of reversibility (Berger 1978). The pathophysiologic mechanism of the syndrome is thought to be a disturbed cholinergic-dopaminergic balance in the basal ganglia (Crane 1973b; Gerlich et al 1974), producing a relative excess of brain dopamine. Long-term antipsychotic therapy will cause a chronic receptor blockade which results in a state of denervation hypersensitivity. Thus, TD reflects dopaminergic hyperactivity (Kobayashi 1977). The phenothiazines and haloperidol are most often associated with TD, which occurs in about 3% to 6% of a mixed population, but up to 40% of the elderly. Some reports state that more than 50% of the elderly, on long-term therapy, will develop TD (Kazamatsuri et al 1972; Crane 1973b; Kobayashi 1977).

TD often first appears on reduction of dosage or withdrawal of an antipsychotic drug, most often the piperazine phenothiazines. The possible hypokinetic or parkinsonism effects of the antipsychotics may mask signs of TD. It is a syndrome of hyperkinetic involuntary movements. In the elderly, TD manifests most often as orofacial dyskinesia and involuntary movements of the extremities and trunk. Speech, manual dexterity, and respiration may be affected (Baldessarini and Tarsy 1978). Although rarely progressive, TD is potentially irreversible. Less than 2% of patients recover, but the recovery rate has also been estimated to range between 19% and 40% (Kobayashi 1977).

Apparently, TD and parkinsonism are reciprocal in their pathophysiology. The functional reciprocal relationship between dopaminergic and cholinergic mechanisms in the basal ganglia indicate that agents which ameliorate parkinsonism can aggravate symptoms of TD (Fann and Lake 1974). In general, anticholinergics tend to worsen TD, even though they are sometimes used to suppress TD (Klawans 1973b). TD is also aggravated by phenytoin (DeVeaugh-Geiss 1978). While it is often recommended that on occurrence of TD a patient should be switched to an antipsychotic with a lower tendency to induce TD, there is no clear evidence that TD is related specifically to any particular antipsychotic. While some antipsychotics may cause TD to appear earlier or more frequently, all agents have been implicated.

Treatment of TD The most effective way to treat tardive dyskinesia is still prevention. Long-term use of antipsychotics, particularly at high doses, should be avoided and the concept of the risk-benefit ratio should govern clinical decisions regarding maintenance therapy with antipsychotics. Periodic drug holidays have been advocated which would serve several purposes. First, without significantly reducing the drug's benefit, they would reduce the total amount of drug administered, and, because TD is thought to be dose-related, would decrease occurrence of TD. Second, the physician would be able to observe whether the patient can be maintained, even for short periods of time, without the antipsychotic. Finally, and most importantly, the period of omission may unmask the first signs of TD. It has been recommended that antipsychotics should be withdrawn at the first sign of TD, if that is possible. Therefore, it is important that patients be examined carefully during periods of omission to detect early signs of TD. Drug withdrawal may initially cause worsening of TD.

Pharmacologically, attempts have been made to modify TD by a reduction of brain dopamine or blockade of dopamine action on receptors. Many drugs have been tried, among them reserpine, tetrabenazine, pimozide, haloperidol, thiopropazate, perphenazine, lithium, methyldopa, alpha-methyl-tyrosine, amantadine, papaverine, physostigmine, deanol, pyridoxine, 5-hydroxytryptophane, and clonazepam. Attempts have been discouraging, and no single drug has yet emerged as the drug of choice.

A new attempt to find an effective treatment for TD involves the use of choline chloride. Choline is the physiologic precursor of acetylcholine, and its oral administration appears to raise brain acetylcholine levels. Therefore, oral doses of choline may be useful in neurologic diseases in which an increase in acetylcholine levels is desirable. Indeed, choline administration has been shown to be able to suppress buccal-lingual masticatory movements in some patients with TD.

Choline has a bitter taste and imparts a fishy body odor to patients to whom it is administered. Therefore, lecithin may be more acceptable to patients. Furthermore, the metabolic fate of choline consumed as lecithin apparently differs from that of free choline. Choline consumed as lecithin causes a much greater increase in plasma choline, per mole consumed, than choline chloride (Cohen and Wurtman 1975, 1976; Wurtman et al 1977; Growdon et al 1977; Davis et al 1977; Betz and Goldstein 1978; Growdon et al 1978; Hirsch and Wurtman 1978). It has also been suggested that administration of choline may be useful when added to existing treatments in such diseases as mania, myasthenia gravis, and psychoses.

The Antidepressants

Depression is a major health problem that often recurs, and suicide is a dangerous consequence of depression (Biggs et al 1977). Depression may be idiopathic, ie, it may be a primary depression. It can also arise secondarily to some other serious medical or psychiatric illness and can also result from some traumatic event (Biggs 1978). Treatment of depression often is based on the appearance of symptoms rather than a diagnosis of depressive illness (Goldstein 1977). Nevertheless, it is important to differentiate between sadness and grief, which often occur as a result of the cumulating losses faced by the elderly, and endogenous depression. Some depressions, especially those related to life experiences, need not necessarily be treated with drugs and should probably never be treated with drugs alone. Psychotherapy or environmental manipulation, which lead to a strengthening of the social support structure, are more clearly indicated.

Endogenous depression apparently is caused by a shortage in the brain of neurotransmitters that are necessary to facilitate conduction of nerve impulses across the synaptic gap between neurons (Diamond et al 1977). Depletion of such amines as norepinephrine and serotonin in the CNS causes depression, and the catecholamine hypothesis proposes that an increase in the transmitters reverses depressive symptoms (Hollister 1973). Depression, frequent among the elderly (Busse and Pfeiffer 1973), particularly the diagnosis of endogenous depression, is sufficient indication for treatment (Talley 1977), the aim of which should be complete remission of symptoms. Treatment of depression in old age is complex and difficult. Effective treatment can be achieved by a careful differential diagnosis between anxiety states and the depressive syndrome; all depressed patients are anxious, but not all anxious patients are depressed. Treatment of depression in the elderly also calls for relief of many diverse symptoms, such as constipation, and aches and pains, which need medical rather than psychiatric attention.

Some treatment modalities   For severely depressed patients, in whom an immediate therapeutic response is necessary, electroconvulsive therapy may be indicated. There is good evidence to indicate its clinical efficacy.

Thioridazine, an antipsychotic drug, has been approved by the FDA for short-term treatment of depression. It should not be used in combination with the tricyclic antidepressants as ventricular tachycardia can occur in patients receiving both drugs simultaneously. The benzodiazepines may have a role as temporary adjunctive therapy for depressed patients with mild anxiety or insomnia. If a patient is primarily anxious and secondarily depressed, the benzodiazepines will most likely elicit a better patient response. However, if the predominating symptom (depression or anxiety) cannot be identified clearly, the tricylcics are preferred for initial treatment, as they have some antianxiety properties (Biggs et al 1977).

Monoamine oxidase levels increase with age, which has been correlated with depressive illnesses. Therefore, it would seem rational to use monoamine oxidase inhibitors (MAOIs) in the treatment of depression. Actually, the MAOIs are excellent antidepressants. However, they are inherently toxic and also predispose the patient to interactive toxicity with other drugs and foods containing tyramine. They appear to be particularly hazardous to the elderly and should, therefore, not be used unless all other treatment modalities have been tried unsuccessfully. The combination of tricyclic antidepressants and MAOIs has been recommended for depression refractory to all other treatments, but most careful attention must be paid to the potential serious side effects of the MAOIs (Goldberg and Thornton 1978). The use of lithium in cyclic affective (manic-depressive) disorders has been proposed but it works best in prevention and not treatment, and is preferred for people with recurrent pyromania (Biggs et al 1977).

Clearly, for practical purposes, only the tricyclic antidepressants can be used safely in the depressions of old age (Charatan 1975). These drugs have a mood-elevating action only in depressed patients. They also affect the somatic manifestations of depression and are effective in counteracting depressive illness in patients in whom mood alterations are not apparent. Their effectiveness is directly related to the severity of the depression, being most effective in patients who are severely depressed (Goldstein 1977). Treatment outcome is also related to the duration of the depression. The tricyclics are most effective in severe, abrupt-onset depression and least effective in patients with long-standing chronic depression.

They are the drugs of choice for the initial therapy for primary depressions or major depressive disorders because of their broad therapeutic range, but should not be given to suicidal patients who should be hospitalized, or to mildly depressed patients without a careful evaluation. Treatment with tricyclics and psychotherapy is compatible and, indeed, pharmacotherapy enhances psychotherapy.

Treatment failure is often related to any of a number of well-recognized factors. Among those is the administration of insufficient doses, the administration of too large a dose of certain tricyclics, and the failure to allow a sufficient time for the therapeutic effects to manifest. It would not be unusual for the therapeutic effects to appear from four to six weeks after the onset of treatment. Frequently, the tricyclics may also be administered concurrently with drugs that can decrease their effectiveness. Initially, the sedating effect of the tricyclics may cause an apparent worsening of the depression, which should be recognized and not treated with increased dosage.

There has been much dispute on the possible misuse of these drugs, particularly in the elderly. In view of the fact that depressive illness often leads to suicide attempts, and in view of the fact that endogenous depression may progress to a more chronic disorder, overuse has been disputed. As a matter of fact, the tricyclics are probably underutilized to the extent that depression has been under-diagnosed (Biggs et al 1977).

The biochemical basis of the action of tricyclics is not yet fully clarified or understood. It is thought that they block, to a variable extent, the reuptake of neurotransmitters. This would tend to restore more normal amounts of these transmitters within the synaptic gap, and, clinically, the patient becomes more normal. It has been suggested that imipramine and desipramine probably inhibit norepinephrine resorption, while amitriptyline, nortriptyline, and protriptyline probably block serotonin reuptake (Diamond et al 1977).

Pharmacokinetically, the tricyclic antidepressants are absorbed completely, but their systemic availability is reduced by a pronounced hepatic first pass elimination. This may vary among individuals but is probably relatively constant during steady state conditions in each individual. Generally, elimination half-lives of the tricyclics average from 20 to 35 hours (Greenblatt and Koch-Weser 1975), but in older patients this may be extended to 80 hours, and the rule that 96% of the steady state is reached by five times the elimination half-life cannot be applied. In the elderly patient, steady state plasma levels may only be reached after two or three weeks. The relatively long half-life is advantageous in the elderly though, as doses can be administered only once or twice a day.

Among a group of patients, there will be a wide variation in steady state plasma levels in response to similar doses. Apparently, individual response is genetically controlled. Nevertheless, for each individual, plasma levels of tricyclics provide a rational approach to improved management in endogenous depression (Ziegler and Biggs 1977). In monitoring plasma levels, both the parent compound and the metabolite must be considered, as well as the fact that nortriptyline responds with an inverted U-shape, while amitriptyline and imipramine apparently respond in a linear fashion. There is no relation between plasma levels and drug effectiveness in depressions other than endogenous depression.

The tricyclics are important in resolving depression but, more importantly, they are potentially life-saving drugs as severely depressed patients may attempt suicide (Berger 1978). Thus, the decision to use a tricyclic is not complicated except in patients with concurrent heart disease. What is difficult is the decision on the particular drug to be used and an estimate of the treatment prognosis. There are still no indicators as to which patient will respond positively to which tricyclic. It has been suggested that good prognosis is expected from the patient who is difficult to cheer up, has early morning insomnia, exhibits decreased energy and a general slowing of speech and movement, and manifests loss of appetite and weight (Hollister 1976; Ayd 1975b; Appleton 1976). A poor prognosis should probably be expected from neurotic, hypochondriacal, or hysterical patients. A history of prior episodes and the presence of delusions also indicate a poor prognosis.

Two major factors may determine successful use of tricyclics. First, the physician must devote more time than usual to a patient. Tricyclic dosages require frequent adjustment. The initial dose should be readjusted after the first, second, and third week and treatment "failure" should not be accepted until at least four to six weeks have elapsed during which time the patient has been closely monitored and adequate dosage levels have been reached (Biggs et al 1977). Successful use also may involve a certain amount of trial and error because of the wide variation in patient response and because there are still no good predictors for response.

In general, 55% to 60% of patients should respond. If the nonresponders then receive an adjusted dose, success can be expected in another 25% to 30% of patients, so that, over all, only about 15% of patients may not respond, even if their plasma levels are normal (Biggs 1978). To be considered adequate, a trial of tricyclics should include the use of the dosage generally recognized as safe for a sufficient period of time. It is important to assure complete patient compliance with the dosage regimen (Paykel 1978). Furthermore, as previously noted, sequential trial of as many as three different agents may be indicated in initially unresponsive patients (Maas 1975; Schildkraut 1974).

Six tricyclic antidepressants are currently approved by the FDA for use in depression (*Medical Letter* 1978). These are presented in Table 22-21. Dosage recommendations for the elderly vary widely and those presented represent a composite of many suggestions. In the very old, serious life-threatening depression has been treated successfully with a dose as low as 5 mg twice daily. As a general rule, it has been suggested that a test dose be one-half the smallest tablet marketed of the particular tricyclic. If there are no adverse effects, one-half of a tablet three times daily should be used and the dosage increased if the patient is unresponsive.

The dosage should be raised to maximum levels only if side effects are tolerable to the patient. In general, elderly patients do not tolerate side effects well, and, therefore, maximum doses are used infrequently. In some instances, amitriptyline for example, a single bedtime dose will be as effective as a three times daily dosage (Biggs 1978). If possible, the initial dosage regimen should include a bedtime dose.

There is still no general agreement as to the need for continuous maintenance therapy. In many patients, continuation of antidepressants apparently does prevent relapse, but withdrawal of the drug is not always followed by a relapse. If withdrawal seems indicated, and in the elderly serious consideration should be given to it as they usually are faced with multiple drug use, symptoms may reappear within 3 to 14 days. Withdrawal should be tapered, probably by 10% of the final maintenance dose every month. If continuous maintenance therapy is decided upon, the elderly patient will probably need reassurance that the drug is not addicting (DiMascio et al 1975). As a general rule, a trial withdrawal is indicated after two months of the start of remission.

The tricyclics appear to be equally effective. Thus, the particular choice often depends on the side effects that the physician wants most to avoid, or use. The sedative effect is often a determining factor, but

Table 22-21
Tricyclics for the Elderly

| Drug | Initial Dose | Side Effects ||||| Comments |
		Sedation	Anti-cholinergic	Sweating	Cardiac Arrhythmias	GI Disturbance	
Amitriptyline	10 mg tid or qid	High	High	Low	Low	Low	Most sedating. Preferred in anxiety depression, and early morning awakening. Alleviates restlessness. Increases normal appetite and causes most weight gain
Nortriptyline	30–50 mg daily in divided doses	Low	High	Low	Low	Low	Less sedating than amitriptyline
Protriptyline	10 mg AM or 5 mg bid	None	High	Low	Low	Low	Mildly stimulating, but of all, most likely to cause stimulation
Imipramine	10–25 mg/day	Medium	Very high	High	Low	Medium	Less sedating than amitriptyline. Preferred in depression with overtones of lethargy. Thought to have some psychomotor activating effect. Does not increase normal appetite

Desipramine	25–50 mg/day	Low	Very high	Very high	Low	Low	Less sedating than amitriptyline and possibly imipramine. Preferred in depressions with overtones of lethargy. Use if patient is hypersomniac. Thought to have marked psychomotor activating effect. Does not tend to increase normal appetite. Least anticholinergic (?)
Doxepin	10 mg tid	High	Low	Low	Low	Low	Most often used to avoid anticholinergic or cardiotoxic effects. Used in anxiety depression. Probably does not inhibit guanethidine with less than 150 mg/day. All others do inhibit guanethidine. Does not tend to increase normal appetite

unless the patient suffers from insomnia, too much drowsiness may result when a sedating antidepressant is chosen. On the other hand, the insomniac patient will appreciate the immediate sedating effect. Imipramine and amitriptyline are probably most often used.

Overdoses of drugs can lead to serious clinical consequences, particularly in the elderly. Thus, the prescriber should limit the number of tablets per prescription to minimize the risk of overdose.

Even though there is no clear difference in the therapeutic effects elicited by these antidepressants, there are differences in response to the tricyclics in different nosological types of depressed patients (Gram 1977). Therefore, it has been suggested that the tricyclics be classified according to the target symptoms that are typical of endogenous depression (Kielholz 1971). Most often, though, different drug actions are related to their chemical structures. A theory has been advanced that some tricyclics are more potent blockers of norepinephrine than others (Maas 1975).

The tertiary amines (the parent compounds) are more potent inhibitors of serotonin uptake (Garattini and Samanin 1978; U'Prichard et al 1978). Specifically, it is thought that imipramine blocks the membrane pump of brain serotonergic neurons and decreases 5-HT turnover. Amitriptyline also blocks this pump, and reduces serotonin turnover in the brain (Valzelli 1978). Based on this action, the tertiary amines are thought to be particularly effective in patients with psychomotor agitation and could ameliorate mood in depressive patients.

The secondary amines are more efficient in blocking the membrane pump of noradrenergic neurons. Treatment with these drugs, therefore, will benefit only patients with noradrenaline depression, since these drugs have little influence on 5-hydroxytryptamine reuptake. Desipramine and protriptyline, in particular, tend to cause psychomotor activation. The secondary amines are thought to be particularly useful for treatment of retarded depression. They are less likely than the tertiary amines to cause either a sedative or hypotensive effect. Thus, it is now believed that the tertiary amines have a predominantly serotonin-potentiating activity, while the secondary amines, the demethylated metabolites, are less potent and have a predominantly noradrenaline-potentiating activity (Gram 1977).

There is no absolute age contraindication to the use of the tricyclics. They should not be given during the acute phase of myocardial infarction. Doxepin is probably the best choice for use in cardiac patients, as it has a low potential for producing arrhythmias. Cardiac effects are more likely to occur in patients with thyrotoxicosis. The elderly are at greater risk to tricyclic antidepressant (TCA) cardiotoxicity because of increased prevalence of underlying cardiac disease and age-related changes in drug elimination (Nies et al 1977). On the other hand, antidepressant serum concentrations of imipramine have a quinidine-like effect on the electrocardiogram and antiarrhythmic effects of both atrial and ventricular arrhythmias (Bigger et al 1977). Therefore, they could be beneficial for patients with a so-called irritable heart, ie, those with premature ventricular contractions or extra beats. If given concurrently with quinidine or another antiarrhythmic, the dose of the antiarrhythmic should probably be reduced.

Side effects may sometimes be difficult to separate from symptoms of the underlying depression (Ziegler et al 1977), but there are some data that adverse effects can be correlated with plasma levels (Petit et al 1977). Major adverse reactions occurred in less than 5% of 260 patients, not necessarily elderly (Boston Collaborative Drug Reaction Surveillance Program 1972). Side effects of all antidepressants are listed in Table 22-22 and those of the tricyclics in Table 22-23. The elderly may be exposed to a particular risk from hypothermia, precipitation of incipient glaucoma, and urinary retention. The

Table 22-22
Frequent Adverse Effects of Antidepressants

Drug	Adverse Effects
Tricyclics	Atropine-like effects (dryness of mouth, tachycardia, mydriasis and cycloplegia, urinary retention, decreased GI motility, deliriform psychotic state with high doses)
	Hypotension
	Drowsiness
MAO inhibitors	Hypotension
	Restlessness
	Insomnia
	Dry mouth
	Nausea
	Anorexia
	Constipation
	Dizziness
	Impotence
Lithium carbonate	
At therapeutic blood levels (0.5–1.5 mEq/liter):	Thirst
	Polyuria
	Fine tremor
	GI irritation
	Diarrhea
At toxic blood levels (about 2.0 mEq/liter):	Vomiting
	Muscular weakness
	Neurologic deficits
	Stupor
	Coma
	Convulsions

Table 22-23
Some Adverse Effects of the Tricyclics in the Elderly

Very frequent	Frequent	Common
Constipation	Blurred vision	Urinary retention
Diaphoresis	Cardiovascular effects	
Dry mouth	Dizziness	
	Drowsiness	

tricyclics may also cause herniation (hiatus hernia) in susceptible individuals. The likelihood that older patients with cardiovascular disease develop more severe grades of postural hypotension is almost three times that in younger healthy patients (Bigger et al 1978). Particularly if given in high doses, these drugs may cause or exacerbate transient confusional states in the elderly. The anticholinergic action of these drugs can also lead to dental problems, which is often overlooked. In general, depressed patients are particularly sensitive to the side effects of the TCAs and, as age increases, their severity increases also. When the tricyclics are withdrawn abruptly, patients may exhibit withdrawal symptoms (Kramer et al 1961).

Blurred vision can be treated with pilocarpine nitrate ophthalmic drops (1%); for the frequent constipation, stool softeners or milk of magnesia are indicated; in hypotension, elastic stockings and patient instructions to avoid sudden changes in condition may be helpful; and for urinary retention, dihydroergotamine, 10 drops three times daily has been tried.

The Antimanics

While depression is caused by a functional underactivity or deficiency of the neurotransmitters serotonin and norepinephrine, mania is associated with their functional hyperactivity (Berger 1978).

Lithium, which has been used since 1967 in the treatment of mania and the prophylaxis of recurrent mania and depressive episodes, has a more specific effect against true mania than the neuroleptics. Lithium exerts its antimanic effect without causing sedation (Gerbino et al 1978). The successful use of lithium carbonate for the treatment of mood disorders, acute mania, and manic-depressive illness is well documented. In order to handle the increasingly numerous clinical reports on lithium use, the University of Wisconsin Center for Health Sciences has now established a computer-oriented program with an up-to-date registry of all lithium references.

When lithium therapy is initiated, there may be a lag time before optimum clinical effect is reached. This has been variously estimated to range from seven to ten days or even from two to three weeks. Therefore, in some instances, mania may be initially managed with neuroleptics. Temporary treatment with chlorpromazine or haloperidol, combined with lithium, is usually suggested for patients who require immediate behavioral control. In depressive periods, tricyclics may also be needed. Lithium prophylaxis becomes increasingly effective in the second and subsequent years of its administration. Conversely, a disproportionate number of treatment failures occur in the first year of lithium administration (Shou 1968). The use of a sustained-release lithium carbonate preparation has been described as successful.

Successful outcome of lithium therapy depends on close control of lithium plasma levels. These should be checked two to three times a week while the patient is being stabilized. When the maintenance dose is reached, weekly levels should be obtained and, later, only monthly levels are necessary, unless other drugs are added to the regimen (Ende 1975).

Normal adult plasma levels have been described to range optimally between 0.9 and 1.4 mEq/liter for therapeutic purposes. For maintenance, levels of 0.6 to 1.0 mEq/liter are desired. Levels above 2 mEq/liter are toxic and those above 5 mEq/liter may be lethal.

For older people, lithium ion levels should range between 0.2 and 0.9 mEq/liter. The geriatric dose may often not exceed 150 mg three times daily and, sometimes, even less (Wharton 1975). Patients on lithium therapy should maintain adequate fluid and sodium intake. Salt depletion, fluid restriction, and diets may precipitate lithium toxicity (Tonks 1977).

Lithium should not be used for patients with significant renal, cardiovascular, or organic brain disease. It should be used with caution in severely debilitated or dehydrated patients and those with thyroid disease, epilepsy, and diabetics. These, and elderly patients in general, should receive lower doses of the drug.

More than 100 side effects have been reported for lithium carbonate therapy (Baylis and Heath 1978), most often nausea, fatigue, tremor, thirst, edema, and weight gain. Lithium may cause thyroid abnormalities which can be severe, and potentially dangerous hypothyroidism can develop rapidly. Parkinsonism-like symptoms have been reported in patients receiving this drug for more than seven years (Johnels et al 1976).

Whenever sodium is decreased, lithium concentration will increase. Lithium tolerance is decreased by any factor which can decrease sodium, such as excessive perspiration, vomiting, and diarrhea. In general, it is recommended that the drug should be withdrawn whenever diarrhea, vomiting, new tremors, or changes in existing tremors occur. The sudden onset of sodium depletion can lead to acutely elevated symptomatic lithium toxicity.

Lithium is excreted almost entirely by the kidneys. In states of sodium depletion, lithium will be reabsorbed by the tubules. Dramatic increases in serum and tissue lithium levels can result. There is much literature on the simultaneous administration of diuretics and lithium (Davis and Fann 1971; Petersen et al 1974; Hurtig and Dyson 1974; McFie 1975; Himmelhoch et al 1977). Diuretics can be used concurrently with lithium; however, there must be an appropriate downward adjustment of the daily lithium dose, lithium levels should be monitored closely, and the patient should be observed for symptoms of lithium toxicity, manifested as tremors, nausea, and mental disorientation. Increasingly large doses of diuretics will cause increasingly high lithium levels. Serious side effects can occur on concurrent administration of lithium with either tetracycline or methyldopa (McGennis 1978; O'Regan 1976). Acetazolamide and aminophylline increase urinary excretion of lithium, haloperidol may increase the neurotoxic reactions, and lithium may lower chlorpromazine plasma levels substantially.

The Antianxiety Agents

Anxiety was formerly called the "psychoneurotic disease" and it has been claimed that this was a better definition as restlessness, irritability, hyperexcitability, fatigue, and other manifestations may be of equal or greater importance than anxiety (Berger 1976a). In any case, anxiety manifests as a constellation of physical complaints (Ack et al 1978).

Anxiety, usually in response to life conditions, is common among the elderly, and functional disorders are treatable. Anxious elderly patients report far fewer somatic complaints than young or middle-aged anxious patients. In the elderly, anxiety is often encountered as body-focused complaints and older patients are likely to deny dysphoria (Epstein 1978).

As anxiety is a normal reaction, it may not require the use of drugs (*Medical Letter* 1976). Whenever possible, a nonpharmacologic approach should first be used in treating the elderly anxious patient. By environmental manipulation, the patient's energy should be channeled into constructive activity. Social activities and exercise may be helpful. Reassurance is often needed.

Antianxiety agents should not be prescribed too lightly, but should be used on a rational basis. They must, of course, be used if anxiety becomes too severe. If an anxious patient apparently cannot function without medication, it should be prescribed, but the patient should be re-evaluated periodically (Ack et al 1978). These drugs are effective in anxiety, hyperactivity, fatigue, psychologic rigidity, and insomnia.

They increase the patient's vigor, but are of little value in anxiety resulting from schizophrenia or hormonal imbalance. It should be remembered that drug therapy will be most effective when used as adjunctive therapy to other treatment modalities.

Antianxiety agents are effective in the elderly, except that the old-old show a lessened response. The decision to treat anxiety with drugs should be based on a clear need, and drug use should not preempt other treatment modalities. Antianxiety drug therapy is most rational when adjusted to the episodic nature of anxiety. Drug dosage should be reduced or drugs could be completely withdrawn during remission, but the dosage should be increased when symptoms are severe or even disabling.

The dosage should be individualized and the initial dose should be small, to be raised if necessary (Greenblatt and Shader 1974a). The lack of need for a fixed daily dosage schedule with time can be turned to an additional advantage. The patient can be included as an active participant in the therapeutic regimen by encouragement to medicate according to need, subject to an upper limit on the daily dose. This gives the patient a feeling of control and self-responsibility (Blackwell 1975).

It is difficult to predict patient response to an antianxiety agent. Treatment of anxiety is purely symptomatic and the complaints are largely subjective. Also, in a large number of cases, anxiety remits spontaneously, or the patient may respond positively to the therapeutic milieu.

Response to antianxiety drugs can differ with personality patterns (Nakano et al 1978; Barrett and DiMascio 1966; DiMascio and Barrett 1965; Hollister 1970). Highly anxious subjects may suffer from a decrease in both speed and accuracy and these patients may respond better to antianxiety agents. In less anxious patients, the drugs may even cause increased anxiety states. Very active persons, oriented to achievement, may respond with increased anxiety as the drug may interfere with their desire to achieve. Those who are more intellectually inclined are likely to respond well to antianxiety agents. Sex of the patient may affect treatment outcome, although this is disputed (McDonald 1967), and the treatment setting can be influential (Salzman et al 1974). If depression overlaps the anxiety state, patients with "hostile" depression will respond to a lesser degree than those with an "anxious" depression (Bowen 1978).

It seems clear that the patient's socioeconomic background influences the response to drug treatment of anxiety (Winokur and Rickels 1977). Good results cannot be expected if a patient lives in disadvantaged socioeconomic circumstances, has little education, and believes the problem to be somatic rather than emotional. On the other hand, these patients may accept the sedating effect of these drugs much more readily than upper social class patients. The latter patients often realize that their problems are emotional. Most likely, they actively seek help and, therefore, a good response can be expected (Fisher 1970; Rickels 1968).

Irrespective of treatment agent, anxiety is more likely to improve with patient's income and education and the patient's acceptance of the emotional nature of the problem. With increasing number of episodes, though, and increasing episodes of drug treatment, prognosis worsens. On the other hand, drugs will work better if treatment is offered in general practice by a physician willing to spend considerable time with the patient (Rickels 1973).

Several classes of drugs are available to treat anxiety. Among those are the propanediols, hydroxyzine, the barbiturates, and the benzodiazepines. Meprobamate, a muscle relaxant, continues to be used, but has no advantage over the benzodiazepines and has many disadvantages. Particularly in the elderly, the propanediols should not be used. The lethal potential from an overdose of meprobamate is considerable and the drug could easily be used in a suicide attempt. Meprobamate also rapidly induces liver microsomal enzymes and, therefore, interferes with the metabolism of many drugs. This is particularly important in the elderly who are usually on multiple-drug regimens. Finally, meprobamate's potential for addiction is considerable.

Some clinicians still favor the use of barbiturates, as they are less expensive than the benzodiazepines. However, their addiction potential is high and so is their lethal potential from an overdose. There may still be a limited place for the barbiturates in the treatment of hospitalized patients with anxiety. Hydroxyzine is less effective than either the propanediols or the barbiturates and there is no longer any indication for its use in the elderly.

The benzodiazepines, on the other hand, are relatively safe for use in the elderly. They do not possess the same abuse potential as do the propanediols, they are almost suicide-proof, they do not depress respiration and are also preferred as they do not interfere with other drugs, an important consideration in treating the elderly (Blackwell 1975). Their margin of safety has been noted (National Institute of Drug Abuse 1977) and, based on these and other considerations, they represent the treatment of choice for most patients.

Contrary to many news reports and popular belief, the benzodiazepines are not most often used by the elderly. As a matter of fact, the median age of those using benzodiazepines is 44 years (Tessler et al 1978; Parr 1971).

Neurotic anxiety is by far the most common indication for the benzodiazepines (Greenblatt and Shader 1974b). They are more valuable for the relief of anxiety in neurotic and depressive anxious states because patients tolerate these drugs better than the antipsychotics. They seem to be especially useful for high-anxiety depressed patients.

They have better antianxiety properties than do antipsychotics and cause fewer and less severe side effects. The broad clinical acceptance of the benzodiazepines is based on their well-established efficacy and their unusual degree of safety (Bookman and Randall 1976). Their use makes the patient more accessible emotionally and more receptive to communication with the physician, perhaps facilitating psychotherapy. The antianxiety action of the benzodiazepines has been related to their "anticonflict" action (Lehmann and Ban 1977). The behavioral action of benzodiazepines, which clearly distinguishes them from other psychotropic drugs, is not depression of behavior but behavioral stimulation (Haefely 1978).

The mode of action of the benzodiazepines is still unclear. It has been postulated that they may exert a primary action on gamma-aminobutyric mechanisms (Guidotti 1978), that they modify the activity of the limbic structures, reduce dopamine and brain 5-HT turnover, as well as change turnover of brain acetylcholine and monoamines. Specific benzodiazepine receptors have been identified in the human brain and binding to these receptors is stereospecific (Moehler and Okada 1977).

Some clinicians have suggested that the antianxiety effects of the benzodiazepines tend to decrease after two to three weeks of steady use, but this has been disputed by other clinicians.

Clearly, the benzodiazepines provide safe and effective treatment for the elderly anxious patient. Much controversy about their use could be eliminated by the recognition that anxiety occurs cyclically and drugs should be used accordingly and not indefinitely.

The currently approved benzodiazepines are listed in Table 22-24 (*Medical Letter* 1977a). As a general rule, the pharmacologically active benzodiazepines are lipophilic compounds that are eliminated from the body almost entirely by biotransformation. The benzodiazepines differ in milligram potency, biotransformation, duration of action, and activity. Chlordiazepoxide, diazepam, prazepam, and clorazepate are first converted to the active metabolite desmethyldiazepam, which is pharmacologically active. The complicated degradative metabolism of prazepam actually produces yet another metabolite, desalkyprazepam and a half-life as long as 78 hours has been reported. Oxazepam and lorazepam do not produce active metabolites, have therefore a shorter duration of action, and would need to be administered in multiple daily dosing (Greenblatt and Shader 1974b). There are indications that diazepam half-life increases with increasing age, from approximately 20 hours at age 20, to 90 hours at age 80 (Rosenberg et al 1976), but in most elderly, its clearance is not impaired (Klotz et al 1975). The absorption rate, clearance, and elimination half-life of chlordiazepoxide change with age (Shader et al 1977). No data appear to be available on the other benzodiazepines. However, one must probably assume a longer duration of action with all these drugs in the elderly. To

Table 22-24
The Benzodiazepines

Drug	Elimination Half-life (hours)	Active Metabolite	Elimination Half-life (hours)	Effect
Chlordiazepoxide	2–12	Yes	20–30	Long-acting
Clorazepate	25–60	Yes	25–60	Steady state in about 7 days
Diazepam	1–10	Yes	25–60	Maximum effect in about 7 days
Lorazepam	8–14	None		
Oxazepam	4–12	None		No accumulation but must give several doses/day
Prazepam	70–120	Yes		Slowly absorbed and metabolized
Flurazepam*	1½–4	Yes	40–100	Steady state in about 7 days

*Only benzodiazepine so far approved and specifically marketed as hypnotic.
Note: Recently, lorazepam has been approved for treatment of insomnia.

minimize disturbing side effects and eliminate possible toxic effects, the dosage of these drugs for the elderly should be lower than the normal adult dose. It is impossible to suggest a fixed starting dose for these drugs, but it must be stressed that in geriatric patients the starting dose should be lower than usual and that the dose should be titrated to the individual patient and should be flexible. Very few dosage recommendations are available. In general, diazepam may be administered as a nighttime dose of 5 mg and chlordiazepoxide as 10 mg. For daytime use, diazepam should be started at no more than 2 mg and chlordiazepoxide at no more than 5 mg. The dosage should not be raised until it is certain that the dose is insufficient. Release of anger may be a side effect.

There is no clinical evidence that any one of the benzodiazepines is more effective than any other, given in appropriate doses. Apparently, though, most clinicians still prefer chlordiazepoxide (*Medical Letter* 1977a), probably as its properties are best known (it was the first benzodiazepine to be marketed) and as the other benzodiazepines do not offer any advantage when used. Daytime administration of benzodiazepines should be avoided when a patient has organic brain syndrome as mental confusion can be worsened. If dosage is not adjusted appropriately, accumulation can lead to disabling effects. Drug complications can be avoided by prescribing diazepam or chlordiazepoxide in the evening. The sedative effect is most pronounced in the first two hours after administration and becomes less after five to seven hours. Except for flurazepam, prazepam is the the most sedating benzodiazepine, which limits its usefulness for many patients. Oxazepam, on the other hand, is least sedating. It also has a relatively short half-life, which mandates more frequent daily administration, often undesirable in the elderly.

Although oxazepam and clorazepate are effective, they are not widely used. Lorazepam, recently approved both as an antianxiety agent and for insomnia, has caused sedation in 20% of a study population and some unsteadiness, disorientation, and autonomic manifestations were noted (Ellison and Cancellaro 1978).

On a weight basis, this newly approved drug is the most potent benzodiazepine so far. Its half-life is approximately 12 hours, and it must, therefore, be given in a three-times-daily schedule. No data on its effect in the elderly are as yet available.

The incidence of side effects to the benzodiazepines increases with age and unwanted depression becomes frequent in the very old. Depression seems to be related to severe hypoalbuminemia (less than 3gm/100 ml) and not to age (Greenblatt and Koch-Weser 1974).

The adverse effects of any of the benzodiazepines may be more severe if the drugs are administered concurrently with barbiturates or any other drugs that depress the CNS.

All benzodiazepines interact to some extent with alcohol and it is important to inform the patient that this can occur even if alcohol is consumed as much as ten hours after administration of the benzodiazepine.

Alcohol is beginning to be used by many clinicians as a therapeutic regimen for the elderly, instead of other CNS drugs. The practice has been roundly condemned by many others, who think alcohol use among the elderly might be dangerous. The exact rate of alcoholism in the elderly is unknown. Possibly 2% to 10% of the elderly suffer from alcohol problems, with a higher rate apparently indicated for widowers and individuals with serious medical problems (Schuckit 1977). Frequent alcohol users who use all types of alcohol, ie, beer, wine, and liquor, comprise less than 20% (Guttman 1977). This may be a way to cope with the various physical stresses and problems, such as boredom and loneliness. Overall, though, the incidence of alcoholism appears to be less in the elderly as compared to younger age groups.

However, older problem drinkers appear to evidence problems significantly different from those of younger problem drinkers (Cahalan 1970). They are likely to be binge drinkers and are less likely to exhibit symptomatic problems or be belligerent while drinking (Horn and Wanberg 1969).

Thus, there appears to be no reason to reject outright the idea that alcohol, used judiciously and in controlled amounts, may well be beneficial. On the other hand, strong support for its therapeutic use has been evidenced (Dock 1963; Kastenbaum and Slater 1964; Lucia 1963, 1968; Sarley and Stepto 1969). Beer sociotherapy may often be more effective than drug therapy (Ching-Piao 1971), as it promotes increased social activity and acts as a facilitator (Ching-Piao et al 1973; Becker and Conn 1978).

Alcohol is also an excellent sedative and deserves a place in the practical treatment of geriatric patients with mental disorders (Kastenbaum 1965; Leake and Silverman 1967; Black 1969; Chien 1970). The patient may also benefit by an increase in appetite. Of course, this type of therapy is probably best used in a somewhat controlled environment, such as a nursing home, where problem drinkers can be identified and handled in an appropriate manner.

Inherent in the use of alcohol as a therapeutic tool is the danger of alcohol-drug interactions. Alcohol interacts with many commonly prescribed drugs (Table 22-25). The severity of alcohol-drug interactions can be greater if alcohol is administered in the form of hard liquor (whiskey or gin) rather than as beer, cider, or wine, even if the total intake does not differ (Lamy 1975). Wine, having a high buffer capacity, is absorbed less rapidly than are distilled liquors, which also can irritate the gastric and duodenal mucosa. Thus, the potential for interaction should be considered when using alcohol therapeutically (Mancini 1970).

Table 22-25
Some Drug Interactions with Alcohol

Drug	Effect	Probable mechanism
Antabuse	Flushing, diaphoresis, hyperventilation, vomiting, confusion, drowsiness	Inhibits intermediary metabolism of alcohol
Anticoagulants, oral	Increased anticoagulant effect with acute intoxication	Reduced metabolism
	Decreased anticoagulant effect after chronic alcohol abuse	Enhanced microsomal enzyme activity
Antihistamines	Increased CNS depression	Additive
Antimicrobials		
Chloramphenicol	Minor Antabuse-like reaction	Inhibits intermediary metabolism of alcohol
Furazolidone	Minor Antabuse-like reaction	Inhibits intermediary metabolism of alcohol
Griseofulvin	Minor Antabuse-like reaction	Inhibits intermediary metabolism of alcohol
Isoniazid	Decreased effect after chronic alcohol abuse	Undetermined
Metronidazole	Minor Antabuse-like reaction	Possible CNS effect
Quinacrine	Minor Antabuse-like reaction	Inhibits intermediary metabolism of alcohol
Hypoglycemics		
Chlorpropamide	Minor Antabuse-like reaction	Inhibits intermediary metabolism of alcohol
	Decreased hypoglycemic effect after chronic abuse	Enhanced microsomal enzyme activity
Tolbutamide	Increased hypoglycemic effect with ingestion of alcohol, particularly in fasting patients	Suppression of gluconeogenesis
	Minor Antabuse-like reaction	Inhibits intermediary metabolism of alcohol

Table 22-25 *(continued)*

Drug	Effect	Probable mechanism
Narcotics	Increased CNS depression with acute intoxication	Additive
Salicylates	Gastrointestinal bleeding	Additive
Sedatives and Psychotropic Drugs		
Barbiturates	Increased CNS depression with acute intoxication	Additive; reduced metabolism
	Decreased sedative effect after chronic alcohol abuse	Enhanced microsomal enzyme activity; decreased CNS sensitivity
Chloral hydrate	Prolonged hypnotic effect	Mutual potentiation
Chlordiazepoxide	Increased CNS depression	Additive
Chlorpromazine	Increased CNS depression	Additive; inhibits oxidation of alcohol
Clorazepate	Increased CNS depression	Additive
Diazepam	Increased CNS depression	Additive; possible increased absorption
Meprobamate	Increased CNS depression with acute intoxication	Additive; reduced metabolism
Oxazepam	Increased CNS depression	Additive
Other*		
Phentolamine	Minor Antabuse-like reaction	Inhibits intermediary metabolism of alcohol
Phenytoin	Increased anticonvulsant effect with acute intoxication	Reduced metabolism
	Decreased anticonvulsant effect after chronic alcohol abuse	Enhanced microsomal enzyme activity

*Many alcoholic beverages contain tyramine, which can cause reactions with MAO inhibitors.
Medical Letter 194:45, 1977. Reprinted with permission.

The Cognitive-acting Drugs

Drug therapy of the effects of senile brain impairment or progressive intellectual deterioration has shown variable results, possibly because of unrealistic goals and evaluation techniques (Gaitz et al 1977). It would be difficult to determine whether or not it is effective in restoring "memory," as memory includes a perceptual, attentional, learning, storage, and recall function. Thus, in general, there is agreement that attempts to manipulate memory and improve it with drugs have been largely unsuccessful.

Possibly, accepted concepts need first to be changed. Memory deficit is often expected in the elderly. It is true that the frequency of errors in learning sets of words (more than eight words) is greater in elderly than in younger persons when time is a factor. However, if time given for responding is lengthened, the difference between older and younger persons diminishes greatly, indicating that it is not memory that is impaired but reaction and concentration time. Resistance to fatigue and ability to concentrate is better in the young than in the old. However, the picture changes with certain disease states and treatment of diseases that masquerade as cognitive disorders has involved the use of cognitive-acting drugs.

Vasodilator therapy, which is now frequently used, is aimed at patients suffering from cerebral arteriosclerosis. The use of vasodilators is based on the assumption that there is neuronal damage due to reduced cerebral blood flow (Caplan 1977; Ban 1978). Cerebral blood flow is significantly reduced in geropsychiatric patients, but cerebral oxygen consumption is reduced only in patients with organic brain syndrome (Sokoloff 1975). The vasodilators are thought to act directly on arterial smooth muscle, but it is not clear that their use can overcome chronic hypoxia in cerebral arteriosclerosis. Concern has also been voiced that the "steal syndrome" may be too powerful.

When these drugs are used, they may actually shunt blood away from ischemic areas, as healthy blood vessels probably dilate better and receive more blood, causing greater hypoxia in the damaged areas. Another concern revolves around the "luxury perfusion syndrome," in which blood supply, stimulated by the vasodilators, may exceed the metabolic demands of the brain.

More recently, the vasodilators have been used to manage the so-called "grey area symptoms of the elderly." This would include confusion, lack of self-esteem, dizziness, mood depression, and unsociability, which may not necessarily be related to cerebrovascular insufficiency, but may be rooted in a large number of organic and psychosocial causes.

Literally hundreds of studies have been published involving the use of cerebral vasodilators such as cyclandelate and papaverine, the two most frequently used such drugs. Evidence of their effectiveness is indeed scanty, and while in some instances their effect is rated better than that of a placebo, in others no positive effect could be discerned (Capote and Parikh 1978; Davies et al 1977; Rao et al 1977). Further studies may show that these drugs do have a place in the therapeutic approach to the organic brain syndrome, particularly if patients to be treated are carefully selected (Branconnier and Cole 1977). Betahistine, a potent cerebral vasodilator, is thought to be somewhat effective in demented geriatric patients (Seipel et al 1977).

Metabolism-stimulating agents have been used to counteract decreased cerebral blood flow that can change brain metabolism. Lessened cerebral metabolism can then cause decreased cerebral blood flow. It has been reasoned that an increase in cerebral metabolism will increase blood flow (Gustafson and Risberg 1974; Obrist 1972).

A dihydrogenated ergot alkaloid preparation (eg, Hydergine) is probably the only drug currently marketed which may be classified as a metabolism-stimulating agent. It has been suggested that it increases the pyruvate-lactate ratio in hypothermic or ischemic brain disease, negating the hypometabolism induced by these states. The biochemical changes are paralleled by a return to normal electroencephalographic energy. This effect on the opening of the cerebral microcirculation is now viewed as a consequence of increased brain metabolism, rather than its cause. Hydergine inhibits phosphodiesterase, which could increase metabolic activity in terms of new protein synthesis (Mongeau 1974; McHenry et al 1971).

A recent review of 12 clinical trials found that this drug consistently produced improvement in 13 symptoms associated with dementia (Hughes et al 1976). The greatest benefit of Hydergine therapy seems to be in the area of intellectual function or cognition (Bazo 1973). Improvement has been noted in confusion, dizziness, unsociability, depressive mood, and mental alertness (Rosen 1975).

Another recent review (Cohen, S. 1978) reported that in the area of confusion, seven investigators reported dihydrogenated ergot alkaloids significantly better than comparative agents. Mood depression was found to respond significantly better to this drug compared to other agents by nine investigators. Similar statistics were reported for impaired self-care, unsociability, and dizziness. Of the total 49 symptom evaluations reviewed, all favored the dihydrogenated ergot alkaloids over the comparative agent, 34 (69%) at a significant level.

Response to this drug typically begins to appear around the sixth to eighth week of treatment and continues to improve throughout week 12.

The drug, which is now available both as a sublingual and an oral tablet, does have a definite place in the treatment of intellectual disorders of the elderly, but must be given in large enough doses for a prolonged period (up to three months) to be effective (Rao and Norris 1972). The new oral tablets are probably more convenient to take, encourage better patient compliance, and require less supervision of administration.

Other drugs and modalities The fact that there is not yet a drug which can be used effectively to manipulate learning and memory is reflected by the large number of drugs that continue to be tried, such as stimulants and depressants, cholinergic and adrenergic drugs, inhibitors of protein synthesis, and polypetides.

Those believing in orthomolecular psychiatry continue to advocate megadoses of vitamins (Hoffer 1977), but a task force of the American Psychiatric Association has concluded that megavitamin therapy for patients with schizophrenia is not helpful (Spector 1977). Dextroamphetamine has been tried (Lipper and Tuchman 1976), and methylphenidate has been recommended for previously unresponsive, oversedated, withdrawn, and apathetic patients (Kaplitz 1975). Physostigmine was very effective in one case of Korsakoff-type memory loss (Peters and Levin 1977).

Hyperbaric oxygen seems to aid some aged patients (*Journal of the American Medical Association* 1976). Hormonal therapy seems to offer promise in facilitating memory retrieval. Investigations involve most often the pituitary peptides and naturally occurring opioids (enkephalins and endorphins) (Jarvik and McGaugh 1978). There is some evidence that a new class of psychotropic drugs may be helpful. These are the nootropic (mind-activating) drugs, of which piracetam is an example. Large-scale studies in Europe and the United States show preliminary results that these experimental antidepressants may be at least as effective as the currently marketed ones in geropsychiatry, but without the side effects of current drugs.

Finally, based on the belief that brain ischemia is a fundamental factor in dementia, both the warfarin and bishydroxycoumarin anticoagulants have been tried with some success. While this type therapy could lead to serious complications and even death, it has been suggested for patients unresponsive to any other treatment modality, even in cases of extreme deterioration (Walsh 1968, 1969; Walsh and Walsh 1972, 1974; Walsh et al 1978).

Sedatives-Hypnotics

Occasional insomnia is universal in any patient population and chronic insomnia is a common complaint. Patients with insomnia are thought to show suppressed REM and non-REM sleep. This is important, as hypnotic agents also suppress REM and non-REM sleep, thus aggravating underlying EEG abnormalities.

The proper place for the traditional sleep medication is in the treatment of acute sleep disturbance secondary to situational stress and not in long-term treatment. All currently marketed drugs suppress REM sleep, but a delayed onset of REM deprivation of one to three weeks is characteristic of the benzodiazepines.

In general, chemopsychotherapeutic agents should be used with caution in patients with pain, fever, thirst, electrolyte imbalance, and a host of other factors which may predispose the patient to drug toxicity. Adverse effects of sedatives tend to be more frequent and more severe in the elderly and severe hypnotic drug intoxications are more dangerous and end lethally four times as often in elderly as in young patients (Summa 1975). Often, complete withdrawal of these drugs in heavily sedated patients leads to improved behavioral disturbances (Prinsley 1973). Side effects of hypnotic therapy may include incontinence, oversedation, hypotension, peripheral neuritis, and liver damage. These drugs may aggravate urinary retention and increase restlessness. Bromides and the belladonna alkaloids, which are found in nonprescription sleep medications, may lead to acute or cumulative toxic effects. Regular use of hypnotics can increase nightly awakenings, abolish deep sleep, and can continue to affect sleep patterns long after the drug is withdrawn (*Journal of the American Medical Association* 1977). Abrupt withdrawal of nonbenzodiazepine hypnotic drugs after prolonged administration may cause "drug-withdrawal insomnia" and an intense form of "rebound insomnia," ie, a worsening of sleep may follow the abrupt withdrawal of the short-acting benzodiazepines (Kales et al 1978). Early administration of sleep medication can lead to a high incidence of negative social behavior (Dittmar and Dulski 1977), while delay of evening administration may drastically curtail the need for hypnotics (Sheerin 1972). It would seem that routine patient care procedures often witnessed in nursing homes should give way to individualized dose administration times.

The barbiturates, as often cited in the abundant literature, should not be used in the elderly. Many elderly are confronted with a dose-related disinhibition, which leads to agitation, insomnia, excitement, and nocturnal restlessness. More serious is the fact that these drugs may be responsible for an unsteady gait (even in low doses), which could lead to falls and fractures. Low body weight seems to heighten the susceptibility of females to the adverse effects of barbiturates. Elderly patients receiving barbiturates as long-term therapy in middle age seem to be more susceptible to adverse effects of these drugs. The use of these drugs is particularly contraindicated in elderly patients with brain damage or poor renal function. Dependency develops rapidly and addiction can occur in about one month. The barbiturates also exhibit a high potential for drug interactions (Tables 22-26 and 22-27). Yet, a recent publication defended the "humble barbiturate"

(Simpson 1976) and barbiturates may be acceptable in doses used for daytime sedation or in moderate doses at bedtime (Cole and Stotsky 1974). Possibly because there are problems with almost all hypnotic drugs, both barbiturates and nonbarbiturates, the barbiturates continue to be used widely and the elderly find them quite useful and helpful. A major reason might well be the cost, as these drugs are much less expensive than are the benzodiazepines.

The benzodiazepines appear to interfere much less with REM sleep than the barbiturates, glutethimide, and others. True addiction to benzodiazepines is rare (Greenblatt and Shader 1974) and these drugs are considered safe for use in geriatric patients (Greenblatt et al 1975).

Flurazepam, if used as a short-term hypnotic, will have the same effectiveness as the barbiturates, but it has a much lower addiction potential than do the barbiturates. It is significantly effective in inducing and maintaining sleep during short, intermediate, and long-term administration (Kales et al 1976a).

While most hypnotics lose effectiveness when used chronically even for short periods of time (Greenblatt and Miller 1974; Kales et al 1977), flurazepam remains effective for at least four weeks, even on a chronic dosing pattern (Greenblatt et al 1975). Following withdrawal of the drug, there is a significant carryover effectiveness for one or two nights.

If flurazepam is used in high doses in the elderly, the incidence of adverse effects increases dramatically and is highest in the old-old. Ataxia, confusion, and hallucination can occur. Therefore, a dose of 15 mg at bedtime, three times weekly has been suggested.

Lorazepam, recently approved for use as a hypnotic, is not affected by aging or liver disease (Kraus et al 1978). Insufficient data at this time do not permit a good comparison of its effectiveness with that of flurazepam. Oxazepam has been suggested as a safe and efficacious

Table 22-26
Probable Clinically Significant Interactions of Phenobarbital with Other Drugs

Interacting drug	Effect
Bilirubin	Decreased serum bilirubin
Dexamethasone	Decreased half-life and increased metabolic clearance of dexamethasone
Doxycycline	Decreased half-life of doxycycline
Folic acid	Blocked uptake of folic acid
Prednisone	Worsening of asthma
Warfarin	Decreased warfarin plasma levels, half-life and prothrombin time

Table 22-27
Drugs That May Interact with Barbiturates

	Effect on pharmacologic action of barbiturates	Effect on clinical action of barbiturates	Untoward reactions
Antacids	Absorption of barbiturates may be decreased	May be decreased	
Antihistamines	Enhance CNS action of barbiturates	Increased	Increased
Benzodiazepines	Pharmacologic effect of barbiturates may be increased	Increased	CNS depression increased
Disulfiram	Metabolism of disulfiram may be decreased	May be increased	CNS depression may be increased
Ethyl alcohol	Pharmacologic effect of barbiturates may be increased	Increased	CNS depression markedly increased
Hypnotics, other	Enhance CNS action of barbiturates	Increased	CNS depression markedly increased
MAO inhibitors	Metabolism of barbiturates may be decreased	May be increased	CNS depression may be increased
Meprobamate	Enhances CNS action of barbiturates	Increased	Increased
Methylphenidate	Metabolism of barbiturates may be decreased	May be increased	CNS depression may be increased
Narcotics	Pharmacologic effect of barbiturates may be increased	Increased	CNS depression increased
Phenothiazines	Pharmacologic effect of barbiturates may be increased	Increased	CNS depression increased
Procarbazine	Pharmacologic effect of barbiturates may be increased	May be increased	CNS depression may be increased
Sulfonylureas	Pharmacologic effect of barbiturates may be increased	May be increased	CNS depression may be increased

drug for the short-term management of insomnia in the elderly (Goldstein et al 1978). Triazolam may be available soon. It is claimed to have a shorter duration of action than flurazepam with side effects similar to those of flurazepam. Drug withdrawal apparently can be followed by significant worsening of sleep (Fabre et al 1977; Leibowitz and Sunshine 1978; Reeves 1977; Kales et al 1976b). Some studies show it to be more effective than flurazepam (Okawa and Bountiful 1978).

Other hypnotics Glutethimide is still used, although it has a dependency liability and the mortality rate among patients taking an overdose is relatively high. It should not be used for elderly ambulatory patients who, in a confused state, may easily take an overdose, as this drug's toxic/therapeutic ratio is very narrow.

There is some ambivalence regarding chloral hydrate. While some clinicians feel it should not be used, others suggest it as the drug of choice, particularly for inducing sleep. A dose of 250 to 500 mg at bedtime has been suggested. The drug, which sometimes may induce a paradoxical reaction in the elderly, is actually widely used, particularly in nursing homes. Finally, diphenhydramine is often effective as a hypnotic in the elderly. Doses as small as 12.5 mg may be effective (Sunshine et al 1978).

REFERENCES

Abuzzahab, F.S. Psychoactive drugs in the elderly. Edited by J.T. Kelly, and J.H. Weir. In *Perspectives of Human Aging.* Minneapolis: Craftsman Press, 1976.

Ack, M., Bulger, J.J., Creson, D.L. et al. Clues to the diagnosis of anxiety. *Patient Care* 13(13):158, 1978.

Adler, S. Methyldopa-induced decrease in mental activity. *JAMA.* 230:1428, 1974.

Alter, M., and Rosenberg, B.S. Are all degenerative neurologic diseases slow virus infections? *Geriatrics* 32(11):77, 1977.

Appleton, W.D. Third psychoactive drug usage guide. *Dis Nerv Syst.* 37:39, 1976.

Ariea, T. Dementia in the elderly: diagnosis and assessment. *Br Med J.* 4:540, 1973.

Ayd, F.J. A survey of drug-induced extrapyramidal reactions. *JAMA.* 175:1054, 1961.

Ayd, F.J. A critical evaluation of molindone (Moban): a new indole derivative neuroleptic. *Dis Nerv Syst.* 35:447, 1974.

Ayd, F.J. Psychotropic drug combinations: good and bad. Edited by M. Greenblatt. In *Drugs in Combination with Other Therapies.* New York: Grune and Stratton, 1975a.

Ayd, F.J. Single daily doses of antidepressants. *JAMA.* 230:263, 1975b.

Bahemuka, M., and Hodkinson, H.M. Screening for hypothyroidism in the elderly inpatient. *Br Med J.* 2:601, 1975.

Baldessarini, R.J. Schizophrenia. *N Engl J Med.* 297:988, 1977.

Baldessarini, R.J., and Lipinski, J.F. Risks vs benefits of antipsychotic drugs. *N Engl J Med.* 289:427, 1973.

Baldessarini, R.J., and Tarsy, D. Tardive dyskinesia. Edited by M.A. Lipton, A. DiMascio, and K.F. Killam. In *Psychopharmacology: A Generation of Progress.* New York: Raven Press, 1978.

Ban, T.A. Vasodilators, stimulants, and anabolic agents in the treatment of geropsychiatric patients. Edited by M.A. Lipton, A. DiMascio, and K.F. Killam. In *Psychopharmacology: A Generation of Progress.* New York: Raven Press, 1978.

Barrett, J.E., and DiMascio, A. Comparative effects of anxiety of the "minor tranquilizers" in "high" and "low" anxious student volunteers. *Dis Nerv Syst.* 27:483, 1966.

Barton, R., and Hurst, L. Unnecessary use of tranquilizers in elderly patients. *Br J Psychiatry.* 112:989, 1966.

Baylis, P.H., and Heath, D.A. Water disturbances in patients treated with lithium carbonate. *Ann Intern Med.* 88:607, 1978.

Bayne, J.R.D. Management of confusion in elderly patients. *Can Med Assoc J.* 118:139, 1978.

Bazo, A.J. An ergot alkaloid preparation (Hydergine) versus papaverine in treating common complaints of the aged: a double-blind study. *J Am Geriatr Soc.* 21:63, 1973.

Beasley, B.A.L., and Ford, D.H. Aging and the extrapyramidal system. *Med Clin North Am.* 60:1315, 1976.

Becker, P.W., and Conn, S.H. Beer and social therapy treatment with geriatric psychiatric patient groups. *Addict Dis.* 3:429, 1978.

Berger, F.M. Therapeutic uses of meprobomate and the propanediols. Edited by L.L. Simpson. In *Drug Treatment of Mental Disorders.* New York: Raven Press, 1976a.

Berger, F.M. Present status of clinical psychopharmacology. *Clin Pharmacol Ther.* 19:725, 1976b.

Berger, P.A. Medical treatment of mental illness. *Science* 200:974, 1978.

Bergmann, K. Assessment of therapy in psychogeriatric illness. *Gerontol Clin.* 16:54, 1974.

Betz, A.L., and Goldstein, G.W. Polarity of the blood-brain barrier: neutral amino acid transport into isolated brain capillaries. *Science* 202:225, 1978.

Bianchine, J.R. Drug therapy of parkinsonism. *N Engl J Med.* 295:814, 1976.

Bianchine, J.R., and Sunyaprikadul, L. Individualization of levodopa therapy. *Med Clin North Am.* 58:1071, 1974.

Bigger, J.T., Giardina, E.G.V., Perel, J.M. et al. Cardiac antiarrhythmic effect of imipramine hydrochloride. *N Engl J Med.* 296:206, 1977.

Bigger, J.T., Kantor, S.J., Glassman, A.H. et al. Cardiovascular effects of tricyclic antidepressant drugs. Edited by M.A. Lipton, A. DiMascio, and K.F. Killam. In *Psychopharmacology: A Generation of Progress.* New York: Raven Press, 1978.

Biggs, J.T. Clinical pharmacology and toxicology of antidepressants. *Hosp Practice.* 13(2):79, 1978.

Biggs, J.T., Davis, J.M., Fann, W.E. et al. *The Tricyclic Antidepressants, Current Issues and Perspectives.* East Hanover, N.J.: Sandoz Pharmacueticals, 1977.

Bignami, G. Effects of neuroleptics, ethanol, hypnotic-sedatives, tranquilizers, narcotics and minor stimulants in adversive paradigms. Edited by H. Anisman, and G. Bignami. In *Psychopharmacology of Aversively Motivated Behavior.* New York: Plenum Press, 1978.

Black, A.L. Altering behavior of geriatric patients with beer. *Northwest Med.* 453, 1969.

Blackwell, B. Psychotropic drugs in use today: the role of diazepam in medical practice. *JAMA.* 225:1637, 1973.

Blackwell, B. Rational drug use in the management of anxiety. *Rational Drug Ther.* 9(6):1, 1975.

Blunk, W., and Gross, D. *Die Schlafstoerung und Ihre Behandlung.* Stuttgart: Hippokrates Verlag, 1971.

Bookman, P.H., and Randall, L.O. Therapeutic uses of the benzodiazepines. Edited by L.L. Simpson. In *Drug Treatment of Mental Disorders.* New York: Raven Press, 1976.

Boston Collaborative Drug Surveillance Program. Psychiatric side effects of nonpsychiatric drugs. *Semin Psychiatry.* 3:406, 1971.

Boston Collaborative Drug Reaction Surveillance Program. Adverse reaction to the tricyclic-antidepressant drugs. *Lancet* 1:529, 1972.

Bowen, D.M. Neurochemistry of senile dementia. Edited by A.N. Davison, and N.A. Hood. In *Action on Aging,* Proceedings of a Symposium, Basle, Switzerland, May 1976. Tunbridge Wells, England: Medical Congresses and Sympsoia Consultants, 1976.

Bowen, R.C. The effect of diazepam on the recovery of endogenously depressed patients. *J Clin Pharmacol.* 18:280, 1978.

Branchey, M.H., Lee, H., Amin, R. et al. High- and low-potency neuroleptics in elderly psychiatric patients. *JAMA.* 239:1860, 1978.

Branconnier, R.J., and Cole, J.D. A memory assessment technique for use in geriatric psycho-pharmacology: drug efficacy trial with naflidrofuryl. *J Am Geriatr Soc.* 25:186, 1977.

British Medical Journal. Depression in old age. 1:1031, 1976.

Brodie, N.H., McGhie, R.L., O'Hara, H. et al. Anxiety/depression in elderly patients. *Practitioner* 215:660, 1975.

Bureau of Drugs. Report of the geriatric neuropsychopharmacology subcommittee. Rockville, Md., 1976.

Busse, E.W. Hypochondriasis in the elderly: a reaction to social stress. *J Am Geriatr Soc.* 24:145, 1976.

Busse, E.W., and Pfeiffer, E. *Mental Illness in Later Life.* Washington, D.C.: American Psychiatric Association, 1973.

Butler, R.N. Psychiatry and the elderly: an overview. *Am J Psychiatry.* 132:893, 1975.

Butler, R.N. Research in organic brain diseases of the elderly. Presented at an Interdisciplinary Conference: Current Concepts in Care of the Elderly, George Washington University. Washington, D.C., 1978.

Butler, R.N., and Lewis, M.I. *Aging and Mental Health.* St. Louis: C.V. Mosby Co., 1973.

Byck, R. Drugs and the treatment of psychiatric disorders. Edited by L.S. Goodman, and A. Gilman. In *The Pharmacological Basis of Therapeutics.* New York: MacMillan Publishing Co., Inc., 1975.

Cahalan, D. *Problem Drinkers.* San Francisco: Jossey-Bass, Inc., 1970.

Calne, D.B. Developments in the treatment of parkinsonism. *N Engl J Med.* 295:1433, 1976.

Cameron, I., Frankel, J., Savitsky, E. et al. Assessing and managing dementia. *Patient Care* 11(20):90, 1977.

Caplan, L.R. Drug therapy reviews: vasodilating drugs and their use in cerebral symptomatology. *Am J Hosp Pharm.* 34:1075, 1977.

Capote, B. and Parikh, N. Cyclandelate in the treatment of senility: a controlled study. *J Am Geriatr Soc.* 26:360, 1978.

Charalampous, K.D. Pharmacotherapy of schizophrenia. Edited by W.E. Fann, I. Karacan, A.D. Pokorny et al. In *Phenomenology and Treatment of Schizophrenia.* New York: Spectrum Publications, Inc., 1978.

Charatan, F.B. Depression in old age. *NY State J Med.* 75:2505, 1975.

Chien, C. Beer more effective than drugs as psychologic prop to elderly. *Geriatr Focus.* 9:5, 1970.

Ching-Piao, C. Psychiatric treatment for geriatric patients: "pub" or drug? *Am J Psychiatry.* 127:110, 1971.

Ching-Piao, C., Stotsky, B.A., and Cole, J.O. Psychiatric treatment for nursing home patients: drug, alcohol, and milieu. *Am J Psychiatry.* 130:543, 1973.

Claveria, L.E., Calne, D.B., and Allen, J.G. On-off phenomena related to high plasma levodopa. *Br Med J.* 2:641, 1973.

Cohen, E.L., and Wurtman, R.J. Brain acetylcholine: increase after systemic choline administration. *Life Sci.* 16:1102, 1975.

Cohen, E.L., and Wurtman, R.J. Brain acetylcholine: control by dietary choline. *Science* 191:561, 1976.

Cohen, G.D. Approach to the geriatric patient. *Med Clin North Am.* 61:855, 1977.

Cohen, G.D. Comment: organic brain syndrome, reality orientation for critics of clinical interventions. *Gerontologist* 18:313, 1978.

Cohen, M.M., and Scheife, R.T. Pharmacotherapy of Parkinson's disease. *Am J Hosp Pharm.* 34:531, 1977.

Cohen, S. Mental impairment in the aged: fable and fact. Scientific Exhibit, 31st Annual Meeting, Gerontological Society. Dallas, Texas, 1978.

Cole, J.O. Phenothiazines. Edited by L.L. Simpson. In *Drug Treatment of Mental Disorders.* New York: Raven Press, 1976.

Cole, J.O., and Stotsky, B.A. Improving psychiatric drug therapy: a matter of dosage and choice. *Geriatrics* 29:74, 1974.

Cole, J.O., Swett, C., and Pope, H.G. Agranulocytosis revisited. *McLean Hosp J.* 1:34, 1976.

Cooper, J.R., Bloom, F.E., and Roth, R.H. *The Biochemical Basis of Neuropharmacology.* New York: Oxford University Press, 1978.

Cooperstock, R. Sex differences in the use of mood-modifying drugs: an explanatory model. *J Health Soc Behav.* 12:238, 1971.

Cotzias, G.C., Miller, S.T., Tang, L.C. et al. Levodopa, fertility and longevity. *Science* 196:549, 1977.

Crane, G.E. Clinical psychopharmacology in its 20th year. *Science* 181:124, 1973a.

Crane, G.E. Persistent dyskinesia. *Br J Psychiatry.* 122:395, 1973b.

Davies, G., Hamilton, S., Hendrickson, E. et al. The effect of cyclandelate in depressed patients: a controlled study in psychogeriatric patients. *Age Ageing.* 6:156, 1977.

Davis, J., and Fann, W. Lithium. *Annu Rev Pharmacol.* 11:285, 1971.

Davis, K.L., Berger, P.A., Hollister, L.E. et al. Choline chloride in the treatment of Huntington's disease and tardive dyskinesia: a preliminary report. *Psychopharmacol Bull.* 13(3):37, 1977.

deGroot, M.H.L. The clinical use of psychotherapeutic drugs in the elderly. *Drugs* 8:132, 1974.

Delaney, J.C., and Ravey, M. Cimetidine and mental confusion. *Lancet* 2:512, 1977.

Dettman, G. Parkinson's disease and ascorbate. *Med J Aust.* 1:131, 1976.

DeVeaugh-Geiss, J. Aggravation of tardive dyskinesia by phenytoin. *N Engl J Med.* 298:457, 1978.

Diamond, S., Goldberg, H.L., Hodge, J.R. et al. Nine experts review an FPs depression regimen. *Patient Care* 11(5):42, 1977.

DiMascio, A., and Barrett, J.E. Comparative effects of oxazepam in "high" and "low" anxious student volunteers. *Psychosomatics* 6:298, 1965.

DiMascio, A., and Demirgian, E. Antiparkinsonian drug overuse. *Psychosomatics* 11:596, 1970.

DiMascio, A., Haskell, D., and Prusoll, B. Rapidity of symptom reduction in depressions treated with amitriptyline. *J New Ment Dis.* 160:24, 1975.

DiMascio, A., and Sovner, R.D. Neuroleptic-induced extrapyramidal side effects. *Drug Ther.* 6(10):99, 1976.

DiMascio, A., Bernardo, D.L., Greenblatt, D.J. et al. A controlled trial of amantadine in drug-induced extrapyramidal disorders. *Psychopharmacol Bull.* 13(3):31, 1977.

Dittmar, S.S., and Dulski, T. Early evening administration of sleep medication to the hospitalized aged: a consideration in rehabilitation. *Nurs Res.* 26:299, 1977.

Dock, W. The clinical value of alcohol. Edited by S.P. Lucia. In *Alcohol and Civilization.* New York: McGraw-Hill Book Co., 1963.

Donlon, P.T., and Stenson, R.L. Neuroleptic-induced extrapyramidal symptoms. *Dis Nerv Syst.* 37:629, 1976.

Dublin, L.I. *Suicide.* New York: Ronald Press, 1963.

Eisdorfer, C. Observations on the psychopharmacology of the aged. *J Am Geriatr Soc.* 23:53, 1975.

Ellison, R.J., and Cancellaro, L.A. A study in the management of anxiety with lorazepam. *J Clin Pharmacol.* 18:210, 1978.

Ende, W. Zur Lithiumdauermedikation bei Manisch Depressiven Erkrankungen im Hoeheren Lebensalter. *Z Alternsforsch.* 30:351, 1975.

Epstein, L.J. Depression in the elderly. *J Gerontol.* 31:278, 1976.

Epstein, L.J. Anxiolytics, antidepressants, and neuroleptics in the treatment of geriatric patients. Edited by M.A. Lipton, A. DiMascio, and K.F. Killam. In *Psychopharmacology: A Generation of Progress.* New York: Raven Press, 1978.

Ernst, P., Badash, D., Beran, B. et al. Incidence of mental illness in the aged: unmasking the effects of diagnosis of chronic brain syndrome. *J Am Geriatr Soc.* 25:371, 1977a.

Ernst, P., Beran, B., Badash, D. et al. Treatment of the aged mentally ill: further unmasking of the effects of diagnosis of chronic brain syndrome. *J Am Geriatr Soc.* 25:466, 1977b.

Fabre, L.F., Gross, L., Pasigajen, V. et al. Multiclinic double-blind comparison of triazolam and flurazepam for seven nights in out-patients with insomnia. *J Clin Pharmacol.* 17:402, 1977.

Fah, S., and Isgree, W.P. Long-term evaluation of amantadine and levodopa combination in parkinsonism by double-blind crossover analyses. *Neurology* 25:695, 1975.

Fann, W.E., and Lake, D.R. On the coexistence of parkinsonism and tardive dyskinesia. *Dis Nerv Syst.* 34:324, 1974.

Fann, W.E., and Wheless, J.C. The new antipsychotics. Edited by W.E. Fann, I. Karacan, A.D. Pokorny et al. In *Phenomenology and Treatment of Schizophrenia.* New York: Spectrum Publications, Inc., 1978.

Faucett, R.L., Litin, E.M., and Achor, R.W.P. Neuropharmacologic action of rauwolfia compounds and its psychodynamic implications. *Arch Neurol Psychiatry.* 77:513, 1957.

Feinberg, I. The ontogenesis of human sleep and the relationship of sleep variables to intellectual function in the aged. *Compr Psychiatry.* 9:138, 1968.

Feinberg, I., and Carlson, V.R. Sleep variables as a function of age in man. *Arch Gen Psychiatry.* 18:239, 1968.

Fisher, S. Nonspecific factors as determinants of behavioral response to drugs. Edited by A. DiMascio, and R.I. Shader. In *Clinical Handbook of Psychopharmacology.* New York: Science House, Inc., 1970.

Frazer, A., and Winokur, A. Psychotropic drugs. Edited by A. Frazer, and A. Winokur. In *Biological Bases of Psychiatric Disorders*. New York: Spectrum Publications, Inc., 1977.

Freeman, H. The therapeutic value of combinations of psychotropic drugs, a review. *Psychopharmacol Bull.* 4:1, 1967.

Freemon, F.R. Evaluation of patients with progressive intellectual deterioration. *Arch Neurol.* 33:658, 1976.

Friedel, R.O. Pharmacokinetics in the geropsychiatric patient. Edited by M.A. Lipton, A. DiMascio, and K.F. Killam. In *Psychopharmacology: A Generation of Progress*. New York: Raven Press, 1978.

Gaitz, C.M., Varner, R.V., and Overall, J.E. Pharmacotherapy for organic brain syndrome in late life. *Arch Gen Psychiatry.* 34:839, 1977.

Garattini, S., and Samanin, R. Physiological regulation and pharmacological action. Edited by W.B. Essman. In *Serotonin in Health and Disease, Volume II, Physiological Regulation and Pharmacological Action*. New York: Spectrum Publications, Inc., 1978.

Gardos, G., and Cole, J.O. Maintenance antipsychotic therapy: is the cure worse than the disease? *Am J Psychiatry.* 133:32, 1976.

Gelenberg, A.J., and Mandel, M.R. Catatonic reactions to high-potency neuroleptic drugs. *Arch Gen Psychiatry.* 34:947, 1977.

Gerbino, L., Oleshansky, M., and Gershon, S. Clinical use and mode of action of lithium. Edited by M.A. Lipton, A. DiMascio, and K.F. Killam. In *Psychopharmacology: A Generation of Progress*. New York: Raven Press, 1978.

Gerlich, J., Reisby, N., and Randrup, A. Dopaminergic hypersensitivity and cholinergic hypofunctions in the pathophysiology of tardive dyskinesia. *Psychopharmacologia* 34:21, 1974.

Ghodse, A.H. Deliberate self-poisoning: a study in London casualty departments. *Br Med J.* 1:805, 1977.

Gilbert, G.J. Quinidine dementia. *JAMA.* 237:2093, 1977.

Glickman, L., and Friedman, S.A. Changes in behavior, mood, or thinking in the elderly. *Med Clin North Am.* 60:1297, 1976.

Godwin-Austen, R.B., and Smith, N.J. Comparison of the effects of bromocriptine and levodopa in Parkinson's disease. *J Neurol Neurosurg Psychiatry.* 40:479, 1977.

Goldberg, R.S., and Thorton, W.E. Combined tricyclic-MAOI therapy for refractory depression: a review with guidelines for appropriate usage. *J Clin Pharmacol.* 18:143, 1978.

Goldfarb, A.J. Masked depression in the old. *Am J Psychotherapy.* 21:791, 1967.

Goldstein, B.J. Drug therapy for the depressed patient. *Hosp Formulary.* 12:855, 1977.

Goldstein, B.J., and Brauger, B. Pharmacologic considerations in the treatment of anxiety and depression in medical practice. *Med Clin North Am.* 55:487, 1971.

Goldstein, S.E., and Birnbom, F. Hypochondriasis and the elderly. *J Am Geriatr Soc.* 24:150, 1976.

Goldstein, S.E., Birnbom, F., Lancee, W.J. et al. Comparison of oxazepam and chloral hydrate as hypnotic sedatives in geriatric patients. *J Am Geriatr Soc.* 26:366, 1978.

Gottlieb, R.M., Nappi, T., and Strain, J.J. The physician's knowledge of psychotropic drugs: preliminary results. *Am J Psychiatry.* 135:29, 1978.

Gram, L.F. Plasma level monitoring of tricyclic antidepressant therapy. *Clin Pharmacokinet.* 2:237, 1977.

Grauer, H. Depression in the aged, theoretical concepts. *J Am Geriatr Soc.* 25:447, 1977.

Greenblatt, D.J., and Miller, R.R. Rational use of psychotropic drugs. I. Hypnotics. *Am J Hosp Pharm.* 31:990, 1974.

Greenblatt, D.J., and Koch-Weser, J. Clinical toxicity of chlordiazepoxide and diazepam in relation to serum albumin concentration: a report from the Boston Collaborative Drug Surveillance Program. *Eur J Clin Pharmacol.* 7:259, 1974.

Greenblatt, D.J., and Shader, R.I. Benzodiazepines. *N Engl J Med.* 291:1239, 1974a.

Greenblatt, D.J., and Shader, R.I. *Benzodiazepines in Clinical Practice.* New York: Raven Press, 1974b.

Greenblatt, D.J., and Koch-Weser, J. Clinical pharmacokinetics, Part II. *N Engl J Med.* 293:964, 1975.

Greenblatt, D.J., Shader, R.I., and Koch-Weser, J. Flurazepam hydrochloride, a benzodiazepine hypnotic. *Ann Intern Med.* 83:237, 1975.

Greenblatt, D.J., DiMascio, A., Harmatz, J.S. et al. Pharmacokinetics and clinical effects of amantadine in drug-induced extrapyramidal symptoms. *J Clin Pharmacol.* 17:704, 1977.

Grøn, V. Bromocriptine versus placebo in levodopa-treated patients with Parkinson's disease. *Acta Neurol Scand.* 56:269, 1977.

Growdon, J.H., Hirsch, M.H., Wurtman, R.J. et al. Oral choline administration to patients with tardive dyskinesia. *N Engl J Med.* 297:524, 1977.

Growdon, J.H., Gelenberg, A.J., Doller, J. et al. Lecithin can suppress tardive dyskinesia. *N Engl J Med.* 298:1029, 1978.

Guidotti, A. Synaptic mechanisms in the action of benzodiazepines. Edited by M.A. Lipton, A. DiMascio, and K.F. Killam. In *Psychopharmacology: A Generation of Progress.* New York: Raven Press, 1978.

Gurland, B.J. The comparative frequency of depression in various adult groups. *J Gerontol.* 31:283, 1976.

Gustafson, L., and Risberg, J. Regional blood flow related to psychiatric symptoms in dementia with onset in the presenile period. *Acta Psychiatr Scand.* 50:516, 1974.

Guttman, D. *A Survey of Drug-Taking Behavior of the Elderly.* Washington, D.C.: Catholic University of America, 1977.

Haefely, W.E. Behavioral and neuropharmacological aspects of drugs used in anxiety and related states. Edited by M.A. Lipton, A. DiMascio, and K.F. Killam. In *Psychopharmacology: A Generation of Progress.* New York: Raven Press, 1978.

Hall, M.R.P. Adverse drug reactions in the elderly. *Gerontol Clin.* 16:144, 1974.

Hanson, H.M., Stone, C.A., and Witoslawski, J.J. Antagonism of antiavoidance effects of various agents by anticholinergic drugs. *J Pharmacol Exp Ther.* 173:117, 1970.

Harrison, M.J.G., and Marsden, C.D. Progressive intellectual deterioration. *Arch Neurol.* 34:199, 1977.

Hartman, E. Drugs for insomnia. *Rational Drug Ther.* 11(12):1, 1977.

Hausner, R. Drugs that reduce efficacy of levodopa. *N Engl J Med.* 295:1538, 1976.

Heilman, K.M., and Fisher, W.R. Hyperlipidemic dementia. *Arch Neurol.* 31:67, 1974.

Henschke, P.J., and Pain, R.W. Thyroid disease in a psychogeriatric population. *Age Ageing.* 6:151, 1977.

Himmelhoch, J.M., Poust, R.I., Mallinger, A.G. et al. Adjustment of lithium dose during lithium-chlorothiazide therapy. *Clin Pharmacol Ther.* 22:225, 1977.

Hirsch, M.J., and Wurtman, R.J. Lecithin consumption increases acetylcholine concentrations in rat brain and adrenal gland. *Science* 202:223, 1978.

Hoehn, M.M. Levodopa-induced postural hypotension: treatment with fluorocortisone. *Arch Neurol.* (Chicago)32:50, 1975.

Hoffer, A. Orthomolecular psychiatry in theory and practice. *Drug Ther.* 7(8):79, 1977.

Hollister, L.E. Methodological considerations in evaluating anti-anxiety drugs. *J Clin Pharmacol.* 10:12, 1970.

Hollister, L.E. Psychiatric syndromes due to drugs. Edited by L. Meyler, and H.M. Peck. In *Drug-Induced Diseases,* Vol. 4. Amsterdam: Excerpta Medica, 1972.

Hollister, L.E. *Clinical Use of Psychotropic Drugs.* Springfield, Ill.: Charles C Thomas, Publisher, 1973.

Hollister, L.E. Clinical use of tricyclic antidepressants. *Dis Nerv Syst.* 37:17, 1976.

Horn, J., and Wanberg, K. Symptom patterns related to excessive use of alcohol. *Q J Stud Alcohol.* 30:35, 1969.

Hughes, J.R., Williams, J.G., and Currier, R.D. An ergot alkaloid preparation (Hydergine) in the treatment of dementia: a critical review of the clinical literature. *J Am Geriatr Soc.* 24:490, 1976.

Hurtig, H.I., and Dyson, W.L. Lithium toxicity enhanced by diuresis. *N Engl J Med.* 290:749, 1974.

JAMA Medical News. Hyperbaric oxygen seems to aid some aged patients. 231:238, 1976.

JAMA Commentary. Chronic insomnia provokes more prescriptions than diagnoses. 237:1569, 1977.

Jarvik, L.F. The aging central nervous system: clinical aspects. Edited by M. Brody, D. Harman, and J.M. Ordy. In *Aging,* Vol. 1. New York: Raven Press, 1975.

Jarvik, M.E., and McGaugh, J.L. Drug influences on learning and memory: progress in research, 1967-1977. Edited by M.A. Lipton, A. DiMascio, and K.F. Killam. In *Psychopharmacology: A Generation of Progress.* New York: Raven Press, 1978.

Joffe, J.R. Functional disorders in the elderly. *Hosp Practice.* 11(6):93, 1976.

Joffe, J.R. Functional psychiatric disorders. Edited by W. Reichel. In *The Geriatric Patient.* New York: H.P. Publishing Co., Inc., 1978.

Johnels, B., Wallin, L., and Walinder, J. Extrapyramidal side effects of lithium treatment. *Br Med J.* 2:642, 1976.

Johns, M.W. Management of insomnia. *Drugs* 4:290, 1972.

Jovanovic, U.J. *Schlaf und Traum.* Stuttgart: G. Fischer Verlag, 1974.

Judge, T.G. Drug treatment of brain failure. *Age Ageing.* 6(suppl):70, 1977.

Kahn, E., and Fisher, C. The sleep characteristics of the normal aged male. *J Nerv Ment Dis.* 148:477, 1969.

Kahn, R.L., Zarit, S.H., Hilbert, N.M. et al. Memory complaint and impairment in the elderly. *Arch Gen Psychiatry.* 32:1569, 1975.

Kales, A., and Kales, J. Recent advances in the diagnosis and treatment of sleep disorders. Edited by G. Usdin. In *Sleep Research and Clinical Practice.* New York: Brunner/Mazel, Publishers, 1973.

Kales, A., Bixler, E.O., Scharf, M.B. et al. Sleep laboratory studies of flurazepam: a model for evaluating hypnotic drugs. *Clin Pharmacol Ther.*

19:576, 1976a.

Kales, A., Kales, J.D., Bixler, E.O. et al. Hypnotic efficacy of triazolam: sleep laboratory evaluation of intermediate-term effectiveness. *J Clin Pharmacol.* 16:399, 1976b.

Kales, A., Bixler, E.O., Kales, J.D. et al. Comparative effectiveness of nine hypnotic drugs: sleep laboratory studies. *J Clin Pharmacol.* 17:207, 1977.

Kales, A., Scharf, M.B., and Kales, J.D. Rebound insomnia: a new clinical syndrome. *Science* 201:1039, 1978.

Kanowski, S., and Paur, R. Psychopharmaka in der Geriatrie. *Therapiewoche.* 26:3822, 1976.

Kaplitz, S.E. Withdrawn, apathetic geriatric patients responsive to methylphenidate. *J Am Geriatr Soc.* 23:271, 1975.

Kartzinel, R., Shoulson, I., and Calne, D.B. Studies with bromocriptine. II. *Neurology* 26:511, 1976.

Kastenbaum, R., and Slater, P. Effects of wine on the interpersonal behavior of geriatric patients: an explanatory study. Edited by R. Kastenbaum. In *New Thoughts on Old Age.* New York: Springer Publishing Co., 1964.

Kastenbaum, R. Wine and fellowship in aging: an explorative action program. *J Hum Rel.* 13:266, 1965.

Kay, D.W.K. Outcome and cause of death in mental disorders of old age. Long-term follow-up of functional and organic psychoses. *Acta Psychiatr Scand.* 38:249, 1962.

Kazamatsuri, H., Chien, C., and Cole, J.O. Treatment of tardive dyskinesia. III. Clinical efficacy of a dopamine-competing agent, methyldopa. *Arch Gen Psychiatry.* 27:824, 1972.

Kelly, J.T., Hanson, R.G., Garetz, F.K. et al. What family physicians should know about treating elderly patients. *Geriatrics* 32:109, 1977.

Kielholz, P. *Diagnose und Therapie der Depression für den Praktiker.* Munich: J.F. Lehmanns Verlag, 1971.

Klawans, H.L. *The Pharmacology of Extrapyramidal Movement Disorders.* Basel: S. Karger Verlag, 1973a.

Klawans, H.L. The pharmacology of tardive dyskinesia. *Am J Psychiatry.* 130:82, 1973b.

Klerman, G.L. Long-term treatment of affective disorders. Edited by M.A. Lipton, A. DiMascio, and K.F. Killam. In *Pyschopharmacology: A Generation of Progress.* New York: Raven Press, 1978.

Klotz, U., Avant, G.R., Hoyumpa, A. et al. The effects of age and liver disease on the disposition and elimination of diazepam in adult man. *J Clin Invest.* 55:347, 1975.

Kobayashi, R.M. Drug therapy of tardive dyskinesia. *N Engl J Med.* 296:257, 1977.

Koeller, W., and Levin, P. (eds). *Sleep.* First European Congress on Sleep Research. Basel, New York: S. Karger Verlag, 1973.

Kramer, J.C., Klein, D.F., and Fink, M. Withdrawal symptoms following discontinuation of imipramine therapy. *Am J Psychiatry.* 118:549, 1961.

Kraus, J.W., Desmond, P.V., Marshall, J.P. et al. Effects of aging and liver disease on disposition of lorazepam. *Clin Pharmacol Ther.* 24:411, 1978.

Kristensen, O., and Hansen, E. Bromocriptine in the treatment of advanced parkinsonism. *Acta Neurol Scand.* 56:274, 1977.

Lader, M.H. Drug-induced extrapyramidal syndromes. *J R Coll Physicians.* 5:87, 1970.

Langsley, D.G., and Martin, L.R. Acute and chronic anxiety. Edited by H.F. Conn, R.E. Rakel, and T.W. Johnson. In *Family Practice.* Philadelphia: W.B. Saunders Co., 1973.

Lamy, P.P. Drug interactions: a growing problem, Part II. *Hosp Formulary Management.* 10:161, 1975.

Lasagna, L. Hypnotic drugs. *N Engl J Med.* 287:1186, 1972.

Leake, C.D., and Silverman, M. The clinical use of wine in geriatrics. *Geriatr Focus.* 6:175, 1967.

Lehmann, H.E., and Ban, T.A. Selecting psychotropic agents by metabolic response. *Drug Ther.* 7(1):32, 1977.

Leibowitz, M., and Sunshine, A. Long-term hypnotic efficacy and safety of triazolam and flurazepam. *J Clin Pharmacol.* 18:302, 1978.

Lennard, H.L., Epstein, L.J., Bernstein, A. et al. Hazards implicit in prescribing psychoactive drugs. *Science* 169:438, 1970.

Lennard, H.L., Epstein, L.J., Bernstein, A. et al. *Mystification of Drug Misuse.* New York: Jossey-Bass, Inc., 1971.

Lennard, H.L., and Bernstein, A. Perspectives on the new psychoactive drug technology. Edited by R. Cooperstock. In *Social Aspects of the Medical Use of Psychotropic Drugs.* Toronto: Addiction Research Foundation of Ontario, 1974.

Leopold, N. Medical management of movement disorders. *Hosp Formulary.* 12:519, 1977.

Lewis, C., Ballinger, B.R., and Presley, A.S. Trial of levodopa in senile dementia. *Br Med J.* 1:550, 1978.

Lewis, W.M. Iatrogenic psychotic depressive reaction in hypertensive patients. *Am J Psychiatry.* 127:1416, 1971.

Lipper, S., and Tuchman, M.M. Treatment of chronic post-trauma organic brain syndrome with dextroamphetamine: first reported case. *J Nerv Ment Dis.* 162:366, 1976.

Livesley, B. Brain failure–pathogenesis and presentation. Edited by A.N. Davison, and N.A. Hood. In *Action on Aging.* Proceedings of a Symposium, Basle, Switzerland, May 1976. Tunbridge Wells, England: Medical Congresses and Symposia Consultants, 1976.

Lloyd, K.G., Davidson, L., and Hornykiewicz, O. Parkinson's disease: activity of L-dopa decarboxylase in discrete brain regions. *Science* 170:1212, 1970.

Lucia, S.P. *A History of Wine as Medicine.* Philadelphia: J.B. Lippincott Co., 1963.

Lucia, S.P. Medicinal values of wine. *Med Digest.* 14(6):40, 1968.

Maas, J.W. Biogenic amines and depression–biochemical and pharmacological separation of two types of depression. *Arch Gen Psychiatry.* 32:1357, 1975.

Mancini, R.T. *Alcohol Interactions.* Philadelphia: Smith Kline and French Laboratories, 1970.

Marsden, C.D., and Harrison, M.J.G. Outcome of investigation of patients with presenile dementia. *Br Med J.* 2:249, 1972.

McDonald, R.L. The effects of personality type on drug response. *Arch Gen Psychiatry.* 17:680, 1967.

McFie, A.C. Lithium poisoning precipitated by diuretics. *Br Med J.* 1:516, 1975.

McGennis, A.J. Lithium carbonate and tetracycline interaction. *Br Med J.* 1:1183, 1978.

McHenry, L.C., Jaffe, M.E., Kawamura, J. et al. Hydergine effect on cerebral circulation in cerebrovascular disease. *J Neurol Sci.* 13:475, 1971.

Medical Letter. Drugs for psychiatric disorders. 18:89, 1976.

Medical Letter. Choice of benzodiazepine for treatment of anxiety of insomnia. 19:49, 1977a.

Medical Letter. Bromocriptine. 19:103, 1977b.
Medical Letter. Drugs for depression. 20:49, 1978.
Mehta, D., Mehta, S., and Mathew, P. Tardive dyskinesia in psychogeriatric patients: a five-year follow-up. *J Am Geriatr Soc.* 25:545, 1977.
Meier-Ruge, W., Enz, A., Gygax, P. et al. Experimental pathology in basic research of the aging brain. Edited by S. Gershon, and A. Raskin. In *Aging,* Vol. 2. New York: Raven Press, 1975.
Meyer, J.S., Welch, K.M.A., Deshmukh, V.D. et al. Neurotransmitter precursor amino acids in the treatment of multi-infarct dementia and Alzheimer's disease. *J Am Geriatr Soc.* 25:289, 1977.
Milliren, J.W. Some contingencies affecting the utilization of tranquilizers in long-term care of the elderly. *J Health Soc Behav.* 18:206, 1977.
Moehler, H., and Okada, T. Benzodiazepine receptor: demonstration in the central nervous system. *Science* 198:849, 1977.
Mon, A., Cryns, A., and Milbrath, K. Personal and social values: concerns of Scandinavian elderly: a multivariate study. *Int J Aging Hum Devel.* 7:221, 1976.
Mongeau, B. The effect of Hydergine on the transit time of cerebral circulation in diffuse cerebral insufficiency. *Eur J Clin Pharmacol.* 7:169, 1974.
Murphy, G.E. Suicide and attempted suicide. *Hosp Practice.* 12(11):73, 1977.
Nakano, S., Ogawa, N., Kawazu, Y. et al. Effects of antianxiety drug and personality on stress-inducing psychomotor performance test. *J Clin Pharmacol.* 18:125, 1978.
National Institute on Drug Abuse. Sedative-hypnotic drugs: risks and benefits. Washington, D.C.: U.S. Department of Health, Education, and Welfare, Alcohol, Drug Abuse and Mental Health Administration, 1977.
Nies, A., Robinson, D.S., Friedman, M.J. et al. Relationship between age and tricyclic antidepressant plasma levels. *Am J Psychiatry.* 134:790, 1977.
Obrist, W.D. Influence of circulatory disorders. Edited by C.M. Gaitz. In *Aging and the Brain.* New York: Plenum Press, 1972.
Okawa, K.K., and Bountiful, U.T. Comparisons of triazolam 0.25 mg and flurazepam 15 mg in treating geriatric insomniacs. *Curr Ther Res.* 23:381, 1978.
O'Regan, J.B. Adverse interactions of lithium carbonate and methyldopa. *Can Med Assoc J.* 115:385, 1976.
Parkes, D. Amantadine. *Adv Drug Res.* 8:11, 1974.
Parr, H.J. Patterns of psychotropic drug use among American adults. *Drug Issues* 1:269, 1971.
Pasker, P., Thomas, J.P.R., and Ashley, J.S.A. The elderly mentally ill–whose responsibility? *Br Med J.* 2:164, 1976.
Pathy, M.S. A comparison of two sedative/hypnotic drugs. Edited by W. Ferguson Anderson, and J.R. Carlton-Ashton. In *Brain Failure in Old Age. Age Ageing.* 6(suppl):91, 1977.
Paykel, E.S. Depression: when to treat, what to use. *Curr Prescribing.* 1:68, 1978.
Peck, A., Wolloch, L., and Rodstein, M. Mortality of the aged with chronic brain syndrome: further observations in a five-year study. *J Am Geriatr Soc.* 26:170, 1978.
Peress, N.S., Kane, W.C., and Aronson, S.M. Central nervous system findings in a tenth-decade autopsy population. *Prog Brain Res.* 40:473, 1973.
Peters, B.H., and Levin, H.S. Memory enhancement after physostigmine treatment in the amnesic syndrome. *Arch Neurol.* 34:215, 1977.
Petersen, V., Hvidt, S., Thomsen, K. et al. Effect of prolonged thiazide treatment of renal lithium clearance. *Br Med J.* 3:143, 1974.

Peterson, D., and Thomas, C.W. Acute drug reactions among the elderly. *J Gerontol.* 30:552, 1975.

Petit, J.M., Spiker, D.G., Ruwitch, J.F. et al. Tricyclic antidepressant plasma levels and adverse effects after overdose. *Clin Pharmacol Ther.* 21:47, 1977.

Pfeiffer, E., and Busse, E. Mental disorders in later life–affective disorders; paranoid, neurotic and situational reactions. Edited by E. Busse, and E. Pfeiffer. In *Mental Illness in Later Life.* Washington, D.C.: American Psychiatric Association, 1975.

Post, F. The outcome of mental breakdown in old age. *Br Med J.* 1:436, 1951.

Postman, J.U., and Van Tilburg, W. Visual hallucinations and delirium during treatment with amantadine (Symmetrel). *J Am Geriatr Soc.* 23:212, 1975.

Powell, C. The use and abuse of drugs in brain failure. Edited by W. Ferguson Anderson, and J.R. Carlton-Ashton. In *Brain Failure in Old Age. Age Ageing.* 6(suppl):83, 1977.

Prien, R.F. A survey of psychoactive drug use in the aged at Veterans Administration hospitals. Edited by S. Gershon, and A. Raskin. In *Aging,* Vol. 2. New York: Raven Press, 1975.

Prien, R.F., Haver, P.A., and Caffey, E.M. The use of psychoactive drugs in elderly patients with psychiatric disorders: a survey conducted in twelve Veterans Administration hospitals. *J Am Geriatr Soc.* 23:104, 1975.

Prinsley, D.M. Psychogeriatric ward for mentally disturbed elderly patients. *Br Med J.* 3:574, 1973.

Raleigh, F.R. Reducing unnecessary antiparkinson medication in antipsychotic therapy. *J Am Pharm Assoc.* NS17:101, 1977.

Rao, D.B., and Norris, J.R. A double-blind investigation of Hydergine in the treatment of cerebrovascular insufficiency in the elderly. *Johns Hopkins Med J.* 130:317, 1972.

Rao, D.B., Georgiev, E.L., Paul, P.D. et al. Cyclandelate in the treatment of senile mental changes: a double-blind evaluation. *J Am Geriatr Soc.* 25:548, 1977.

Raskin, M.A., and Eisdorfer, C. When elderly patients can't sleep. *Drug Ther.* 7(8):44, 1977.

Reeves, R.L. Comparison of triazolam, flurazepam and placebo as hypnotics in geriatric patients with insomnia. *J Clin Pharmacol.* 17:319, 1977.

Regenstein, Q.R. Treating insomnia: a practical guide for managing chronic sleeplessness. *Compr Psychiatr.* 17:517, 1976.

Reichel, W. Organic brain syndromes. Edited by W. Reichel. In *The Geriatric Patient.* New York: H.P. Publishing Co., Inc., 1978.

Rickels, K. (ed). *Non-Specific Factors in Drug Therapy.* Springfield, Ill.: Charles C Thomas, Publishers, 1968.

Rickels, K. Predictors of response to benzodiazepines in anxious outpatients. Edited by S. Garattini, E. Mussini, and L.O. Randall. In *The Benzodiazepines.* New York: Raven Press, 1973.

Rickels, K. Drug treatment of anxiety. Edited by M.E. Jarvick. In *Psychopharmacology in the Practice of Medicine.* New York: Appleton-Century-Crofts, 1977.

Rifkin, A., Quitkin, F., and Klein, D.F. Akinesia: a poorly recognized drug-induced extrapyramidal behavioral disorder. *Arch Gen Psychiatry.* 32:672, 1975.

Rifkin, A., Quitkin, F., Kane, J. et al. Is prophylactic procyclidine necessary? *Psychopharmacol Bull.* 13(3):33, 1977.

Rivera-Calimlim, L., Nasrallah, H., Strauss, J. et al. Clinical response and plasma levels: effect of dose, dosage schedule, and drug interactions on plasma chlorpromazine. *Am J Psychiatry.* 133:6, 1976.

Rivera-Calimlim, L. The pharmacology and therapeutic application of the phenothiazines. *Rational Drug Ther.* 11(4):1, 1977.

Rosen, H.J. Mental decline in the elderly: pharmacotherapy (ergot alkaloids versus papaverine). *J Am Geriatr Soc.* 23:169, 1975.

Rosenberg, J.M., Simon, W.A., Sangkachand, P. et al. Benzodiazepines for the elderly. *Hosp Pharm.* 11:308, 1976.

Rosenhan, D.L. The contextual nature of psychiatric diagnosis. *J Abnorm Psychol.* 84:467, 1975.

Roth, M. The psychiatric disorders of later life. *Psychiatr Ann.* 6(9):57, 1977.

Salzman, C., Kochmansky, G.E., Shader, R.I. et al. Chlordiazepoxide-induced hostility in a small group setting. *Arch Gen Psychiatry.* 31:401, 1974.

Salzman, C., Shader, R.I., and Van der Kolk, B.A. Clinical psychopharmacology and the elderly patient. *NY State J Med.* 76:71, 1976.

Salzman, C., and Shader, R.I. Depression in the elderly. I. Relationship between depression psychologic defense mechanism and physical illness. *J Am Geriatr Soc.* 26:253, 1978a.

Salzman, C., and Shader, R.I. Depression in the elderly. II. Possible drug etiologies; differential diagnostic criteria. *J Am Geriatr Soc.* 26:303, 1978b.

Samorajski, T. Central neurotransmitter substances and aging: a review. *J Am Geriatr Soc.* 25:337, 1977.

Sarley, V., and Stepto, R.C. Wine is fine for patients' morale and helps stimulate their appetite. *Mod Nurs Home.* 23(1):7, 1969.

Schallert, T., Whishaw, I.Q., Ramirez, V.D. et al. Compulsive, abnormal walking caused by anticholinergics in akinetic, 6-hydroxydopamine-treated rats. *Science* 199:1461, 1978.

Schildkraut, J.J. Biogenic amines and affective disorders. *Ann Rev Med.* 25:333, 1974.

Schmidt, C.W. Psychiatric problems of the aged. *J Am Geriatr Soc.* 22:355, 1974.

Schuckit, M.A. Geriatric alcoholism and drug abuse. *Gerontologist* 17:168, 1977.

Seipel, J.H., Fischer, R., Floam, J.E. et al. Rheoencephalographic and other studies of betahistine in humans. II. Improved methods of diagnosis and selection in arteriosclerotic dementia. *J Clin Pharmacol.* 17(1):63, 1977.

Seligman, M.E.P. *Helplessness: On Depression Development and Death.* San Francisco: W.H. Freeman Co., 1975.

Shader, R.I., Greenblatt, D.J., Sharmatz, J.S. et al. Absorption and disposition of chlordiazepoxide. *J Clin Pharmacol Ther.* 17:709, 1977.

Sheerin, E. A programme which led to a reduction in night sedation at a major hospital. *Med J Aust.* 2:678, 1972.

Shou, M. Lithium in psychiatric therapy and prophylaxis in young and elderly male volunteers. *J Psychiatr Res.* 6:67, 1968.

Simpson, R.G. In defence of barbiturates. Letter to the Editor *Br Med J.* 1:1147, 1976.

Snyder, S., Greenberg, D., and Yamamaru, H.I. Antischizophrenic drugs and brain cholinergic receptors. *Arch Gen Psychiatr.* 31:58, 1974.

Sokoloff, L. Cerebral circulation and metabolism in the aged. Edited by S. Gershon, and A. Raskin. In *Aging,* Vol. 2. New York: Raven Press, 1975.

Special Committee on Aging, U.S. Senate, Mental Health Care and the Elderly. *Shortcomings in Public Policy.* Washington, D.C.: U.S. Government Printing Office, 1971.

Spector, R. Vitamin homeostasis in the central nervous system. *N Engl J Med.* 296:1393, 1977.

Stotsky, B. Use of psychopharmacologic agents for geriatric patients.

Edited by A. DiMascio, and R.I. Shader. In *Clinical Handbook of Psychopharmacology.* New York: Science House, 1970.

Summa, J.D. Erfolge der Intensivetherapie in der Geriatrie. *Aktuel Gerontol.* 5:655, 1975.

Sunshine, A., Zighelboim, I., and Laska, E. Hypnotic activity of diphenhydramine, methapyrilene, and placebo. *J Clin Pharmacol.* 18:425, 1978.

Sweet, R.D., and McDowell, F.H. Five years' treatment of Parkinson's disease with levodopa. *Ann Intern Med.* 83:456, 1975.

Swett, C. Drug-induced dystonia. *Am J Psychiatry.* 132:532, 1975a.

Swett, C. Adverse reactions to chlorpromazine in medical patients. *Curr Therap Res.* 18:199, 1975b.

Talley, J.H. Treat depression as the curable disease it is. *Patient Care* 11(5):20, 1977.

Tessler, R., Stokes, R., and Pietras, M. Consumer response to Valium. *Drug Ther.* 8(2):178, 1978.

Tonks, C.M. Lithium intoxication induced by dieting and saunas. *Br Med J.* 2:1396, 1977.

U'Prichard, D.C., Greenberg, D.A., Sheehan, P.P. et al. Tricyclic antidepressants: therapeutic properties and affinity for alpha-noradrenergic receptor-binding sites in the brain. *Science* 199:197, 1978.

Valzelli, L. Clinical pharmacology of serotonin. Edited by W.B. Essman. In *Serotonin in Health and Disease, Volume II. Physiological Regulation and Pharmacologic Action.* New York: Spectrum Publications, Inc., 1978.

Van der Kolk, B.A., Shader, R.I., and Greenblatt, D.J. Autonomic effects of psychotropic drugs. Edited by M.A. Lipton, A. DiMascio, and K.F. Killam. In *Psychopharmacology: A Generation of Progress.* New York: Raven Press, 1978.

Verwoerdt, A. *Clinical Geropsychiatry.* Baltimore: Williams and Wilkins Co., 1976.

Walsh, A.C. Senile dementia: a report on the anticoagulant treatment of thirteen patients. *Penn Med.* 71:65, 1968.

Walsh, A.C. Hypochondriasis associated with organic brain syndrome: a new approach to therapy. *J Am Geriatr Soc.* 24:430, 1976.

Walsh, A.C. Prevention of senile and presenile dementia by bishydroxycoumarin (Dicumarol) therapy. *J Am Geriatr Soc.* 17:477, 1969.

Walsh, A.C., and Walsh, B.H. Senile and presenile dementia: further observations on the benefits of a Dicumarol-psychotherapy regimen. *J Am Geriatr Soc.* 22:127, 1972.

Walsh, A.C., and Walsh, B.H. Presenile dementia, further experience with an anticoagulant-psychotherapy regimen. *J Am Geriatr Soc.* 22:467, 1974.

Walsh, A.C., Walsh, B.H., and Melaney, C. Senile-presenile dementia: follow-up data on an effective psychotherapy-anticoagulant regimen. *J Am Geriatr Soc.* 26:467, 1978.

Wechsler, D. *The Measurement of Adult Intelligence.* Baltimore: Williams and Wilkins Co., 1944.

Wells, C.E. Stroke in dementia. *Stroke* 9:1, 1978.

Werner, J., Rosenberg, G., Grad, B. et al. Cardiovascular effects of levodopa in aged versus younger patients with Parkinson's disease. *J Am Geriatr Soc.* 24:185, 1976.

Wershow, H.J. Comment: reality orientation for gerontologists: some thoughts about senility. *Gerontologist* 17:297, 1977.

Wharton, R. Geriatric doses. *JAMA.* 233:22, 1975.

Williams, R.L., and Karacan, I. Clinical disorders of sleep. Edited by G. Usdin. In *Sleep Research and Clinical Practice.* New York: Brunner/Mazel, Publishers, 1973.

Williamson, J. Summary of workshop activities: treatment and management of brain failure. *Age Ageing.* 6(suppl):121, 1977.

Willington, W.R., and Vance, M.A. Treatment of Parkinson's disease since levodopa. *Hosp Pharm.* 12:377, 1977.

Winkelman, A.C., and DiPalma, J.R. Drug treatment of parkinsonism. *Semin Drug Treat.* 1:10, 1971.

Winokur, A., and Rickels, K. Clinical evaluation of psychotropic drugs. Edited by A. Frazer, and A. Winokur. In *Biological Bases of Psychiatric Disorders.* New York: Spectrum Publications, Inc., 1977.

Wolstenholme, G.E.W., and O'Connor, M. *Alzheimer's Disease and Related Conditions.* London: J. and A. Churchill, 1970.

Wurtman, R.J., Hirsch, M.J., and Growdon, J.H. Lecithin consumption elevates serum-free choline levels. *Lancet* 2:68, 1977.

Yahr, M.D. The treatment of parkinsonism. *Med Clin North Am.* 57:1377, 1972.

Yahr, M.D. Variations in the on-off effect. Edited by F.H. McDowell, and A. Barbeau. In *Advances in Neurology.* New York: Raven Press, 1974.

Yahr, M.D., and Duvoisin, R.C. Pyridoxine and levodopa in the treatment of parkinsonism. *JAMA.* 220:861, 1972.

Zarit, S.H., Miller, N.E., and Kahn, R.L. Brain function, intellectual impairment and education in the aged. *J Am Geriatr Soc.* 26:58, 1978.

Ziegler, V.E., Clayton, P.J., and Biggs, J.T. A comparison study of amitriptyline and nortriptyline with plasma levels. *Arch Gen Psychiatry.* 34:607, 1977.

Ziegler, V.E., and Biggs, J.T. Tricyclic plasma levels. Effect of age, race, sex, and smoking. *JAMA.* 238:2167, 1977.

23 Management of Respiratory Problems

In the aging person, there is a reduction of vital capacity and an increase in residual volume, a reduction of pulmonary diffusing capacity, and a loss of lung recoil, among other respiratory decrements. Even in healthy elderly persons, there seems to be a significant impairment of the mucociliary transport apparatus. These changes can be correlated with an alteration of the fibrous proteins collagen and elastin, which make up the lung matrix. Old patients with reduced lung function are more at risk to respiratory problems, particularly infections of the bronchopulmonary system, than younger people (Schubert and Horbaschk 1974). The increased incidence with age of some chronic respiratory conditions is depicted in Table 23-1. In general, treatment of respiratory problems in the old is similar to the treatment younger patients would receive (Reichel 1978), but the problem of respiratory infections in the elderly is more acute and these infections may be difficult to treat. Infections are mainly the result of lowered resistance. The bedfast patient is particularly at risk, being

Table 23-1
Incidence of Some Chronic Respiratory Conditions*

	All ages	45–64 years	65 years and over
Emphysema			
Male	10	22	59
Female	3	7	12
Asthma			
Male	32	30	42
Female	29	37	31
Chronic Sinusitis			
Male	93	150	122
Female	113	167	147
Chronic Bronchitis			
Male	31	29	47
Female	34	42	37

*Conditions per 1000 persons per year
Source: Prevalence of selected chronic respiratory conditions, U.S., 1970. DHEW Publ. No. (HRA) 74-1511, Rockville, Md.: National Center for Health Statistics, 1973.

predisposed to stasis. This may be exacerbated by generalized weakness or cerebrovascular disease, both of which may suppress cough and predispose the patient to atelectasis (airlessness of the lung). Dehydration, not unusual in the elderly, adversely affects the patient, but management of dehydration may be difficult in patients with ischemic heart disease, who must be protected from fluid overload which could lead to pulmonary congestion and edema. Attention to cough, dehydration, and antibiotics are all part of patient management in respiratory infections.

Finally, the elderly are often exposed chronically to some drugs which can produce pulmonary disease (Table 23-2) and their use should be established by a careful drug history.

Table 23-2
Some Drugs Which Can Produce Pulmonary Disease

Aspirin	Nitrofurantoin
Corticosteroids	Para-aminosalicylic acid
Cromolyn sodium	Penicillin
Gentamicin	Phenytoin
Isoniazid	Propranolol
Kanamycin	Propoxyphene
Mineral oil	Sulfonamides
Neomycin	Vitamin D

Pneumonia

Gram-negative pneumonia is an important problem among elderly institutionalized patients (Valenti et al 1978). Susceptibility is linked to impaired pulmonary defense mechanisms and mortality with this type of pneumonia in the elderly approaches 80%.

The elderly, in general, but particularly those who are chair-bound or bedfast, suffer from an impaired clearance mechanism. Decreased desquamation of epithelial cells, a decreased salivary flow, and decreased swallowing adversely affect the clearance mechanism.

The elderly are very sensitive to sedatives and hypnotics. These drugs, if absolutely necessary, should be used with great caution in the elderly patient with pneumonia. Their use can lead to respiratory depression and depression of the cough reflex. Good coughing and sputum production are basic to pneumonia therapy, and it is clear that these drugs could negate efforts to achieve these goals. Physical therapy is important for pneumonia patients who should not remain in bed longer than absolutely necessary. If necessary, bronchodilators are used.

Chronic Obstructive Pulmonary Disease

The major respiratory or pulmonary problem facing the elderly is chronic bronchitis, emphysema, or chronic obstructive pulmonary disease (COPD). The first signs of the disease can appear in the fourth decade, the disease becoming disabling in the sixth decade. The disease is irreversible and will demand life-long care. COPD is manifested by severe dyspnea. Treatment is directed toward reversing the current symptomatology and possibly some of the inflammatory components. In general, treatment is palliative and often ineffective (Williams 1974).

Patients with COPD need a fairly well-controlled environment in terms of temperature and humidity and must become adept at the use of home health care devices, such as inhalation therapy devices.

Maintenance of bronchial hygiene is most important. Patients must be taught techniques for promoting cough and drainage from the lung. Reinforcement of the natural cough reflex with purposeful coughing is important. Most persons with COPD have assumed inefficient breathing patterns and breathing retraining will probably be necessary. A graded amount of daily exercise is also necessary.

Steam or an aerosol generator provides hydration, which is necessary to permit liquefaction of the sputum so that it can be expelled more easily.

The basic treatment program usually starts with a bronchodilator such as isoproterenol, delivered by a simple bulb or pump-driven nebulizer. Usually, a patient is started off with one inhalation every three hours, using the medication equally diluted with water. Side effects that may be expected are light-headedness, palpitations, or tachycardia, and these will determine whether or not a dosage adjustment is necessary. At times, oral administration of ephedrine, 25 mg four times daily, is used. In this case, the patient should be carefully monitored for possible urinary retention, which is a particular problem in elderly males. This drug, furthermore, may have a cerebral stimulating effect, and then aminophylline may be administered.

Early and aggressive treatment of pulmonary infection is mandatory (Bates et al 1971). If sputum changes to a more yellowish or green color, and if consistency and volume of sputum change, antibiotic therapy is indicated. In anticipation of this, the patient may have a supply of antibiotic at home, either ampicillin or tetracycline. Patients can be instructed as to when to start antibiotic therapy, and to use antibiotic therapy for at least seven days. Immediately following start of antibiotic therapy, the patient must contact the physician.

The use of corticosteroids should only be considered after careful consideration of the benefit/risk ratio, as patients tend to "feel better" and often will refuse to stop treatment. If used, a one-week course of treatment may be indicated, and the dose is tapered for the next 10 days. Patients with right heart failure may require cardiac glycosides, but in lower than usual maintenance doses, such as 0.125 mg of digoxin. As influenza can be particularly serious for the elderly, especially those with diabetes, heart, lung, or kidney disease, yearly use of influenza vaccine is mandatory for elderly with COPD. If the patient's oxygen tension falls below 50 to 55 mm Hg on room air, the physician may wish to consider home use of oxygen. This can be beneficial in many instances, but cost is a factor. Tranquilizers, sedatives, or hypnotics should only be given with extreme caution, if at all.

Bronchial Asthma

It is not uncommon to see onset of asthma in the sixth or seventh decade. Patients will suffer from reversible bronchospasms, dyspnea, shortness of breath, wheezing, and cough. Secretions are thick and tenacious and inflammation is common.

Atopic asthma patients seem to have a genetic predisposition to sensitization to environmental antigens. This leads to increased levels of IgE and release of histamine and other substances. On the other hand, the nonatopic patients develop asthma after prolonged and intensive exposure to a single antigen. Finally, some patients do not fit into either of these two categories. They seem to become sensitized during bacterial or viral infections.

In the elderly, asthma is generally more chronic and sustained, with continuing airway obstruction.

Traditionally, the ephedrines were the basic drugs most often used in the treatment of bronchial asthma, partly because they could be administered orally. However, the use of ephedrine is no longer recommended (Wilson and McPhillips 1978; *Medical Letter* 1978). Epinephrine raises blood pressure and high doses of it or isoproterenol can precipitate attacks of angina pectoris and cause cardiac arrhythmias. If isoproterenol is used, the patient must be closely monitored if there is heart disease. The patient must be taught proper technique if inhalation products are to be used.

Metaproterenol causes less cardiac stimulation than isoproterenol and little change in blood pressure. However, tremor is a common side effect.

Among the other and newer sympathomimetic agents which have less beta-1 activity (cardiac effect) and no alpha-adrenergic stimulation, terbutaline, given orally, causes relatively little cardiac stimulation. Its use effectively prevents acute exacerbation of asthma in patients with significant coronary disease (Weinberger and Hendeles 1977). Terbutaline has a longer duration of action than metaproterenol. This drug, too, often causes tremor.

Theophylline is most frequently used. It has the same indications as the sympathomimetics, and is efficiently absorbed when given orally or intravenously, but not when given in the form of a rectal suppository.

The therapeutic index of theophylline is relatively low. Blood levels above 20 mcg/ml are often associated with abdominal pain, anorexia, nausea, vomiting, headaches, irritability, nervousness, or tachycardia. For theophylline, the steady-state volume of distribution ranges from 0.45 to 0.50 liters/kg of body weight. Protein binding is about 55% to 63% at therapeutic serum concentrations. The drug is extensively metabolized in the liver, and only a small amount is excreted unchanged in the urine. The half-life in adult patients ranges from three to nine hours and 50% of the drug will be eliminated within that period (Mitenko and Ogilvie 1973; Piafsky and Ogilvie 1975). Clearance of the drug is affected by age, liver disease, cardiac failure, and other diseases. Intercurrent diseases can increase the half-life of the drug considerably.

In addition, metabolic clearance rates differ from patient to patient and, therefore, dosages must be individualized based on blood levels. Toxicity is usually encountered when serum concentrations exceed 20 mcg/ml. Optimal therapeutic response is usually expected with serum levels ranging between 10 and 20 mcg/ml.

It is customary to start with relatively low doses and increase the dosage as necessary, based on patient response and blood level data.

The equivalent content of anhydrous theophylline is the factor which determines blood concentrations and clinical response. High protein diets can decrease the half-life of theophylline significantly. If necessary, corticosteroids can be used. They are useful in cases of mucosal edema and secretions of bronchi and bronchioles during asthmatic attacks. However, their adverse effects limit their clinical usefulness. Their use also produces a rather high incidence of posterior polar cataracts. Patients receiving corticosteroids should be closely followed to see whether dosage can be reduced and if the drug can be withdrawn. The patient should probably be started with 10 to 20 mg/day. When maximum effect has been reached, the dose should be reduced by 2.5 mg or 5 mg every five to seven days. Often, administration on alternate days is effective. Beclomethasone dipropionate, a potent topical corticosteroid, is an alternate to systemic corticosteroid therapy.

Cromolyn sodium is neither a bronchodilator nor a corticosteroid. It is thought to prevent the release of the mediators of immediate allergic reactions. It is also thought to prevent histamine release by direct liberators. The drug does not prevent fixation of IgE or IgA to the cell surface, nor does it prevent the antibody-antigen combination. Cromolyn sodium has no direct effect on bronchial smooth muscle and does not act as an antihistamine. It is, therefore, ineffective in the treatment of acute asthmatic attacks, but is used to prevent acute attacks. It is usually used in combination with theophylline and, sometimes, the steroids. Its correct use must be carefully explained to the patient. While the drug is remarkably free of adverse effects, it is a very fine powder and, thus, can cause increased bronchospasms and throat irritation.

Inefficient or exhaustive breathing efforts and mechanical impairment of lung function may necessitate the use of a respirator (Crocco et al 1978). The primary goal of respiratory therapy should be the correction of the underlying cause of the respiratory problem. The machine helps the patient by improving ventilation, oxygenation, and mechanical lung function. A reasonable reversal of the respiratory problem, alleviation of acute bronchospasms, improved cardiac function in CHF patients with pulmonary edema, or control of infection in COPD patients mandates respirator withdrawal. Sometimes, the physician must persuade the patient to stop respirator treatment.

Iatrogenic and nosocomial infections accompany respirator use. A strict program of cleaning and sterilization of the equipment keep them to a minimum.

REFERENCES

Bates, D.V., Macklem, P.T., and Christie, R.V. *Respiration Function in Disease*. Philadelphia: W.B. Saunders Co., 1971.

Crocco, J.A., Rooney, J.J., Westfall, R.E. et al. When your patient needs a respirator. *Patient Care* 12(6):134, 1978.

Medical Letter. Drugs for asthma. 20:69, 1978.

Mitenko, P.A., and Ogilvie, R.I. Pharmacokinetics of intravenous theophylline. *Clin Pharmacol Ther*. 14:509, 1973.

Piafsky, K.M., and Ogilvie, R.I. Dosage of theophylline in bronchial asthma. *N Engl J Med*. 292:1218, 1975.

Reichel, J. Pulmonary problems. Edited by W. Reichel. In *Clinical Aspects of Aging*. Baltimore: Williams and Wilkins Co., 1978.

Schubert, R., and Horbaschk, G. Intensivetherapie bei Akuten Erkrankungen des Bronchopulmonalen System im Alter. *Aktuel Gerontol*. 4:591, 1974.

Valenti, W.M., Trudell, R.G., and Bentley, D.W. Factors predisposing to oropharyngeal colonization with gram-negative bacilli in the aged. *N Engl J Med*. 298:1108, 1978.

Weinberger, M., Hendeles, L. Management of asthma-antiasthmatic drugs. *Postgrad Med*. 61:95, 1977.

Williams, M.H. Special problems in respiratory diseases. *Geriatrics* 29:67, 1974.

Wilson, A.F., and McPhillips, J.J. Pharmacologic control of asthma. *Ann Rev Pharmacol Toxicol*. 18:541, 1978.

24 Skin Problems of the Elderly

The incidence of skin disorders increases with age. It reaches a peak between the ages of 65 and 74 years. Skin disorders are more prevalent in men than in women and men are substantially more likely to have fungal conditions or folliculitis than women (Johnson and Roberts 1977). Some degenerative and proliferative skin disorders of the aged have been described (Hodgson 1968), and general as well as specific data are presented in Table 24-1 and Figures 24-1 and 24-2. A bewildering array of etiologic factors is often listed for certain conditions, such as skin ulcers (Table 24-2). Sometimes, it may be totally unexpected and hard to elucidate a cause. For example, the elderly, particularly the bedbound elderly, may be prone to textile dermatitis, after wearing new, unwashed clothing or lying on sheets having been treated with formaldehyde resins (Uehara 1978). Some suggested treatment modalities are outlined in Table 24-3.

Table 24-1
Skin Conditions*

Condition	All ages (A)	65 years and over (B)	B/A
Inflammatory conditions	7.2	20.0	2.8
Corns and callosities	41.5	109.9	2.6
Hypertrophic and atrophic	8.8	14.5	1.6
Psoriasis	6.5	10.6	1.6
Eczema, dermatitis, urticaria	30.2	25.7	0.85

*Rate per 1000 persons
Source: Prevalence of chronic skin and musculoskeletal conditions, U.S. 1969. DHEW Publ. No. (HRA) 75-1519, Rockville, Md.: National Center for Health Statistics, 1974.

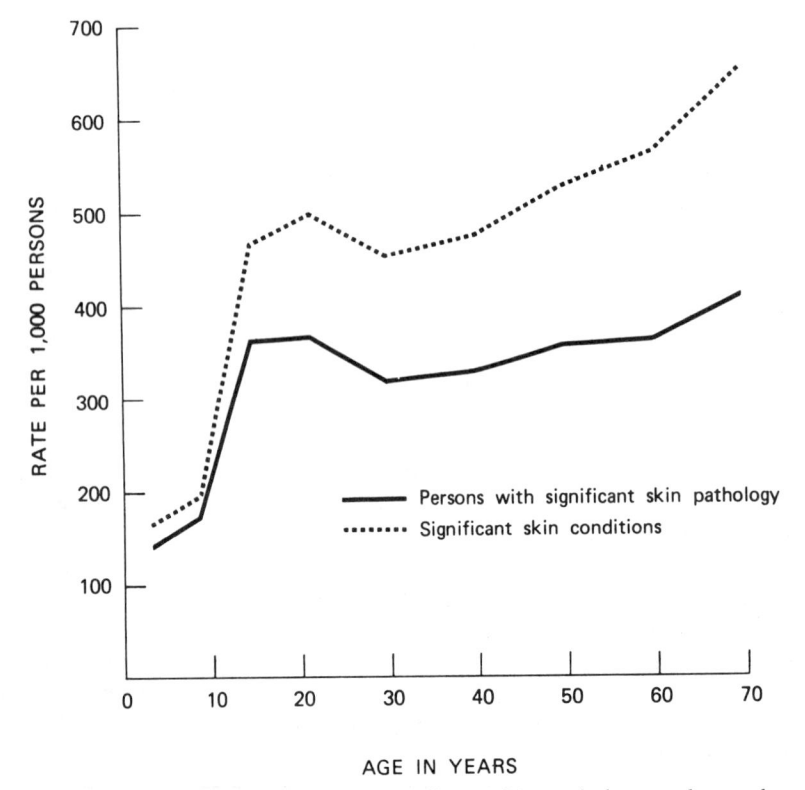

Figure 24-1 Prevalence rates for significant skin pathology and prevalence rates of significant skin conditions among persons 1-74 years by age: United States, 1971-74. M.L.T. Johnson, and J. Roberts. Prevalence of dermatological disease among persons 1-74 years of age: United States. *Adv Data.* 4:1, 1977.

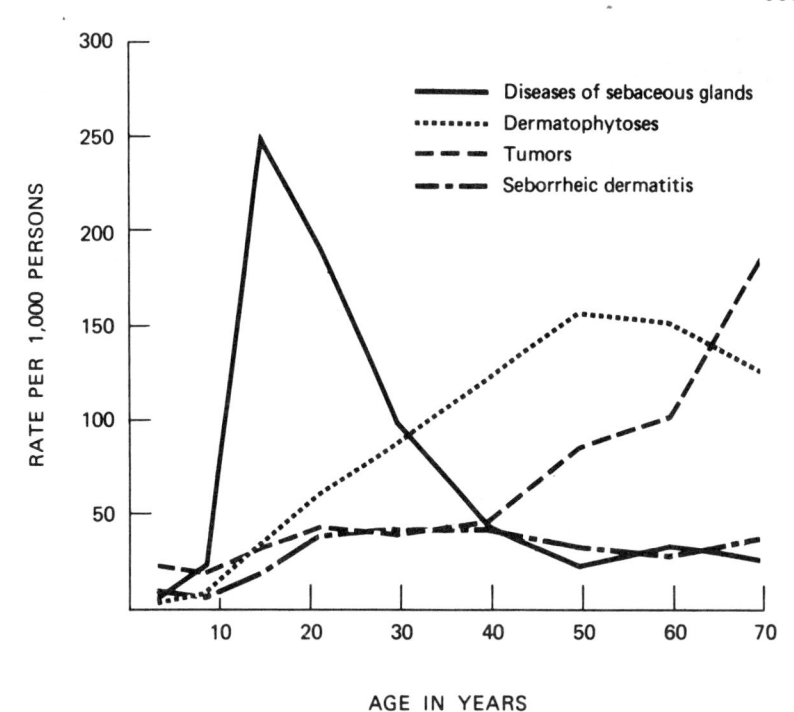

Figure 24-2 Prevalence rates for the four leading types of significant skin pathology among persons 1-74 years by age: United States, 1971-74. M.L.T. Johnson, and J. Roberts. Prevalence of dermatological disease among persons 1-74 years of age: United States. *Adv Data.* 4:1, 1977.

Table 24-2
Some Possible Causes of Skin Ulcers

Collagen disease
Drug toxicity
  Bromides
  Iodides
Hematologic disorders
  Anemia
  Proteinemia
Infections
  Bacterial
  Fungal
Metabolic disorders
Pyoderma
Syphilis
Tumors
Vascular disorders
  Arterial insufficiency
  Vasculitis
  Venous stasis

Table 24-3
Suggested Treatment of Dermatitis and Skin Ulcers

Dermatitis	Eliminate possibility of sensitizing agent
	Use compresses 3-4 times daily for about 1 hour each. Use Burow's solution (1:20 or 1:40) or 0.5% saline. Can use 1% hydrocortisone cream
	Reduce edema by leg elevation, elastic bandages, or support stockings
Ulcer	If necessary, debride with compresses and povidone-iodine or 1% gentian violet
	Cover clean ulcer with these antiseptics and absorbable gelatin powder
	Cover leg and ulcer with Unna's boot (zinc gelatin) from foot to below knee. Initially, change boot every 24 hours, then increase interval gradually

Source: D.J. Cripps. Skin care and problems in the aged. *Hosp Practice.* 12(4):119, 1977.

Pruritus

One of the most common geriatric complaints is itching or pruritus. A number of diseases, commonly found among the elderly, can be responsible for pruritus. Among those are psychiatric disturbances, hyperthyroidism, diabetes, gout, and liver disease. Itching associated with chronic renal disease often is very severe and does not respond to the most commonly employed methods of treatment. Even parathyroidectomy may give only transient relief (Thorne 1978; Hampers et al 1968). Drug reactions are often responsible for itching and, in those cases, moisturizing creams or lotions are of no benefit. Stress most often is responsible for localized pruritus (Cripps 1977) that occurs commonly in the perianal areas, and the back of the neck. Hydrocortisone cream may be helpful, but the more potent topical steroid preparations may cause skin atrophy, particularly if used for prolonged periods of time. Itching is intensified when external stimuli are reduced, for example just prior to sleep. Most often though, when elderly patients complain about itching, dry skin is responsible, particularly in the lower legs. There is a greater need to moisturize the aging skin. Aging skin is dry. The horny layers of the stratum corneum of young individuals contain about 13% of water, the level diminishes to about 7% with advanced age (Ward 1976). Moreover, the aging skin has less capacity to take up water from the environment and bind it to the stratum corneum. Environmental influences contribute importantly to the development of dry skin, and thus, itching. Overexposure to sun must be avoided (Lubowe 1976); sunlight is probably the most dangerous influence on the skin. Extremes of temperature should also be avoided. Extreme heat can cause heat rash, while extreme cold is often accompanied by very low humidity. Low humidity, either associated with extreme cold or found in the homes of the elderly, increases itching (Johnson 1975); the atmosphere must be adequately humidified. In an effort to cope with dry skin and itching, the elderly patient may resort to frequent baths, which will only exacerbate the dry skin conditions, particularly if the bath water is hot. Ultimately, frequent baths will result in more skin dehydration, unless the skin is lubricated immediately after, before the skin is dried.

In general, all elderly should follow certain suggestions:

1. Avoid the use of soaps. Use soap only in axillary, anal, and pubic areas.
2. Do not use soapy water to rinse.
3. Use moisturizing preparations, day and night.

When following certain guidelines carefully, bathing can be beneficial. It is often recommended twice daily. The water should be warm, not hot. Sparing use of a mild soap, such as Basis soap or Lowilla soap, is recommended. While bath oils, such as Alpha-Keri can often be beneficial, their use for geriatric patients is disputed. They tend to make the bathtub slippery and, in the elderly already prone to falls and resulting fractures, they may pose a problem. Additions to the bath, such as bubble bath, are absolutely contraindicated, as they tend to make the skin drier.

Of greater importance is the treatment after the bath. Before the skin is dried, a lotion such as Lubriderm or a petrolatum-based ointment such as Eucerin should be applied to the wet skin. These trap moisture, which creams cannot do. Drying should be done gently, as vigorous toweling may lead to increased pruritus. Finally, the patient should be instructed to protect the skin from irritation by woolen garments or synthetic fibers. Nighttime, but not daytime, sedation is sometimes helpful.

Other Skin Problems

Although dry skin is the major geriatric skin problem, moisture which collects in the groin area, under breasts, and in skin creases is a common problem, particularly in the bedbound or institutionalized elderly patients. Baby powder, particularly after bathing, is recommended.

The incontinent patient presents a special skin care problem. The effects of occlusion from lying on a waterproof mattress, wet clothing, or from body folds touching each other, can cause skin irritation and disease. It can also cause enhanced cutaneous absorption of externally applied medications. Fungal and bacterial problems increase manyfold in these patients.

The water content of the skin and the blood flow in a particular area of the skin, among other factors, may affect the penetration of drugs through the intact skin. These parameters may change with age. The FDA OTC Panel on External Analgesics felt that penetration through the geriatric skin differs from drug penetration through skin of younger adults, and may warrant special consideration. Unfortunately, the panel failed to obtain information which would have permitted it to reach a definitive conclusion on this issue.

REFERENCES

Cripps, D.J. Skin care and problems in the aged. *Hosp Practice.* 12(4):119, 1977.

Hampers, C.L., Katz, A.I., and Wilson, R.E. Disappearance of "uremic" itching after subtotal parathyroidectomy. *N Engl J Med.* 279:695, 1968.

Hodgson, A.G. Some degenerative and proliferative skin disorders of the aged. *Gerontol Clin.* 10:201, 1968.

Johnson, M.L.T., and Roberts, J. Prevalence of dermatological disease among persons 1-74 years of age: United States. *Adv Data.* 4:1, 1977.

Johnson, S.A.M. Problems of aging: relieving itching in the geriatric patient. *Postgrad Med.* 58(7):105, 1975.

Lubowe, I. Treatment of the aging skin by dermatologic methods. *J Am Geriatr Soc.* 24:25, 1976.

Thorne, E.G. Coping with pruritus-a common geriatric complaint. *Geriatrics* 33(7):47, 1978.

Uehara, M. Follicular contact dermatitis due to formaldehyde. *Dermatologia* 156:48, 1978.

Ward, J.B. A cosmetic chemist's view on aging. *Drug Cosmet Ind.* 115:55, 1976.

25 Pressure Sores

The problem of pressure sores is serious. These sores are not benign entities and should not be treated as such. It is imperative that all health care providers who care for the aged are fully aware of the procedures involved in the prevention and treatment of pressure sores.

The terms "bedsore" and "decubitus ulcer" are misnomers since "decubitus" means "lying down" and "bedsore" implies that these wounds occur in patients confined to bed. Many ulcers do result from the patient's lying in one position too long, but others can arise from sitting, from prolonged standing on tilt boards or electric beds, or even from tight-fitting casts or dressings. All sores, though, result from pressure, especially prolonged pressure against a bony prominence. In turn, the term "prolonged" may be misleading, as the first stage of pressure sore development, hyperemia, may occur in as short a period of time as 30 minutes (Table 25-1) (Enis and Sarmiento 1973).

Table 25-1
Development of Pressure Sores

Stage	Manifestation	Comments
1	Hyperemia	Redness of skin, rapidly appears and disappears if pressure is removed
2	Ischemia	Redness of skin which takes longer to develop (up to 6 hours) and disappear (36 hours)
3	Necrosis	Blueness of skin. Lump similar to boil. Can occur after unremittent pressure of 6 hours
4	Ulceration	Follows necrosis if pressure is not relieved. Infection may occur, muscles and bony prominences may become involved

Source: J.E. Enis, and A. Sarmiento. The pathophysiology and management of pressure sores. *Orthoped Rev.* 2(10):25, 1973.

The minimum pressure for keeping capillaries open is about 25 mm Hg, and the usual intracapillary pressure is about 40 mm Hg (Dowling 1970). Thus, it follows that exogenous pressure in excess of these levels, exerted on susceptible bony areas, will produce ischemia. Even when a patient is sitting quietly, pressure can build up to 300 mm Hg, and sores can develop in most patients with pressure of 100 mm Hg. The amount and duration of applied force are the most important etiologic factors in the development of pressure sores. There is an inverse relationship between pressure and time, but high pressure exerted over a short period of time is probably less damaging than low pressure exerted over a prolonged period of time. When a patient is allowed to remain in the same position for an extended period of time, blood flow is diminished or obstructed by pressure. This will result in tissue anoxia, increased capillary permeability, tissue edema, and finally cell death. Necrosis of the entire epidermis, dermis, and subdermal tissues can be the end result. Signs of skin irritation may occur early and at any site. Most frequently, though, those sites are involved where a high proportion of body weight is constantly placed on a small skin area covering bony prominences, such as the sacrum, greater trochanter, dorsal convexity, or heels. The least susceptible areas are the abdomen, thighs, and posterior calves.

The prognosis depends on the action taken when evidence of pressure sore development first presents itself. The presence of pressure sores is a poor prognostic sign and their presence is often the most common event associated with the terminal stages of life (Howell 1969). Mortality rates of between 60% and 75% have been reported (Vasile and Chaitin 1972; Michocki and Lamy 1976a); thus, early detection and prompt and vigorous action are mandatory. Even very early signs of redness of the skin should be treated immediately, as erythema on the overlying skin may mean that the underlying subcutaneous tissue has already been severely damaged.

Many factors contribute to the development of pressure sores. Immobility, which may be exaggerated by the administration of sedatives, general malnutrition, and vitamin C deficiency, debilitated conditions with anemia, hypoproteinemia and other metabolic disorders, low blood pressure, peripheral vascular disease, prolonged dampness from urine and feces, maceration of the skin, loss of sensations, and poor nursing care have all been identified as contributory factors. The practice of maintaining the supine patient with the head of the bed elevated at a high degree also increases the likelihood of pressure sores.

Thus, healing depends not only on the specific treatment modality selected but also on the patient's clinical state. As many as half of elderly patients may indeed be anemic and may be maintained on tube feeding (Michocki and Lamy 1976a).

Advanced age, itself, seems to be a significant factor in the development of pressure sores. About 40% of geriatric patients in nursing homes have pressure sores (Edberg et al 1973), and depending on the number and severity of the sores, the estimated cost of treating a patient with sores is between $15,000 and $30,000, mainly caused by enormous increase in required nursing time (Sather et al 1977; Spira et al 1969; Schell and Wolcott 1966; Gerson 1975; Berecek 1975; Gruis and Innes 1976).

Classification of Pressure Sores

Several different classifications have been proposed, among them a thermographic classification (Barton and Barton 1973). According to this system, a normal pressure sore has a temperature differential of approximately 2.5 °C between the ulcer margin and the surrounding skin. This type of sore has a reasonable prognosis and may heal within four to six weeks if treated early and vigorously. In the indolent pressure sore, there is a temperature differential of about 1 °C and debridement will be necessary to achieve healing. Finally, the terminal type of sore, which occurs in terminally ill patients, is characterized by alternate contraction and retraction of the ulcer margin at short intervals.

Sores are also classified according to the degrees of tissue involvement (Shea and Merlino 1975) into superficial or deep lesions (Walker 1971; Moolten 1972; Binks 1968). Deep sores, in turn, may be open or closed (Bliss and McLaren 1967).

Superficial sores A superficial sore involves damage to the superficial layers of the skin. It does not extend into subcutaneous tissue or muscle. Treatment is conservative and directed toward cleanliness, relief of pressure, and exposure to air. A superficial sore, which is clean and not draining, will heal quickly if those procedures are performed diligently (Weiss 1960; Edberg et al 1973; Michocki and Lamy 1976b). The decision to use a dressing depends, in part, upon the location of the sore. In an exposed area, such as the knee or hip, it probably is best to let the sore dry without any dressing. In areas that are in contact with bedclothes, such as buttocks or elbows, the patient may feel more comfortable and the new granulation tissue may be protected if the sore is covered with a single layer of gauze.

Superficial debridement is far superior to proteolytic enzymes in removing deep fibrotic tissue (Bailey 1967). However, proteolytic enzymes may aid in the dissolution of fibrin, liquefaction of pus, and removal of coagula and purulent exudate (Kahn 1960). Proteolytic enzymes may be necessary as a treatment adjunct until surgical debridement can be performed.

Deep sores A deep sore is one in which all the layers of the skin, subcutaneous tissue, or superficial fascia, and sometimes even muscle, have been damaged by pressure or subsequent infection. An open sore originates from the surface and extends downward through the various layers of tissue. A closed sore originates in the subcutaneous tissues and proceeds toward the surface, allowing degenerative changes to spread in all directions, possibly involving bone. The surface of a closed deep sore may show only a small opening with a persistent discharge of pus.

An open deep sore involves the necrosis of a great deal of tissue. The wound must be debrided and the necrotic tissue must be removed. Removal of necrotic tissue is necessary because this is the substance upon which bacteria thrive. Removal also shortens the lag phase of wound healing and permits the underlying normal tissue to start the proliferative phase. Once surgical debridement has been performed, the clean wound can be maintained with normal saline dressings applied four times daily (Guthrie and Goulian 1973). If the wound is a cavity, it should be loosely packed and the dressing should be allowed to dry for six hours. The dressing is then removed without rewetting. This aspect is extremely important, as the dry gauze will adhere to the necrotic material, removing it from the wound. If the cavity is extremely dirty, and a large amount of necrotic tissue is present, modified Dakin's solution may be substituted for saline. After the wound has been thoroughly debrided, irrigation with a cleansing agent such as hydrogen peroxide can be performed. If extensive purulent drainage is present, a wet dressing of modified Dakin's solution or a solution of sodium oxychlorosene should be used. When the purulent discharge has become serous, saline dressing may be substituted.

Modified Dakin's solution is very irritating and may dissolve clots or delay clotting in the same way it dissolves necrotic tissue. Solutions must be freshly prepared, to avoid deterioration on exposure to air or elevated temperatures. Sodium oxychlorosene solution, in concentrations of 0.5%, should be tried more frequently. It appears to have a high degree of activity against most resistant microorganisms and is said to be effective against gram-negative and gram-positive organisms, yeasts, fungi, mold, viruses, and spores. It appears to lack many of the irritating properties of modified Dakin's solution. This solution, too, is very labile, being stable for only about eight hours.

If the color of the purulent discharge is blue-green or green, this may indicate contamination by *Pseudomonas*. A 4% boric acid solution has been recommended (Walker 1971), as well as acetic acid. Acetic acid is effective against *Pseudomonas aeruginosa* in superficial wounds (Phillips et al 1968). Concentrations ranging between 0.5% and 4% have been suggested, sometimes administered as a continuous drip (Sather et al 1977). Closed deep sores usually occur on the hips of patients lying on their sides. Treatment is very difficult because only a small opening on the surface of the skin may be visible, yet extensive sinus tracking may be present. The removal of necrotic tissue and treatment of infection become especially troublesome. Ribbon gauze soaked in modified Dakin's solution or solution of sodium oxychlorosene or physiologic saline may be inserted deeply into the opening by means of sinus forceps. Vigorous mechanical debridement, application of medicinal soaks (hydrogen peroxide or Epsom salts), and careful attention to the general nutritional status of the patient represent the key to successful therapy (Harris 1965). For treatment of closed deep sores, the use of iodoform gauze or silver nitrate sticks introduced deeply into the sinus tracks has been recommended (Harris 1965). Usually, the presence of a deep closed sore means a poor prognosis in relation to therapeutic management, and surgical intervention is often necessary.

PATIENT MANAGEMENT

Treatment usually consists of combined measures involving patient care measures and drug treatment. Lack of response is often caused by a lack of protocol and/or lack of persistence. Many protocols have been developed in different institutions (Appendices A, B, and C).

Antibiotics Frequently, pressure sores are routinely treated with systemic antibiotics. In general, systemic antibiotics are of little value as they may not reach the site of infection because of poor tissue perfusion of ulcerated areas (Herceg and Harding 1971). On the other hand, pressure sores may be the focus of serious local sepsis or bacteremia. Thus, if there is evidence of cellulitis of the surrounding area or severe infections, for example, in Grade III or Grade IV sores (see Appendix B), systemic antibiotics may be indicated.

Topical administration of antibiotics is probably not necessary in most instances, if the sore is properly irrigated and packed sufficiently often to keep the wound clean. Nevertheless, topical antibiotics are widely used, but their effectiveness is questionable. Such drugs as neomycin, chloramphenicol, gentamicin, carbenicillin, and combinations of bacitracin, neomycin, and polymyxin continue to be used. Neurotoxicity and nephrotoxicity may easily develop with the use of some of these drugs.

Proteolytic enzymes Enzymatic debridement is effective when it follows surgical debridement. It is not a substitute for surgical debridement. Most proteolytic enzymes belong to three main groups, ie, originating from animal, vegetable, or bacterial precursors (Table 25-2). There are some major disadvantages to the use of these agents. Among those are the need for frequent daily applications, the inability to affect large amounts of dead collagenous tissue, and the expense. These enzymes may also cause excessive local irritation and, because of their animal origin, allergic reactions. Routine use is inadvisable, especially if it leads to the neglect of more important patient care measures.

Products for granulation-epithelialization Once an ulcer has been properly debrided and a healthy granular bed has been created, re-epithelialization can begin. Gelfoam powder or a 10% Mercurochrome solution, among other products, have been used with varying degrees of success.

Gold leaf The therapeutic rationale for using gold leaf is believed to be its ability to cause epithelialization of cells (Smith et al 1967), to elicit a mild foreign-body reaction (Gallagher and Geschickter 1964), and to promote healing (Wolf et al 1966).

The use of gold leaf was first reported in 1688 to prevent scarring of smallpox lesions (Robertson 1925) and its effectiveness has been investigated in a number of studies (Kanof 1964; Chick 1969; Risbrook et al 1973). These studies, unfortunately, differ greatly in the duration of treatment, controls, use of occlusive devices, and other measures, thereby not permitting definite conclusions about its effectiveness.

Oxygen Oxygen, under pressure, also has been used to stimulate granulation tissue (Rosenthal and Schurman 1971; Gorecki 1964; Ursu 1970). It is very difficult, if not impossible, to assess the validity of this treatment method. Adequate controlled trials are not available. Reported healing rates and progress are based upon subjective data and thus lack significance. Nevertheless, oxygen is being used in the treatment of pressure sores. Sometimes this is accomplished by using an intranasal oxygen catheter to direct the flow to the site of the sore, usually for periods of 15 to 20 minutes, three or four times daily.

Table 25-2
Enzymatic Debriding Agents in Common Use

Vegetable Product:
  Panafil ointment (Rystan Company, Inc.)
    Ingredients—standardized papain 10%; urea USP 10%; water-soluble chlorophyl derivates 0.5%
    Application—once or twice daily
    Precautions—hydrogen peroxide may inactivate papain.

Animal Products:
  Biozyme ointment (Armour Pharmaceutical Company)
    Ingredients—neomycin 0.35%; trypsin-chymotrypsin concentrate 10,000 Armour Units per gm.
    Application—one to three times daily.
    Derivation—mammalian pancreas.

  Elase ointment (Parke, Davis and Company)
    Ingredients—fibrinolysin 30 units/30 gm; desoxyribonuclease 20,000 units/30 gm; thimerosal (mercury derivative) 0.12 mg/30 gm.
    Application—two to three times daily.
    Derivation—bovine plasma; bovine pancreas.
    Precautions—mercury allergy; hypersensitivity to products of bovine origin.

Bacterial Products:
  Travase ointment (Flint Laboratories)
    Ingredients—sutilains, 82,000 casein units of proteolytic activity per gm.
    Application—three to four times daily.
    Derivation—*Bacillus subtilis.*
    Precautions—optimal pH 6.0-6.8; inactivation by: 1) detergents, 2) antiseptics, 3) germicides, 4) Burow's solution (pH 3.6-4.4), 5) metallic ions (hexachlorophene, iodine, thimerosal, silver nitrate, nitrofurazone).

  Collagenase ABC Ointment (Advance Biofactures Corp.) Santyl Ointment (Knoll Pharmaceutical Company)
    Ingredients—collagenase activity 250 units per gm.
    Application—once daily or every other day.
    Derivation—*Clostridium histolyticum.*
    Precautions—optimal pH 7-8; inactivation by: 1) detergents, 2) hexachlorophene, 3) heavy metals (mercury, silver), 4) Burow's solution (aluminum acetate).

No adverse effects have been reported, but proof of therapeutic effectiveness is lacking. Oxygen therapy should, therefore, not be viewed as a treatment entity. The wound must be debrided, cleansed, and the external pressure must be relieved. Oxygen therapy may complement these measures, but cannot replace them.

    Dry heat Dry heat has also been used in the treatment of pressure sores (Smigel and Russell 1962; Nyquist 1959; Williams 1968); heat is thought to improve circulation, tissue oxygenation, and possibly retard infection. Dry heat is usually employed for superficial sores or early ulcers. Treatment will have no beneficial effect whatsoever if sloughs and necrotic tissue are present because it is impossible to improve circulation in an area harboring necrosis.

Electric lamp therapy consists of focusing a lighted 60-watt bulb on the involved body area for ten minutes at a distance of no closer than 18 inches nor farther than 24 inches. Morning and evening treatment is suggested.

Sugar A special sugar paste was at one time recommended for treatment of ulcerated lesions (Rostenberg et al 1958) and it has been rationalized that cane sugar is an inexpensive fermenting agent that can be substituted for the more expensive enzymes. It may stimulate the growth of granulation tissue and may serve as a matrix around which the new granulation tissue can form. While, theoretically, these factors may sound appealing, the "logic of this packing of an unsterile, nonabsorbable form of nutrient which is more liable to act as an irritant seems doubtful. It would appear better to feed such substances to the patient" (Walker 1971).

New modalities New products continue to be marketed for the treatment of ulcers and old products, approved for other uses, are tried in the treatment of pressure sores. For most of these, sufficient clinical experience is still lacking, so that no recommendations can be made at this time.

For example, a silver-sulfadiazine combination, approved for use in burn patients, has been tried. It has been suggested that massaging the skin around the edges of the sores and applying a karaya gum ring, normally used with ostomy appliances, and application of karaya powder directly to the ulcer, is effective. On the other hand, vigorous massage, once strongly advocated, is now strongly deemphasized, and there are several reports that karaya gum is not effective. A 1% silver-zinc-allantoinase cream (AZAC) has been suggested as an effective treatment for chronic leg ulcers (Margraf and Covey 1977). According to one preliminary study, the average healing time for a leg ulcer was about ten weeks, but the average bacterial count in the ulcer was reduced by 99% within one week of treatment initiation. Heel ulcers have been treated with a solution of tri-iodide (saturated solution of potassium iodide and iodine). The solution is applied to a dressing that is covered on both sides with dry gauze so the solution does not come into direct contact with the ulcer. It has been postulated that the liberated iodine would control the ulcer (Friedman 1976).

A new product, which is being promoted for use in the debridement of secreting wounds, consists of a highly hydrophilic dextran polymer. Each gram is claimed to be able to absorb about 4 ml of fluid. As the beads absorb wound exudates, they help to prevent crust formation, and reduce inflammation and edema. Crust formation is prevented as the beads absorb protein, particularly fibrin/fibrinogen degradation products. The material is poured into the wound, which is prepared by cleansing and application of vaseline around the edges. A compress is then applied and taped in place. If the wound is draining profusely, three or four changes daily may be necessary. The preparation is expensive and sufficient clinical studies have not yet been reported to judge its effectiveness (*Medical Letter* 1978).

Finally, a recent concept suggests that corticotrophin should be a part of the standard premedication for surgical procedures with a high risk for postsurgical development of pressure sores. In a study, patients over 65 years of age who received 89 IU of corticotrophin four hours before surgery to the upper shaft of the femur and hip joint developed significantly fewer pressure sores than those patients who did not receive this drug as a presurgical medication (Barton and Barton 1976).

PREVENTIVE AND SUPPORTIVE MANAGEMENT

Preventive measures are mandatory for good patient care. All other measures focus on early detection of possible skin damage. The patient at risk must be identified and, if skin damage occurs, the treatment success is a function of efficient medical and nursing care. The major current concepts in prevention and supportive treatment revolve around immediate relief of pressure, provision of adequate nutrition, cleanliness, and dryness.

Even a person with intact skin sensation may develop pressure sores if confined to one position over prolonged periods. If inspection identifies any reddened skin area, pressure must be relieved until the redness disappears. A regular program should be maintained so that the patient is turned at least once every one to two hours. Mattresses or pads should be used which exert minimal contact pressure. The patient should not be elevated in bed more than 30° to prevent forward sliding. Circulation should be increased with a program of active and passive range of movements. Vulnerable heels and ankles should be raised with wedge-shaped foam pads placed under the calves. A heavy patient should not sit in a chair or wheelchair for more than one hour without moving and a frail patient should be moved at least every two hours.

Maintenance of adequate nutrition is important. Large, weeping ulcers can cause loss of protein, vitamins, and minerals. Chronic disease is often responsible for anemia in older patients, and general malnutrition and lack of vitamins and minerals affect wound healing adversely. Thus, a high-protein diet is indicated, high in caloric value and rich in vitamins and minerals. Many patients, however, may be maintained by tube feeding and others may lack proper dentition or find the diet unacceptable and unpalatable. Iron, vitamin B-12, or folic acid should not be given indiscriminately without attempting to determine whether or not a deficiency exists and the etiology of the deficiency. Anabolic steroids prevent a negative nitrogen balance.

The role of zinc in wound healing, particularly in relation to the healing of pressure sores, has been discussed for some time. Zinc plays an important part in protein synthesis. Because of protein loss in the presence of pressure sores, it has been suggested that zinc could hasten wound healing (Greaves 1972; Flynn et al 1973; Henkin 1974). Plasma zinc levels appear to be decreased in patients with a variety of protein-losing states and atherosclerosis (Volkow 1963). It has been shown safe for use in geriatric patients (Czerwinski et al 1974) and is therefore suggested for patients with lowered (not normal) zinc plasma levels (Pories et al 1967; Husain 1969). For those patients, it may be safely administered as an oral dosage form.

It is of paramount importance that cleanliness and dryness be maintained in order to insure adequate healing or to prevent further deterioration. If the skin is unbroken, cleanliness can be achieved with gentle washing, using a mild, nonirritating soap like Ivory. Washing removes urine, excreta, and perspiration and leaves the skin more absorbent, which allows for proper secretory function.

It is difficult to justify the application of pastes and ointments to ulcerated lesions because these agents might encourage bacterial growth and impede re-epithelialization (Adams and Bluefarb 1968). The indiscriminate use of ointments and bandages may promote sweating and excoriating discharges, which can irritate the ulcer, retard healing, and often induce extension of the ulceration (Smigel and Russell 1962). Alcohol removes essential fatty constituents from the skin, while rubbing may cause dryness, allergic inflammation, fissures, or desiccation, and abrasion of the skin (Rudd 1962). After cleansing of the sores with soap and water, a nonalcoholic, antiseptic, mildly fatted lotion may be used.

The problem of keeping the patient clean and dry may not be too complicated if dealing with a cooperative, ambulant patient. However, patients being treated for pressure sores are chiefly those in high-risk situations, unable or unwilling to cooperate or ambulate. Furthermore, these patients are often incontinent. Thus, it may be exceedingly difficult to assure that the patient has a clean and dry skin. A methylbenzethonium powder dusted and rubbed into the texture of draw sheets, helps to delay the decomposition of urine by ammonia-producing (urea-splitting) organisms, delaying the onset of ammoniacal dermatitis. However, caution must be exercised in using powders because of caking and additional irritation. If necessary, a cream containing methylbenzethonium chloride may be used. This type of product is among the most effective in the care of aged, incontinent patients.

Fecal incontinence is difficult to control. It may be caused by overuse of stool softeners. Control of fecal incontinence can be achieved, it has been suggested, by inducing constipation to the point of obstipation. This is followed by administration of an enema at a predetermined time every second day (Smigel and Russell 1962). The sphincters then become habituated to a certain timing, thus preventing prolonged contact of fecal matter with the skin.

Since its introduction (Davis 1959), the sheepskin has been used extensively to prevent and treat bedsores. Bed linen, if not kept dry, clean, and wrinkle-free, may act as an abrasive or irritant. Conversely, sheepskin is soft and resilient, does not wrinkle, and distributes pressure evenly. It provides a smooth surface, reduces friction, and permits free circulation of air. The dense cushion of wool also allows for the absorption and dissipation of moisture and prevents it from remaining on the skin. If the sheepskin is to work properly, the patient must lie on it without any intervening material. Yet this elementary fact is often overlooked. Many patients are permitted to wear hospital gowns or pajamas, which prevent direct contact and negate any advantage of the sheepskin.

Numerous mechanical devices and specially designed mattresses are available to reduce pressure by means of cyclical alteration or redistribution of weight. Among these are large-celled ripple mattresses, polyurethane foam, Stryker frames, rocking beds, water beds, and air mattresses. For example, a flotation mattress has recently been marketed which contains three baffled water chambers said to prevent water pooling when the patient's bed is adjusted.

REFERENCES

Adams, L.A., and Bluefarb, S.M. How we treat decubitus ulcers. *Postgrad Med.* 44:269, 1968.

Bailey, B.N. *Bedsores.* Baltimore: Williams and Wilkins, Co., 1967.

Barton, A.A., and Barton, M. The clinical and thermographical evaluation of pressure sores. *Age Ageing.* 2:55, 1973.

Barton, A.A., and Barton, M. Drug-based prevention of pressure sores. *Lancet* 2:443, 1976.

Berecek, K. Etiology of decubitus ulcers. *Nurs Clin North Am.* 10:157, 1975.

Binks, F.A. Pathogenesis and treatment of pressure sores. *Physiotherapy* 54:281, 1968.

Bliss, M.R., and McLaren, R. Preventing pressure sores in geriatric patients. *Nurs Mirr.* 123:434, 1967.

Chick, N. Treatment of ischemic and stasis ulcers with gold leaf and polyethylene film: preliminary report. *J Am Geriatr Soc.* 17:605, 1969.

Czerwinski, A.W., Carck, M.L., Serafetinides, E.A. et al. Safety and efficacy of zinc sulfate in geriatric patients. *Clin Pharmacol Ther.* 15:436, 1974.

Davis, L. Sheepskins and decubitus ulcers. *J Med Assoc Ala.* 29:164, 1959.

Dowling, A.S. Pressure sores–their cause, prevention and treatment. *Md State Med J.* 19:131, 1970.

Edberg, E.L., Cerny, K., and Stauffer, E.S. Prevention and treatment of pressure sores. *Phys Ther.* 53:246, 1973.

Enis, J.E., and Sarmiento, A. The pathophysiology and management of pressure sores. *Orthop Rev.* 2(10):25, 1973.

Flynn, A., Pories, W.J., Stain, W.H. et al. Zinc deficiency with altered adrenocortical function and its relation to delayed healing. *Lancet* 1:789, 1973.

Friedman, S.A. Common manifestations of degenerative arterial disease. *Med Clin North Am.* 6:1079, 1976.

Gallagher, J.P., and Geschickter, C.F. The use of charged gold leaf in surgery. *JAMA.* 189:928, 1964.

Gerson, L.W. The incidence of pressure sores in active treatment hospitals. *Int J Nurs Stud.* 12:201, 1975.

Gorecki, Z. Oxygen under pressure applied directly to bedsores: case report. *J Am Geriatr Soc.* 12:1147, 1964.

Greaves, M.W. Zinc in cutaneous ulceration due to vascular insufficiency. *Am Heart J.* 83:716, 1972.

Gruis, M., and Innes, B. Assessment: essential to prevent pressure sores. *Am J Nurs.* 1762:64, 1976.

Guthrie, R.H., and Goulian, D. Decubitus ulcers: prevention and treatment. *Geriatrics* 28:67, 1973.

Harris, C. Decubitus ulcers in the sick aged. *J Am Geriatr Soc.* 13:538, 1965.

Henkin, R.I. Zinc in wound healing. *N Engl J Med.* 291:675, 1974.

Herceg, S.J., and Harding, R.L. Surgical treatment of pressure sores. *Pa Med.* 74(8):45, 1971.

Howell, T.H. Some terminal aspects of disease in old age: a clinical study of 300 patients. *J Am Geriatr Soc.* 17:1034, 1969.

Husain, S.L. Oral zinc sulfate in leg ulcers. *Lancet* 1:1069, 1969.

Kahn, S. A guide to the treatment of decubitus (pressure) ulcers in paraplegia. *Surg Clin North Am.* 40:1657, 1960.

Kanof, N.M. Treatment of cutaneous ulcers. *J Invest Dermatol.* 43:441, 1964.

Margraf, H.W., and Covey, T.H. A trial of silver-zinc-allantoinase in the treatment of leg ulcers. *Arch Surg.* 112:699, 1977.

Medical Letter. Debrisan. 20:47, 1978.

Michocki, R.J., and Lamy, P.P. The problem of pressure sores in a nursing home population: statistical data. *J Am Geriatr Soc.* 24:323, 1976a.

Michocki, R.J., and Lamy, P.P. The care of decubitus ulcers (pressure sores). *J Am Geriatr Soc.* 24:217, 1976b.

Moolten, S.E. Bedsores in the chronically ill patient. *Arch Phys Med Rehab.* 53:430, 1972.

Nyquist, R.H. Brine bath treatments for decubitus ulcers. *JAMA.* 169:927, 1959.

Phillips, I., Lobo, A.Z., Fernandes, R. et al. Acetic acid in the treatment of superficial wounds infected by *Pseudomonas aeruginosa. Lancet* 56:12, 1968.

Pories, W.J., Henzel, J.H., Rob, C.G. et al. Acceleration of wound healing in man with zinc sulfate given by mouth. *Lancet* 1:121, 1967.

Risbrook, A.T., Goodfriend, S.S., and Reiter, J.M. Gold leaf in the treatment of leg ulcers. *J Am Geriatr Soc.* 21:325, 1973.

Robertson, W.G. Digby's receipts. *Ann Med Hist.* 7:216, 1925.

Rosenthal, A.M., Schurman, A. Hyperbaric treatment of pressure sores. *Arch Phys Med Rehab.* 52:413, 1971.

Rostenberg, A., Medansky, R., and Wasserman, E. Sugar paste in the treatment of leg ulcers. *Arch Dermatol.* 78:94, 1958.

Rudd, T.N. The pathogenesis of decubitus ulcers. *J Am Geriatr Soc.* 10:48, 1962.

Sather, M.R., Weber, C.E., and George, J. Pressure sores and the spinal cord injury patient. *Drug Intell Clin Pharm.* 11:155, 1977.

Schell, V., and Wolcott, L. The etiology, prevention and management of decubitus ulcers. *Mod Med.* 63:100, 1966.

Shea, J.D., and Merlino, A. *Patient Care* 8:236, 1975.

Smigel, J.O., and Russell, A. The do's and dont's of therapy for decubitus lesions, with emphasis on use of the electric lamp. *J Am Geriatr Soc.* 10:975, 1962.

Smith, K.W., Oden, P.W., and Blaulock, W.K. A comparison of gold leaf and other occlusive therapy. *Arch Dermatol.* 96:703, 1967.

Spira, M., Moore, J., Herdy, S.B. et al. Care of the decubitus ulcer patient. *GP.* 39(4):78, 1969.

Ursu, G. Bedsores treated with negative air-ions. *Paraplegia* 8:182, 1970.

Vasile, J., and Chaitin, H. Prognostic factors in decubitus ulcers of the aged. *Geriatrics* 21:126, 1972.

Volkow, N.F. Cobalt, manganese and zinc content in the blood of atherosclerosis patients. *Fed Proc.* 22:1897, 1963.

Walker, K.A. *Pressure Sores: Prevention and Treatment.* London: Butterworth, 1971.

Weiss, A. Management of decubitus ulcers. *NY State J Med.* 60:79, 1960.

Williams, R.W. Report on the WCPT investigation into the treatment of pressure sores. *Physiotherapy* 54:288, 1968.

Wolf, N., Wheeler, P.C., and Wolcott, L.E. Gold leaf treatment of ischemic skin ulcers. *JAMA.* 196:105, 1966.

APPENDIX A

DECUBITUS CARE PROTOCOL

Operating Principles

1. All new admissions will have predilection scores done by staff on each floor. For scores of 7 or over, an aggressive prevention program will be instituted.
2. All decubiti will be evaluated weekly or bi-weekly by the designated physician and the decubitus team to determine grade and/or change in treatment plan.
3. The team will debride the decubitus at the appropriate time if they are following your patient. If you specifically do not wish decubiti with hard eschar to be debrided, please indicate in the orders and/or integrated progress notes.
4. Patients who arrive with decubiti will be photographed on admission and periodically thereafter. Please view these serial pictures at any time.
5. Cultures and sensitivity of decubiti will be taken on admission and, when positive, orders will be written for 7-10 days of systemic antibiotic therapy if there is evidence of systemic infection. The antibiotic to which the organism is sensitive will be selected, providing the patient is not allergic to it.
6. An adequate nutritional level must be maintained with high protein diet and good hydration.
7. Vitamin deficiencies will be corrected when identified.
8. Blood tests and blood chemistries will be done if indicated (total protein, A/G ratio, serum zinc, hematocrit and hemoglobin).
9. Decubitus care will be provided daily by the team until the lesions are stable and healed. Those with high predilection scores (ie, over 7) will continue to receive aggressive preventive care.
10. If you wish the decubitus team to follow your patient, please write or telephone an order to that effect.
11. These procedures are being carried out throughout the Institution.
12. Changes in protocol will be made depending upon functional utility and experience.

The John L. Deaton Medical Center, Baltimore, Md. Reproduced with permission.

APPENDIX B

DECUBITUS CARE PROTOCOL

Treatment Principles

Grade I
    A. Pressure areas — the presence of erythema, cyanosis or vesicle formation, usually over a bony prominence, with no break in the skin.

    B. Treatment —
1. Antipressure padding.
2. Good skin care.
3. Maintain adequate nutritional and hydration levels.
4. Turning and positioning, every two (2) hours.

Grade II
    A. Early decubitus — the presence of any break in the skin, which contains no necrosis.

    B. Treatment —
1. Light cleansing with normal saline solution.
2. Topical antibiotic therapy— Neosporin powder or Terramycin powder
3. Antipressure padding or air.

Grade III
    A. Moderate decubitus — a well circumscribed area of inflammation and tissue necrosis which extends through the dermis and into the subcutaneous fat.

    B. Treatment —
1. Cleansing with peroxide, thorough rinsing with normal saline.
2. Chemical debridement—Panafil, Santyl.
3. Manual debridement if indicated.
4. Topical antibiotic therapy after debridement and when granulation is well established. Example: Neosporin powder.
5. Sterile dressings.
6. Antipressure padding.
7. Water mattress.

Grade IV
- A. Advanced decubitus — a necrotic excavating ulceration which extends through skin, fat and muscle, down to and usually including periosteum and bone, with a moderate amount of debris and purulent exudate.
- B. Treatment —
  1. Cleansing with peroxide and thorough rinsing with normal saline solution.
  2. Chemical and/or manual debridement.
  3. Pack cavities or fistulas—with 4×3s and/or iodoform gauze.
  4. Sterile dressings.
  5. Antipressure padding.
  6. Water mattress.

The John L. Deaton Medical Center, Baltimore, Md. Reprinted with permission.

APPENDIX C

DECUBITUS CARE PROTOCOL

Record and Progress Report

Predilection Score on _____ Was _____

Condition	Mental state	Activity	Mobility in bed	Incontinence
0 Good	0 Alert	0 Ambulant	0 Full	0 Not
1 Fair	1 Confused	1 Walks with help	1 Slightly limited	1 Occasional
2 Poor	2 Apathetic	2 Chairfast	2 Very limited	2 Usually of urine
3 Bad	3 Stuporous	3 In bed all day	3 Immobile	3 Doubly incontinent

NOTE: A score of 7 or more is considered a "high-risk score" for the development of decubiti. Special attention to regular turning, protection padding over areas most vulnerable, meticulous skin care and good intake of protein foods are especially indicated in those with a "high-risk score."

Referred to Ulcer Treatment Room on

_____

Cultures taken   _____

Pictures taken   _____

Debridement done   _____

The John L. Deaton Medical Center, Baltimore, Md. Reprinted with permission.

26 Drugs and Surgery

Any surgical procedure entails some degree of danger to the patient. Various sources have reported a threefold increase in mortality related to surgical procedures in patients older than 70 years. Many surgeons are still hesitant to operate on a patient who is older than 70 or 80 years of age (Ballard 1969). Yet, it has been shown, for example, that the elderly female can tolerate surgery very well in a modern-day hospital setting (McKeithern 1975). Surgical risks can be significantly reduced by adequate and careful preoperative management (Sehhati and Sarvestani 1976). Equally important is early mobilization and rehabilitation, which reduces the risk of surgical correction of the geriatric hip fracture considerably (Liss and Wylie 1978). Thus, the evidence indicates that careful attention to preoperative and postoperative procedures reduces the risk of surgery for the elderly. Elective surgery is preferred to emergency surgery, which should be performed only when absolutely necessary. The need for care is particularly heightened if a patient is senile, semi-invalid, or hesitant about surgery.

PREOPERATIVE CONSIDERATIONS

These revolve around two major concerns, ie, patient's health status, and a careful, detailed drug history. Particular care should be given to an evaluation of the patient's cardiovascular, central nervous, circulatory, and respiratory systems (Cowdry and Steinberg 1971; Anderson 1971; Stanaszek 1974).

Various stages of brain failure may increase a patient's vulnerability to anesthesia, and necessitate lower doses of anesthetic drugs. These patients, too, will probably be managed with one or more of the psychotropic drugs, which may reduce the need for preoperative medication. A patient history of stroke will influence anesthetic selection, as will the etiology of the stroke, either hemorrhage or thrombosis.

Surgical procedures are likely to cause electrolyte disturbances, which could cause toxic reactions in patients on digitalis therapy. Congestive heart failure patients or patients with a history of atrial fibrillation with a rapid ventricular response should be stabilized with preoperative digitalis therapy.

Patients who require nitroglycerin for angina pectoris on slight exercise and those who are awakened at night by anginal pain are poor surgical risks. Antihypertensives are potentiated by many anesthetics. Guanethidine should be discontinued two weeks before surgery, methyldopa seven to ten days, and ganglionic blocking agents 24 hours before surgery. There are conflicting recommendations regarding propranolol. It has been said that propranolol should be continued, but it has also been recommended that it be withdrawn slowly over a two-week period. Clonidine, if it is to be withdrawn, must be discontinued over a two- to four-day period. If the patient suffers from moderate or severe hypertension, a rebound effect must be expected on withdrawl of the antihypertensive drug. If this is suspected, the drug may have to be continued. Anesthetics that produce myocardial depression should not be used.

Even minor office procedures are sometimes contraindicated in patients on anticoagulant therapy. Protamine sulfate counteracts heparin promptly. If heparin is discontinued prior to surgery, its effect will be eliminated within eight hours (its half-life is only 1.5 hours).

Vitamin K is used to reverse the effect of oral anticoagulants. Vitamin K, though, remains active for about seven days, and the patient will be resistant to anticoagulant action for approximately that time. Administration of plasma, 200 ml to 500 ml, may then be necessary (Lain and Shinn 1976).

Asthmatic patients need particular care, both preoperatively and postoperatively. Marked pulmonary obstruction would necessitate administration of bronchodilators via intermittent positive pressure breathing (IPPB). The physician may wish to consider steroid therapy prior to any thoracic or abdominal surgery. If the patient has been receiving corticosteroids for chronic therapy, their sudden withdrawal preoperatively may induce serious hypotension.

Patients on oral hypoglycemics should probably receive intravenous glucose during surgery and during the postoperative period. Administration of small doses of insulin before and after surgery may also be necessary.

Preanesthetic medications pose certain problems in the elderly, who may exhibit increased sensitivity. Geriatric patients probably need less sedation and less anesthetics. Narcotic and sedative dosages are usually given at one-half the usual adult dose. Anticholinergic drugs, such as atropine or scopolamine make secretion removal difficult (Niesenbaum 1968).

Because of extracellular fluid deficit in the elderly, the patient may receive a balanced isotonic salt solution preoperatively. There may also be an indication for adrenocorticosteroid use for several days before surgery to increase ability to withstand stress.

ANESTHETICS

Traditionally, it is believed that elderly patients require less anesthesia than younger patients. Yet some anesthetics are difficult to adjust because their dose is expressed as concentration of one gas dispersed in another gas.

Also, physiologic changes of advancing age affect anesthesia. Older patients have a lowered oxygen tension and a lowered response to inhaled carbon dioxide. Spinal anesthesia may be difficult to administer in patients with degenerative joint and bone disease. The altered homeostatic mechanisms concomitant to old age heighten the elderly's vulnerability to stress. Finally, an impaired cardiovascular system alters the circulation. Anesthetics can also interact with many drugs (Table 26-1). For example, the aminoglycoside antibiotics can potentiate the action of neuromuscular blocking agents used for anesthesia.

The choice of an anesthetic agent and the route of administration will be determined largely by the patient's physiologic state. The danger of hypoxia must always be considered carefully.

Cyclopropane seldom produces nausea and, if administered in a mixture with oxygen, does not produce hypoxia. On the other hand, it is contraindicated in patients with cardiac disorders because it affects the conduction mechanism of the heart.

For patients judged fair or poor surgical risks, block anesthesia is usually recommended. Otherwise, anesthetics will be selected which are primarily eliminated via the lungs. If thiopental sodium is used for

Table 26-1
Drugs That Might Interact with Anesthetic Agents

Anticoagulants
Antimicrobials
Cardiovascular agents
Corticosteroids
CNS drugs
  Anticonvulsants
  Antidepressants (Tricyclics)
  Phenothiazines
  Sedatives-Hypnotics
Hypoglycemic agents
  Insulin
Levodopa
Miotics

Adapted from: J. Dancey. List of drugs that may interact with anesthetic agents. *Can J Hosp Pharm.* 28(1):26, 1975.

induction of anesthesia, patients with advanced cardiac or respiratory diseases should receive oxygen before and during its administration.

It is important to note that if local anesthesia is used, solutions containing epinephrine are contraindicated because of possible cardiac stimulation and blood vessel spasticity (Pratt 1978).

POSTOPERATIVE CONSIDERATIONS

Early mobilization and rehabilitation are vital. The usual monitoring procedures should be followed, in addition to fluid and electrolyte replacement.

Total parenteral nutrition may be considered. This is the intravenous administration of sufficient nutrients above the usual basal requirements to achieve tissue synthesis, positive nitrogen balance, and anabolism.

Catheter placement requires an additional surgical procedure and maintenance of the administration site is demanding. Furthermore, as the elderly may be particularly sensitive to swings in potassium concentrations, it is important to note that the basic protein solution may contain up to 18 mEq of potassium without addition of exogenous potassium. If there is evidence of impaired renal function, retention of excess amounts of potassium or nitrogenous substances may be a problem. A formulation containing a low potassium concentration may be ordered, or the use of the total parenteral nutrition may be deferred until an adequate urinary flow is assured.

REFERENCES

Anderson, H.C. *Newton's Geriatric Nursing.* St. Louis: C.V. Mosby Co., 1971.

Ballard, L.A. Gynecologic surgery in the aged. *Geriatrics* 24:172, 1969.

Cowdry, E.V., and Steinberg, F.U. (Eds.). *The Care of the Geriatric Patient.* St. Louis: C.V. Mosby Co., 1971.

Lain, D., and Shinn, A.F. Adjusting medications for preoperative patients on long-term drug therapy. *Hosp Pharm.* 11:458, 1976.

Liss, S.E., and Wylie, W.J. Practical aspects of mobilizing the elderly patient following hip fracture. *Tex Med.* 74:69, 1978.

McKeithern, W.S. Major gynecologic surgery in elderly females 65 years of age and older. *Am J Obstet Gynecol.* 123:59, 1975.

Niesenbaum, L. Problems of pulmonary disease in the elderly. *Geriatrics* 23:127, 1968.

Pratt, G.H. Elderly patient as surgical problem. *NY State J Med.* 78:271, 1978.

Sehhati, G.H., and Sarvestani, M. Möglichkeiten und Probleme der Anesthesia und Operationsvorbereitung beim Alten Menschen. *Therapiewoche* 26:2765, 1976.

Stanaszek, W.F. The hospital pharmacist and the geriatric patient. *Hosp Form Management.* 9(8):18, 1974.

27 Patient Counseling and Compliance

The physician's labors do not end with the writing of a prescription; rather, they have just begun (Lamy and Vestal 1978). Patient counseling and follow-up, both of which should be a part of the patient's medical record, are necessary if the prescribed regimen is to achieve its desired effect. Although nobody would disagree that it is important to achieve patient cooperation so that the treatment plan will be followed, nobody would disagree either that this may be a time-consuming and uncertain process. Elderly patients, in particular, may simply seek a physician for companionship, for sympathy regarding financial, domestic or personal problems, or for confirmation or refutation of their fears. Others may have little drive to continue a struggle with life and still others, living alone, may lack the necessary support, both economic and psychosocial (Lamy 1979). The difficulties in achieving patient compliance and the uncertainties about the methods used to achieve compliance have recently been highlighted (Currie and Currie 1978).

The responsibility for drug treatment has been shifted from the physician to the patient. This implies good cooperation between physician and patient or strict "compliance" by the patient with the provider's directions. The term "compliance" has been interpreted to mean the extent to which a patient adheres to a treatment regimen as prescribed, which places the burden of "compliance" on the patient (Sackett 1974). It also implies that compliance is a consistent trait in a given individual. In contrast, it is recognized that it is cooperation that is needed and not compliance, and the establishment of basic trust is the keystone to success. Without it, the patient may reject any counseling efforts (Lamy 1971). Thus, the goal of any patient education effort is to instill a desire in the patient to cooperate fully and intelligently with the mutually agreed upon therapeutic regimen and, in so doing, maintain or improve health (Morris et al 1975). Patient education, therefore, encompasses a greater acceptance of the responsibilities of self-care (Task Force Committee on Patient Education 1972).

A review of the health literature underscores the need for effective patient education, if recommended health behaviors are to be adopted. Patients need to understand their susceptibility to the illness in question, the severity of that illness, the consequences of inaction, and the efficacy of the recommended action. Unless these conditions are met, it is unlikely that patients will alter their behavior to adopt the prescribed course of therapy. This is the dilemma of the compliance problem. The lack of understanding by the health provider of the need to assess a patient's health beliefs and to deal with those that are dissonant with desired health practices should not be labeled in terms that connote patient blame or failure. More appropriately, much of the responsibility lies with the practitioner, and patient passivity is not to be encouraged or condoned (Becker 1974).

COMMUNICATIONS

Most patient education activities stress teaching, not learning. Information dissemination is stressed, and it has become apparent that health care personnel should not overly rely on information dissemination (Knowles 1970). A learning process should be used where the material presented is problem-oriented and where there is active participative learning and mutual respect between provider and patient. Yet a patient may apparently understand and comprehend the material presented and then not adhere to the prescribed regimen (McGuire 1972, 1974). Anyone involved in direct patient care has encountered this phenomenon. What went wrong?

Basic to any understanding is good communication. Communication is a dynamic process involving both the provider and the patient (Lively 1978). It is an interpersonal relationship (Kron 1972) in which one person attempts to understand the other person's point of view and feelings about a particular situation (Lewis 1973). Communication is a process of mutual influence in which meanings are not contained in the message but in the translation of the message by the receiver (Welk et al 1974).

A message leading to a cooperative effort will only be successful if the patient's attention has been won, the patient understands and comprehends the message and, importantly, accepts the meaning of the message (Insko 1967). The persuasive effect of the message, which ultimately leads to patient cooperation, will depend entirely on patient acceptance. The function of persuasive communication is to suggest reasons why the message should be accepted. Verbal and positive reinforcements are needed during the encounter to help evoke the desired response (Insko 1965; Hildum and Brown 1956; Krasner et al 1965). The patient must not only be exposed to the information, but must understand and comprehend its meaning, accept the intent of the message, and must remember the information. Exposure, attention, comprehension, acceptance, and retention are necessary to achieve cooperation. All of this is based on good communication.

PATIENT COMPLIANCE

The patient-provider encounter can be disappointing and fruitless in terms of achieving the therapeutic goal (Korsch and Negrete 1969). Patients are dissatisfied with physicians and physicians are dissatisfied with the lack of patient cooperation. Complete failure to take medications occurs in up to 50% of patients (Blackwell 1973), which may simply reflect a patient's dislike of being told what to do (Van Putten 1974). Compliance data fluctuate widely. Physicians overestimate their patient's adherence by about 100% (Roth and Caron 1978). It seems that about one-third of patients always comply, one-third never comply, and one-third sometimes comply. Reports of compliance range from 7% to 87% (Hobby and Deuschle 1959; Wilson 1973; Gillum and Barsky 1974), and can vary with the prescribed drug (Stewart and Cluff 1972). About 40% of patients may stop taking their medication within the first year (Hogarty and Goldberg 1973), and compliance with one regimen does not mean that the patient will automatically comply with another one. Unfortunately, it is not possible to identify a potential drug defaulter; compliance should never be assumed. People who are socially isolated, the poorly educated, and those treated in outpatient clinics, are most likely not to comply (Porter 1969).

Compliance by the Elderly

Some time ago, it was shown that despite the time spent by a physician with an elderly patient, in general, their record of compliance is poor (Schwartz et al 1962). Since then, it has been established that the elderly do not, in general, differ from other patients in their drug-taking behavior and compliance with established treatment regimens (Weintraub 1978). There is no indication that the elderly comply more or less than other patients (Lundin 1978a). In fact, elderly patients have demonstrated surprising accuracy in self-administration (Libow and Mehl 1970). However, concern with lack of compliance by the elderly is more than justified. Because of chronic diseases, the elderly are likely to receive a variety of complex and potent drugs. In addition to adverse effects, these drugs also exhibit a tendency to interact with other drugs, and the elderly are more susceptible to adverse and interaction effects than younger patients (Wynne and Heller 1973). Nearly 20% of patients entering the geriatric service of one general hospital displayed disorders attributable to the effects of prescribed drugs.

Specific compliance problems of the elderly Whether or not a particular patient will comply with a particular set of instructions depends on a variety of factors, and the uncooperative patient will only be identified when lack of cooperation becomes apparent. Nevertheless, noncompliance by the elderly could be reduced if certain factors are kept in mind. Foremost among these may be lack of frequent contact between provider and patient (Brocklehurst and Shergold 1969), which may depend on the patient's ability to meet transportation and economic demands. Misuse or incorrect use of drugs by the elderly is often caused by a lack of practical information or instructions on appropriate use. Although it appears self-evident, counseling of the elderly requires care in the selection of a specific modality. Failing sensory systems (sight and hearing) may mandate increased use of communications by touch. There must be patience and willingness to extend the counseling period beyond the "normal" time.

Still, older and disadvantaged people often have difficulties with compliance despite good intentions. In addition, the heaviest drug users, which are the elderly (particularly the elderly, white female), are known to be at risk to noncompliance (Lech et al 1975) as well as patients with chronic illnesses who require long-term maintenance therapy with suppressive or preventive treatment (Blackwell 1973). Medication compliance diminishes sharply with the passage of time, and much of the medication the elderly must take is given on a long-term basis (Sackett et al 1978). Specifically, instructions for the elderly may be written in print that is too small to be deciphered by those with an impaired vision. Complete directions may not have been given. The fact that a patient does not question any instructions should not be taken to mean that the patient understands them. The attitude that "the doctor will tell me what I need to know" still persists (Lundin 1978b). The patient may hesitate to ask any questions. Later, the patient may forget verbal instructions or misinterpret poorly written instructions. For example, one elderly woman, who received a prescription for tolbutamide "to be taken two times a day" took one tablet at 9 AM and the other at 10 AM—complying with the instructions as written but facing potentially serious clinical consequences. In one study, 62% of 170 prescriptions reviewed had similarly ambiguous instructions (Lundin 1978b). In another study, 67 patients misinterpreted directions on each of ten labels. Not once was a label interpreted uniformly by all patients (Mazzullo et al 1974), thus demonstrating how poorly-worded prescription directions increase medication errors (Powell et al 1973). Even more potentially hazardous is the common practice of writing "Take as Directed" (Lundin 1978b), which places the burden of both decision-making and recall on the patient. "Take with Meals" is a similar and confusing instruction. Does the patient eat two, three, or more times a day? The tea-and-toast syndrome, often observed with the elderly, indicates that they may well eat less (or frequently more) than three times a day. Vague instructions, which refer to "before meals" and "after meals," are not much more helpful. Some tablets must be taken before or after meals (one or two hours) (Appendix A). Thus, the physician, when prescribing, should recognize the time a patient usually eats and goes to sleep (Mazzullo 1976). Directions given verbally and reinforced by "Take as Directed" are useless and even hazardous. With advancing age, it takes longer and is more difficult to recall verbal information, especially recently acquired information (Waugh et al 1978).

The physician must also establish whether the elderly patient can properly open and close the medication container (Sherman 1978). Many elderly patients may discontinue the use of a medication because of the difficulty encountered in opening a child-proof container. It is not at all unusual to visit patients at home and find that prescription containers have been smashed in order to gain access to the medication.

Elderly patients, like others, seek help from different physicians. One physician may prescribe a drug by its trade name, while a second may prescribe the same drug, but by its generic name. Thus, the elderly, in no position to identify the duplication, may take both and be at risk to serious clinical consequences. Use of many physicians also often leads to a larger number of prescribed drugs, and thus greater risk to adverse and interaction effects.

Other factors, which might not be as easily discernible, center on the shape, color, or size of the medication (Arthur 1974). Elderly patients may react differently than younger patients to different formulation colors.

Error frequency is a function of the number of drugs prescribed and the dosage number (Vere 1965; Crooks et al 1965; Caron and Roth 1968; Davis 1966). Compliance decreases significantly with an increasing number of prescriptions and with an increasing number of doses administered per day. Higher cost causes a pronounced effect on noncompliance (Brand et al 1977). The complexity of the differing administration schedules confuses elderly patients; and those who err are likely to make multiple mistakes (Wandless and Davis 1977). The complexity of the drug administration schedule can be increased even further by dietary instructions (Table 27-1).

Finally, the results of patient behavior in noncompliance should be carefully considered. Many patients deviate from instructions, including the elderly. They may reduce a dose or cease taking a drug because a disease has abated or because they feel that they could obtain adequate relief by using fewer doses. Elderly patients with arthritis or hypertension may do so. A large number of patients probably cease to cooperate because of side effects that were not explained, or because of unexpected adverse effects. Patients receiving antidepressants may react in this fashion because the expected side effects start almost immediately, but the full therapeutic effects may be delayed for four to six weeks. The particular difficulty with this behavior, and one that can be especially hazardous in the elderly, is the tendency by elderly patients to discontinue all drugs if they are unable to identify the drug with the undesirable effect.

Table 27-1
Dietary Suggestions for Some Diseases

Disease	Diet	Fluid intake
Asthma, bronchial	Certain foods may cause attacks	8 oz fluid/hr
Bronchitis, acute		8 oz/hr
Congestive heart failure	Avoid salt, use salt substitute	Avoid carbonated fluids including beer, and OTC drugs
Constipation	Use high-fiber foods, stewed fruits, raw and cooked fruits	Fruit juices
Diarrhea, acute	Ice chips for nausea, gelatin	Small volumes of clear liquids
Emphysema	Weight control	8 oz 8 times/day
Fatigue	Weight control if indicated. Eat several small meals a day	
Gout (acute attack)	No liver, sweetbreads, kidney, sardines	8–10 glasses/day

Methods to Increase Compliance

The unexpected difficulties that may be encountered by those wishing to establish compliance can be understood by citing one dramatic example. In one study, all glaucoma patients who had sought help when they noticed a loss of vision were asked to use eye drops three times a day, or "go blind." The prescribers purposely added that last phrase, thinking it would bring about excellent compliance. Yet, 58% of the patients did not comply, probably operating on the principle that if no attention is paid to the problem, it is likely to go away. At the point at which the subjects became legally blind in one eye, compliance improved, but only by 17% (Vincent 1971). Many variables have been studied in an effort to increase patient compliance (Becker 1976); some are listed in Table 27-2. Onset of illness, type of illness, patient attitude toward the provider, the illness or death, family interaction with the patient, the setting of the provider-patient interaction, and certain personality measures have all been investigated and found to lack correlation with compliance and behavior (Davidson 1976). There is no agreement as to the effect of patient surveillance. The social science literature seems to indicate that strong surveillance reduces compliance, while the medical literature seems to indicate the opposite effect (Davidson 1976). In general, there appears to be a negative relationship between the amount of pressure exerted and the amount of change produced.

Table 27-2
Summary of Studies Examining Sociodemographic Variables on Patient Compliance

Sociodemographic Variables	Positive	No Correlation	Negative
Age	7	30	0
Sex	3	25	3
Education	8	24	0
Social class	4	9	0
Occupation	6	12	0
Income	2	11	1
Marital status	6	11	0
Race and ethnicity	7	11	0
Religion	0	4	0
"Demographic variables"	0	1	0
	43	138	4

Number of Studies by Type of Correlation

Reprinted with permission from M.H. Becker. The role of the patient: social and psychological factors in non-compliance. Edited by G.F. McMahon. In *Principles and Techniques of Human Research and Therapeutics,* Vol. 10. Mt. Kisco, N.Y.: Futura Publishing Company, 1976.

The physician and other health care providers often fail to communicate with patients in easily understood language. These shortcomings in verbal provider-patient communication reflect a common pattern in health care in need of reform and innovation. Social and religious beliefs are other barriers to patient compliance. For example, suggested use of wine instead of a hypnotic may not be accepted because of religious concerns. Yet, physicians may actually spend very little time acquiring information about a patient's social and family history (McKelvey and Lamy 1972). Also operating against compliance is the patient and physician-accepted meaning of the sick-role, which implies and often demands abrogation of personal responsibility.

Thus, it is clear that there are many barriers to patient compliance (Powell and Lamy 1977). It is also clear that noncompliance to a therapeutic regimen in a clinical setting may have important clinical consequences for the patient. Therefore, those who prescribe and dispense drugs to the elderly have an increased responsibility to find and use any means possible to increase patient compliance (Lamy and Kitler 1971; Lamy 1978). Attitudes and expectations of both patient and provider affect outcome and compliance (Isaacs 1973). The provider's behavior may be just as important as the patient's motivation in achieving adherence to a particular drug regimen. Therapy can be significantly more effective when given by a physician who shows "confidence" in the treatment offered (Uhlenhuth et al 1966), who has enthusiasm for the proposed treatment and communicates that to the patient (Hollister 1973), and who is rated "warm" by the patient (Rickels et al 1971).

Ambulatory patients usually remember less than one-half of instructions concerning the proposed regimen and about one-third of the explanations about the particular illness to be treated. Recall can be increased if material is organized into categories. Information presented first is remembered best, possibly because the elderly have a shortened attention span.

Verbal information should be reinforced by written instructions, keeping in mind the possibility that the patient may not be able to read, may be visually impaired, and may not understand carelessly chosen, technical words.

Repeated exposures to the same message may aid in acquiring and maintaining newly accepted attitudes, which are necessary if the patient is to accept the responsibility for the therapeutic regimen. Therefore, instructions should always be reinforced on repeat encounters and the patient should be asked, at every encounter, to demonstrate familiarity with the instructions and their meaning. This is a time-consuming effort and, unfortunately, the physician does not always give enough time for it (Lamy and Riley 1978). It is assumed that the patient fully understands and reacts correctly to the instructions. The number of medication errors can be significantly reduced when verbal and written instructions are backed up by other memory aids, such as administration calendars (Wandless and Davis 1977).

In the counseling process, it is important to convey to the patient knowledge and understanding of the illness to be treated, but this is not always sufficient (Matthews and Hingson 1977), and at times has no effect at all. Teaching a group of middle-aged men the dangers of hypertension to the target organs, to health and life expectancy, the benefits of treatment, and the need for compliance did not increase compliance (Sackett et al 1978).

It is necessary to allay the patient's possible anxiety and fear of the disease and its consequences. The possible influence of the selected therapeutic regimen on the patient's remaining independence must be assessed. If drug taking interferes too much with the patient's activity, noncompliance will follow. It is probably best to tailor administration times to specific activities which the patient always undertakes and to require regular administration times, which encourages recollection (Gibson 1974). Self-management programs should involve the patient. The patient may participate in the regimen by daily weighing, for example, to measure the effect of a diuretic. The program should be as straightforward as possible; simple programs encourage compliance (Mahoney and Thoresen 1974). Any counseling session should not be considered complete unless the patient has been asked to reformulate the advice and the instructions given and has been given the opportunity to ask questions, which should not be a negative process.

A recent proposal suggests that patients fall into one of two categories; they may either be capricious compliers or intelligent noncompliers (Weintraub 1976). The drug-taking behavior of the capricious complier is unpredictable and may vary from day to day. The intelligent noncomplier, on the other hand, may have an important message to convey. Elderly patients, for example, may not take a dose when they feel a particular undesirable effect. As a matter of fact, elderly who are on strict regimens may do more poorly than those who are on a more flexible regimen and can adjust, within limits, to unanticipated or anticipated side effects of a drug. Based on this consideration, the concept of "creative compliance" has been suggested. In this model, the patient will continue to "elect" what to do with a particular regimen, but the provider effort will be directed toward improving the basis for the patient's choice. The characteristics of creative compliance include the following major components:

1. The patient becomes an aide-therapist, ie, the patient assumes an active role in assessing response to therapy.
2. Information is exchanged between patient and therapist.
3. The therapy is modified, if necessary, on the basis of new data.

If the patient is permitted to actively participate in this manner in the management of the disease and is, indeed, not only permitted but encouraged to do so, then this would most likely lead to a number of beneficial effects:

1. The patient is more likely to make rational compliance decisions.
2. There is going to be a likely decrease in serious dose-related toxicities.
3. The prescriber will have the opportunity to increase his knowledge of the disease and its therapy.

This system, it has been suggested, invites and permits the patient to become a part of the therapeutic team. In turn, the patient will be less restrained about raising questions regarding the medication regimen. This information interchange is central to creative compliance because it leads to better targeting of the therapeutic plan.

REFERENCES

Arthur, M.B. Formulation of drugs for the elderly. *Gerontol Clin.* 16:25, 1974.

Becker, M.H. The role of the patient: social and psychological factors in non-compliance. Edited by G.F. McMahon. In *Principles and Techniques of Human Research and Therapeutics,* Vol. 10. Mt. Kisco, N.Y.: Futura Publishing Co., 1976.

Becker, M.H. The health belief model and sick role behavior. *Health Education Monographs* 2(4):409, 1974.

Blackwell, B. Patient compliance. *N Engl J Med.* 289:249, 1973.

Brand, F.N., Smith, R.T., and Brand, P.A. Effect of economic barriers to medical care on patients' noncompliance. *Public Health Rep.* 92(1):72, 1977.

Brocklehurst, J.C., and Shergold, M. Old people leaving hospital. *Gerontol Clin.* 11:115, 1969.

Caron, H.S., and Roth, H.P. Patients' cooperation with a medical regimen: difficulties in identifying the non-cooperator. *JAMA.* 203:911, 1968.

Crooks, J., Clark, C.G., Caie, H.B. et al. Prescribing and administration of drugs in hospital. *Lancet* 1:383, 1965.

Currie, B.E., and Currie, M.N. (eds). Patient education in the primary care setting. Proceedings of a Conference held in Madison, Wis., Madison, Wis.: Department Family Medicine and Practice, 1978.

Davidson, P. Therapeutic compliance. *Can Psychol Rev.* 17:247, 1976.

Davis, M.S. Variations in patients' compliance with doctors' orders: analysis of congruence between survey response and results of empirical investigations. *J Med Educ.* 41:1037, 1966.

Gibson, I.I.J.M. Hospital drugs in the home. *Gerontol Clin.* 16:10, 1974.

Gillum, R.F., and Barsky, A.J. Diagnosis and management of patient compliance. *JAMA.* 228:1563, 1974.

Hildum, D., and Brown, R. Verbal reinforcement and interview bias. *J Abnorm Soc Psychol.* 53:108, 1956.

Hobby, G., and Deuschle, K. The use of riboflavin as an indicator of isoniazid ingestion in self-medication patients. *Am Rev Respir Dis.* 80:415, 1959.

Hogarty, G.E., and Goldberg, S.C. Drug and sociotherapy in the aftercare of schizophrenic patients. *Arch Gen Psychiatry.* 28:54, 1973.

Hollister, L.E. *Clinical Use of Psychotherapeutic Drugs.* Springfield, Ill.: Charles C Thomas, Publisher, 1973.

Insko, C.A. Verbal reinforcement of attitude. *J Pers Soc Psychol.* 2:621, 1965.

Insko, C.A. *Theories of Attitude Change.* New York: Appleton-Century-Crofts, 1967.

Isaacs, B. Medicine in old age: treatment of the "irremediable" elderly patient. *Br Med J.* 3:526, 1973.

Knowles, M. *The Modern Practice of Adult Education.* New York: Association Press, 1970.

Korsch, B., and Negrete, V. Doctor-patient communication. *Sci Am.* 220:21, 1969.

Krasner, L., Knowles, J., and Ullman, L. Effects of verbal conditioning of attitudes on subsequent motor performance. *J Pers Soc Psychol.* 1:407, 1965.

Kron, T. *Communication in Nursing.* Philadelphia: W.B. Saunders Co., 1972.

Lamy, P.P. Audio-visual aids in patient instruction. *J Am Pharm Assoc.* NS11:486, 1971.

Lamy, P.P. Therapeutics and the elderly. *Addict Dis.* 3:311, 1978.

Lamy, P.P. Considerations in drug therapy of the elderly. *J Drug Issues.* 9(1):27, 1979.

Lamy, P.P., and Kitler, M.E. Drugs and the geriatric patient. *J Am Geriatr Soc.* 19:23, 1971.

Lamy, P.P., and Riley, A.N. Considerations for a Pediatric pharmaceutical patient care service. *Drug Intell Clin Pharm.* 12:89, 1978.

Lamy, P.P., and Vestal, R.E. Drug prescribing for the elderly. Edited by W. Reichel. In *The Geriatric Patient.* New York: H.P. Publishing Co., Inc., 1978.

Lech, S.V., Friedman, G.D., and Ury, H.K. Characteristics of heavy users of outpatient prescription drugs. *Clin Toxicol.* 8:599, 1975.

Lewis, G.K. *Nurse-Patient Communication.* Dubuque, Ia.: William C. Brown Co., Publisher, 1973.

Libow, L.S., and Mehl, B. Self-administration of medications by patients in hospital or extended care facilities. *J Am Geriatr Soc.* 18:81, 1970.

Lively, B.T. Communication as a transactional process–basic tools of the community pharmacist. *Contemp Pharm Practice.* 1:81, 1978.

Lundin, D.V. Medication-taking behavior of the elderly: a pilot study. *Drug Intell Clin Pharm.* 12:518, 1978a.

Lundin, D.V. Must taking medication be a dilemma for the independent elderly? *J Gerontol Nurs.* 4(3):25, 1978b.

Mahoney, M.J., and Thoresen, C.E. *Self-control: Power to the Person.* Monterrey, Calif.: Brooks/Cole Publishing Co., 1974.

Matthews, D., and Hingson, R. Improving patient compliance. A guide for physicians. *Med Clin North Am.* 64:879, 1977.

Mazzullo, J.M. Methods of improving patient compliance. Edited by G.F. McMahon. In *Principles and Techniques of Human Research and Therapeutics,* Vol. 10. Mt. Kisco, N.Y.: Futura Publishing Co., 1976.

Mazzullo, J.M., Cohn, R., Lasagna, L. et al. Variations in interpretation of prescription instruction: the need for improved prescribing habits. *JAMA.* 227:929, 1974.

McGuire, W.J. Attitude change: the information-processing paradigm. Edited by C.G. McClintock. In *Experimental Social Psychology.* New York: Holt, Rinehart, and Winston, 1972.

McGuire, W.J. Communication-persuasion models for drug education. Edited by M.S. Goodstadt. In *Research Methods on Programs of Drug Education.* Toronto: Alcohol Drug Addict Research Foundation, 1974.

McKelvey, C.P., and Lamy, P.P. Patient care information in an ambulatory environment. *Am J Hosp Pharm.* 29:401, 1972.

Morris, R.W., Burkhart, V.P., and Lamy, P.P. Patient counseling. *Drug Intell Clin Pharm.* 9:485, 1975.

Porter, A.M.W. Drug defaulting in general practice. *Br Med J.* 1:218, 1969.

Powell, M.F., and Lamy, P.P. Compliance obstacles to the insulin-dependent diabetic. *Md Pharm.* 53(3):10, 1977.

Powell, R.J., Cali, T.J., and Linkewich, J.A. Inadequately written prescriptions. *JAMA.* 226:999, 1973.

Rickels, K., Lipman, R.S., Park, L.C. et al. Drug, doctor warmth, and clinic setting in the symptomatic response to minor tranquilizers. *Psychopharmacologia* 20:128, 1971.

Roth, H.P., and Caron, H.S. Accuracy of doctors' estimates and patients' statements on adherence to a drug regimen. *Clin Pharmacol Ther.* 23:361, 1978.

Sackett, D.L. *Compliance with Therapeutic Regimens.* Hamilton, Ontario: McMaster University Medical Center, 1974.

Sackett, D.L., Haynes, R.B., Gibson, E.S. et al. Patient compliance with antihypertensive regimens. *Patient Counsel Health Ed.* 1(1):18, 1978.

Schwartz, D., Wang, M., Zeitz, L. et al. Medication errors made by elderly, chronically ill patients. *Am J Publ Health.* 52:2018, 1962.

Sherman, F.T. Geriatric generic prescription form. *NY State J Med.* 78:1292, 1978.

Stewart, R.B., and Cluff, L.E. Review of medication errors and compliance in ambulatory patients. *Clin Pharmacol Ther.* 13:463, 1972.

Task Force Committee on Patient Education. Concepts of planned hospital-based patient education programs. Presented to the President's Committee on Health Education, Washington, D.C., 1972.

Uhlenhuth, E.H., Rickels, K., Fisher, S. et al. Drug, doctors' verbal attitude and clinic in the symptomatic response to pharmacotherapy. *Psychopharmacologia* 9:392, 1966.

Van Putten, T. Why do schizophrenic patients refuse to take their drugs? *Arch Gen Psychiatry.* 31:67, 1974.

Vere, D.W. Errors of complex prescribing. *Lancet* 1:370, 1965.

Vincent. P. Factors influencing patient non-compliance: a theoretical approach. *Nurs Res.* 20:509, 1971.

Wandless, I., and Davis, J.W. Can drug compliance in the elderly be improved? *Br Med J.* 1:359, 1977.

Waugh, N.C., Thomas, J.C., and Fozard, J.L. Retrieval time from different memory stores. *J Gerontol.* 33:718, 1978.

Weintraub, M. Intelligent noncompliance and capricious compliance. Edited by G.F. McMahon. In *Principles and Techniques of Human Research and Therapeutics,* Vol. 10. Mt. Kisco, N.Y.: Futura Publishing Company, 1976.

Weintraub, M. Toward creative compliance: improving therapeutics in the elderly. Edited by C.R. Beber, and P.P. Lamy. In *Medication Management and Education of the Elderly.* Princeton, N.J.: Excerpta Medica, 1978.

Welk, P.G., Burkhart, V.P., and Lamy, P.P. The technology of patient counseling. *Hosp Pharm.* 9:224, 1974.

Wilson, J.T. Compliance with instructions in the evaluation of therapeutic efficacy. *Clin Pediatr.* 12:333, 1973.

Wynne, R.D., and Heller, F. Drug overuse among the elderly. *Perspectives on Aging.* Mar/April 15, 1973.

APPENDIX A

DRUG ADMINISTRATION AND FOOD

Take with no food	Ampicillin and Ampicillin trihydrate (Alpen, Amcill, Omnipen, Penbritin, Polycillin, Principen, Totacillin)
	Cloxacillin (Tegopen)
	Dicloxacillin and Dicloxacillin sodium (Dynapen, Veracillin)
	Erythromycin base (Erythrocin, E-Mycin)
	Hetacillin (Versapen)
	Lincomycin (Lincocin)
	Nafcillin (Unipen)
	Penicillamine (Cuprimine)
	Penicillin G potassium (Pentids)
	Penicillin V (Compocillin V, Pen-Vee, V-Cillin)
	Pentaerythritol tetranitrate (Duotrate, Peritrate)
	Phenethicillin (Darcil, Maxipen, Ro-Cillin, Syncillin)
	Phenmetrazine (Preludin)
	Rifampin (Rifadin, Rimactane)
	Sitosterols, Beta and Dihydrobeta (Cytellin)
	Tetracyclines and derivatives (Achromycin, Panmycin, Steclin, Tetrex, Urobiotic, etc) EXCEPT: Doxycycline (Vibramycin)
Take ½–1 hour before meals	Atropine sulfate
	Belladonna alkaloids and Phenobarbital (Donnatal)
	Belladonna tincture and extract
	Chlordiazepoxide with Clidinium bromide (Librax)
	Dimenhydrinate (Dramamine)
	Diethylpropion (Tenuate)
	Ethoxazene (Serenium)
	Propantheline bromide (Pro-Banthine)

Take with food or milk

Acetohexamide (Dymelor)
Acetylsalicylic acid (aspirin and some combinations
Allopurinol (Zyloprim)
Aminophylline
Antihistamines (some)
APC
Azapetine phosphate (Ilidar)
Bethanechol chloride (Urecholine)
Biperiden (Akineton)
Bismuth sodium triglycollomate (Bistrimate)
Chloral hydrate
Chlorphenoxamine HCl (Phenoxene)
Chlorpromazine (Thorazine)
Chlorpropamide (Diabinese)
Chlorthalidone (Hygroton, Regroton)
Cycrimine HCl (Pagitane)
Cyproheptadine (Periactin)
Diphenhydramine HCl (Benadryl)
Doxycycline (Vibramycin)
Ephedrine, Hydroxyzine, and Theophylline (Marax)
Ephedrine, Phenobarbital, Theophylline, and KI (Quadrinal)
Ethacrynic acid (Edecrin)
Ethionamide (Trecator SC)
Ethotoin (Peganone) AFTER FOOD
Ferrous Salts
  Among them:
  Ferrous fumarate (various)
  Ferrous gluconate (Fergon)
  Ferrous sulfate (Feosol)
Furazolidone (Furoxone)
Griseofulvin (Fulvicin, Grisactin)
Hydrochlorothiazide (Esidrix, Hydrodiuril, Oretic)
Hydrocortisone (Cortef, Hydrocortone)
Hypoglycemics, oral
Indomethacin (Indocin)
Iron salts and preparations
Isoniazid (INH, Niconyl, Nydrazid, Rimifon, Tyvid)
Isosorbide dinitrate (Isordil)
Levodopa (Bendopa, Dopar, Larodopa, Levopa)

Mefenamic acid (Ponstel)
Metronidazole (Flagyl)
Nalidixic acid (Neg Gram)
Nitrofurantoin (Furadantin, Macrodantin)
Oxyphenbutazone (Tandearil)
Para-aminosalicylic acid (PAS)
Phenformin (DBI)
Phenylbutazone (Azolid, Azolid A, Butazolidin, Sterazolidin)
Phenytoin (Dilantin)
Piperidolate, Pancreatin, Taurocholic acid, etc (Dactilase)
Potassium salts and/or preparations
  Among them:
  Potassium bicarbonate
  Potassium chloride (Kay Ciel, K-Lor)*
    *DO NOT TAKE WITH MILK
  Potassium citrate solution
  Potassium gluconate (Kaon)
Prednisolone (Meticortelone, Sterane)
Prednisone (Delta Dome, Deltasone, Deltra, Meticorten, Paracort, Prednis, Servisons)
Procyclidine HCl (Kemadrin)
Quinine and Aminophylline (Quinamm)
Rauwolfia (Raudixin)
Reserpine (Serpasil)
Salicylates
Salicylazosulfapyridine (Salazopyrin)
Sulfamethoxypyridazine (Midicel, Kynex)
Sulfinpyrazone (Anturane)
Theophylline and Glyceryl guaiacolate (Quinbrom)
Thiabendazole (Mintezol)
Tolazamide (Tolinase)
Tolbutamide (Orinase)
Triamterene (Dyrenium)
Trihexyphenidyl (Artane, Pipanol, Tremin)
Trimeprazine (Temaril)
Triprolidine HCl (Actidil)
Tubercular (oral) drugs
Vitamins B (Troph-Iron, Trophite)

Take with large volume of water	Aspirin Natural vegetable compounds Psyllium hydrophilic mucilloid (Metamucil) Sulfonamides

Take no milk or milk products	Bisacodyl (Dulcolax)
	Demeclocycline (Declomycin)
	Ferrous salts and/or preparations
	  Among them:
	    Ferrous fumarate (various)
	    Ferrous gluconate (Fergon)
	    Ferrous sulfate (Feosol)
	Oxytetracycline (Terramycin)
	Potassium salts and/or preparations
	  Among them:
	    Potassium chloride (Kay Ciel, K-Lor)
	    Potassium iodide
	Tetracyclines (Achromycin, Panmycin, Steclin, Tetracyn, Tetrex, Urobiotic, etc)
	  EXCEPT: Doxycycline (Vibramycin)

Take no fruit juice	Erythromycin base (Erythrocin) Penicillin G (Pentids)

28 A New Care System is Needed

The United States allocates more resources to the aged relative to any other country in the Western World (Anderson 1972). Yet the results in terms of the health status of the elderly are unsatisfactory. Many possible reasons can be cited, but it is probably the combination of a number of factors. The elderly, for example, may not receive the vigorous care and consideration they deserve, as they may have been judged economically unproductive. Their diseases may seem to carry only a poor prognosis. The problems of the aged surely have been addressed in a case-by-case disjointed manner.

The currently operative medical model of health care defines "disease" in terms of somatic parameters. It delivers primarily disease care, and not health care. Moreover, the current system lacks effective market controls (Kristein et al 1977). Health care professionals are mainly in the business of minimizing the effects of disease (Fielding 1977), and do not focus on an individual's ability to function in a particular environment nor on the need to help sustain the quality of life of the care-seeker. Not infrequently, patients, particularly elderly patients, who take psychotropic drugs because their physician has prescribed them, are characterized later as "drug abusers," focusing attention on the victim of a problem rather than the problem itself. Adherence to this model is thus no longer adequate, especially for the elderly.

The holistic notion of health holds that individual illness may be a reflection of many external factors (Health Resources Administration 1977). The problems of the aged can be cataloged in terms of money, health, and psychosocial dislocation. Poor housing, poor nutrition, and poor health are too often cohorts of old age. Some impairment, lack of cleanliness, lack of a warm meal, immobility, deafness, or loss of vision may be more important than a heart murmur. On the other hand, benevolent, overzealous care may aggravate functional disability. Life-change events impose stress on the elderly, in particular (Rahe and Arthur 1978), and there is a relationship between life events and onset of illness. It is now thought possible that specific types of diseases are strongly related to certain life changes (Lundberg and Theorell 1976; Schless et al 1974; Mechanic 1975). Yet, with advancing age stresses increase and it is, therefore, important that a feeling of self-reliance and independence be fostered in the elderly (Nordlicht 1975). This is important, as even adequate provision of food, shelter, and clothing will not necessarily relate to a successful outcome, because the elderly, like everyone else, need to relate to other people, plans, and opportunities. In short, maintenance of an effective self-concept is an important component of successful aging (Cohen and O'Flynn-Comiskey 1976; Havighurst 1968; Blank 1971).

The new care system should provide multiple interventions. It should be a people-oriented system, rather than one that deals with case studies, case reports, and simply cases, all of which call for a caseworker and not a health-care professional. The major objective of health care for the elderly is to improve the quality of life by preventing and controlling disease so that the person receiving care can continue to function for as long as possible. Quality of life will be improved or at least sustained by alleviating the distress of disease and impairment. Life can be worthwhile even though it may be accompanied by some undesirable conditions.

Medical management of a patient should span four phases, control of the underlying disease, prevention of secondary disabilities such as bedsores, restoration (as much as possible) of the patient's functional ability, all leading to an effort to maximize residual functional capabilities, including manipulation of the environment (Hunt 1977). Throughout this process, it must be realized by those delivering care to the elderly, that lung cancer and coronary heart disease require a different approach from that developed against typhoid fever and poliomyelitis.

Obviously, to attain these goals, changes are necessary in the current health care system, and alternate behavior patterns for everyone connected with the health care system must be formed (National Commission 1977). A psychosocial model of health care is needed (Engel 1977) to explain why some patients experience illness conditions that others might regard as problems of living, "be they emotional reactions to life circumstances or somatic symptoms." Disease must be viewed in terms of psychological, social, and cultural, as well as anatomic, physiologic, and biochemical terms (Peterson 1977). Similar suggestions have been made in the past (Dubos 1961). A system of human services is needed that will span organizational boundaries in order to achieve integrated human services, of which health care services are only one part.

As most major chronic illnesses in America have environmental and behavioral components that play important parts in their etiology, systems of preventive care should be developed. A Life-Time Health-Monitoring Program (LHMP) has been proposed that would bring together epidemiologic and clinical approaches to health, a public health approach and a medical approach (Breslow and Somers 1977). Several preventive services proposed for older adults are listed in Table 28-1 (Health Resources Administration 1977). The Department of Health, Education and Welfare also addresses the issue of necessary changes in health care delivery and has issued health planning goals, many of which address the problems of the elderly:

1. The health status should be improved in all parts of the country and among all population groups, especially among medically underserved populations.
    a. Preventable morbidity and mortality from noncommunicable diseases and conditions should be reduced to the lowest rates reported in comparable populations.
    b. The incidence and prevalence of mental illness should be reduced.
    c. An increasing portion of persons with chronic disabilities should be enabled to function to their fullest capabilities.
    d. Oral health should be improved so that at least 90% of persons 55-64 years of age have not lost all of their natural teeth.
2. Health promotion and disease prevention should be extended through both individual and community actions.
    a. Individuals should have enhanced capabilities to make informed choices about styles of living and health

practices that maximize well-being and minimize risks of avoidable diseases, disability, stress, and premature death.
  b. Preventive health services should be strengthened as an integral and important part of community and personal health services.
3. Every person should have access to emergency and primary health care services and to appropriate specialized, long-term, and rehabilitative services.
  a. The knowledge and capabilities of persons to obtain needed health care, including self-care, in an appropriate and economical manner, should be increased.
  b. Health care services should be linked closely to other social and human services.
4. The rate of increases in expenditures for health care should be reduced.
  a. Lack of income should not be a barrier to needed health care.
  b. Health care financing systems should facilitate accessibility to appropriate care for all populations and encourage efficient methods of providing and managing services.

Table 28-1
Preventive Services Proposed for Older Adults

	FIC*	ASPH ATPM†	APHA‡	TF§
History	x		x	x
Height and weight	x	x	x	x
Blood pressure	x	x	x	x
EKG	x	x	x	x
Vision	x	x		x
Tonometry		x	x	
Hearing	x	x		x
Spirometry			x	
Physical examination	x	x	x	x
Breast examination (females)	x			x
Rectal examination	x	x	x	
Sigmoidoscopy			x	
Podiatric examination	x			
Dental examination	x			

Table 28-1 (continued)

	FIC*	ASPH ATPM†	APHA‡	TF§
Laboratory examinations				
Cholesterol	x		x	
Triglycerides	x		x	
Glucose/Blood sugar	x	x		x
Uric acid	x			
SGOT	x			
Hemoglobin/Hematocrit	x			x
Blood count, complete			x	
BUN			x	
Creatinine			x	
Urinalysis	x		x	
VDRL			x	
Tuberculin			x	
Pap smear (females)	x	x		x
Stool guaiac	x	x	x	x
Mammography (females)		x		x
Chest x-ray			x	
Tetanus and diphtheria boosters	x			x
Influenza immunization	x			x
Counseling				
Nutrition	x	x	x	
Smoking	x		x	
Alcohol and drugs	x	x		x
Social habits	x			
Exercise		x	x	
Sleep		x		
Housing	x			
Retirement plans		x		
Depression/Suicide				x
Accidents				x

*Preventive medical services for National Health Insurance. Report of a Fogarty International Center Task Force prepared under the auspices of the Office of the Assistant Secretary for Health, DHEW, May 1974.
†Incorporation of preventive medical services into National Insurance. A paper prepared for the Office of Management and Budget by Lester Breslow on behalf of the Association of Schools of Public Health and Association of Teachers of Preventive Medicine.
‡Proposed preventive benefits to be covered on a first-dollar basis under National Health Insurance. The American Public Health Association, July 16, 1974.
§The preventive procedures proposed in the task force report. The task force recommended that its procedures be offered several times during pregnancy and infancy, again at school entry and adolescence, thereafter every five years during early and middle adult life and every two years during later life.
Source: The Priorities of Section 1502, Health Resources Administration, Hyattsville, Md., 1977.

The Central Maryland Health Systems Agency suggests health education as one means to bring about change in the pattern of mortality among the elderly (Table 28-2).

Table 28-2
Three Leading Causes of Mortality in Central Maryland 1974 (65–79 Years)

Age group	Cause of death	Death in age group (%)*	Suggested health education
65–69 years	Diseases of the circulatory system	51.8	Understanding of alcohol and drug abuse symptoms
	Neoplasms	26.3	Individual responsibility for health
	Diseases of the respiratory system	5.0	
70–74 years	Diseases of the circulatory system	56.2	Seeking diagnosis and treatment for suspicious emotional disorders
	Neoplasms	23.6	
	Diseases of the respiratory system	5.5	
75–80 years	Diseases of the circulatory system	60.6	Self-care
	Neoplasms	18.7	
	Diseases of the respiratory system	5.9	

*Percentages for each age group do not total 100 because only the three leading causes of death in these categories have been selected.
Source: Data were compiled from Maryland Center for Health Statistics.

Thus, there is emerging a range of community health and medical services such as the collection and dissemination of health information, environmental management, and delivery of community medicine services. As these develop and care for the elderly changes, the results must be evaluated carefully. It is not yet clear what the role of preventive medicine will be and, more importantly, what the responsibility of an individual will be for maintaining health (Abelin 1976). There have already been warnings that the "optimism generated by the idea of prevention in an era of high cost may lead us to divert resources from caring for the sick to 'preventing illness,' to the detriment of both care and prevention" (Eisenberg 1977).

Changes in health care delivery to the aged can be seen in the 23,000 nursing homes in the United States. The physician, who may visit the patient in such institutions only at long intervals, is no longer the primary-care provider, and much of the day-to-day care and evaluation of therapeutic regimens has been delegated to nurses, pharmacists, and social workers.

Nurses and other health care professionals, in this setting, should not blindly comply with any medical orders; they have a more intimate and better knowledge of the patient and the patient's response to drugs than the physician (Rank and Jacobson 1977).

Day treatment centers are slowly developing in this country. Day treatment is aimed at adults who do not require 24-hour institutional care but who are, because of physical and/or mental impairment, not capable of full-time, independent living. The centers are alternatives to institutionalization. The day treatment setting may be looked upon as a "controlled" setting, which assures correct drug use for the elderly patient. However, it must be realized that patients often receive less than half their drugs under supervision and are responsible themselves for the remainder of drug therapy (Boykin and Lamy 1978). The potential for drug misuse among mentally impaired patients must be realized in the continued assessment of patient response to drug therapy.

Finally, the relationship between the formal health care system and its supportive parts, such as home care, needs to be re-examined and re-evaluated (Anderson 1977).

Other serious re-evaluations of current concepts and methods are needed. While patient care is the primary issue, economics of patient care will play an increasingly important role. Economic rewards for efficiency and cost-reducing innovations are lacking under the current system. Health insurance of any type ordinarily includes few if any incentives for either the consumer or the provider to economize. Health conservation seems to offer some hope of containing costs, as well as improving the well-being of patients.

Acceptance of the need for a new health care model will also demand far-reaching changes in medical education. In a testimony to the United States Senate (Butler 1976), it was stated that "perhaps less than 15 of an estimated 25,000 faculty members of the American medical schools have any genuine expertise in geriatric medicine." In response to a survey by the American Medical Association in 1972 only 300 physicians classified themselves as geriatricians. Geriatric medicine is taught in only a few American medical schools. A survey in 1976 revealed only 32 electives in geriatric medicine in 114 medical schools.

REFERENCES

Abelin, T. *Selbstverantwortung für die Gesundheit.* Geneva: Sandoz Institut, 1976.

Anderson, O.W. *Health Care: Can There Be Equity? The United States, Sweden, and England.* New York: John Wiley & Sons, 1972.

Anderson, O.W. Reflections on the sick and aged and the helping system. *J Gerontol Nurs.* 3(2):14, 1977.

Blank, M.L. Recent research findings on practice with the aging. *Soc Casework.* 52:382, 1971.

Boykin, S.P., and Lamy, P.P. Day treatment–a new care modality. *Hosp Formulary.* 13:683, 1978.

Breslow, L., and Somers, A.R. The lifetime health-monitoring program. *N Engl J Med.* 296:601, 1977.

Butler, R.N. *Medicine and Aging.* Washington, D.C.: National Institute on Aging, 1976.

Cohen, S., and O'Flynn-Comiskey, A.I. A treatment model for the institutionalized elderly. *J Gerontol Nurs.* 2(5):26, 1976.

Dubos, R. *Mirage of Health.* New York: Doubleday & Co., 1961.

Eisenberg, L. The perils of prevention: a cautionary note. *N Engl J Med.* 22:1230, 1977.

Engel, G.L. The need for a new medical model: a challenge for biomedicine. *Science* 196:132, 1977.

Fielding, J.E. Health promotion–some notions in search of a constituency. *Am J Public Health.* 67:1082, 1977.

Havighurst, R.J. A social-psychological perspective on aging. *Gerontologist* 8:67, 1968.

Health Resources Administration. *The Priorities of Section 1502.* DHEW Publ. No. (HRA) 77-641. Hyattsville, Md., 1977.

Hunt, T.E. Rehabilitation of the elderly. *Hosp Practice.* 12(1):89, 1977.

Kristein, M.M., Arnold, C.B., and Wynder, E.L. Health economics and preventive care. *Science* 195:457, 1977.

Lundberg, Y., and Theorell, T. Scaling of life changes: differences between three diagnostic groups and between recently experienced and nonexperienced events. *J Hum Stress.* 2:7, 1976.

Mechanic, D. Some problems in the measurement of stress and social readjustment. *J Hum Stress.* 1:43, 1975.

National Commission on the Cost of Medical Care. Summary report. Chicago, Ill.: American Medical Association, 1977.

Nordlicht, S. Stress, aging, and mental health. *NY State J Med.* 75:2135, 1975.

Peterson, H. Who'll sponsor a biopsychosocial model of disease? *Patient Care* 11(15):8, 1977.

Rahe, R.H., and Arthur, R.J. Life change and illness studies: past history and future directions. *J Hum Stress.* 4(1):3, 1978.

Rank, S.G., and Jacobson, C.K. Hospital nurses' compliance with medication overdose orders: a failure to replicate. *J Health Soc Behav.* 18:188, 1977.

Schless, A.P., Schwartz, L., and Mendels, J. How depressives view significance of life events. *Br J Psychiatry.* 125:406, 1974.

BIBLIOGRAPHY

PAPERBACK BOOKS ON AGING

American Association of Homes for the Aging. *Social Components of Care.* 1966.

American Hospital Association. *Winds of Change: Report of a Conference on Activity Programs for Long Term Care Institute.* 1971. $1.00.

American Psychiatric Association. *Reality Orientation.* 1969. $1.00.

Blumberg, J., and Drummond, E. *Nursing Care of the Long-Term Patient.* New York: Springer-Verlag, 1963. $2.75.

Bromley, D.B. *The Psychology of Human Aging.* Baltimore: Penguin Books, 1966. $1.45.

Burnside, I.M. *Psychosocial Nursing Care of the Aged.* New York: McGraw Hill Co., 1973. $4.95.

Felstein, I. *Later Life: Generations Today & Tomorrow.* Baltimore: Penguin Books, 1969. $1.25.

Gibson, A. *The Remotivators Guide Book.* Philadelphia: F.A. Davis. $1.95.

Gorer, G. *Death, Grief, and Mourning.* Garden City, New York: Doubleday, Anchor Books Edition, 1967. $1.25.

Group for the Advancement of Psychiatry. *Psychiatry and the Aged: An Introductory Approach,* Report #59. New York, 1965. $1.00.

Group for the Advancement of Psychiatry. Report #81: *The Aged and Community Mental Health.* 1971. $2.00.

Hinton, J. *Dying.* Baltimore: Penguin Books, 1967. $0.95.

Hodkinson. A. *Nursing the Elderly.* Oxford: Pergamon Press, 1966. $2.95.

Irvine, Bagnall, and Smith. *The Older Patient,* 2nd ed. London: English University Press, $2.50.

Kalish, R. *The Dependencies of Old People: Occasional Papers in Gerontology #6.* University of Michigan Gerontology Institute, 1969. $2.00.

Kastenbaum, R. (Ed.) *Contributions to the Psychobiology of Aging.* New York: Springer-Verlag, 1965. $3.00.

Kubler-Ross, E. *On Death and Dying.* New York: Macmillan Co., 1969. $1.95.

Larsen, D. *Dialogue on Aging.* New York: Teachers College Press, 1966. $1.50.

Loether, H.J. *Problems of Aging.* Belmont, Calif.: Dickenson Publishing Company, 1967. $1.95.

McKain, W.C. *Retirement Marriage.* University of Connecticut Press. $1.00.

Pearson, L. *Death & Dying: Current Issues in the Treatment of Dying Person.* Cleveland: Case Western Reserve Press, 1969. $1.95.

Post, F. *The Clinical Psychiatry of Late Life.* Oxford: Pergamon Press, 1968. $2.95.

Rothenberg, R.E. *Health in the Later Years and a Complete Manual on New Medical and Social Security Benefits.* New York: New American Library, 1967. $1.25.

Rubin, I. *Sexual Life After Sixty.* New York: New American Library, 1967. $1.25.

Rudd, T.N. *The Nursing of the Elderly Sick.* London: Faber & Faber, 1966. $2.10.

Rudd, T.N. *Human Relations in Old Age.* London: Faber & Faber, 1967. $2.00.

Simon, A., and Epstein, L. *Aging in Modern Society.* Psychiatric Research Report #23, A.P.A., Washington, D.C., 1968. $5.00.

Smith, Kline, and French Laboratories. *Remotivation Technique: A Manual for Use in Nursing Homes.* (For free copies write to Smith, Kline, and French Laboratories, Remotivation Project, 1500 Spring Garden Street, Philadelphia, Pa.)

Stevens, M. K. *Geriatric Nursing for Practical Nurses.* Philadelphia: W.B. Saunders, 1965. $3.50.

U.S. Department of Health, Education and Welfare, Public Health Service, Division of Nursing. *Elementary Rehabilitation Nursing Care.* PHS Publication #1436. Washington, D.C.: U.S. Government Printing Office, 1967. $0.55.

U.S. Department of Health, Education and Welfare, Social and Rehabilitation Service Administration on Aging. *The Fitness Challenge in the Later Years: An Exercise Program for Older Americans.* AoA Publication No. 802. Washington, D.C.: U.S. Government Printing Office, 1968. $0.30.

U.S. Department of Health, Education and Welfare, Public Health Service, Division of Chronic Diseases, Gerontology Branch (prepared by the Gerontological Society, St. Louis, Missouri, under contract PH 86-63-184 with the Public Health Service). *Working with Older People, A Guide to Practice, Volume 1: The Practitioner and the Elderly,* PHS Publication No. 1459, Vol. 1, Washington, D.C.: U.S. Government Printing Office, Revised 1969. $0.65.

Vol. 2 *Biological, Psychological and Sociological Aspects of Aging.* 1970. $0.65.

Vol. 3 *The Aging Person: Needs and Services.* 1970. $1.00.

Vol. 4 *Clinical Aspects of Aging.* 1971. $3.50.

INDEX

Absorption of drugs, 255–257
  antacids affecting, 323–324
  and drug interactions, 305–306
  nutrition affecting, 225
Acetaminophen, 315, 319
  absorption of, 256
    nutrition affecting, 225
  clearance of, hepatic, 265
  hepatic effects of overdose, 266
  interaction with
    anticoagulants, 340
  interval extension administration
    in renal failure, 276
  nephrotoxicity of, 57
  pharmacokinetics affected by
    bed rest, 253–254
  protein binding of, 262
  therapeutic plasma levels of, 279
Acetanilid, and hemolysis in
  G-6-PD deficiency, 154
Acetazolamide, 449
  interaction with other drugs,
    379, 562
  interval extension administration
    in renal failure, 276
  protein binding of, 261
  site of action of, 448
Acetohexamide
  affecting diagnostic test for
    diabetes, 479
  affecting laboratory test values,
    483
  food intake with, 646
  interaction with other drugs, 480
Acetophenazine, 531
  adverse effects of, 538
  potency of, 535
Acetophenetidin, and hemolysis in
  G-6-PD deficiency, 154
Acetylation of drugs, 263
  variations in, 153
Acetylcysteine, in dry eye, 497
Acetylsalicylic acid. *See* Salicylates
  or aspirin
Achlorhydria, 46
  and absorption of drugs, 257
Acid secretion, in aging, 46
Acidosis, diabetic, 472
Acrogeria, 21
ACTH. *See* Corticotropin

Activity limitations, from chronic
  disease, 115–117
Actol Expectorant, 326
Acute illnesses, disability from,
  118–119
Adrenal steroids, aging affecting,
  50
Adrenalin Chloride, for inhalation,
  328
Adrenergic blockers, interaction
  with other drugs, 482
Adverse effects of drugs, 293–309.
  See also specific drugs
  and age as risk factor, 296–297
  and assessment of hazards, 173
  disease affecting, 300–302
  dose relationship in, 299
  drugs responsible for, 297–298
  genetic factors in, 302
  in hemopoietic system, 50–51
  incidence of, 295–296
  and interactions of drugs, 304–309
  and multiple medications,
    172–173, 299–300
  nephrotoxicity, 57, 369, 373
  with nonprescription drugs, 97,
    298–299
  ototoxicity, 64, 282, 373–374
  risk in females, 125, 134
  tissue sensitivity changes in,
    303–304
  types of reactions in, 302–303
Affective disorders, 515–526
Age classifications, 14–16
Ageism, 74, 76
Aging process, description of,
  20–21
Akathisia, from antipsychotic
  drugs, 541, 542
  treatment of, 545
Akinesia
  from antipsychotic drugs, 541,
    542
  treatment of, 545
  paradoxica, from levodopa,
    547–548
Albumin, serum levels of, 214
Alcohol
  in Brompton's Mixture, 349, 350
  consumption by elderly, 74, 568

661

in cough and cold remedies, 326
hepatic effects of, 266
interaction with other drugs, 320,
  437, 480, 539, 540, 568–570, 576
ocular effects of, 490
therapeutic uses of, 568
vitamin deficiency from, 339, 340
Alcoholism, 568
Alconefrine, 328
Alka-Seltzer, 323
Allerest, 328
Allopurinol
  food intake with, 646
  interaction with other drugs, 437
  protein binding of, 262
Aloe, as stimulant laxative, 330
Aluminum hydroxide, in antacids, 322, 324
Alzheimer disease, 40, 505, 507
Amantadine
  adverse effects of, 546
  in parkinsonism, 528, 544, 545–546
Amikacin
  excretion of, 369
  interval extension administration in renal failure, 277
  ototoxicity of, 64, 374
  protein binding of, 260
  toxic blood levels of, 373
Amino acids, affecting urine glucose tests, 478
Aminoglycosides, 372–374
  adverse effects of, 301, 372, 373–374
  dosage reduction in renal failure, 274
  interval extension administration in renal failure, 277
  nephrotoxicity of, 57, 369, 373
  ototoxicity of, 64, 373–374
  protein binding of, 260
  therapeutic plasma levels of, 373
  toxic blood levels of, 373
  in urinary tract infections, 382
Aminophylline
  food intake with, 646
  interaction with other drugs, 562
Aminopyrine
  affecting urine glucose tests, 478
  age-related pharmacokinetic changes in, 251
p-Aminosalicylic acid
  affecting urine glucose tests, 478

food intake with, 647
and hemolysis in G-6-PD deficiency, 155
interaction with other drugs, 318
interference with nutrients, 230
interval extension administration in renal failure, 277
protein binding of, 260
pulmonary disease from, 594
vitamin deficiency from, 340
Amitriptyline
  absorption of, 257
  contraindicated in glaucoma, 495
  in depression, 531
  dosage reduction in renal failure, 275
  dosage and side effects of, 556
  protein binding of, 262
  therapeutic plasma levels of, 279, 280, 281
Amobarbital
  in anxiety, 523
  metabolism affected by age, 267
Amoxicillin
  interval extension administration in renal failure, 277
  protein binding of, 260
  in urinary tract infections, 376, 381
Amphetamines
  in Brompton's Mixture, 349
  contraindicated in glaucoma, 495
Amphojel, 321, 322
Amphotericin
  interaction with other drugs, 368
  interval extension administration in renal failure, 277
  nephrotoxicity of, 369
  protein binding of, 260
Ampicillin
  absorption of, 256
  excretion of, 369
    in anuria, 269
  food intake with, 645
  interaction with other drugs, 367
  interval extension administration in renal failure, 277
  nephrotoxicity of, 57
  sodium in, 372
  in urinary tract infections, 376, 380, 381
Amyl nitrite, contraindicated in glaucoma, 495
Anabolic agents, oral, hepatic

effects of, 266
Analgesics, 345-350
  aspirin and other salicylates, 347-348
  combinations of drugs, 348
  dosage reduction in renal failure, 274
  and hemolysis in G-6-PD deficiency, 154
  interaction with other drugs, 540
  interference with nutrients, 230
  interval extension administration in renal failure, 276
  narcotic, 348-350
  as nonprescription drugs, 315-319
  ocular effects of, 490
  protein binding of, 262
Anatuss Syrup, 326
Androgen therapy, heart failure from, 399
Anemia
  drug-induced, 50, 154-155
    hemolytic, 154-155
  incidence of, 113
  iron deficiency, 204-206
    from aspirin, 316
  and metabolism of drugs, 267
Anesthetics, 629-630
  interaction with other drugs, 628, 630
  ocular effects of, 490
Angina pectoris, 389
  in surgical patients, 628
  treatment of, 395-398
Anisotropine, contraindicated in glaucoma, 495
Anorexiants, interfering with nutrients, 230
Anthelmintics, ocular effects of, 490
Antabuse (disulfiram), interaction with other drugs, 569, 576
Antacids, 320-325
  and absorption of drugs, 257
  adverse effects of, 298, 323-325
  aluminum and magnesium in, 322, 324
  calcium carbonate in, 322
  constipation from, 333
  interaction with other drugs, 306, 323-325, 337, 539, 576
  as nonprescription drugs, 315
  palatability of, 321-322
  potency of, 320-321

sodium in, 322-323
  vitamin deficiency from, 339, 340
Antagonism, and drug interactions, 304
Antianxiety agents, 522, 523, 531, 532, 562-570
  factors affecting responses to, 563-564
Antiarrhythmic agents, 416-420, 438,
  adverse effects of, 416-417
  dosage reduction in renal failure, 275
  interval extension administration in renal failure, 276
  ocular effects of, 490
  properties of, 417
  protein binding of, 261
Antiarthritic drugs, protein binding of, 262
Antibiotics. *See* Antimicrobials
Anticholinergic agents
  affecting intraocular pressure, 494
  constipation from, 333
  in cough and cold remedies, 327
  interaction with other drugs, 306, 539, 548
  interference with nutrients, 230
  in parkinsonism, 544
  urine retention from, 374
Anticholinesterase agents
  in glaucoma, 493, 496
  lens opacities from, 496
  ocular effects of, 490
Anticoagulants, 434-438
  adverse reactions to, 172, 298, 436
  in dementia, 573
  interaction with other drugs, 307, 308, 318, 320, 324, 337, 340, 367, 419, 436-438, 480, 540, 569, 630
  pharmacokinetics of, 435
  in surgical patients, 628
Anticonvulsants, 363-364
  hepatic effects of, 266
  interaction with other drugs, 630
  interference with nutrients, 230
  ocular effects of, 490
Antidepressants, 520, 531, 532, 551-560
  adverse effects of, 559-560
  experimental, 573
  hepatic effects of, 266

interference with nutrients, 230
ocular effects of, 490
tricyclic. See Tricyclic
 antidepressants
urine retention from, 374
Antifungal agents
 interval extension administration
  in renal failure, 277
 ocular effects of, 490
 protein binding of, 260
Antigout drugs, protein binding
 of, 262
Antihistamines
 affecting intraocular pressure, 494
 constipation from, 333
 in cough and cold remedies,
  326-327
 food intake with, 646
 interaction with other drugs, 548,
  569, 576
 in parkinsonism, 544-545
Antihypertensive agents, 403-416,
 420-434
 adverse effects of, 298, 406,
  432-434
 characteristics of, 413-415
 depression from, 518
 dosage reduction in renal failure,
  275
 hemodynamic effects of, 423
 interaction with other drugs,
  432-434, 540, 548
 interval extension administration
  in renal failure, 276
 ocular effects of, 490
 protein binding of, 261
 in surgical patients, 628
 treatment failure with, 416
Antiinflammatory agents, 350-359
Antimalarials, ocular effect of, 490
Antimicrobials, 365-382
 adverse effects of, 172, 298
 aminoglycosides, 372-374. See
  also Aminoglycosides
 bactericidal, 371
 bacteriostatic, 371
 cephalosporins, 372. See also
  Cephalosporins
 dosage reduction in renal failure,
  274
 excretion of, 368-369
 interaction with other drugs,
  367-368, 374, 437, 569, 629, 630
 interference with nutrients, 230

interval extension administration
 in renal failure, 277
nephrotoxicity of, 369
ocular effects of, 490
penicillins, 371-372. See also
 Penicillins
in pressure sores, 611-612
protein binding of, 260
response of elderly to, 370-374
urinary pH affecting, 378-379
in urinary tract infections,
 380-382
Antiparkinsonism drugs, 527-528,
 543-549
 affecting intraocular pressure, 494
 constipation from, 333
 urine retention from, 374
Antipsychotic agents, 532-551
 classification of, 534
 extrapyramidal side effects of,
  540-549
  treatment of, 543-549
 indications for, 534-547
 interaction with other drugs,
  539-540
 potency of, 535
 tardive dyskinesia from, 549-551
Antipyrine
 adverse effects of, 301
 age-related pharmacokinetic
  changes in, 251
 clearance of, hepatic, 265
 and hemolysis in G-6-PD
  deficiency, 154
 interaction with anticoagulants,
  340
 metabolism of
  age affecting, 267
  malnutrition affecting, 266-267
Antirheumatic drugs
 adverse reactions to, 172
 hepatic effects of, 266
Antithyroid drugs, hepatic effects
 of, 266
Antituberculars
 food intake with, 647
 hepatic effects of, 266
 interval extension administration
  in renal failure, 277
 ocular effects of, 490
 protein binding of, 260
Antitussives, 326. See also Cough
 and cold remedies
Anuria, and excretion of drugs, 269

Anxiety, 521-522
  alcohol in, 568
  antianxiety agents, 522, 523, 531, 532, 562-570
  factors affecting responses to, 563-564
  symptoms with, 521-522
Anxiolytics, 532
APC, food intake with, 646
Aphasia, 62
Arcus senilis, 491
Arrhythmias, 35
  treatment of, 416-420, 438. See also Antiarrhythmic agents
Arteries, aging affecting, 33
Arteriosclerosis obliterans, 87
  in diabetes, 484
Arthritis, 350-359
  osteoarthritis, 357-358
  and protein binding of antiarthritic drugs, 262
  rheumatoid, 352-357
Ascorbic acid. See Vitamin C
Aspidium oleoresin, affecting urine glucose tests, 478
Aspirin, 347-348. See also Salicylates or aspirin
Asthma, 596-598
  diet in, 638
  drug-induced, 59
  incidence of, 594
  in surgical patients, 628
AsthmaNefrin, 328
Astigmatism, 491
Ataractics, 532
Atherosclerosis, 87
  and cholesterol intake, 200-201
  of coronary arteries, 389
  factors in development of, 387
Atrophy
  muscular, 52
  neural, 63
Atropine
  anticholinergic potency of, 530
  and carbohydrate absorption, 229
  contraindicated in glaucoma, 495
  in cough and cold remedies, 327
  food intake with, 645
  urine retention from, 374
Attitudes toward elderly persons, 74-77
Auditory dysfunction in aging, 62-64
Auditory system, drugs affecting, 64, 282, 373-374
Auranofin, in rheumatoid arthritis, 356
Autoimmune theory of aging, 24
Azapetine phosphate, food intake with, 646
Azaphenothiazines, 534

Bacteriuria. See also Urinary tract infections
  asymptomatic, 376, 377
Barbiturates
  absorption of, 257
  adverse effects of, 574
  age-related pharmacokinetic changes in, 251
  in anxiety, 523, 531, 564
  dosage reduction in renal failure, 275
  interaction with other drugs, 324, 437, 480, 482, 539, 570, 576
  interference with nutrients, 230
  metabolism affected by age, 267
  protein binding of, 261
  vitamin deficiency from, 339, 340
Basaljel, 321, 322
Beclomethasone dipropionate, in asthma, 598
Bed rest, effects of, 85-86, 395
  and pharmacokinetics, 253-254
Behavioral disturbances, 74
Bell-Ans, 323
Belladonna
  contraindicated in glaucoma, 495
  food intake with, 645
  urine retention from, 374
Bendroflumethiazide
  dosage of, 451
  reserpine with, 426
  site of action of, 448
Benzodiazepines
  adverse effects of, 567
  age-related pharmacokinetic changes in, 251
  in anxiety, 522, 523, 564-568
  characteristics of, 566
  in depression, 552
  dosage reduction in renal failure, 275
  hepatic effects of, 266
  as hypnotics, 523, 526, 575
  interaction with other drugs, 576
  metabolism affected by age, 267
  protein binding of, 261

Benzphetamine, contraindicated in glaucoma, 495
Benzthiazide, site of action of, 448
Benztropine
 anticholinergic potency of, 530
 in parkinsonism, 544
Beta-blocking agents
 bronchoconstriction from, 59
 in glaucoma, 493
 in hypertension, 427
 interaction with other drugs, 482
Betahistine, in dementia, 572
Bethanechol chloride, food intake with, 646
Bilirubin, interaction with phenobarbital, 575
Biofeedback therapy, in hypertension, 408
Biologic aging, 28–31
Biologic factors, in responses to drugs, 152–155
Biozyme ointment, 613
Biperiden
 contraindicated in glaucoma, 495
 food intake with, 646
 in parkinsonism, 544
Birthrate, in United States, 7, 11, 13
Bisacodyl, 330
 adverse effects of, 335
 food intake with, 648
 interaction with other drugs, 337
Bismuth, affecting urine glucose tests, 478
Bismuth sodium triglycollomate, food intake with, 646
Bisodol, 323
Blacks, health problems in, 162–163, 216, 390
Bladder, aging affecting, 56
Blood flow
 cerebral, in aging, 41
 hepatic
  and clearance of drugs, 265
  and metabolism of drugs, 267
 intestinal, and absorption of drugs, 257
 renal, and excretion of drugs, 268
Blood levels of drugs
 therapeutic. See Therapeutic plasma levels of drugs
 toxic levels of aminoglycosides, 373

Blood pressure. See also Hypertension; Hypotension
 changes with aging, 147, 404
Blood tests. See Laboratory test values
Blood vessels, aging affecting, 33
Bone, aging affecting, 30, 52–54
Brain
 changes in aging, 37–41
 organic syndrome, 504–515. See also Dementia
Breacol, 326
Breads, nutrient content of, 194–195
Breatheasy, 328
Brioschi, 323
Bromocriptine, in parkinsonism, 528, 546
Bromo-Quinine, 328
Bromo-Seltzer, 323
Brompton's Mixture, 349–350
Bromsulphthalein excretion, diet affecting, 226
Bronchitis
 acute, diet in, 638
 chronic, 595–596
 incidence of, 594
 drug-induced, 59
Bronchodilators, 595–596
 in cough and cold remedies, 327–328
Broncho-Tussin, 326
Bronitin, 328
Bronkaid, 328
Bronkaid Mist, 328
Butaperazine, potency of, 535
Butyrophenones, 531, 534
 muscarinic affinity of, 542

Cadmium, effects of, 33
Calcium
 absorption of, 256
 deficiency of, 215, 218
 intake of, 202–203
  recommended daily allowances, 192
 serum levels of, 214
Calcium carbonate, in antacids, 322
Callosities and corns, 602
Caloric intake, 186, 216, 219, 231–232

Camalox, 321, 322
Carbachol, in glaucoma, 496
Carbamazepine
  contraindicated in glaucoma, 495
  therapeutic plasma levels of, 279
Carbamine, 323
Carbenicillin
  coagulation disorders from, 367
  dosage reduction in renal failure, 274
  excretion of, 369
  interaction with other drugs, 368
  interval extension administration in renal failure, 277
  protein binding of, 260
  sodium in, 372
  in urinary tract infections, 376, 381
Carbidopa, 549
Carbohydrate, dietary, 200
Carbonic anhydrase inhibitors, 449
  in glaucoma, 493
  ocular effects of, 490
Cardiovascular drugs, 385-454
  adverse effects of, 172, 298
  antiarrhythmics, 416-420. See also Antiarrhythmic agents
  anticoagulants, 434-438. See also Anticoagulants
  antihypertensives, 403-416, 420-434. See also Antihypertensive agents
  diuretics, 445-454. See also Diuretics
  dosage reduction in renal failure, 275
  glycosides, 438-445. See also Glycosides, cardiac
  interaction with other drugs, 630
  interval extension administration in renal failure, 276
  protein binding of, 261
Cardiovascular system
  aging affecting, 30, 33-36, 84, 385-389
  diseases of, and effects of antimicrobials, 367
  heart diseases, 389-395
  hypertension, 390-394
Carisoprodol, therapeutic plasma levels of, 279
Carphenazine, potency of, 535
Cascara sagrada, 330
  adverse effects of, 335
Castor oil, 330
  adverse effects of, 335
Cataracts, 491-493, 495-496
Catecholamines, aging affecting, 25, 35
Cathartics. See Laxatives
Catheterization, urinary, bacteriuria from, 375
Cefamandole, 372
Cefazolin, 372
Cell counts, 214
Cell division
  finite limit of, 23
  mitotic capacity in aging, 32
Cell population, decrease in, 28, 29
Central nervous system
  drugs affecting. See also Psychopharmacologic drugs
    dosage reduction in renal failure, 275
    interval extension administration in renal failure, 276
  neurologic disorders, 527-528
Cephalexin, 372
Cephaloridine, 372
  nephrotoxicity of, 369
Cephalosporins, 372
  dosage reduction in renal failure, 274
  excretion of, 369
  in anuria, 269
  interaction with other drugs, 368, 372
  interval extension administration in renal failure, 277
  neurotoxicity of, 367
  protein binding of, 260
  in urinary tract infections, 376, 380, 381
  and urine glucose tests, 367
Cephalothin, 372
  affecting urine glucose tests, 478
Cephapirin, 372
Cephradine, 372
Cereals, nutrient content of, 194-195
Cerebrovascular disease
  and adverse drug reactions, 302
  effects of antimicrobials in, 367, 370
  effects of antimicrobials in, 367, 370

Chelating agents, ocular effects of, 490
Cheracol Cold Capsules, 328
Chexit, 328
Chloral hydrate
 affecting urine glucose tests, 478
 food intake with, 646
 as hypnotic, 523, 526, 577
 interaction with other drugs, 437, 570
Chloramphenicol
 adverse effects of, 372
 affecting urine glucose tests, 478
 aplastic anemia from, 50
 clearance of, hepatic, 265
 dosage reduction in renal failure, 274
 excretion of, 369
 in anuria, 269
 and hemolysis in G-6-PD deficiency, 154
 interaction with other drugs, 307, 366, 367, 370, 437, 569
 interference with nutrients, 230
 protein binding of, 260
 and urine glucose tests, 367
 vitamin deficiency from, 339
Chlordiazepoxide, 565, 566
 absorption of, 256, 257
 in anxiety, 523, 531, 567
 dosage of, 567
  reduction in renal failure, 275
 food intake with, 645
 interaction with other drugs, 324, 570
 metabolism affected by age, 267
 protein binding of, 261
 sensitivity to, in aging, 250
 therapeutic plasma levels of, 279
Chloride levels in serum, 214
Chlormezanone, in anxiety, 523
Chloroform, affecting urine glucose tests, 478
Chloroform water, in Brompton's Mixture, 349
Chlorophenoxamine, food intake with, 646
Chloroquine
 dosage reduction in renal failure, 274
 hearing loss from, 64
 interaction with other drugs, 437
 protein binding of, 260

Chlorothiazide
 characteristics of, 449
 dosage of, 451
 site of action of, 448
 thrombocytopenic purpura from, 51
Chlorpheniramine, interaction with other drugs, 433
Chlorphenoxamine
 contraindicated in glaucoma, 495
 in parkinsonism, 544
Chlorphentermine, contraindicated in glaucoma, 495
Chlorpromazine, 531, 534
 adverse effects of, 538, 539
 with Brompton's Mixture, 350
 in depression, 537
 dosage of, 538
  reduction in renal failure, 275
 food intake with, 646
 hepatic effects of, 266
 interaction with other drugs, 324, 437, 539, 540, 562, 570
 lens opacities from, 492
 potency of, 535
 protein binding of, 261
 therapeutic plasma levels of, 279, 281-282
Chlorpropamide, 471
 affecting diagnostic test for diabetes, 479
 affecting laboratory test values, 483
 food intake with, 646
 interaction with other drugs, 480, 569
Chlorprothixene, 531
 contraindicated in glaucoma, 495
 potency of, 535
Chlortetracycline
 affecting urine glucose tests, 478
 excretion in anuria, 269
Chlorthalidone, 449
 affecting diagnostic test for diabetes, 479
 characteristics of, 449
 dosage of, 452
 food intake with, 646
 in heart failure, 401
 interaction with other drugs, 480
 interval extension administration in renal failure, 276
 protein binding of, 261

reserpine with, 426
site of action of, 448
Chlortrimeton, 329
Cholesterol
  intake of, 200–201
  serum levels of, and heart disease, 387
Cholestyramine
  interaction with other drugs, 437
  vitamin deficiency from, 339, 340
Choline chloride, in tardive dyskinesia, 551
Choline magnesium trisalicylate, 348, 353
Choline salicylate, as antiinflammatory agent, 353, 355
Cholinergic agents, in glaucoma, 493, 496
Cholinesterase inhibitors. *See* Anticholinesterase agents
Chromium, recommended daily allowances for, 202
Chronic diseases and disabilities, 113–117
  and activity limitation, 115–117
  prevalence of, 113–115
Cimetidine, mental confusion from, 506
Cirrhosis, 47
Citrisum, 328
Citrocarbonate, 323
Claudication, intermittent, 394
Clindamycin
  clearance of, hepatic, 265
  dosage reduction in renal failure, 274
  excretion of, 369
  protein binding of, 260
Clinistix, 477, 478
Clinitest, 477, 478
Clofibrate, interaction with other drugs, 307, 437, 482
Clonazepam, therapeutic plasma levels of, 279
Clonidine
  adverse effects of, 433
  characteristics of, 414
  dosage reduction in renal failure, 275
  effects with impaired kidney or liver function, 410
  hemodynamic effects of, 423
  in hypertension, 411, 430

dosage of, 424
interaction with other drugs, 434
Clorazepate, 565, 566
  in anxiety, 523, 531, 567
  interaction with other drugs, 570
  therapeutic plasma levels of, 279
Cloxacillin
  food intake with, 645
  interval extension administration in renal failure, 277
  protein binding of, 260
Clozapine, 534
Coagulation. *See also* Anticoagulants
  antimicrobials affecting, 367
Cobalt, effects of, 33
Cocaine, in Brompton's Mixture, 349–350
Codeine, 348–349, 355
  dosage reduction in renal failure, 274
Cognitive-acting drugs, 571–573
Colchek, 328
Colchicine
  and carbohydrate absorption, 229
  and folic acid depletion, 306
  in gout, 358
  interaction with other drugs, 437
  interference with nutrients, 230
  protein binding of, 262
  vitamin deficiency from, 339, 340
Cold remedies. *See* Cough and cold remedies
Coldene, 328
  Adult Cough Formula, 326
Colistimethate
  dosage reduction in renal failure, 274
  excretion of, 369
  protein binding of, 260
Colistin
  excretion in anuria, 269
  in urinary tract infections, 380
Collagen, changes in, 30, 52, 65, 593
Collagenase ABC ointment, 613
Colors, for drug preparations, 179
Communication with patients, 634–635
Compliance of patients, 634, 635–642
  with antihypertensive therapy, 416

with diabetic therapy, 468
methods for improvement of, 639-642
with potassium supplements, 444
problems in, 636-638
variables in, 639
Conduction velocity in nerves, aging affecting, 36-37
Confusional states, acute, 506-507
Conjunctivitis, 490
Connective tissue, changes in, 30, 52
Consotus Antitussive, 326
Constipation, 46, 47, 331-333
 from calcium carbonate, 322
 diagnosis of, 333
 diet in, 638
 laxatives in. See Laxatives
 possible causes of, 332-333
Contac, 328
Contraceptives, oral
 affecting diagnostic test for diabetes, 479
 interaction with other drugs, 480
Convulsions, management of. See Anticonvulsants
Coping mechanisms in aging, 74
Copper
 effects of, 33
 recommended daily allowances for, 202
 serum levels of, 214
Coricidin, 328, 329
Cornea, aging affecting, 491
Corns and callosities, 602
Coronary artery disease, 389
Corticosteroids
 adverse reactions to, 172, 357
 affecting diagnostic test for diabetes, 479
 affecting urine glucose tests, 478
 in asthma, 598
 cataracts from, 492
 heart failure from, 399
 interaction with other drugs, 318, 480
 and opportunistic infections, 59
 pulmonary disease from, 594
 in rheumatoid arthritis, 357
 topical, ocular effects of, 497
Corticotropin
 affecting diagnostic test for diabetes, 479
 affecting urine glucose tests, 478
 and prevention of pressure sores, 615
Cortisone, and carbohydrate absorption, 229
Coryban-D, 328
Cost of health care, 89-96
 and cost of drugs, 104-107
 in nursing homes, 125
Cough and cold remedies, 325-329
 alcohol in, 326
 antihistamines in, 326-327
 bronchodilators and decongestants in, 327-328
 as nonprescription drugs, 315
 sugar in, 328-329
Coumarins
 interaction with other drugs, 340, 482
 vitamin deficiency from, 339
Counseling of patients, 633-635
Cranberry juice, and urinary pH, 379
Creatinine
 affecting urine glucose tests, 478
 clearance of, and renal function, 270-271
Cromolyn sodium
 in asthma, 598
 pulmonary disease from, 594
Cross-linking theory of aging, 23-24
Cyanocobalamin deficiency, 210
Cybernetic pacemaker theory of aging, 24
Cyclophosphamide, in rheumatoid arthritis, 356
Cycloserine
 adverse effects of, 370, 372
 vitamin deficiency from, 340
Cyclothiazide
 dosage of, 451
 site of action, 448
Cycrimine
 contraindicated in glaucoma, 495
 food intake with, 646
 in parkinsonism, 544
Cyproheptadine
 contraindicated in glaucoma, 495
 food intake with, 646

Cystitis, 375, 376
Cytotoxic drugs, hepatic effects of, 266

Dairy products, nutrient content of, 196
Dakin's solution, modified, in pressure sores, 610-611
Danthron, as stimulant laxative, 330
Death rates. *See* Mortality rates
Debridement, in pressure sores, 610
Deceleration of aging, 81-87
Decongestants, in cough and cold remedies, 327-328
Decubitus ulcers. *See* Pressure sores
Definition of elderly, and age classifications, 14-15
Delcid, 321, 322
Delirium, 506-507
 drug-induced, 506-507
Demecarium bromide, lens opacities from, 496
Dementia, 505-506, 507-515
 causes of, 512-513
  reversible, 510
  treatable, 509
 cognitive-acting drugs in, 571-573
 diagnostic process in, 510-511
 incidence of, 507-508
 manifestations of, 513, 514
 presenile, 505
 senile, 40, 505
 treatment of, 514-515
Demethylchlortetracycline, food intake with, 648
Demographic data, 1-13
Demulcents, ocular effects of, 490
Dentures, fitting of, 44-45
Depression, 515-520
 agitated, 518
 antidepressants in, 520, 531, 532, 551-560. *See also* Antidepressants
 bipolar, 516
 drug-induced, 425, 518
 endogenous, 516-518, 552
 and insomnia, 524, 525
 involutional, 518
 in nutritional deficiency, 188, 224

 in parkinsonism, 518
 prognosis of, 554
 psychoneurotic, 517
 reactive, 516, 517
 retardive, 516
 symptoms with, 519
 unipolar, 516
Dermatitis, 602
 treatment of, 603
Desipramine
 contraindicated in glaucoma, 495
 in depression, 531
 dosage and side effects of, 557
 interaction with other drugs, 434
 therapeutic plasma levels of, 280
Desmethylimipramine
 dosage reduction in renal failure, 275
 protein binding of, 262
Dexamethasone, interaction with other drugs, 575
Dextroamphetamine
 contraindicated in glaucoma, 495
 in psychiatric disorders, 573
Diabetes mellitus, 463-485
 adverse drugs reactions in, 299, 300
 cough and cold remedies in, 327, 328
 diagnosis of, 465-466
 dietary regimen in, 469-470
 drug interactions in, 479-483
 and effects of antimicrobials, 366-367
 foot care in, 484-485
 and immune response, 366
 incidence of, 113, 463-464
 insulins in, 474-477. *See also* Insulin
 manifestations of, 466-467
 oral hypoglycemic agents in, 470-474. *See also* Hypoglycemic agents, oral
 self-care activities in, 468
 skin care in, 483-484
 treatment of, 467-485
 urine testing in, 477-478
  drugs affecting, 367, 381, 478
Diagnosis of disorders, 143-149
 and abnormal clinical presentation, 145-146
 laboratory test values in,

146-148. See also Laboratory test values
Diarrhea, diet in, 638
Diazepam, 565, 566
  absorption of, 257
  in anxiety, 523, 531, 567
  clearance of, hepatic, 265
  dosage of, 567
    reduction in renal failure, 275
  indomethacin with, 357
  interaction with other drugs, 570
  protein binding of, 261
  sensitivity to, in aging, 250
  therapeutic plasma levels of, 279, 281, 282
Diazoxide
  dosage reduction in renal failure, 275
  heart failure from, 399
  interaction with other drugs, 437
Dibenzodiazepine derivatives, 534
  muscarinic affinity of, 542
Dibenzoxazepine, 531
Dibenzoxepines, in anxiety, 531
Dicloxacillin
  food intake with, 645
  interval extension administration in renal failure, 277
  protein binding of, 260
Dicoumarol, 435
  interaction with other drugs, 324
  metabolism affected by age, 267
Diet. See Nutrition
Diethazine, in parkinsonism, 544
Diethylpropion
  contraindicated in glaucoma, 495
  food intake with, 645
Di-Gel, 321, 322
Digestive system, aging affecting, 30, 43-48
Digitalis, 399-400, 438-443
  in arrhythmias, 417
  dosage in thyroid disorders, 254
  in heart failure, 438
  interaction with thiazide diuretics, 309, 320, 434
  mental confusion from, 506
  in surgical patients, 628
  toxicity of, 298, 399-400, 441-443
    affected by drugs, 254
    from antimicrobials, 368
    and potassium levels in serum, 443

quinidine affecting, 419
Digitoxin, 399, 439-441
  and carbohydrate absorption, 229
  dosage reduction in renal failure, 275
  effects with impaired kidney or liver function, 410
  excretion in anuria, 269
  pharmacokinetics of, 440
  protein binding of, 261
  therapeutic plasma levels of, 279
Digoxin, 399, 439-441
  absorption of, 256, 257
    neomycin affecting, 254
  dosage reduction in renal failure, 275
  effects with impaired kidney or liver function, 410
  excretion in anuria, 269
  interaction with other drugs, 324, 327, 368, 419
  pharmacokinetics of, 283, 440
    age-related changes in, 251
  protein binding of, 261
  therapeutic plasma levels of, 279, 282
Dihydroindolone, 531
Dihydrostreptomycin, age-related pharmacokinetic changes in, 251
Dilantin. See Phenytoin
Dimenhydrinate, food intake with, 645
Dimercaprol, and hemolysis in G-6-PD deficiency, 155
Dimethindene, contraindicated in glaucoma, 495
Dioctyl sodium sulfosuccinate, 330
  adverse effects of, 335, 336
  interaction with other drugs, 336, 337
Diphemanil, contraindicated in glaucoma, 495
Diphenidol, contraindicated in glaucoma, 495
Diphenhydramine
  food intake with, 646
  as hypnotic, 577
  in parkinsonism, 544
Diphenylhydantoin. See Phenytoin
Disopyramide, in arrhythmias, 420
Distribution of drugs, in elderly persons, 258-263
Disulfiram (Antabuse), interaction

with other drugs, 569, 576
Diuretics, 445-454
  adverse effects of, 450
  carbonic anhydrase inhibitors, 449. *See also* Carbonic anhydrase inhibitors
  characteristics of, 449
  chlorthalidone, 449. *See also* Chlorthalidone
  and digitalis toxicity, 254
  dosage reduction in renal failure, 275
  electrolyte imbalance from, 400
  in heart failure, 400-401, 445
  in hypertension, 445
  interaction with other drugs, 368, 374, 480, 482, 562
  interval extension administration in renal failure, 276
  loop, 401, 447, 453-454. *See also* Ethacrynic acid; Furosemide
  ocular effects of, 490
  potassium-sparing, 447
  protein binding of, 261
  rauwolfia-diuretic combinations, 426
  site of action of, 448
  spironolactone, 449-453. *See also* Spironolactone
  thiazide, 446-449. *See also* Thiazide diuretics
  treatment failure with, 446
  triamterene, 449. *See also* Triamterene
Diverticula, intestinal, 46
Dondril, 328
L-Dopa
  absorption of, 257
  adverse effects of, 547-548
  contraindications in glaucoma, 495
  depression from, 518
  food intake with, 646
  interaction with other drugs, 324, 548, 630
  mental confusion from, 506
  in parkinsonism, 228, 528, 546-549
Dopamine levels in brain, aging affecting, 25
Dosage of drugs, 170-172
  and adverse reactions, 299
  and interval extension in renal failure, 273, 276-277
  reduction in renal failure, 273, 274-275
Doxepin
  contraindicated in glaucoma, 495
  in depression, 531
  dosage and side effects of, 557
Doxycycline
  adverse effects of, 301
  dosage reduction in renal failure, 274
  food intake with, 646
  interaction with other drugs, 575
  protein binding of, 260
Drilitol, 328
Dristan
  capsules, 328
  Liquid, 326
  sugar in, 329
Drug interactions, 304-309
Drug use by elderly, 96-107
  cost of, 104-107
  in institutions, 100-104
  nonprescription drugs, 97
  prescription drugs, 98
Dry eye, 494, 497
Dry skin, 605
Ducon, 321, 322
Duodenum, changes in, 46
Dysarthria, 62
Dysgraphia, 61
Dyskinesias
  from antipsychotic drugs, 541
  tardive, 226
    from antipsychotic drugs, 549-551
Dyslexia, 61
Dysphasia, 62
Dystonias, from antipsychotic drugs, 541, 543
  treatment of, 545

Echothiophate, lens opacities from, 496
Economic status of elderly, 4-5
  changes in, 73-74
  and food intake, 158
Ectropion, senile, 490
Eczema, 602
Edathamil, affecting urine glucose tests, 478
Educational status of elderly persons, 5
Eggs, nutrient content of, 193
Elase ointment, 613

Elastic recoil of lungs, changes in, 58, 593
Elastin, changes in, 33, 52, 65
Electroencephalogram, aging affecting, 40
Electrolyte balance
 changes in, 57
 diuretics affecting, 400
 and drug interactions, 309
Emphysema, 58, 368, 595–596
 diet in, 638
 incidence of, 594
Endocrine function in aging, 24–25, 48–50
 in females, 50
 in males, 50
Endocrine therapy. See Hormone therapy
Eno, 323
Entropion, senile, 491
Enzymes
 activity in aging, 32–33, 47
 and metabolism of drugs, 264, 265–266
 proteolytic, in pressure sores, 612, 613
Ephedrine
 affecting urine glucose tests, 478
 in asthma, 597
 food intake with, 646
Epilepsy
 anticonvulsants in, 363–364. See also Anticonvulsants
 effects of antimicrobials in, 370
Epinephrine
 affecting diagnostic test for diabetes, 479
 and carbohydrate absorption, 229
 in glaucoma, 493
 ocular effects of, 496
 solution for inhalation, 328
Ergot alkaloids, dihydrogenated, in dementia, 572
Error catastrophe theory of aging, 23
Erythrityl tetranitrate, contraindicated in glaucoma, 495
Erythrocytes, binding to drugs, 263
Erythromycin
 dosage reduction in renal failure, 274
 excretion of, 369
 in anuria, 269
 food intake with, 645, 648
 hepatic effects of, 266
 interaction with other drugs, 306, 325
 protein binding of, 260
 urinary pH affecting, 378
Escherichia coli, and urinary tract infections, 376
Esophageal problems, in aging, 45
Estrogen-dependent cells, atrophy of, 24
Estrogen production, in aging, 50
Estrogen therapy
 heart failure from, 399
 interaction with other drugs, 437, 480, 539
 in osteoporosis, 53
Ethacrynic acid, 453–454
 adverse effects of, 450
 affecting diagnostic test for diabetes, 479
 affecting urine glucose tests, 478
 and carbohydrate absorption, 229
 characteristics of, 449
 food intake with, 646
 hearing loss from, 64
 interaction with other drugs, 368, 374, 437, 480
 interval extension administration in renal failure, 276
 protein binding of, 261
 site of action of, 448
Ethambutol
 interval extension administration in renal failure, 277
 protein binding of, 260
Ethchlorvynol
 dosage reduction in renal failure, 275
 as hypnotic, 523
 interaction with other drugs, 437
 protein binding of, 261
Ethinamate, as hypnotic, 523
Ethionamide, food intake with, 646
Ethnic groups
 health status in, 159
 nutritional needs in, 158
 prescription of drugs in, 163–164
 responses to drugs in, 155–158
 use of health facilities, 160–164
Ethopropazine
 contraindicated in glaucoma, 495
 in parkinsonism, 544
Ethosuximide, therapeutic plasma levels of, 279
Ethotoin, food intake with, 646

Excretion of drugs, 267-278
  in antimicrobial therapy, 369
  in anuria, 269
  drug interactions affecting, 308-309
Exercise, effects of, 52, 84-87
Expectorants, 326
Expenditures for health care, 89-96
  and drug costs, 104-107
  for nursing home care, 125
Extracellular fluid, 253
Extrapyramidal symptoms, from antipsychotic drugs, 540-549
  treatment of, 543
Eyes
  aging affecting, 60-61, 490-495
  cataracts in, 491-493, 495-496
  drugs affecting, 490, 496
  dry eye, 494, 497
  glaucoma, 493-494, 496
  macular degeneration, 493, 496
  treatment of problems in aged, 495-498

Fat, dietary, 200-201
Fatigue, dietary suggestions in, 638
Fatty tissue in body, and distribution of drugs, 258-259
Fedrazil, 328
Females
  adverse reactions to drugs, 125, 134
  blood pressure in, 147, 404
  endocrine function in aging, 50
  nutritional deficiencies in, 216
Fenoprofen, 353, 355, 358
  hearing loss from, 64
Ferritin, 204
Ferrous salts, food intake with, 646, 648
Ferrous sulfate, nephrotoxicity of, 57
Fever. See Hyperthermia
Fiber, dietary, 213, 246, 334-335
Fish, nutrient content of, 193-194
Fizrin, 323
Flavoxate, contraindicated in glaucoma, 495
Floaters, ocular, 491
Fluid balance, and drug interactions, 309. See also Water content of body
Fluid compartments of body, 253
Fluid intake, 213, 246, 648

and sodium in water, 446
5-Fluorocytocine
  interval extension administration in renal failure, 277
  protein binding of, 260
Fluphenazine, 534, 543
  adverse effects of, 538
  contraindicated in glaucoma, 495
  potency of, 535
Flurazepam, 566
  adverse effects of, 299
  dosage reduction in renal failure, 275
  as hypnotic, 523, 526, 575
  sensitivity to, in aging, 250
  therapeutic plasma levels of, 279
Folic acid, 211-212
  deficiency of
    drug-induced, 306, 340
    and drug metabolism, 266
  excessive intake of, 337
  interaction with other drugs, 575
  recommended daily allowance, 191
  serum levels of, 214
Follicle stimulating hormone levels, 50
Foot problems, 54
  in diabetes, 484-485
Formaldehyde, affecting urine glucose tests, 478
Formula 44-D, 326
4-Way Cold Tablets, 328
Fractures, incidence of, 52-53
Free-radical theory of aging, 24
Fruits, nutrient content of, 196-197
Fungus diseases, therapy in. See Antifungal agents
Furazolidone
  food intake with, 646
  and hemolysis in G-6-PD deficiency, 154
  interaction with other drugs, 569
Furmethonol, and hemolysis in G-6-PD deficiency, 154
Furosemide, 453-454
  adverse effects of, 450
  affecting diagnostic test for diabetes, 479
  characteristics of, 449
  dosage reduction in renal failure, 275
  hearing loss from, 64
  in heart failure, 401

in hypertension, 411
interaction with other drugs, 364, 368, 374, 379, 480
protein binding of, 261
site of action of, 448

Ganglionic blocking agents
constipation from, 332
interference with nutrients, 230
Gastric emptying rate
and absorption of drugs, 257
and drug interactions, 306
Gastritis, 46
Gastrointestinal tract
aspirin-induced bleeding in, 317, 347
changes in aging, 30, 43-48
Gelfoam powder, in pressure sores, 612
Gelusil, 321, 322
Gelusil Lac, 323
Gene redundancy, and error theory of aging, 23
Genetic factors
in adverse drug reactions, 302
in responses to drugs, 152-155
Genitourinary system, aging affecting, 30, 56-57
Gentamicin
adverse effects of, 373, 374
dosage guides in renal disease, 273, 274
excretion of, 369
in anuria, 269
fever affecting pharmacokinetics of, 254
interaction with other drugs, 325
interval extension administration in renal failure, 277
ototoxicity of, 64, 374
protein binding of, 260
pulmonary disease from, 594
therapeutic plasma levels of, 282
toxic blood levels of, 373
urinary pH affecting, 378
in urinary tract infections, 380, 382
Gerokinesiatrics, 86
Gerontophobia, 74
Gerovital, 82
GG-Cen Syrup, 326
Glaucoma, 493-494, 496
anticholinergic agents affecting, 327

drugs contraindicated in, 495
Glomerular filtration rate
and effectiveness of drugs, 271
and excretion of drugs, 267-268
Glucagon, interaction with other drugs, 437
Gluconates, affecting urine glucose tests, 478
Glucose
serum levels in diabetes, 468-469
tolerance test, 48, 465
in urine, testing for, 477-478
drugs affecting, 367, 381, 478
Glucose-6-phosphate dehydrogenase (G-6-PD) deficiency, 154
Glutethimide
constipation from, 333
dosage reduction in renal failure, 275
as hypnotic, 523, 577
interaction with other drugs, 437
protein binding of, 261
therapeutic plasma levels, 279
Glycopyrrolate, contraindicated in glaucoma, 495
Glycosides, cardiac, 438-445
dosage reduction in renal failure, 275
ocular effects of, 490
protein binding of, 261
Gold leaf therapy, in pressure sores, 612
Gold salts
bronchitis from, 59
nephrotoxicity of, 57
protein binding of, 262
in rheumatoid arthritis, 356
Gonadotrophic agents, ocular effects of, 490
Gout, 351, 353, 358
and protein binding of antigout drugs, 262
diet in, 638
Griseofulvin
absorption of, 256
nutrition affecting, 225
food intake with, 646
interaction with other drugs, 306, 367, 437, 569
Guanethidine
adverse effects of, 429, 433
characteristics of, 413
effects with impaired kidney or liver function, 410

in hypertension, 411, 412,
   429-430
      dosage of, 424
   interaction with other drugs, 307,
      416, 430, 434
   interval extension administration
      in renal failure, 276
   protein binding of, 261
   in surgical patients, 628

Hair, graying or loss of, 28
Halls Cough Syrup, 326
Haloperidol, 531, 534
   adverse effects of, 538
   in dementia, 514
   dosage reduction in renal failure,
      275
   interaction with other drugs, 562
   potency of, 535
Halothane, hepatic effects of, 266
Headache, 346
   migraine, 113, 346
Health care
   expenditures for, 89-96
   goals for improvements in,
      649-666
   and hospitalization, 122-123
   in institutions. *See* Institutional
      care
Health professionals, attitudes of,
   76
Health status of elderly persons,
   109-136
   acute conditions in, 118-119
   chronic diseases and disabilities
      in, 113-117
   ethnic factors in, 159
   and housebound patients, 121
   and mortality, 129-135
   nutritional deficiencies in,
      214-221
   religious beliefs affecting,
      161-162
   and visits to physicians, 119-120
Hearing loss, 62-64
   drug-induced, 64, 282, 373-374
Heart
   aging affecting, 33-36
   congestive failure of, 389
      diet in, 638
      digitalis in, 438
      diuretics in, 445
      drug-induced, 398-399
      interaction of drugs in, 368

   pharmacokinetics in, 254
   in surgical patients, 628
   treatment of, 398-403
ischemic disease of, 389
myocardial infarction, 395
thyrotoxic heart disease, 394-395
Heat treatments
   dry heat in pressure sores,
      613-614
   precautions with, 358-359
Height, loss of, 27
Hematocrit, 214
Hemochromatosis, 204
Hemoglobin, 214
Hemolytic anemia, drug-induced,
   154-155
Hemopoietic system
   aging affecting, 50-51
   and normal values for blood tests,
      214
Heparin, 435
Hepatitis, 47
Heptabarbital, interaction with
   other drugs, 306
Herb remedies, 158
Hernia, hiatal, reflux esophagitis
   with, 45
Heroin, in Brompton's Mixture,
   349
Hexocyclium, contraindicated in
   glaucoma, 495
Hiatal hernia, reflux esophagitis
   with, 45
Hippuric acid, affecting urine
   glucose tests, 478
Homatropine, contraindicated in
   glaucoma, 495
Home care for elderly persons, 121
Homogentisic acid, affecting urine
   glucose tests, 478
Hormonal factors in aging, 24-25,
   48-50
Hormone therapy
   androgen, heart failure from, 399
   estrogen. *See* Estrogen therapy
   in memory disorders, 573
   ocular effects of, 490
Hospitalization, 122-123
   cost of, 89-93
   and length of stay, 93
Hot flashes, 50
Hutchinson-Gilford disease, 21-22
Hydantoins, interference with
   nutrients, 230

Hydergine, in dementia, 515, 572
Hydralazine, 401, 402
  adverse effects of, 57, 431, 434
  characteristics of, 414
  effects with impaired kidney or liver function, 410
  hemodynamic effects of, 423
  in hypertension, 412, 430-431
    dosage of, 424
  interval extension administration in renal failure, 276
  nephrotoxicity of, 57
  protein binding of, 261
  reserpine with, 426
  vitamin deficiency from, 340
Hydrochlorothiazide
  characteristics of, 449
  dosage of, 451
  food intake with, 646
  in heart failure, 401
  reserpine with, 426
  site of action of, 448
Hydrocortisone, food intake with, 646
Hydroflumethiazide
  dosage of, 452
  site of action of, 448
Hydrogen peroxide, affecting urine glucose tests, 478
Hydropres-50, 426
Hydroxychloroquine, in rheumatoid arthritis, 356
Hydroxyzine, in anxiety, 531
Hypertension, 169-170
  antihypertensives in, 403-416, 420-434. See also Antihypertensive agents
  diuretics in, 445
  guidelines for therapy in, 408-410, 422
  incidence of, 390-392
  ocular, 494
  as risk factor in diseases, 404-405
  in surgical patients, 628
Hyperthermia, 65
  and gentamicin concentrations, 254
  in salicylate intoxication, 317
Hypnotic drugs, 523, 525-526, 573-577
  adverse effects of, 573
  interaction with other drugs, 630
  protein binding of, 261

Hypochlorites, affecting urine glucose tests, 478
Hypocholesterolemic agents, ocular effects of, 490
Hypochondriasis, 503-504
Hypoglycemia, 472-473
Hypoglycemic agents, oral, 470-475. See also Sulfonylureas
  food intake with, 646
  hepatic effects of, 266
  interaction with other drugs, 320, 479-483, 569, 630
  in surgical patients, 629
Hyponatremia, dilutional, 57
Hypotension, 35
  drug-induced, 406
  from guanethidine, 429
  from prazosin, 431
Hypothermia, 65
  and adverse drug reactions, 301
  aspirin-induced, 317

Ibuprofen, as antiinflammatory agent, 353, 355, 358
Imipramine
  anticholinergic potency of, 530
  contraindicated in glaucoma, 495
  in depression, 531
  dosage reduction in renal failure, 275
  dosage and side effects of, 556
  protein binding of, 262
  therapeutic plasma levels of 280, 281
Immobilization, and osteoporosis, 52
Immune system, aging affecting, 24, 51, 365-366
Immunosuppressive therapy, infections in, 370, 371
Inactivity, effects of, 85-86, 395
Income sources in aging, 5, 73-74
Incontinence
  fecal, 617
  and skin problems, 606, 616-617
Indomethacin
  affecting diagnostic test for diabetes, 479
  affecting urine glucose tests, 478
  age-related pharmacokinetic changes in, 251
  as antiinflammatory agent, 353, 356-357, 358

diazepam with, 357
food intake with, 646
hearing loss from, 64
interaction with other drugs,
    306, 357, 437
metabolism affected by age, 267
protein binding of, 262
Infections
  antimicrobials in, 365-382
  in diabetes, 484
  in immunosuppressive therapy,
    370, 371
  and intercurrent conditions,
    366-370
  and malnutrition, 222-223
  ocular, 495
  respiratory, 593-594
  susceptibility to, 51
  of urinary tract, 374-382
Inflammation, control of, 350-359
Influenza vaccination, 174
Insomnia, 523-526
  hypnotics in, 525-526, 573-577.
    See also Hypnotic drugs
Institutional care
  drug use in, 100-104
  eye care in, 497-498
  in hospitals. See Hospitalization
  laxatives used in, 330-331
  and length of stay, 93
  negative attitudes in, 75
  in nursing homes, 124-129
  time spent in, 93, 96
  use by ethnic groups, 160
  and nutritional deficiencies,
    220-221
  and urinary tract infections, 374
Insulin
  synthesis and release of, 48
  therapy, 474-477
    affecting diagnostic test for
      diabetes, 479
    affecting laboratory test values,
      483
    and digitalis toxicity, 254
    interaction with other drugs, 327,
      480, 630
    mixtures in, 476-477
    response to, in aging, 464-465
    in surgical patients, 629
    types of insulins in, 475
Intellectual function
  aging affecting, 41-43, 501

causes of deterioration in, 508
cognitive-acting drugs affecting,
    571-573
loss of. See Dementia
Interactions of drugs, 304-309
  affecting excretion of drugs,
    308-309
  affecting liver metabolism,
    307-308
  displacement interactions,
    306-307
  electrolyte or fluid balance in, 309
  at end-organ receptor site, 307
Intestines, changes in, 46-47
Intracellular fluid, 253
Iodine
  deficiency of, 215, 218
  protein-bound, in serum, 214
  recommended daily allowances,
    192
Iron
  absorption of, 256
  binding capacity of blood, 214
  deficiency of, 204-206
    from aspirin, 316
  hepatic effects of overdose, 266
  intake of, 203-206
  recommended daily allowances,
    192
  serum levels of, 214
Iron salts
  constipation from, 333
  food intake with, 646, 648
Ischemic heart disease, 389
Isocarboxazid, contraindicated in
    glaucoma, 495
Isoflurophate, lens opacities from,
    496
Isoniazid
  adverse effects of, 370, 372
  affecting diagnostic test for
    diabetes, 479
  affecting urine glucose tests, 478
  food intake with, 646
  and hemolysis in G-6-PD
    deficiency, 155
  interaction with other drugs, 308,
    324, 336, 370, 419, 569
  interference with nutrients, 230
  interval extension administration
    in renal failure, 277
  protein binding of, 260
  psychiatric side effects of, 507

pulmonary disease from, 594
and urine glucose tests, 367
vitamin deficiency from, 340
Isopropamide, contraindicated in glaucoma, 495
Isoproterenol, as bronchodilator, 595, 597
Isosorbide dinitrate, 402
in angina pectoris, 397
contraindicated in glaucoma, 495
food intake with, 646
Itching, 604-605

Kanamycin
adverse effects of, 373
dosage guides in renal disease, 273, 274
excretion of, 369
in anuria, 269
interaction with other drugs, 325
interval extension administration in renal failure, 277
ototoxicity of, 64, 374
protein binding of, 260
pulmonary disease from, 594
therapeutic plasma levels of, 282
urinary pH affecting, 378
in urinary tract infections, 380
vitamin deficiency from, 339, 340
Keratoconjunctivitis sicca, 494
Kidney
drugs affecting, 57
and excretion of drugs, 267-278
function changes in aging, 54-56
Kidney disease
and adverse drug reactions, 301, 302
and effects of antihypertensives, 410
incidence of, 113
pharmacokinetics in, 254-255
and protein binding of drugs, 263
and response to antimicrobials, 368-369
Kolantyl, 321, 322, 323
Kudrox, 322

Laboratory test values
antimicrobials affecting, 367
and diagnostic problems, 146-148
hypoglycemic agents affecting, 483

normal blood tests, 214
salicylates affecting, 317-318
urine tests in diabetes, 477-478
drugs affecting, 367, 381, 478
vitamins affecting, 338
Laxatives, 329-337
and absorption of drugs, 257
abuse of, 333
adverse effects of, 335-337
appropriate use of, 333-335
bulk, 330, 334
adverse effects of, 336
and digitalis toxicity, 254
interaction with other drugs, 306, 336, 340
as nonprescription drugs, 315
saline, 330, 334
adverse effects of, 336
stimulant, 330, 334
adverse effects of, 336
Lecithin, in tardive dyskinesia, 551
Lens of eye, aging affecting, 491-493
Levodopa. See L-Dopa
Lidocaine
in arrhythmias, 419
clearance of, hepatic, 265
dosage reduction in renal failure, 275
mental confusion from, 506
metabolism affected by age, 267
properties of, 417
protein binding of, 261
therapeutic plasma levels, 279, 417
Life expectancy, in United States, 6-9
Life-style of elderly persons, 3-5
Lincomycin
excretion in anuria, 269
food intake with, 645
interval extension administration in renal failure, 277
protein binding of, 260
Lipofuscin accumulation, in aging, 24
Lipoprotein, low density, and atherosclerosis development, 387
Lithium, 560-562
adverse effects of, 559, 561
dosage reduction in renal failure, 275

interaction with other drugs, 324, 434, 539
protein binding of, 261
therapeutic plasma levels of, 279, 561
Liver
 changes in aging, 47
 metabolism of drugs, 263-265
  age affecting, 267
  drug interactions affecting, 307-308
Liver disease
 and adverse drug reactions, 301
 and effects of antihypertensives, 410
 pharmacokinetics in, 255
Lorazepam, 565, 566
 in anxiety, 523, 531, 567
 as hypnotic, 575
Lotions, skin, 605
Loxapine, 531, 534, 537
 potency of, 535
Ludotherapy, 86
Lungs
 changes in aging, 59
 drugs affecting, 59
 and respiratory problems, 593-598
Luteinizing hormone levels, 50

Maalox, 321, 322, 325
Macular regeneration, retinal, 493, 496
Magnesium
 in antacids, 322, 324
 recommended daily allowances for, 192
 serum levels of, 214
Magnesium citrate, 330
 adverse effects of, 335
Magnesium hydroxide, interaction with other drugs, 438
Magnesium salicylate, as antiinflammatory agent, 353
Magnesium sulfate, as saline laxative, 330
Magnesium trisilicate, as antacid, 322
Males
 blood pressure in, 147, 404
 endocrine function of aging, 50
 nutritional deficiencies in, 216

Malnutrition, 187-190. *See also* Nutrition
Manganese, recommended daily allowances for, 202
Mannitol, in glaucoma, 496
Marblen, 322
Meat, nutrient contents of, 193-194
Mechlorethamine, hearing loss from, 64
Medicaid, and nursing home costs, 125
Medihaler-Epi, 328
Mefenamic acid
 food intake with, 647
 interaction with other drugs, 437
Megavitamin therapy, 208, 573
 toxicity of, 337
Memory loss, 42
 cognitive-acting drugs in, 571-573
Menopause, and osteoporosis, 52
Mepenzolate, contraindicated in glaucoma, 495
Meperidine, 348
 age-related pharmacokinetic changes in, 251
 clearance of, hepatic, 265
 constipation from, 333
 dosage reduction in renal failure, 274
 protein binding of, 262
Meprobamate
 in anxiety, 523, 531, 564
 interaction with other drugs, 576
 interval extension administration in renal failure, 276
 protein binding of, 261
Mercaptomerin sodium, site of action of, 448
Mercurial diuretics, interval extension administration in renal failure, 276
Mesoridazine, 531
 interaction with other drugs, 539
 potency of, 535
Mestranol, and hemolysis in G-6-PD deficiency, 155
Metabolic changes in aging, 32-33
Metabolism of drugs, 263-267
 drug interactions affecting, 307-308
 factors affecting, 153-154
 nutrition affecting, 225-226

Metacillin, food intake with, 645
Metageria, 21
Metals, heavy
  hepatic effects of, 266
  interaction with other drugs, 306
  ocular effects of, 490
Metaproterenol
  affecting urine glucose tests, 478
  in asthma, 597
Metaxalone, affecting urine glucose tests, 478
Metformin, affecting diagnostic test for diabetes, 479
Methadone, in Brompton's Mixture, 349
Methamphetamine, contraindicated in glaucoma, 495
Methantheline, contraindicated in glaucoma, 495
Methaqualone
  dosage reduction in renal failure, 275
  as hypnotic, 523
  protein binding of, 261
Methenamine
  dosage reduction in renal failure, 274
  interaction with other drugs, 324
  urinary pH affecting, 379
  in urinary tract infections, 377, 378, 379
Methicillin, 371
  excretion of, 369
  in anuria, 269
  interval extension administration in renal failure, 277
  nephrotoxicity of, 57
  protein binding of, 260
Methixene, contraindicated in glaucoma, 495
Methotrexate
  interaction with other drugs, 318
  interference with nutrients, 230
  vitamin deficiency from, 340
Methscopolamine, contraindicated in glaucoma, 495
Methylatropine, contraindicated in glaucoma, 495
Methylbenzethonium, in skin care, 616
Methylcellulose
  as bulk laxative, 330
  solutions for dry eye, 497

Methylclothiazide
  dosage of, 452
  site of action of, 448
Methyldopa
  adverse effects of, 406, 430, 433
  characteristics of, 414
  effects with impaired kidney or liver function, 410
  hemodynamic effects of, 423
  and hemolysis in G-6-PD deficiency, 155
  hemolytic anemia from, 50
  hepatic effects of, 266
  in hypertension, 411, 412, 430
    dosage of, 424
  interaction with other drugs, 434, 562
  interval extension administration in renal failure, 276
  protein binding of, 261
  psychiatric side effects of, 507
Methylene blue, and hemolysis in G-6-PD deficiency, 155
Methylphenidate
  contraindicated in glaucoma, 495
  interaction with other drugs, 437, 576
  in psychiatric disorders, 573
Methyltestosterone, hepatic effects of, 266
Methyprylon, as hypnotic, 523
Metolazone
  dosage reduction in renal failure, 275
  protein binding of, 261
  site of action of, 448
Metoprolol tartrate, in hypertension, 429
Metronidazole
  food intake with, 647
  interaction with other drugs, 437, 569
  interval extension administration in renal failure, 277
  protein binding of, 260
Migraine, 113, 346
Milk of magnesia, 325, 330, 334
  adverse effects of, 335
Mineral(s), dietary, 201-207
  recommended daily allowances for, 192
  and trace elements, 33, 202

Mineral oil
  adverse effects of, 335, 336
  interaction with other drugs, 337, 340, 437
  pulmonary disease from, 594
  vitamin deficiency from, 339
Minocycline
  interval extension administration in renal failure, 277
  protein binding of, 260
Minoxidil
  dosage reduction in renal failure, 275
  in hypertension, 432
  protein binding of, 261
Miotics, interaction with other drugs, 630
Mobility limitation, from chronic disease, 115-117
Molindone, 531, 534, 537
  potency of, 535
Molybdenum, recommended daily allowances for, 202
Monoamine oxidase inhibitors
  adverse effects of, 559
  in depression, 520, 552
  interaction with other drugs, 480, 482, 548, 576
  ocular effects of, 490
  and reactions from tyramine, 570
Morphine, 348
  age-related pharmacokinetic changes in, 251
  in Brompton's Mixture, 349
  clearance of, hepatic, 265
  dosage reduction in renal failure, 274
  protein binding of, 262
  sensitivity to, in aging, 250
Mortality rates, 129-135, 152
  in cardiovascular diseases, 386-387
  in dementia, 507
  in hypertension, 393
  leading causes in, 654
Multiple medications, 172-173
  and adverse reactions, 299-300
  and interactions of drugs, 304-309
  and protein binding of, 263
Muscle relaxants, ocular effects of, 490
Musculoskeletal system
  aging affecting, 52-54
  disorders in, 351
Mutations, somatic, and aging process, 22-23
Mylanta, 321, 322
Mylanta II, 321, 322

Nafcillin, 371
  food intake with, 645
  interval extension administration in renal failure, 277
  protein binding of, 260
Nail growth, changes in, 28
Nalidixic acid
  affecting urine glucose tests, 478
  dosage reduction in renal failure, 274
  food intake with, 647
  and hemolysis in G-6-PD deficiency, 155
  interaction with other drugs, 324, 367, 370, 437
  protein binding of, 260
Naloxone, dosage reduction in renal failure, 274
Naphthalene, and hemolysis in G-6-PD deficiency, 155
Naproxen, as antiinflammatory agent, 353, 356, 358
Narcotics, 348-350
  constipation from, 333
  interaction with other drugs, 539, 570, 576
Nausea and vomiting, 48
Negative attitudes toward aging, 75
Neoarsphenamine, and hemolysis in G-6-PD deficiency, 154
Neomycin
  and carbohydrate absorption, 229
  and digoxin absorption, 254
  interaction with other drugs, 368
  interval extension administration in renal failure, 277
  ototoxicity of, 64, 374
  pulmonary disease from, 594
  urinary pH affecting, 378
  vitamin deficiency from, 339, 340
Neo-Synephrine, 328
Nephrotoxic drugs, 57, 369, 373
Nervous system, aging affecting, 24-25, 30, 36-41
Neuralgia, incidence of, 113
Neurofibrillary tangles, in brain, 39

Neuroleptics, 531, 532
Neurologic disorders, 526-528
Neuromuscular blocking agents,
  ocular effects of, 490
Niacin
  deficiency of, 215, 217
  excessive intake of, 337
  recommended daily allowances
    for, 191
Nialamide, contraindicated in
  glaucoma, 495
Nickel, effects of, 33
Nicotinic acid
  affecting urine glucose tests, 478
  interaction with other drugs, 480
Nitrazepam, sensitivity to, in aging,
  250
Nitrofurans
  in urinary tract infections, 380
  and urine glucose tests, 367
Nitrofurantoin
  food intake with, 647
  and hemolysis in G-6-PD
    deficiency, 155
  hemolytic anemia from, 50
  interaction with other drugs, 324
  pulmonary disorders from, 59,
    594
  urinary pH affecting, 379
  in urinary tract infections, 378
  vitamin deficiency from, 340
Nitrofurazone, and hemolysis in
  G-6-PD deficiency, 155
Nitroglycerin, 402
  in angina pectoris, 396-397
  contraindicated in glaucoma, 495
  in heart failure, 403
  in surgical patients, 628
Nocturia, 55
Nonprescription drugs, 313-328
  adverse effects of, 97, 298-299
  analgesics, 315-319
  antacids, 320-325
  cough and cold remedies,
    325-329
  interaction with anticoagulants,
    340
  laxatives, 329-337
  salicylates in, 173
  use by elderly, 314-315
  vitamins, 337-340
Norepinephrine, and carbohydrate
  absorption, 229

Nortriptyline
  contraindicated in glaucoma, 495
  in depression, 531
  dosage reduction in renal failure,
    275
  dosage and side effects of, 556
  protein binding of, 262
  therapeutic plasma levels of,
    279-280
Nose drops, 327, 328
Novahistine, 328
Novahistine DMX Liquid, 326
Novobiocin, urinary pH affecting,
  378
NTZ, 328
Nucleoproteins, affecting urine
  glucose tests, 478
Nurses, attitudes of, 76, 77
Nursing homes, 124-129. *See also*
  Institutional care
  and rights of patients, 139-141
  time spent in, 93, 96
  use by ethnic groups, 160
Nutrition, 183-232
  and American diet, 184-186
  and caloric intake, 186, 216, 219,
    231-232
  carbohydrates in, 200
  in diabetes, 469-470
  and disease, 221-225
  and drug action, 225-226
  drugs affecting, 226-231
  ethnic factors in, 158
  fats in, 200-201
  fiber in, 213, 246, 334-335
  fluid intake in, 213, 246, 648
  food intake with drug adminis-
    tration, 645-648
  and immune response, 366
  in institutionalized elderly,
    220-221
  and malnutrition, 187-190,
    214-221
  drug metabolism in, 266-267
  primary, 187-189
  secondary, 189-190
  signs of, 213-214
  minerals and trace elements in,
    201-207
  and needs of elderly persons,
    186-187
  and nutrient content of foods,
    193-197

potassium-rich foods, 445
and prevention of pressure sores,
  615-616
proteins in, 198-199
and psychological functioning,
  224-225
recommendations for, 231-232,
  245-247
and recommended daily allowances, 191-192
and salt content of foods, 408
suggestions in some diseases, 638
and urinary pH, 226, 227, 272
vitamin K content of foods, 437
vitamins in, 207-212
Nyquil, 326

Ocular conditions. See Eyes
Odors of drugs, 179-180
Ophthalmic conditions. See Eyes
Opiates, constipation from, 333
Oral mucosa, changes in, 45
Organic brain syndrome, 504-515
Orphenadrine
  contraindicated in glaucoma, 495
  in parkinsonism, 544
Orthoxicol, 328
Osmotic agents, heart failure
  from, 399
Osteoarthritis, 353, 357-358
Osteomalacia, 53, 203
Osteoporosis, 52-53, 202-203
Ototoxicity of drugs, 64, 282,
  373-374
Over-the-counter drugs. See
  Nonprescription drugs
Oxacillin, 371
  excretion in anuria, 269
  interval extension administration
    in renal failure, 277
  protein binding of, 260
  sodium in, 372
  in urinary tract infections, 380
Oxalic acid, affecting urine glucose
  tests, 478
Oxazepam, 565, 566
  in anxiety, 523, 531, 567
  as hypnotic, 526
  interaction with other drugs, 570
Oxolinic acid, in urinary tract
  infections, 381
Oxychlorosene solutions,
  in pressure sores, 610-611

Oxygen therapy
  hyperbaric, in psychiatric
    disorders, 573
  in pressure sores, 612-613
Oxyphenbutazone
  as antiinflammatory agent, 353,
    356, 358
  food intake with, 647
  interaction with other drugs, 481
Oxyphencyclimine, contraindicated in glaucoma, 495
Oxyphenonium, contraindicated in
  glaucoma, 495
Oxytetracycline
  affecting urine glucose tests, 478
  food intake with, 648

Paget disease of bone, 53
Pain
  analgesics in. See Analgesics
  chronic, 346
  general management of, 346-347
  perception of
    and diagnostic problems,
      145-146
    ethnic factors in, 161
  in terminal illness, Brompton's
    Mixture in, 349-350
Pamaquine, and hemolysis in
  G-6-PD deficiency, 154
Panafil ointment, 613
Pangeria, 21, 22
Papaverine, contraindicated in
  glaucoma, 495
Para-aminosalicylic acid. See
  p-Aminosalicylic acid
Paranoid disorders, 526
Parasympatholytics, ocular effects
  of, 490
Parasympathomimetics
  in glaucoma, 493
  ocular effects of, 490
Pargyline, affecting diagnostic
  test for diabetes, 479
Parkinsonism, 228, 527-528
  antiparkinsonism drugs, 527-528,
    544-549
  depression in, 518
  drug-induced, 527, 540-549
  treatment of, 543, 545
  effects of antimicrobials in, 370
Paromomycin, hearing loss from,
  64

Pathologic aging, 31
Penicillamine
  food intake with, 645
  vitamin deficiency from, 340
Penicillins, 371-372
  adverse effects of, 371, 372
  affecting urine glucose tests, 478
  age-related pharmacokinetic changes in, 251
  asthma from, 59
  dosage reduction in renal failure, 274
  excretion of, 369
  in anuria, 269
  food intake with, 645, 648
  interaction with other drugs, 308, 324, 368
  interference with nutrients, 230
  interval extension administration in renal failure, 277
  nephrotoxicity of, 57
  neurotoxicity of, 367
  protein binding of, 260
  pulmonary disease from, 594
  sodium in, 372
  urinary pH affecting, 378
  in urinary tract infections, 376, 380, 381
Pentaerythritol tetranitrate
  contraindicated in glaucoma, 495
  food intake with, 645
Pentapiperide, contraindicated in glaucoma, 495
Pentaquine, and hemolysis in G-6-PD deficiency, 14
Pentazocine
  absorption of, 257
  dosage reduction in renal failure, 274
  for pain relief, 355
  protein binding of, 262
Penthienate, contraindicated in glaucoma, 495
Pentobarbital
  in anxiety, 523
  dosage reduction in renal failure, 275
  protein binding of, 261
Peptic ulcers, 46
Perphenazine, 531
  dosage of, 538
  potency of, 535
Perspiration volume, changes in, 65

pH
  gastric, antacids affecting, 320-321
  intestinal, antacids affecting, 323
  urinary
    and activity of antimicrobials, 378-379
    affecting excretion of drugs, 308-309
    antacids affecting, 324-325
    diet affecting, 226, 227, 272
Pharmacodynamics
  aging affecting, 249-250
  and drug interactions, 304
Pharmacokinetics, 251-284
  basic principles of, 251-253
  and drug interactions, 304
  in elderly persons, 250-251, 255-278
    absorption of drugs, 255-257
    distribution of drugs, 258-263
    excretion of drugs, 267-278
    metabolism of drugs, 263-267
  factors causing variations in, 253-255
  nutrition affecting, 225-226
  and steady state concentration, 252
  and therapeutic plasma levels of drugs, 278-283
  two-compartment model of, 251-252
Phenacetin, in analgesics, 315
Phenazopyridine, interval extension administration in renal failure, 276
Phendimetrazine, contraindicated in glaucoma, 495
Phenelzine, contraindicated in glaucoma, 495
Phenethicillin, food intake with, 645
Phenformin
  affecting diagnostic test for diabetes, 479
  affecting laboratory test values, 483
  and carbohydrate absorption, 229
  food intake with, 647
  interaction with other drugs, 480, 481
Phenindione, 435
  nephrotoxicity, 57
Phenmetrazine

contraindicated in glaucoma, 495
food intake with, 645
Phenobarbital
  as anticonvulsant, 363
  in anxiety, 523, 531
  food intake with, 645
  interaction with other drugs, 306, 307, 318, 575
  interval extension administration in renal failure, 276
  protein binding of, 261
Phenol, affecting urine glucose tests, 478
Phenolphthalein
  adverse effects of, 298, 335
  as stimulant laxative, 330
Phenothiazines, 531, 534, 537-539
  adverse effects of, 538
  affecting intraocular pressure, 494
  with Brompton's Mixture, 350
  cataracts from, 492
  constipation from, 333
  dosage reduction with renal failure, 275
  interaction with other drugs, 306, 327, 432-433, 434, 539-540, 548, 576, 630
  muscarinic activity of, 542
  protein binding of, 261
Phentermine, contraindicated in glaucoma, 495
Phentolamine, interaction with other drugs, 570
Phenylbutazone
  absorption of, 256
  adverse effects of, 358
  age-related pharmacokinetic changes in, 251
  as antiinflammatory agent, 353, 356, 358
  aplastic anemia from, 50
  food intake with, 647
  hepatic effects of, 266
  interaction with other drugs, 307, 318, 371, 437, 481, 482
  metabolism affected by age, 267
  nephrotoxicity of, 57
  protein binding of, 262
  thrombocytopenic purpura from, 51
Phenylephrine
  interaction with other drugs, 430
  ocular effects of, 494
Phenylhydrazine, and hemolysis in

G-6-PD deficiency, 155
Phenylpropanolamine, interaction with other drugs, 481
Phenyramidol, interaction with other drugs, 481
Phenytoin, 364
  adverse effects of, 262
  affecting diagnostic test for diabetes, 479
  age-related pharmacokinetic changes in, 251
  in arrhythmias, 419
  clearance of, hepatic, 265
  interaction with other drugs, 318, 324, 364, 370, 380, 419, 437, 570
  mental confusion from, 506
  nephrotoxicity of, 57
  properties of, 417
  pulmonary disease from, 594
  therapeutic plasma levels of, 279, 417
  vitamin deficiency from, 339, 340
Phillips's Milk of Magnesia, 325
Phosphorus
  affecting diagnostic test for diabetes, 479
  recommended daily allowances for, 192
  serum levels of, 214
Photopsia, 491
Physical changes in aging, 27-28
Physicians
  attitudes of, 76
  visits to, rate of, 119-120
Physostigmine
  affecting diagnostic test for diabetes, 479
  in memory loss, 573
Philocarpine, in glaucoma, 493, 496
Pipenzolate, contraindicated in glaucoma, 495
Piperacetazine, potency of, 535
Piperadine derivatives, 531
  muscarinic affinity of, 542
Piperazine derivatives, 531
  and hemolysis in G-6-PD deficiency, 155
  muscarinic affinity of, 542
Piperidolate
  contraindicated in glaucoma, 495
  food intake with, 647
Piracetam, 573

Plasma levels of drugs, therapeutic, 278-283
Pneumonia, 58, 368, 595
Poldine, contraindicated in glaucoma, 495
Poloxalkol, interaction with other drugs, 337
Polymyxin
  excretion of, 369
  in anuria, 269
  in urinary tract infections, 380
  vitamin deficiency from, 339
Polythiazide, dosage of, 452
Polyvinyl alcohol, in dry eye, 497
Population statistics, 1-13
  and birthrate in United States, 7, 11, 13
  and projections for elderly persons, 10-13
Posture, changes in, 27
Potassium
  depletion from diuretics, 448-449
  intake of, 206-207
    recommended daily allowances for, 192
  serum levels of, 214
  and digitalis toxicity, 443
Potassium chloride, affecting diagnostic test for diabetes, 479
Potassium oxalate, affecting diagnostic test for diabetes, 479
Potassium preparations, food intake with, 647, 648
Potassium-sparing diuretics, 447
Potassium supplements, 443-445
Potentiation, and drug interactions, 304
Prazepam, 565, 566
  in anxiety, 523, 567
Prazosin, 401-403
  characteristics of, 415
  dosage reduction in renal failure, 275
  hemodynamic effects of, 423
  in hypertension, 431-432
  protein binding of, 261
Prednisolone, food intake with, 647
Prednisone
  food intake with, 647
  psychiatric side effects of, 507
Prejudice against aged people, 74, 76
Presbycolon, 333
Presbycusis, 62-64

Prescription of drugs
  and assessment of hazards, 173
  dosage form in, 180-181
  dosage levels in, 170-172
  ethnic factors, 163-164
  in hyptertension, 169-170
  and multiple medications, 172-173
  and nonpharmacologic basis of therapeutics, 177-181
  and physical appearance of drugs, 178-180
  vaccines in, 174
Pressure sores, 607-617
  classification of, 609-611
  deep, 610-611
  factors in development of, 609
  preventive management of, 615-617
  prognosis of, 608
  protocol for care of, 621-625
  superficial, 609-610
  treatment of, 611-615
Preventive measures in aging, 81-87
  and pressure sores, 615-617
Primaquine, and hemolysis in G-6-PD deficiency, 154
Primatene Mist, 328
Primidone, vitamin deficiency from, 339, 340
Privine, 328
Probenecid
  affecting urine glucose tests, 478
  interaction with other drugs, 308, 318, 320, 437
  protein binding of, 262
Procainamide
  in arrhythmias, 419
  interaction with other drugs, 433
  interval extension administration in renal failure, 276
  properties of, 417
  protein binding of, 261
  therapeutic plasma levels of, 279, 417
Procarbazine, interaction with other drugs, 576
Prochlorperazine, 531
  with Brompton's Mixture, 350
  potency of, 535
Procyclidine
  contraindicated in glaucoma, 495

food intake with, 647
in parkinsonism, 544
Progeria, 21-22
Progesterone production, in aging, 50
Promazine, 531
  potency of, 535
Propanediols, in anxiety, 523
Propantheline
  contraindicated in glaucoma, 495
  food intake with, 645
  urine retention from, 374
Propionic acid derivatives, as antiinflammatory agents, 355
Propoxyphene
  clearance of, hepatic, 265
  dosage reduction in renal failure, 274
  protein binding of, 262
  pulmonary disease from, 594
Propranolol
  adverse effects of, 428, 433
  age-related pharmacokinetic changes in, 251
  in arrhythmias, 420
  characteristics of, 415
  clearance of, hepatic, 265
  dosage reduction in renal failure, 275
  heart failure from, 399
  in hypertension, 411, 412, 427-429
  interaction with other drugs, 307, 482
  mental confusion from, 506
  metabolism affected by age, 267
  protein binding of, 261
  pulmonary disease from, 594
  in surgical patients, 628
  therapeutic plasma levels, 279, 427
Propylthiouracil, nephrotoxicity of, 57
Prostatism, 56
Prostatitis, and urinary tract infections, 377
Protein
  affecting urine glucose tests, 478
  binding by drugs, 259-263
  deficiency of, 215, 217
  dietary, 198-199
  serum levels of, 214
Proteolytic enzymes, in pressure sores, 612, 613

Proteus, and urinary tract infections, 376
Prothrombin time, 214
Protriptyline
  contraindicated in glaucoma, 495
  in depression, 531
  dosage and side effects of, 556
  therapeutic plasma levels of, 280
Pruritus, 604-605
Pseudodementia, 506
Pseudomonas
  and pressure sores, 611
  and urinary tract infections, 376
Psoriasis, 602
Psychoactive drugs, 531
Psychological disorders
  affective disorders, 515-526
  anxiety, 521-522
  delirium, 506-507
  dementia, 505-506, 507-515
  depression, 515-520
  insomnia, 523-526
  paranoid disorders, 526
Psychological function
  aging affecting, 73-79
  nutrition affecting, 224-225
Psychopharmacologic drugs, 528-577
  adverse effects of, 528-530, 533
  antianxiety agents, 522, 523, 531, 532, 562-568
  antidepressants, 520, 531, 532, 551-560. *See also* Antidepressants
  antipsychotics, 532-551
  cognitive-acting drugs, 571-573
  considerations in use of, 532
  geropsychiatric drugs, 531
  lithium, 560-562. *See also* Lithium
  sedatives-hypnotics, 573-577. *See also* Hypnotic drugs; Sedatives
Psychotomimetic drugs, 532
Psychotropic drugs, 531-532
  adverse effects of, 172
Psyllium
  adverse effects of, 335
  as bulk laxative, 330
  fluid intake with, 648
  interaction with anticoagulants, 340
Pyelonephritis, 56, 375, 376
Pyrazolone derivatives
  affecting urine glucose tests, 478

in rheumatoid arthritis, 356
Pyridoxine, 209-210. *See also*
    Vitamin B-6
Pyrimethamine
    dosage reduction in renal failure, 274
    vitamin deficiency from, 340

Quench, for dry mouth, 544
Quiet-Nite Syrup, 326
Quinacrine
    and hemolysis in G-6-PD deficiency, 154
    interaction with other drugs, 569
Quinethazone
    affecting diagnostic test for diabetes, 479
    affecting urine glucose tests, 478
    dosage of, 452
    site of action of, 448
Quinidine
    adverse effects of, 418
    in arrhythmias, 417-419
    and hemolysis in G-6-PD deficiency, 155
    interaction with other drugs, 419, 433, 437
    interval extension administration in renal failure, 276
    properties of, 417
    protein binding of, 261
    therapeutic plasma levels of, 279, 417
    thrombocytopenic purpura from, 51
Quinine
    hearing loss from, 64
    and hemolysis in G-6-PD deficiency, 155
    interaction with other drugs, 437
    interval extension administration in renal failure, 277
    nephrotoxicity of, 57
    protein binding of, 260

Radiodiagnostic agents, ocular effects of, 490
Rate-of-living theory of aging, 22
Rauwolfia/reserpine
    adverse effects of, 425, 433
    as antipsychotic agent, 531
    characteristics of, 413
    depression from, 518
    diuretic-rauwolfia combinations, 426
    dosage reduction in renal failure, 275
    effects with impaired kidney or liver function, 410
    food intake with, 647
    in hypertension, 411, 412, 425
        dosage of, 424
    interaction with other drugs, 437
    protein binding of, 261
Rauzide, 426
Regroton, 426
Religious beliefs, and health status, 161-162
Reserpine. *See* Rauwolfia/reserpine
Respirator therapy, in asthma, 598
Respiratory problems, 593-598
    chronic obstructive pulmonary disease, 595-596
    drug-induced, 594
    and effects of aging, 30, 58-59
    pneumonia, 58, 368, 595
Responses to drugs
    aging affecting, 249-250
    in antimicrobial therapy, 370-374
    ethnic factors in, 155-164
    genetic or biologic factors in, 152-155
    patient factors in, 151-164
    in renal failure, 272-278
Reticuloendothelial system, and immune response, 51
Retina, macular degeneration in, 493, 496
Rheumatism, 350-351
    and antirheumatic drugs
        adverse reactions to, 172
        hepatic effects of, 266
Rheumatoid arthritis, 352-357
Riboflavin, 209. *See also*
    Vitamin B-2
Rickets, adult, 53. *See also*
    Osteomalacia
Rifampin
    dosage reduction in renal failure, 274
    food intake with, 645
    interaction with other drugs, 367, 437
    nephrotoxicity of, 57
    protein binding of, 260

Rigidity, from antipsychotic drugs, 541
  treatment of, 545
Riopan, 321, 322
Robalate, 325
Robitussin, 328, 329
Rolaids, 323
Romilar CF, 328
Romilar II Syrup, 326

Saccharides, and carbohydrate absorption, 229
St. Joseph Nose Drops for Children, 328
Salicylates or aspirin, 347-348
  absorption of, 256
  adverse effects of, 298, 316-317, 347, 354-355
  affecting diagnostic test for diabetes, 479
  affecting urine glucose tests, 478
  as antiinflammatory agents, 353, 354-355
  buffered aspirin, 319
  and digitalis toxicity, 254
  fluid intake with, 648
  food intake with, 646, 647
  hearing loss from, 64
  and hemolysis in G-6-PD deficiency, 154
  interaction with other drugs, 306, 307, 318, 320, 324, 340, 357, 434, 437, 438, 481, 482, 570
  interval extension administration in renal failure, 276
  nephrotoxicity of, 57
  in nonprescription drugs, 173, 315, 316-318
  protein binding of, 262
  pulmonary disease from, 594
  therapeutic plasma levels of, 279, 354
  vitamin deficiency from, 340
Salicylazosulfapyridine, food intake with, 647
Saliva flow, aging affecting, 45
Salsalate, as antiinflammatory agent, 353
Salt substitutes, potassium in, 207, 444-445
Sciatica, incidence of, 113
Scopolamine, anticholinergic potency of, 530

Sebaceous glands, aging affecting, 64
Secobarbital
  in anxiety, 523
  dosage reduction in renal failure, 275
  protein binding of, 261
Secondary aging, 31
Sedatives, 573-577
  constipation from, 333
  interaction with other drugs, 539, 570, 630
  ocular effects of, 490
  protein binding of, 261
Seizures, anticonvulsants in. See Anticonvulsants
Selenium, recommended daily allowance for, 202
Self-medication. See Nonprescription drugs
Senility. See Dementia
Senna, 330
  adverse effects of, 336
Sensory deprivation, effects of, 31, 42
Sensory system, aging affecting, 30, 59-64
Ser-Ap-Es, 426
Serenium, food intake with, 645
Sexual activity, in aging, 50
Silver-sulfadiazine, in pressure sores, 614
Silver-zinc-allantoinase cream, in pressure sores, 614
Sinex, 328
Sinusitis, incidence of, 594
Sitosterols, food intake with, 645
Skeletal system, aging affecting, 30, 52-54
Skin
  aging affecting, 27-28, 64-65
  care in diabetes, 483-484
  pressure sores of, 607-617
  problems with, 601-606
Sleep
  and insomnia, 523-526
  treatment of, 573-577
  patterns in aging, 41
Soaps, effects of, 605
Sociogenic aging, 73-79
Soda Mint, 323
Sodium
  in antacids, 322-323

in antibiotics, 368
depletion of, 57
and lithium toxicity, 561
in drinking water, 446
in drugs, heart failure from, 399
in foods, 408
in penicillins, 372
serum levels of, 214
Sodium phosphate, 330
adverse effects of, 335
Somatic mutation theory of aging, 22–23
Sorbitol, laxative effects of, 467
Spanish-speaking patients, and problems in health care, 162
Speech, changes in aging, 52
Spinal cord, aging affecting, 37
Spironolactone, 449–453
adverse effects of, 450
characteristics of, 449
in hypertension, 411
interaction with other drugs, 434, 437
interval extension administration in renal failure, 276
protein binding of, 261
site of action of, 448
Spleen, changes in aging, 51
Spondylitis, ankylosing, 353, 358
Sprue, 46
Stereotypes of elderly problems, 75
and diagnostic problems, 144
Stomach, changes in aging, 46
Stool softeners, 330, 334
adverse effects of, 336
Streptomycin
affecting urine glucose tests, 478
asthma from, 59
excretion in anuria, 269
interval extension administration in renal failure, 277
ototoxicity of, 64, 374
protein binding of, 260
toxic blood levels of, 373
Stress, adaptation to, 31
Sudafed, 328
Sugar(s)
absorption of, 256
in cough and cold remedies, 328–329
nutrient content of, 195
paste in pressure sores, 614
Sulfamethizole
absorption of, 256

age-related pharmacokinetic changes in, 251
Sulfamethoxazole-trimethoprim
internal extension administration in renal failure, 277
protein binding of, 260
in urinary tract infections, 377, 378, 380, 381
Sulfamethoxypyridazine, food intake with, 647
Sulfaphenazole, affecting diagnostic test for diabetes, 479
Sulfasalazine, vitamin deficiency from, 340
Sulfinpyrazone
food intake with, 647
interaction with other drugs, 318, 320
Sulfisoxazole
interval extension administration in renal failure, 277
protein binding of, 260
Sulfonamides
affecting urine glucose tests, 478
fluid intake with, 648
and hemolysis in G-6-PD deficiency, 154
hemolytic anemia from, 50
hepatic effects of, 266
interaction with other drugs, 307, 324, 366, 367, 380, 437, 481, 482
interference with nutrients, 230
interval extension administration in renal failure, 277
nephrotoxicity of, 57, 369
protein binding of, 260
pulmonary disease from, 594
urinary pH affecting, 379
in urinary tract infections, 376, 379–380
and urine glucose tests, 367
vitamin deficiency from, 339
Sulfonylureas, in diabetes, 470–474
affecting laboratory test values, 483
interaction with other drugs, 318, 366, 380, 480, 482, 576
thrombocytopenic purpura from, 51
Sunlight affecting skin, 65
Super Anahist Cough Syrup, 328
Surgical procedures, 627–630

anesthetics in, 629–630
postoperative considerations in, 630
preoperative considerations in, 628–629
Sweat glands, changes in aging, 64
Sympathomimetic agents
 in asthma, 597
 in cough and cold remedies, 327–328
 interaction with other drugs, 307, 482, 548
 ocular effects of, 490
Synergism, and drug interactions, 304

Tardive dyskinesia, 226
 from antipsychotic drugs, 549–551
Taste of drugs, 179–180
Tear drainage, aging affecting, 495
Teeth, loss of, 44–45
 and malnutrition, 187
Temperatue of body, regulation of, 65
 aspirin affecting, 317
Terbutaline, in asthma, 597
Terpin Hydrate Elixir, 326
Testape, 477, 478
Testosterone production, in aging, 50
Tetracyclines
 absorption affecting by nutrition, 225
 ashtma from, 59
 dosage reduction in renal failure, 274
 excretion of, 369
  in anuria, 269
 food intake with, 645, 648
 hepatic effects of, 266
 interaction with other drugs, 306, 324, 367, 370, 562
 interference with nutrients, 230
 interval extension administration in renal failure, 277
 protein binding of, 260
 urinary pH affecting, 379
 and urine glucose tests, 367, 478
 vitamin deficiency from, 339
Tetrahydrazoline, ocular effects of, 494
Theophylline
 in asthma, 597

clearance of, hepatic, 265
therapeutic plasma levels of, 597–598
Theories of aging, 22–25
Thephorin-Ac, 328
Theracin, 328
Therapeutic plasma levels of drugs, 273, 278–283
 and minimum effective concentration (MEC), 273
 and minimum inhibitory concentration (MIC), 273
Thermoregulation, 65
 aspirin affecting, 317
Thiabendazole
 affecting diagnostic test for diabetes, 479
 food intake with, 647
Thiamine, 209. See also Vitamin B-1
Thiazide diuretics, 446–449
 adverse effects of, 412, 450, 446–449
 affecting diagnostic test for diabetes, 479
 characteristics of, 413
 dosage of, 451–452
  reduction in renal failure, 275
 effects with impaired kidney or liver function, 410
 in heart failure, 401
 hemodynamic effects of, 423
 hepatic effects of, 266
 in hypertension, 411–412
 interaction with other drugs, 309, 379, 480
 protein binding of, 261
 rauwolfia-diuretic combinations, 426
 and urine glucose tests, 478
Thioridazine, 531, 534
 adverse effects of, 538
 anticholinergic potency of, 530
 in dementia, 514
 in depression, 537, 552
 dosage of, 538
 potency of, 535
 therapeutic plasma levels of, 279
Thiothixene, 531
 potency of, 535
Thioxanthenes, 531, 534
Thirst, and fluid intake, 213
Thrombocytopenic purpura, drug induced, 51

Thromboembolic disease, venous, 394
Thymoleptics, 532
Thymus, changes in aging, 51
Thyroid disorders
  diagnostic problems in, 146
  and digitalis dosage, 254
  incidence of, 113
Thyroid function changes, in aging, 48-49
Thyrotoxic heart disease, 394-395
Thyroxine, interaction with other drugs, 437, 480
Ticarcillin
  dosage reduction in renal failure, 274
  excretion of, 369
  interaction with other drugs, 368
  interval extension administration in renal failure, 277
  protein binding of, 260
Timolol, in glaucoma, 493
Tinnitus, in aspirin toxicity, 347, 354
Tissue changes, in aging, 30, 32
Tissue sensitivity to drugs, aging affecting, 303-304
Titralac, 321, 322, 325
Tobramycin
  excretion of, 369
  ototoxicity of, 64, 374
  toxic blood levels of, 373
  in urinary tract infections, 380, 382
Tolazamide
  affecting diagnostic test for diabetes, 479
  affecting laboratory test values, 483
  food intake with, 647
  interaction with other drugs, 480
Tolbutamide, 471
  absorption of, 256
  affecting laboratory test values, 483
  food intake with, 647
  and hemolysis in G-6-PD deficiency, 155
  interaction with other drugs, 307, 437, 480, 569
  therapeutic plasma levels of, 279
Tolmetin, as antiinflammatory agent, 353, 356

Trace substances, 33
  recommended daily allowances for, 202
Tranquilizers, 531, 532
  ocular effects of, 490
  protein binding of, 261
Transferrin, 214
Travase ointment, 613
Tremor
  from antipsychotic drugs, 541
    treatment of, 545
  in parkinsonism, 527
Triaminic, 328, 329
Triaminicin, 328
Triaminicol, 328
Triamterene, 449
  characteristics of, 449
  food intake with, 647
  in hypertension, 411
  interval extension administration in renal failure, 276
  protein binding of, 261
  site of action of, 448
Triazolam, as hypnotic, 577
Trichlormethiazide
  characteristics of, 449
  dosage of, 452
  site of action of, 448
Triclofos sodium, as hypnotic, 523
Tricyclamol, contraindicated in glaucoma, 495
Tricyclic antidepressants, 530, 531, 553-560
  adverse effects of, 559-560
  affecting intraocular pressure, 494
  constipation from, 332-333
  dosage of, 554-555
    reduction in renal failure, 275
  interaction with other drugs, 306, 307, 320, 416, 430, 433, 434, 437, 539, 630
  interference with nutrients, 230
  mechanisms in action of, 553-554
  in parkinsonism, 528
  protein binding of, 262
  therapeutic effects of, 558-559
  therapeutic plasma levels of, 279, 554
  treatment failure with, 553
Tridihexethyl, contraindicated in glaucoma, 495
Trifluoperazine, 531

adverse effects of, 538
dosage of, 538
potency of, 535
vitamin deficiency from, 340
Triflupromazine, potency of, 535
Trihexyphenidyl
  anticholinergic potency of, 530
  contraindicated in glaucoma, 495
  food intake with, 647
  interaction with other drugs, 539
  in parkinsonism, 544
Trimeprazine, food intake with, 647
Trimethoprim. *See also* Sulfamethoxazole-trimethoprim
  vitamin deficiency from, 340
Trind, 328, 329
Trind Syrup, 326
Trinitrotoluene, and hemolysis in G-6-PD deficiency, 155
Trioxazine
  affecting diagnostic test for diabetes, 479
  affecting urine glucose tests, 478
Triprolidine
  contraindicated in glaucoma, 495
  food intake with, 647
Tri-Span, 328
Trolnitrate, contraindicated in glaucoma, 495
Tuberculosis, 59
  drugs in. *See* Antituberculars
Tussagesic, 328
Tussend Expectorant, 326
Tybamate, in anxiety, 523
Tyramine, intraction with MAO inhibitors, 570

Ulcers
  decubitus. *See* Pressure sores
  peptic, 46
    antacids in, 320
  skin, 603
    treatment of, 603
Urea nitrogen in blood, 55, 214
Urea therapy, in glaucoma, 496
Uremia
  and adverse drug reactions, 302
  pharmacokinetics in, 254
Ureteral diseases, incidence of, 113
Urethritis, 375
Uric acid, affecting urine glucose tests, 478
Urinary tract infections, 374-382
  antibiotics in, 380-382
  and effects of urinary pH, 378-379
  diagnosis of, 375-376
  incidence of, 113
  organisms in, 376
  recurrent or persistent, 377-378
  treatment of, 376-382
Urine
  drug-induced retention of, 57-58, 374
  testing in diabetes, 477-478
    drugs affecting, 367, 381, 478
Ursinus Inlay-Tabs, 328
Urticaria, 602

Vaccines, 174
  adverse reactions to, 172
Vaginitis, atrophic, 50
Vancomycin
  excretion of, 369
  hearing loss from, 64
  interval extension administration in renal failure, 277
  nephrotoxicity of, 369
  protein binding of, 260
  therapeutic plasma levels of, 282
  in urinary tract infections, 380
Vascular disease, and effects of antimicrobials, 367
Vasculature, aging affecting, 33
Vasoconstrictors, ocular effects of, 494
Vasodilators
  cerebral, 571-572
  characteristics of, 414-415
  in heart failure, 401-403
  in hypertension, 412
Vasopressors, ocular effects of, 490
Vasoxyl, 328
Vegetables, nutrient content of, 196-197
Vegetarians, 198, 226
Viomycin, hearing loss from, 64
Vision, changes in aging, 60-61
Vitamin(s), 207-212, 337-340
  absorption of, 257
  affecting laboratory test values, 338
  drug-induced deficiency of, 339-340

excessive intake of, 337
interaction with other drugs, 324, 337
megavitamin therapy, 208, 573
toxicity of, 337
as nonprescription drugs, 315
ocular effects of, 490
recommended daily allowances for, 191–192
Vitamin A, 209
  deficiency of, 215, 218
    drug-induced, 339
  and drug metabolism, 266
  excessive intake of, 337
  interaction with anticoagulants, 340
  recommended daily allowance for, 191
  serum levels of, 214
Vitamin B-1 (thiamine), 209
  absorption of, 256
  deficiency of, 215, 217
    drug-induced, 340
  recommended daily allowance for, 191
  serum levels of, 214
Vitamin B-2 (riboflavin), 209
  deficiency of, 215, 217
  excessive intake of, 357
  recommended daily allowance for, 191
  serum levels of, 214
Vitamin B-3. See Niacin
Vitamin B-6 (pyridoxine), 209–210
  drug-induced deficiency of, 340
  excessive intake of, 337
  interaction with other drugs, 548
  recommended daily allowance for, 192
Vitamin B-12, 210
  drug-induced deficiency of, 340
  recommended daily allowance for, 192
  serum levels of, 214
Vitamin B complex, food intake with, 647
Vitamin C (ascorbic acid), 210
  affecting urine glucose tests, 478
  deficiency of, 215, 218
    drug-induced, 340
  and drug metabolism, 266
  excessive intake of, 337
  and hemolysis in G-6-PD deficiency, 154, 155
  interaction with daily allowance for, 191
  serum levels of, 214
  and urinary pH, 379
Vitamin D, 210–211
  deficiency of, 215, 218
    drug-induced, 339
  excessive intake of, 337
  in osteoporosis, 53
  pulmonary disease from, 594
  recommended daily allowance for, 191
Vitamin E, 83, 211
  recommended daily allowance for, 191
  serum levels of, 214
Vitamin K
  content of foods, 437
  deficiency of
    and anticoagulant action, 435–436
    drug-induced, 339
  and hemolysis in G-6-PD deficiency, 155
  interaction with other drugs, 437
  recommended daily allowance for, 191
  in surgical patients, 628
Voice changes, in aging, 62

Warfarin, 435–436
  clearance of, hepatic, 265
  interaction with other drugs, 306, 307, 540, 575
  metabolism affected by age, 267
  sensitivity to, in aging, 250
Water content of body, 253
  decrease in, 28, 29
  and drug interactions, 309
  and distribution of drugs, 258
Water intake, 213, 246, 648
  and sodium in water, 446
Werner's syndrome, 21, 22
Willard's antacid, 323
Wound healing, in aging, 32

Xerophthalmia, 494

Yager's Liniment, 346

Zantrate, 328
Zinc
  intake of, 206
  recommended daily allowances for, 192
  and wound healing, 616

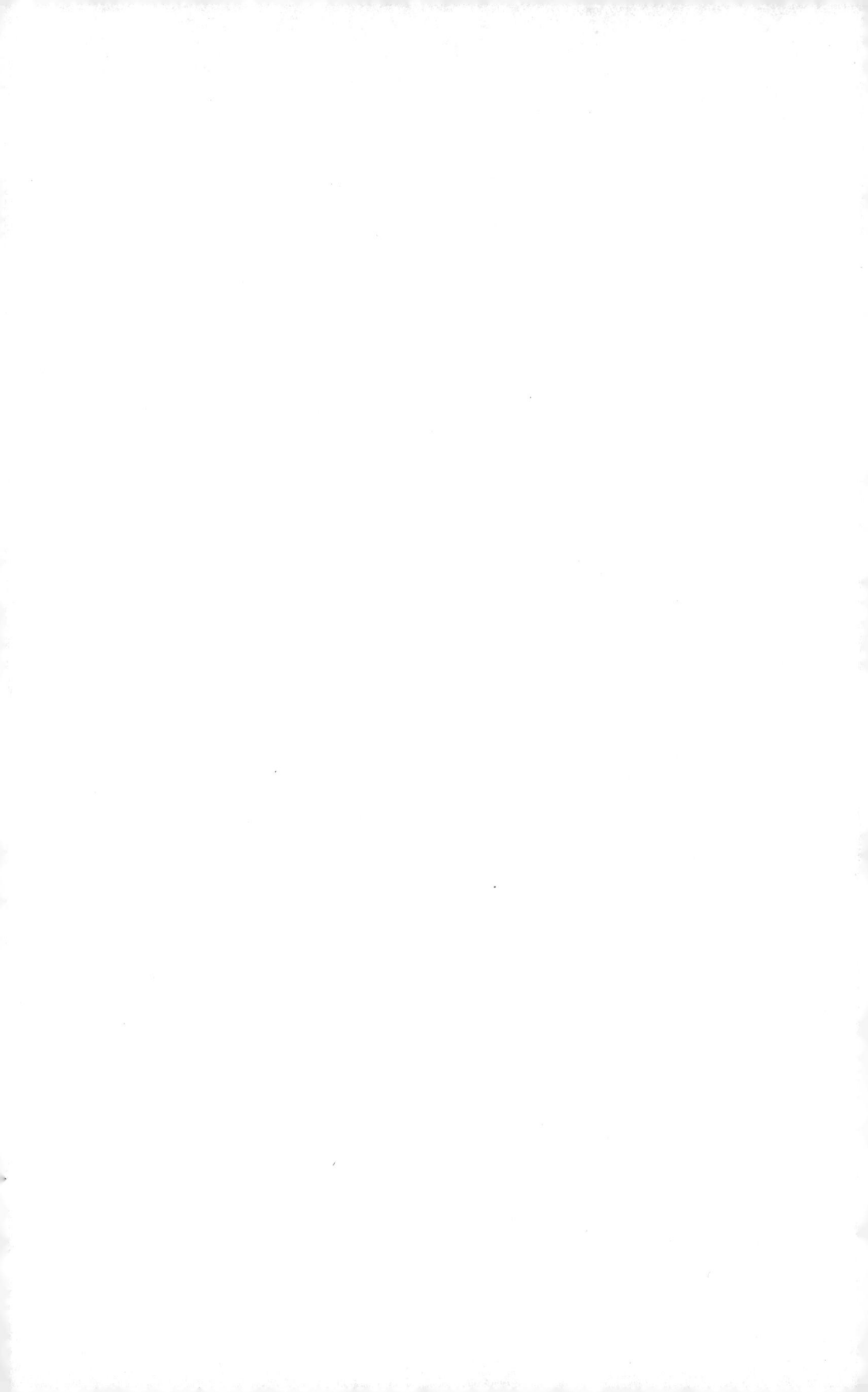